TRAUMA- AND STRESSOR-RELATED DISORDERS

PRIMER ON SERIES

Anxiety Disorders
Kerry J. Ressler, Daniel S. Pine, Barbara Olasov Rothbaum

Autism Spectrum Disorder
Christopher J. McDougle

Schizophrenia and Psychotic Spectrum Disorders
S. Charles Schulz, Michael F. Green, Katharine J. Nelson

Mental Health Practice and the Law
Ronald Schouten

Borderline Personality Disorder
Barbara Stanley, Antonia S. New

TRAUMA- AND STRESSOR-RELATED DISORDERS

EDITED BY

FREDERICK J. STODDARD JR., MD

Professor, Part-time, Department of Psychiatry
Harvard Medical School, at the
Massachusetts General Hospital and the
Shriners Hospital for Children
Boston, MA

DAVID M. BENEDEK, MD

Professor & Chair, Department of Psychiatry
Uniformed Services University School of Medicine
Bethesda, MD

MOHAMMED R. MILAD, PHD

Professor, Department of Psychiatry
University of Illinois at Chicago
Chicago, IL

ROBERT J. URSANO, MD

Director, Center for the Study of Traumatic Stress
Professor of Psychiatry and Neuroscience
Chair, Department of Psychiatry
Uniformed Services University School of Medicine
Bethesda, MD

OXFORD
UNIVERSITY PRESS

OXFORD
UNIVERSITY PRESS

Oxford University Press is a department of the University of Oxford. It furthers the University's objective of excellence in research, scholarship, and education by publishing worldwide. Oxford is a registered trade mark of Oxford University Press in the UK and certain other countries.

Published in the United States of America by Oxford University Press
198 Madison Avenue, New York, NY 10016, United States of America.

CIP data is on file at the Library of Congress
ISBN 978–0–19–045713–6

9 8 7 6 5 4 3 2 1

Printed by Webcom, Inc., Canada

In memory of my parents, F Jackson Stoddard M.D. (1911-1968) and Annette Dods Stoddard Freeman (1916-2017), with gratitude for their inspiration in medical education, translational science, and compassionate patient care (F.J.S.).

For my friends and colleagues who continue to care for those in harm's way, and for all who strive to improve their ability to do so (D.M.B).

A remembrance of all refugees: for your strength and power to stand; albeit with pierced knees, for all that we have learned from you and for inspiring us to stay the course. For you father (M.R.M).

To our patients who educate us and to whom we strive to show and give care (R.J.U.).

CONTENTS

FOREWORD

SCOTT L. RAUCH, MD

It is a privilege to provide the foreword to this outstanding volume. The editors, Drs. Stoddard, Benedek, Milad, and Ursano, all experts in their respective domains, have collaborated to create a book that is thoughtfully organized; each chapter is prepared by authors wisely selected for their perspectives, skills, and expertise. Named a primer, while no essential prior knowledge is assumed, the reader can be brought by this accessible scholarly work to a relatively sophisticated level of understanding.

This is undoubtedly a topic of profound importance. Stress and emotional trauma are endemic to the human condition as they have been from time immemorial. Yet it has been progressively appreciated that severe or extreme exposures, titrated against some diathesis (vulnerability vs. capacity for resilience) in the host conveys tremendous burden of disease globally. These illnesses are highly prevalent, potentially disabling, and treatable.

Whether in health care, science, or policy, there are few things more gratifying than successfully easing suffering, or better yet achieving prevention or cure. While those battles are often waged one patient or family member, one experiment, or one regulation at a time, there is something captivating and enormously compelling about witnessing the maturation of a field such as this over a generation or more.

This past century has seen remarkable progress. The hallmarks of how this field has evolved in some respects serve as a template for the sections of this book. Remote history reminds us of the ubiquity of these conditions, how vexing they have been over the ages, and the degree to which some basic truths currently accepted were long obscured or denied. The fundamental frameworks of nosology remain dynamic. At once the establishment of a separate category in the *Diagnostic and Statistical Manual of Mental Disorders* (fifth edition; American Psychiatric Association, 2013) for this array of conditions was meaningful and groundbreaking; whereas the disruptive approach of Research Domain Criteria represents a healthy alternative scheme, as we devise, test, and refine novel or prevailing models. There is a rich story to be told for each of these conditions. All of them must be viewed from the developmental perspective, through every phase of life—youth, adulthood, and older age. Moreover, there is a diversity of trauma types as well as special populations to be investigated, to discover which dimensions are salient to etiology, pathogenesis, pathophysiology, presentation, course, and intervention.

Beyond these elements, the harbingers of revolutionary advancements in medicine and health care are reflected in the translational cascade from basic science to clinical trials to broader dissemination, in order to ultimately impact public health. In this regard, it is not mere coincidence that psychiatric genetics, cognitive-affective neuroscience, psychiatric neuroimaging, and neurostimulation therapeutics have all come of age in the past three decades. More specifically, the study of fear and threat-related learning (principally through studies of fear conditioning and extinction) have provided some of the very best examples of translational neuroscience—including a vehicle for the most transformational advances in epigenetics to date. Likewise, over a similar time frame, the advent and proliferation of studies employing highly structured or manualized cognitive behavioral therapies have largely defined the psychotherapy evidence base for these as well as other disorders in psychiatry.

Looking forward, there is still much work to do. One crucial agenda will be to take current activities to scale. This includes large research data collection as is essential for psychiatric genetics and gene x environment studies. Likewise, it will be critical to leverage the established evidence base to ensure that at-risk populations are screened for early detection and intervention. In this regard, development of cost-efficient modes of assessment and therapy represent pressing public health concerns.

It is exciting to consider what new tools may emerge to transform the landscape with regard to translational neuroscience, just as the innovative capabilities for functional imaging, optogenetics, gene editing, and induced pluropotential stem cells have burst on the scene in recent years. Already there is promise in leveraging mobile/wearable devices, the web, and teletechnologies to cost-efficiently gather behavioral data in situ, as well as extend therapeutics to enhance access and reduce barriers to care.

In fact, in this volume, the authors beautifully articulate the historical context, current state of the art, and future opportunities for this complex and vastly consequential field of trauma and stressor-related disorders As epitomized in the final chapter, the editors provide a vision for future directions that is a worthwhile compass and blueprint for clinicians, scientists, policymakers, funding agencies, and advocates as well as students in this realm.

REFERENCE

American Psychiatric Association. *Diagnostic and Statistical Manual of Mental Disorders.* 5th ed. Arlington, VA: American Psychiatric Association, 2013.

PREFACE

For persons who have endured serious trauma or stress, diagnosis of a "trauma- and stressor-related disorder" (TSRD) can carry multiple meanings. For some, a specific diagnostic label may provide validation for their symptoms. Others may not readily embrace the notion that present emotional or behavioral symptoms are the result of an event that occurred long ago. Still others may worry about the social or occupational implications of receiving such a diagnosis. Regardless of personal beliefs or biases, as with most medical disorders, it is also common for people not to fully comprehend what is meant when clinicians use terms such as posttraumatic stress disorder (PTSD), acute stress disorder (ASD), adjustment disorder, or reactive attachment disorder to define the constellations of concerns they share with their care providers. It may take an extended period of time for patients to learn where and how they may obtain assistance once a diagnosis is rendered.

Clinicians rely on evidence-based and evidenced-informed approaches to patient care. In the long term, prevention of traumatic exposures and management of stressors requires broad public health and governmental planning and cooperation (Bronfenbrenner, 2005; Shonkoff, Boyce, & McEwen, 2009; Shonkoff, Radner, & Foote, 2017). We hope this primer will aid in the care of those confronting these disorders.

Section I provides an overview of each of the TSRDs of the fifth edition of the *Diagnostic and Statistical Manual of Mental Disorders* (DSM-5). Within the DSM-5, the TSRD are the only disorders necessitating specific etiological requirements (i.e., exposure to traumatic or stressful events) for diagnosis. In prior editions of the DSM, PTSD and ASD were categorized within "anxiety disorders" and as having anxiety- or fear-based symptoms. However, their classification in this new and separate category (i.e., the impetus for this volume) stems from a recognition that in the case of *ASD* and *PTSD* that "many individuals who have been exposed to a traumatic or stressful event exhibit a phenotype in which, rather than anxiety- or fear-based symptoms, the most prominent clinical characteristics are anhedonic and dysphoric symptoms [negative mood], externalizing angry and aggressive symptoms, or dissociative symptoms"(American Psychiatric Association, 2013). Social neglect is a diagnostic requirement in both *reactive attachment disorder* and *disinhibited social engagement disorder* included in this classification scheme, but symptoms in the former are "expressed as an internalizing disorder with depressive symptoms and withdrawn behavior" while the latter is marked by "disinhibition and externalizing behavior." *Adjustment disorders* are now also recognized as TSRD diagnoses, with emotional or behavioral symptoms in response to a stressor within three months. The degree to which any particular environmental occurrence may be considered traumatic, though specifically defined in the DSM-5, remains debatable in that adjustment disorder symptoms (as opposed to PTSD symptoms) have also been documented in the aftermath of DSM-5 "traumatic experiences." Finally, *other specified trauma and stressor related disorder* encompasses five types, two variants of adjustment disorder, two cultural syndromes of distress, and *persistent complex bereavement disorder* (or complicated grief), an important and common condition characterized by persistent grief and mourning reactions that is listed under "Conditions for Further Study" due to insufficient evidence to support a diagnosis (DSM-5,

p. 265). These are also described in Section I of this primer.

EPIDEMIOLOGY AND SPECIAL POPULATIONS

While each of the TSRDs share the requirement of environment precipitant for their diagnosis, the constellations of symptoms representing ASD, PTSD, and the various subcategories of adjustment disorder present with different rates of prevalence, incidence, and associated comorbidity in the general population and in various subpopulations. Section II of the volume summarizes epidemiologic data in the United States and internationally with regard to the TSRD diagnosed in adults and presents epidemiological, diagnostic, and treatment considerations for special populations including culture-specific issues and those particularly related to children, the elderly, and disaster-afflicted populations.

ETIOLOGY

The neurobiological underpinnings and trajectory of response to traumatic experiences are addressed in Section III. Key aspects of this include impacts of early trauma, progress in neurochemistry, genetics, epigenetics, neuroimaging, and emerging understanding of sex differences in PTSD. While the effects of "adverse childhood events" on later development are described throughout the chapters of this volume, Section III focuses on the neurochemistry, genetics, and effects of physical injury and illness on the various trajectories of response. In this section protective factors and mechanisms are also summarized.

PREVENTION AND TREATMENT

Section IV summarizes evidence-based and emerging treatment for TSRD. While clinical trials have focused primarily on PTSD, clinical practice—and, to a lesser extent, scientific study—also inform the treatment of ASD, adjustment disorders, and the TSRD diagnosed in childhood. In addition to traditional psychotherapeutic and psychopharmacological treatments, complementary and alternative approaches to TSRD as well as new technology (device) based interventions are addressed here.

CARE DELIVERY SERVICES AND PERSPECTIVES

As we learn more about the etiology, neurobiology, and management of TSRDs, still new questions emerge. Diverse challenges related to the management and mitigation of traumatic events in the workplace, in at-risk communities (including the military), and within families as well as ethical questions arising from the assessment of disability or criminal responsibility in the aftermath of trauma are discussed in Section V. The final chapter highlights areas where future investigations are likely to change the terms used to define response to trauma and stressors, to enhance understanding of the mechanisms underlying the range of responses, and to refine and target our treatments to the disabling cognitive, emotional, or behavioral symptoms domains for a specific patient or population.

Trauma- and Stressor-Related Disorders begins with a summary of the historical events and accounts shaping our understanding of trauma, and leading to the DSM-5 conceptualization of TSRDs. Recognition of the tremendous disease burden associated with these disorders historically and through the present day should encourage us to strive to reduce risk for all and minimize the experience of trauma for those most at risk. Thus we must continue to focus efforts on mitigating the effects of traumatic experience, reduce the burden of TSRD though traditional pharmacological and psychotherapeutic modalities, and develop new and evolving approaches. We hope the pages that follow contribute to this ongoing effort.

REFERENCES

American Psychiatric Association. *Diagnostic and Statistical Manual of Mental Disorders*. 5th ed. Arlington, VA: American Psychiatric Association, 2013.

Bronfenbrenner U. *Making Human Beings Human: Bioecological Perspectives on Human Development*. Thousand Oaks, CA: SAGE, 2005.

Shonkoff JP, Boyce WT, McEwen BS. Neuroscience, molecular biology, and the childhood roots of health disparities: Building a new framework for health promotion and disease prevention. *JAMA*. 2009; 301(21):2252–2259. [PubMed: 19491187]

Shonkoff JP, Radner JM, Foote N. Expanding the evidence base to drive more productive early childhood investment. *Lancet*. 2017 Jan 7;389(10064):14–16. doi:10.1016/S0140-6736(16)31702-0.

CONTRIBUTORS

David M. Benedek, MD
Professor & Chair, Department of Psychiatry
Uniformed Services University School of Medicine
Bethesda, MD

Ryan Bottary, BS
Department of Psychiatry
Massachusetts General Hospital
Boston, MA

Adam D. Brown, PsyD
Department of Child and Adolescent Psychiatry
New York University School of Medicine
New York, NY

Richard A. Bryant, M.Clin.Psych., PhD
Scientia Professor
School of Psychology
University of New South Wales, Sydney
Sydney, NSW, Australia

Meredith E. Charney, PhD
Instructor in Psychiatry, Harvard Medical School Assistant in Psychology, Massachusetts General Hospital Director of Psychotherapy and Training, MGH Center for Anxiety & Traumatic Stress Disorders Staff Psychologist, Red Sox Foundation and Massachusetts General Hospital Home Base Program
Boston, MA

Stephen J. Cozza, MD
Professor, Department of Psychiatry
Uniformed Services University of the Health Sciences
Bethesda, MD

Alexandra C. De Young, PhD
Centre for Children's Burns and Trauma Research
University of Queensland
Brisbane, QLD, Australia

Brian Flynn, MD
Department of Psychiatry
Uniformed Services University
Associate Director, Center for the Study of Traumatic Stress
Bethesda, MD

Shannon C. Ford, MD
Psychiatrist
Walter Reed National Military Medical Center
Bethesda, MD

Hannah Gartner, BA
Department of Child and Adolescent Psychiatry
New York University School of Medicine
New York, NY

Sheila Gaynor, BS, AM
Department of Psychiatry
McLean Hospital
Harvard Medical School
Boston, MA

Samuel Gazecki
Department of Psychiatry
Massachusetts General Hospital
Boston, MA

Guia Guffanti, PhD
Department of Psychiatry
McLean Hospital
Harvard Medical School
Boston, MA

Jessica L. Hamblen, PhD
National Center for PTSD–Executive Division
White River Junction, VT
Geisel School of Medicine at Dartmouth
Hanover, NH

Juliette M. Harik, PhD
National Center for PTSD–Executive Division
White River Junction, VT
Geisel School of Medicine at Dartmouth
Hanover, NH

Ilan Harpaz-Rotem, PhD
Associate Professor of Psychiatry
VA-Yale Clinical Neurosciences PDS Research Program
Yale University School of Medicine
New Haven, CT

Ryan Herringa, MD, PhD
Assistant Professor of Child & Adolescent Psychiatry
University of Wisconsin–Madison
Madison, WI

Devon E. Hinton, MD, PhD
Department of Psychiatry
Massachusetts General Hospital
Harvard Medical School
Boston, MA

Edmund G. Howe, MD, JD
Department of Psychiatry
Uniformed Services University
Bethesda, MD

Derek Hursey, PharmD, RPh
Adjunct Clinical Assistant Professor
Northeastern University
Director of Pharmacy Services
Shriner's Hospital for Children
Boston, MA

Suni Jani, MD, MPH
Child and Adolescent Psychiatry
Massachusetts General/McLean Hospital
Boston, MA

Natalie Jones, BA
Yale Department of Psychiatry
National Center for PTSD
Yale University School of Medicine
New Haven, CT

Christopher Keary, MD
Massachusetts General Hospital
Boston, MA

Jennifer M. King, MD
Department of Internal Medicine
Indiana University School of Medicine
Indianapolis, IN

Torsten Klengel, MD
Department of Psychiatry
McLean Hospital
Harvard Medical School
Boston, MA

Nicole Leblanc, MA
Department of Psychology
Harvard University
Boston, MA

Lauren A. M. Lebois, PhD
Department of Psychiatry
McLean Hospital
Harvard Medical School
Boston, MA

Roberto Lewis-Fernández, MD
Department of Psychiatry
Columbia University
New York State Psychiatric Institute
New York, NY

Meng-chen Lo, PhD
Department of Psychiatry
Massachusetts General Hospital
Charlestown, MA
Department of Psychiatry
Harvard Medical School
Boston, MA

Lisa Y. Maeng, PhD
Department of Psychiatry
Massachusetts General Hospital
Harvard Medical School
Boston, MA

Marie-France Marin, PhD
Research Center of the Montreal Mental Health University Institute
Department of Psychiatry
Faculty of Medicine
Université de Montréal
Montreal, QC, Canada

Christopher J. McDougle, MD
Department of Psychiatry
Massachusetts General Hospital
Harvard Medical School
Boston, MA

Mohammed R. Milad, PhD
Professor, Department of Psychiatry
University of Illinois at Chicago
Chicago, IL

Kylie N. Moore, BS
Department of Psychiatry
Massachusetts General Hospital
Boston, MA

James E. Nininger, MD
Clinical Associate Professor of Psychiatry
Weill/Cornell Medical College
New York, NY

Sonya B. Norman, PhD
National Center for PTSD–Executive Division
White River Junction, VT
VA San Diego Healthcare System
San Diego, CA

Kevin O'Brien, PhD
Chief, Disaster Mental Health
Department of Behavioral Health
Washington, DC

Edward F. Pace-Schott, MS, MA, PhD
Department of Psychiatry
Massachusetts General Hospital
Harvard Medical School
Boston, MA

Robert H. Pietrzak, PhD, MPH
Associate Professor of Psychiatry
Director, Translational Psychiatric Epidemiology Laboratory
Clinical Neurosciences Division
US Department of Veterans Affairs National Center for PTSD
Yale University School of Medicine
New Haven, CT

Robert M. Post, MD
Clinical Professor of Psychiatry
George Washington University School of Medicine
Bipolar Collaborative Network
Bethesda, MD

Nadia Quijije, MD
Department of Psychiatry
Massachusetts General Hospital
Boston, MA

Elspeth Cameron Ritchie, MD, MPH
Colonel (retired)
Chief, Mental Health
Community Based Outpatient Clinics
Washington, DC VA
Washington, DC

Kenneth Sakauye, MD
Emeritus Professor of Psychiatry
University of Tennessee Health Science Center
Memphis, TN

Patcho N. Santiago, MD, MPH
Commander, Medical Corps, US Navy
Program Director, National Capital Consortium—Psychiatry
Walter Reed National Military Medical Center
Center for the Study of Traumatic Stress
Uniformed Services University
Bethesda, MD

Glenn N. Saxe, MD
Department of Child and Adolescent Psychiatry
New York University School of Medicine
New York, NY

Michael S. Scheeringa, MD, MPH
Department of Psychiatry & Behavioral Sciences
Tulane University School of Medicine
New Orleans, LA

Paula P. Schnurr, PhD
National Center for PTSD–Executive Division
White River Junction, VT
Geisel School of Medicine at Dartmouth
Hanover, NH

Eric L. Scott, PhD
Associate Professor of Pediatrics and Communicable Diseases
Associate Professor of Anesthesia
University of Michigan
Ann Arbor, MI

Naomi Simon, MD
Associate Professor, Harvard Medical School
Director, Center for Anxiety & Traumatic Stress Disorders
Chief Medical Officer, Red Sox Foundation and MGH Home Base Program
Massachusetts General Hospital
Boston, MA

Steven M. Southwick, MD
Glenn H. Greenberg Professor of Psychiatry
Yale University School of Medicine
New Haven, CT

Frederick J. Stoddard Jr., MD
Professor, part-time, Department of Psychiatry
Harvard Medical School
Psychiatrist, Massachusetts General Hospital
Shriners Hospital for Children
Boston, MA

Jack Tsai, PhD
Assistant Professor of Psychiatry
Director, Yale Division of Mental Health Services and Treatment Outcomes Research
Yale University School of Medicine
New Haven, CT

Robert J. Ursano, MD
Director, Center for the Study of Traumatic Stress
Professor of Psychiatry and Neuroscience
Chair, Department of Psychiatry
Uniformed Services University School of Medicine
Bethesda, MD

Allison M. B. Webb, MD, MAT
Walter Reed National Military Medical Center
Bethesda, MD

Alik S. Widge, MD
Department of Psychiatry
Massachusetts General Hospital
Charlestown, MA
Department of Psychiatry
Harvard Medical School
Boston, MA

Sarah Wieman, BA
Clinical Research Coordinator
Center for Anxiety and Traumatic Stress Disorders
Complicated Grief Program
Massachusetts General Hospital
Boston, MA

Gary H. Wynn, MD
Center for the Study of Traumatic Stress
Department of Psychiatry
Uniformed Services University
School of Medicine
Bethesda, MD

Charles H. Zeanah, MD
Department of Psychiatry & Behavioral Sciences
Tulane University School of Medicine
New Orleans, LA

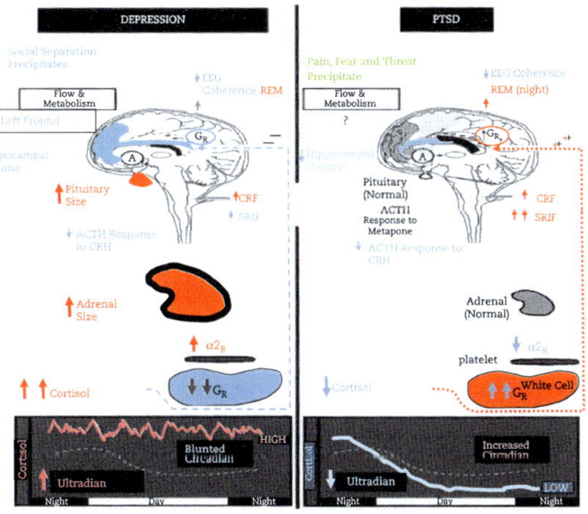

FIGURE 14.1 Gaultier, after Meurisse, Descriptio, Houghton Library, Harvard University, *FB6.M5718614a (artwork in the public domain; photograph provided by Houghton Library)

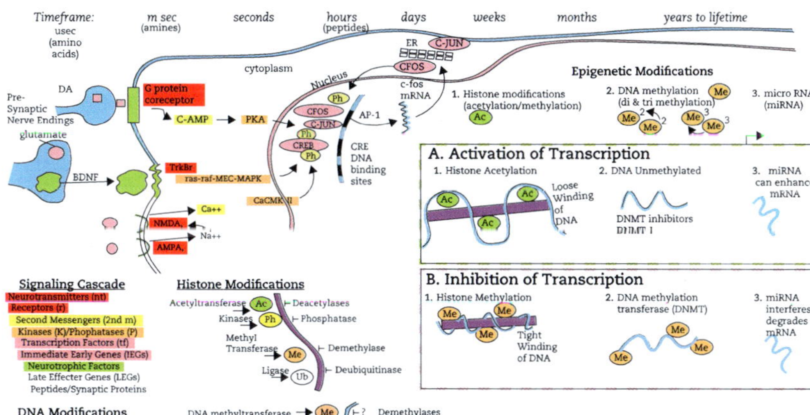

FIGURE 14.2 Gaultier, after Chéron, Typus (detail showing man fleeing from a blindfolded siren), Princeton University Library, Broadside 120 (artwork in the public domain; photograph provided by Princeton University Library)

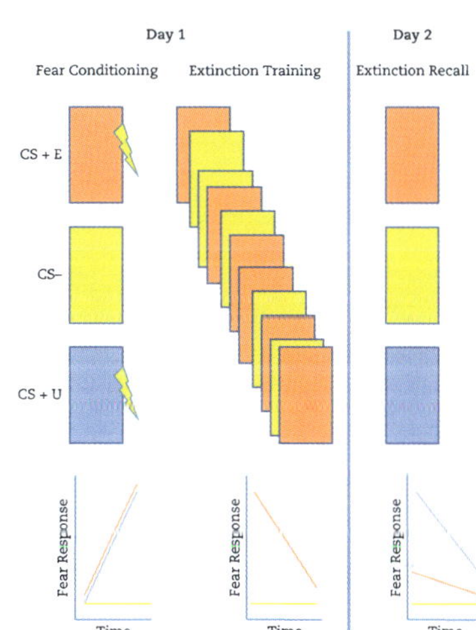

FIGURE 15.1 Gaultier, after Meurisse, Tableau (detail showing a "Siren of concupiscence"), Bibliothèque nationale de France, Paris, Cabinet des Estampes, Réserve QB-201 (21) (artwork in the public domain; photograph provided by Bibliothèque nationale de France)

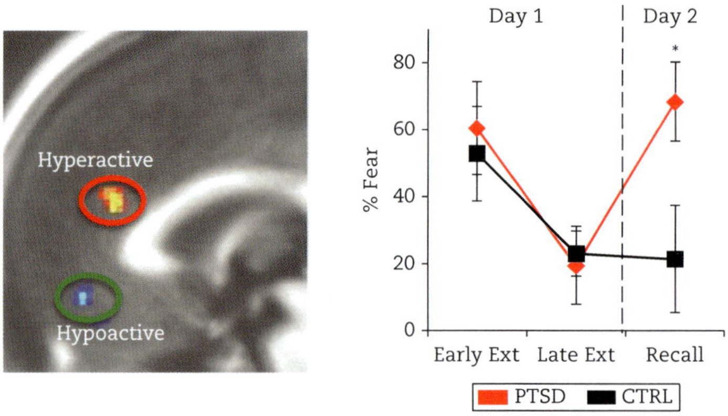

FIGURE 15.2 Gaultier, after Meurisse, Tableau (detail showing a "monster of ignorance"), Bibliothéque nationale de France, Paris, Cabinet des Estampes, Réserve QB-201 (21) (artwork in the public domain; photograph provided by Bibliothéque nationale de France)

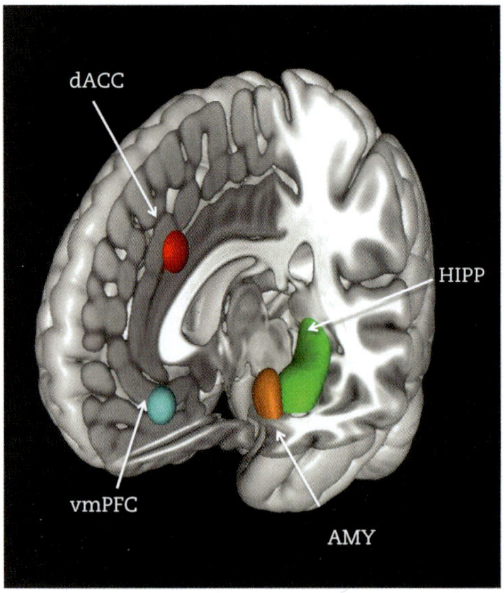

FIGURE 15.3 Gaultier, after Meurisse, Tableau (detail showing Venus, Mars, and the individual Sensitive Appetites), Bibliothéque nationale de France, Paris, Cabinet des Estampes, Réserve QB-201 (21) (artwork in the public domain; photograph provided by Bibliothèque nationale de France)

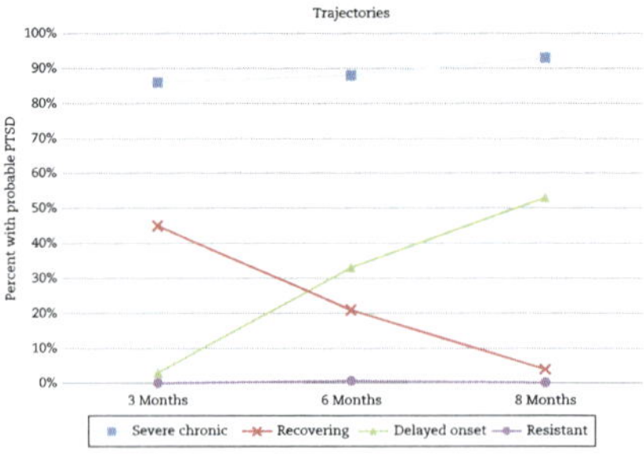

FIGURE 19.1 Gaultier, after Meurisse, Tableau (detail showing Venus, Mars, and the individual Sensitive Appetites), Bibliothéque nationale de France, Paris, Cabinet des Estampes, Réserve QB-201 (21) (artwork in the public domain; photograph provided by Bibliothèque nationale de France)

1

History and Evolution of the Trauma- and Stressor-Related Disorders

FREDERICK J. STODDARD JR., DAVID M. BENEDEK, MOHAMMED R. MILAD, AND ROBERT J. URSANO

Doctor [of Physic]
Foul whisp'rings are abroad. Unnatural deeds
Do breed unnatural troubles; infected minds
To their deaf pillows will discharge their secrets.
More needs she the divine than the physician.
God, God forgive us all! Look after her.
Remove from her the means of all annoyance,
And still keep eyes upon her. So, good night.
My mind she has mated, and amazed my sight.
I think, but dare not speak.

(SHAKESPEARE, 2006, Act 5, Scene 1)

INTRODUCTION: THE MEANING OF "TRAUMA- AND STRESSOR-RELATED DISORDER"

Traumatic events are tragically common worldwide and across all ages. The recognition of trauma- and stressor-related disorders (TSRDs) is important to inform clinical care both in primary care and mental health specialty care. Traumatic exposures may occur in many contexts including life-threatening accidents, physical or sexual violence, natural or manmade disasters, war, or terrorism. Symptoms following such exposures are highly variable. Some individuals who endure even the most extreme trauma never develop symptoms sufficient to meet criteria for a TSRD or experience relatively brief symptoms. Others demonstrate symptoms consistent with the diagnosis of debilitating TSRD resulting in considerable morbidity for weeks or months. Still others may be chronically burdened by symptoms of TSRD, another mental disorder (e.g., depression), or both.

Diagnostic and clinical management challenges and questions confront those who treat persons with trauma- and stressor-related symptoms. While some, like the doctor in *Macbeth* quoted above, may hope for a priest's "divine" intervention, most clinicians rely increasingly on evidence-based approaches to patient care. The clinical and scientific observations summarized in the chapters that follow synthesize the environmental, neurobiological, and genetic processes underpinning the range of responses to trauma and stressors, as well as provide rationale for current treatment and emerging treatments, and in so doing, may help clarify the meaning of these diagnoses to patients and care providers. This chapter provides the historical context leading to our present conceptualization of TSRDs. As an introduction to the chapters that follow, it describes examples of the range of traumatic experience through history and reviews the manner in which the cognitive, emotional, and behavioral effects of traumatic experience have been subsequently classified in global medical nosology.

DESCRIPTIONS OF TRAUMA- AND STRESSOR-RELATED SYMPTOMS THROUGH THE AGES

World history, literature, and art are rife with examples of trauma and posttraumatic sufferings and often contrast with those celebrating conquest and triumph. Examples are paintings (Sargent: *Gassed*; Picasso: *Guernica*), sculpture (Michelangelo: *The Dying Slave*), and both fictional and documentary films (*Apocalypse Now, Schindler's List, Sophie's Choice, The Invisible War, I Am Not Your Negro, Spotlight, After Spring*). Historians, artists, and other commentators describe trauma and stress on individuals from varying vantage points in children, women, and soldiers from the earliest writings of disciplines including religion, sociology, science, law, and public policy. The Bible, the Koran, and Indian, Buddhist, and other sacred texts describe trauma and suffering from disease, pestilence, social rejection, and loss of status. In the Bible and Torah, Job's faith in God sustains him representing a common theme in sacred texts that religious faith allows the individual to endure and survive adversity. Homer's *Iliad* and the *Odyssey* describe symptoms now listed within the framework of the TSRDs—and are also the subjects of Jonathan Shay's (1994, 2002) books describing the symptomatology of suffering from posttraumatic stress disorder (PTSD) of the warrior in battle and on his return home, with poignant parallels with soldiers in Vietnam and on their return to America. Virgil and Roman authors portray a glorious history yet describe the suffering of those conquered as well as ordinary life, heroism, defeat, and conflicts of Rome's leaders. Shakespeare called upon historical themes to depict, for a wide audience, emotional reactions to violence and sudden death, shades of inner psychological conflict among royalty, and the wisdom of "fools" observing and reflecting on suffering like a Greek chorus.

Throughout history, colonialism, slavery, and war have caused massive physical and psychological trauma to world populations. Spanish, British, and other colonial military power, religious crusades, and the spread of disease led to immense psychological and physical traumatization and subjugation of peoples worldwide. In America, the westward expansion decimated the tribes of Native Americans. The full extent of the posttraumatic sequelae of slavery in America continues to be explored (Davis, 2006). This includes history of bondage in the South and North and the transgenerational posttraumatic impacts which continue to divide society. Death and suffering caused by "brother fighting against brother" in the Civil War is described in medical-surgical records and histories, by Drew G. Faust (2008) in *This Republic of Suffering*, and by many others. Slavery remains an international scourge, with few effective controls over it, causing chronic immense suffering to women, children, and men (Bales, 2012). In the 20th century World War I caused millions to be traumatized, die or be wounded, described in Erich Maria Remarque's *All Quiet on the Western Front*.

Scientific understanding of "war neuroses," a precursor to the diagnosis of PTSD, began in Europe during and after the devastations of World War I (Mott, 1916). The suffering from wounds and death early in World War II was informed by detailed descriptions of neuropsychiatric complications in the survivors of burns from the Cocoanut Grove Fire in Boston in 1942 which killed 592 people (Adler, 1943; Cobb & Lindemann, 1943). Erich Lindemann's (1944) classic paper explored acute grief and its management. "Combat fatigue" and "shell shock" secondary to soldiers' combat exposure in World War II were described by Grinker and Spiegel (1945). Robert Lifton (1967) and others described the emotional aftermath of the nuclear bombings of Hiroshima and Nagasaki: terror, death, disfiguring burns, and the effects of radiation. PTSD, the central diagnosis in the TSRD category, was brought to prominence during the Vietnam war, due to its devastating trauma to soldiers and civilians (Camp, 2015).

Until the avoidance, denial, numbing and guilt during and after the terrors of the Holocaust, inflicted mainly on Jews and also others, were forced into public awareness, these avoidance reactions to the Holocaust and to genocide, interfered with acceptance, understanding, and bereavement. Once the avoidance, denial, numbing and guilt about the Holocaust were confronted, spoken and written about, memorials and active responses have informed ongoing personal, national and international efforts to honor the dead, those who survived, and to condemn perpetrators, protect human rights, and prevent recurrence (Arendt, 1951; Wiesel, 1962). Psychotherapies of trauma, and historical understandings of suffering from those traumatic experiences continue to be transformed by writings and testimonials music, and art, of Holocaust survivors and by some who perished. These works were most important in the gradual awareness of the tremendous suffering caused by the Holocaust and its sequelae, including disorders we now describe as trauma- and stressor-related.

The psychological sequelae of traumatic events experienced by children, women, and elders are better understood and prevention and intervention efforts are increasing. Advocates for women and children in social work, psychology and psychiatry led in efforts to acknowledge the broad extent of psychological and physical abuse and its posttraumatic sequelae, including the International Society for Traumatic Stress Studies, professional mental health organizations, and legislatures which passed laws to prevent abuse. Neglect and abuse of children by parents, caretakers, clergy (Keenan, 2011), teachers, coaches and others are increasingly combatted with laws and services to protect children (Crosson-Tower, 2013).

THE DIMENSIONALITY OF TRAUMATIC STRESS RESPONSE

While historians provide abundant descriptions of posttraumatic symptoms, the parsing of such symptoms into one or more psychiatric diagnoses through medical history taking and mental status examination by a clinician is the method called for by the *Diagnostic and Statistical Manual of Mental Disorders* (fifth ed. [DSM-5], American Psychiatric Association, 2013). Yet when clinicians treat those who have experienced stressful life events, they often find that these patients have disabling symptoms but do not meet diagnostic full criteria. Hence patients are noted to have "partial," "spectrum," or "subsyndromal" conditions, for which there may be genetic determinants. This phenomenon illustrates the dimensional manifestations of exposure to trauma.

This raises theoretical and practical questions involving the categorical ("yes" vs. "no") diagnosis of disorders on the basis of specific symptoms and course rather than a dimensional perspective on illness based on brain science (Kendler & Engstrom, 2017), and whether or what specific treatment may be indicated for individuals meeting some but not all of the DSM diagnostic criteria. In fact this limitation not only applies to the TSRD or psychiatric disorders but also reflects the categorical nature of most diagnoses in medicine.

Eleven indicators served as empirical guidelines in the clustering of the DSM disorders: "shared neural substrates, family traits, genetic risk factors, specific environmental risk factors, biomarkers, temperamental antecedents, abnormalities of emotional or cognitive processing, symptom similarity, course of illness, high comorbidity, and shared treatment response." The DSM-5 Task Force expected "that dimensional approaches to diagnosis will likely supplement or supersede current categorical approaches in coming years" (American Psychiatric Association, 2013, pp. 12–13). This comment acknowledges the reality that the present edition of the DSM-5 is not the only diagnostic classification in widespread use. There are three different, and occasionally conflicting, systems of diagnosis for mental disorders, one primarily for clinical use in the United States: the DSM-5; one recognized internationally and by many US insurance companies: the International Classification of Diseases, 10th revision (ICD-10); and the conceptual framework for research from the National Institute of Mental Health (NIMH): the NIMH Research Domain Criteria (RDoC; Maj, 2016).

The ICD-10 is the tenth revision of the International Statistical Classification of Diseases and Related Health Problems (ICD), a medical classification list by the World Health Organization (1992). It has codes for diseases including mental disorders, signs and symptoms, abnormal findings, complaints, social circumstances, and external causes of injury or diseases. There is generally speaking a logical "crosswalk" from DSM to ICD diagnoses, but differences in diagnostic criteria have hindered transnational epidemiological surveys.

The NIMH RDoC is a matrix representing functional constructs or dimensions of behavior which aggregate the molecules, genes, and circuits, used to measure or otherwise quantify observable symptoms. These constructs are then grouped into five higher domains reflecting knowledge of major systems of emotion, cognition, motivation, and social behavior, which are Negative Valence Systems, Positive Valence Systems, Cognitive Systems, Systems for Social Processes, and Arousal/Regulatory Systems. The RDoC is dimensional and represents a fundamental departure from the categorical diagnostic systems of the DSM and ICD, which classify disorders on constellations of symptoms frequently observed together.

TRAUMA- AND STRESSOR-RELATED DISORDERS IN THE DSM

In 1980, the diagnosis of PTSD was introduced in the American Psychiatric Association's (1980) third edition of the DSM. This occurred largely as a result of recognition of the pattern of persistent psychiatric symptoms observed in Vietnam veterans. The first DSM conceptualizations of PTSD required that the traumatic event be "outside the range of normal human experience," but this requirement was eliminated at the turn of the century in the fourth edition of the DSM (DSM-IV; American Psychiatric Association, 2004) as epidemiological studies of what the artists and historians had already observed: that disaster, violence, and war—though traumatic—were hardly outside the range of normal human experience. Since veterans of recent military operations recalled their reactions to fire-fights as "automatic and emotionless narrowing of focus" (i.e., without a conscious experience of fear), the DSM diagnostic requirement for PTSD of fear, hopelessness, or horror during the traumatic event was also eliminated in the fifth edition of the DSM (DSM-5; American Psychiatric Association, 2013). Additional DSM-5 revisions include the expansion of PTSD symptoms observed in the aftermath of trauma and recognition of entities such as a subtype with dissociative symptoms of depersonalization or derealization, subthreshold PTSD, other specified TSRDs, and an increasingly nuanced discussion of the broad range of psychopathological responses to military operations and war.

TRAUMA- AND STRESSOR-RELATED DISORDERS IN THE DSM-5

The DSM-5 carefully specifies that its diagnoses are primarily intended for use by clinicians, rather than for third-party insurance companies or forensic (legal) use, although it is used for those purposes. The DSM-5 also explains that the diagnoses are not linked in the DSM to specific treatments. Nonetheless, in psychiatry as well as other medicine, evidence-based practice guidelines link treatment to specific diagnoses, and in this book we describe the evidence-based treatments for patients with TSRDs. The DSM-5 was a "massive undertaking" over 12 years, which involved physicians, psychologists, social workers, nurses, counselors, epidemiologists, statisticians, neuroscientists, and neuropsychologists, as well as patients, families, lawyers, consumer organizations, and advocacy groups. It summarizes (p. 5) its aim, for children and for adults, as

> DSM-5 is designed to better fill the need of clinicians, patients, families and researchers for a clear and concise description of each mental disorder organized by explicit diagnostic criteria, supplemented when appropriate, by [Level 1 and Level 2] dimensional [cross-cutting symptom] measures [and a disability measure] that cross diagnostic boundaries, and a brief digest of information about the diagnosis, risk factors, associated features, research advances, and various expressions of the disorder. (American Psychiatric Association, 2013, p. 5; see also pp. 733–748)

A work group of the DSM-5 Task Force concluded that TSRDs were distinct from anxiety disorders (Friedman et al., 2011), and this category was accepted.

Hence, the TSRD chapter is a new addition to the DSM. It recognizes that PTSD in particular has symptoms which are not only anxiety related. The TSRDs are the only psychiatric diagnoses that require a link between environmental precipitants to the development of symptoms. This chapter in the DSM-5 implicitly provides for the inclusion of additional disorders in the future as we are better able to link environment and neurobiology with specific mental disorders over the lifespan.

REFERENCES

Adler, A. Neuropsychiatric complications in victims of Boston's Cocoanut Grove disaster. *JAMA, 123*, 1098–1101, 1943.

American Psychiatric Association. *Diagnostic and Statistical Manual of Mental Disorders*, 3rd ed. Washington, DC: Author, 1980.

American Psychiatric Association. *Diagnostic and Statistical Manual of Mental Disorders*, 4th ed. Washington, DC: Author, 2004.

American Psychiatric Association. *Diagnostic and Statistical Manual of Mental Disorders*, 5th ed. Arlington, VA: American Psychiatric Publishing, 2013.

Arendt, H. *The Origins of Totalitarianism*. New York: Schocken Books, 1951.

Bales, K. *Disposable People*. Berkeley: University of California Press, 2012.

Brown, D. *Bury My Heart at Wounded Knee*. New York: Holt, Rinehart and Winston, 1970.

Camp, N. M. *U.S. Army Psychiatry in the Vietnam War: New Challenges in Extended Counterinsurgency Warfare*. Pittsburgh, PA: Borden Institute, 2015.

Cobb, S., & Lindemann, E. Neuropsychiatric observations. *Ann Surg, 117*, 814–824, 1943.

Crosson-Tower, C. *Understanding Child Abuse and Neglect*, 9th ed. Boston: Pearson, 2013.

Davis, D. B. *Inhuman Bondage: The Rise and Fall of Slavery in the New World*. New York: Oxford University Press, 2006.

Faust, D. G. *This Republic of Suffering: Death and the American Civil War*. New York: Alfred A. Knopf, 2008.

Friedman, M. J., Resick, P. A., Bryant, R. B., et al. Classification of trauma and stressor--related disorders in DSM-5. *Depress Anxiety*, *28*, 737–749, 2011.

Fromm, M. G., Ed. *Lost in Transmission: Studies of Trauma Across Generations*. London: Karnac, 2012.

Grinker, R., & Spiegel, J. *Men Under Stress*. New York: McGraw-Hill, 1945.

Herman, J. *Trauma and Recovery: The Aftermath of Trauma: From Domestic Violence to Political Terror*. New York: Basic Books, 1992.

Keenan, M. *Child Sexual Abuse and the Catholic Church*. New York: Oxford University Press, 2011.

Kendler, K. S., Engstrom, E. J. Kahlbaum, Hecker, and Kraepelin and the transition from psychiatric symptoms complexes to empirical disease forms. *Am J Psychiatry*, *174*, 102–109, 2017. doi:10.1176/appi.ajp2016.16030375

Lifton, R. J. *Survivors of Hiroshima*. New York: Random House, 1967.

Lindemann, E. Symptomatology and management of acute grief, 1944. *Am J Psychiatry*, *151*(Suppl.), 155–160, 1944.

Maj, M. Current Developments in refining diagnoses: Narrowing the gap between ICD/DSM and RDoC constructs: possible steps and caveats. *World Psychiatry*, *15*(3), 193–194, 2016.

Mott, F. W. The effects of high explosives upon the central nervous system. *Lancet*, *1*(12), 331–338, 1916.

Shakespeare, W. Macbeth. In S. Wells & G. Taylor (Eds.), *The Oxford Shakespeare: The Complete Works*, 2nd ed. New York: Oxford University Press, 2006.

Shay, J. *Achilles in Vietnam: Combat Trauma and the Undoing of Character*. New York: Scribner, 1994.

Shay, J. *Odysseus in America: Combat Trauma and the Trials of Homecoming*. New York: Scribner, 2002.

Wiesel, E. *The Night Trilogy*. New York: Farrar, Straus and Giroux, 1972.

World Health Organization. *International Statistical Classification of Diseases and Related Health Problems*, 10th rev. Geneva: Author, 1999.

2

Reactive Attachment Disorder and Disinhibited Social Engagement Disorder

ERIC L. SCOTT,* CHRISTOPHER KEARY, JENNIFER M. KING, CHARLES H. ZEANAH, AND CHRISTOPHER J. MCDOUGLE

INTRODUCTION

Although social abnormalities in young children raised in abnormal environments have been described for many years, it was not until the publication of *Diagnostic and Statistical Manual of Mental Disorder* (third edition; American Psychiatric Association, 1980) that reactive attachment disorder (RAD) appeared in psychiatric nosologies. The disorder described aberrant social behaviors in young children that were believed to derive from being reared in caregiving environments lacking in species-typical nurturance and stimulation, such as in instances of maltreatment or institutional rearing. Subsequent to the original description of the disorder, criteria in the *Diagnostic and Statistical Manual of Mental Disorders* (fifth edition [DSM-5]; American Psychiatric Association, 2013) have been revised bifurcating RAD into separate diagnoses (Table 2.1). This chapter describes features, characteristics, and treatment considerations for RAD and disinhibited social engagement disorder (DSED).

HISTORY OF DIAGNOSES

A systematic, multiyear, longitudinal study in 1975 by Tizard and Rees of children raised in institutionalized care described two behavioral phenotypes: one characterized by "indiscriminate sociability" with familiar and unfamiliar adults and another by emotional withdrawal and unresponsiveness to comfort given from adults when distressed. Their atypical patterns of behavior with caregivers were thought to reflect their severe early social deprivation despite adequate nutrition and physical care.

Attachment disorders take their name from concepts in attachment theory which have their basis in work by the British psychoanalyst John Bowlby. Attachment theory sought to examine the qualities of behaviors in toddler-age children toward parental figures, highlighting the importance of interpersonal relationships with caregivers to social and emotional development. Mary Ainsworth would further these concepts in her formation of a research paradigm, the Strange Situation Protocol (SSP), that elicits attachment behaviors in children during the early years. In the SSP, consistent patterns of children's behavior following a moderately stressful separation from their caregivers were identified over time and interpreted by Ainsworth as reflecting the child's strategy of seeking comfort from a specific caregiver (Ainsworth, Blehar, Waters, & Wall, 1978).

Ainsworth's research identified secure patterns of attachment as compared to insecure patterns of attachment characterized by either indifferent response to the absence and reunification of child with caregiver (*avoidant/insecure*) or intense levels of distress at separation with persistent difficulty with soothing upon reunification (*resistant/insecure*). Longitudinal studies of insecure patterns of attachment were found to place the infant at higher risk for psychiatric disorders as well as increase the chance for functional difficulties within relationships. An additional category of *disorganized* attachment was identified by Mary Main who found a cohort of children who lacked a coherent response to separation and unification

* Corresponding author: University of Michigan, Pediatric Psychology, 1500 E. Medical Center Drive, MPB D2234–SPC 5718, Ann Arbor, MI 48109-5718. Phone: 734-763-7535. Fax: 734-936-6897. Email: erlscott@med.umich.edu

TABLE 2.1. CRITERIA OF REACTIVE ATTACHMENT DISORDER AND DISINHIBITED SOCIAL ENGAGEMENT DISORDER

Diagnosis	Early experience of extremes of insufficient care	Attachment behaviors	Response to sensitive, emotionally available caregiving environment	Differential diagnosis
Disinhibited Social Engagement Disorder	Yes	Expressed nonselectively toward strangers in risky ways: overly trusting or physically close	Variable response to intervention	Attention deficit hyperactivity disorder Williams syndrome Bipolar disorder
Reactive Attachment Disorder	Yes	Absent/rare seeking or response to comfort from primary caregiver when distressed; Reduced emotional responsiveness with or without social interest in primary caregiver	Expected complete or near-complete resolution of symptoms	Depressive disorder Autism spectrum disorder Posttraumatic stress disorder

(Main & Solomon, 1990), a profile seen especially frequently in institutionalized populations (Vorria et al., 2003).

While both share a theoretical underpinning, attachment disorders are distinguished from patterns of attachment in that disorders describe pervasive and impairing disturbances in relationships with caregivers and unfamiliar adults. Attachment patterns in contrast, as identified in the SSP, are specific to a given child–caregiver relationship and understood as *risk factors* for greater social dysfunction and psychopathology. Moreover, longitudinal assessments of institutionalized child populations have demonstrated consistent symptoms of both RAD and DSED across a four-year period (Gleason et al., 2011a). In contrast, patterns of attachment have not necessarily shown such consistency throughout early childhood development on sequential testing (Rutter et al., 2009).

REACTIVE ATTACHMENT DISORDER

Diagnostic Features

According to the DSM-5, RAD is a pattern of absent or aberrant attachment behaviors in infancy or in early childhood, evident after reaching the age at which selective attachments should be made (7 to 9 months). Though children with the disorder are thought to possess the capacity to form attachments, because of limited opportunities to form selective attachments, either due to social neglect of the child or frequent changes in caregiving environments (e.g., foster placements), they do not form attachments. The critical period for attachment typically ranges from 9 months to just before 5 years of age. While lack of selective attachment is the essential criterion for RAD, problems with emotional regulation also exist. Withdrawn behavior toward caregivers is typical, whereby the child may not seek comfort or respond to comfort when distressed. Limited positive emotions are expressed around caregivers, and children with RAD may express negative emotions in nonthreatening circumstances. Examples of deprivation sufficient to cause RAD include mistreatment or perhaps institutionalized care where formation of attachment was not possible. If signs of the disorder have been present for more than 12 months, a diagnosis of persistent RAD is given. Severe RAD is noted if all criteria are met and symptoms are present at high levels.

Autism spectrum disorder (ASD) [ASD in other chapters is Acute Stress Disorder.] must be ruled out before giving a diagnosis of RAD. Ruling out pervasive developmental disorders or ASD has remained somewhat controversial. Zeanah and Gleason (2010) had previously argued that since individuals with intellectual disability (ID) and ASD can develop normal attachment relationships and pathogenic relationships, they can indeed develop RAD in addition to their ASD. Their argument is supported by more recent data from Giltaij, Sterkenburg, and Schuengel (2015) demonstrating a considerable co-occurrence of the two disorders among individuals with ID. Indeed, 14% (of 102 individuals diagnosed with ID) met criteria for both a diagnosis of RAD and ASD. They conclude that, "Important for the ongoing discussion of diagnostic criteria, the findings do not support using PDD as an exclusion criterion for the diagnosis of RAD." (p. 145).

Assessment Issues

Individuals at highest risk for psychopathology should be screened with instruments sensitive and specific to attachment disorders. These instruments have not existed until recently, when Minnis et al. (2007) created the Relationship Problems Questionnaire (RPQ). Vervoort, De Schipper, Bosmans, and Verschueren (2013) tested the RPQ as a screening instrument among school-aged children and found good psychometric qualities. Factor analytic results confirmed that the instrument can measure symptoms consistent with Inhibited (internal consistency α=.63) and Disinhibited (internal consistency α=.77) behavioral constellations. Multi-informant, parallel forms analyses of the RPQ demonstrated that the instrument can be effectively used by both parents and teachers, yielding similar results. Finally, there was convergent validity between results of the RPQ and interview and observational procedures known to measure RAD symptoms. Overall, this instrument and others like it can be a boon for both clinicians and researchers looking to rapidly screen individuals suspected to have RAD within clinical settings.

As with most other disorders of early childhood, RAD is best diagnosed through a combination of interviewing and direct-behavioral observation. A detailed history of the child's caregiving experiences is important in order to establish that deficiencies were sufficient to account for the child's social abnormalities. Therefore, details of the child's caregiving history, with attention to neglect, changes in primary caregiving relationships, or significant losses of primary caregivers should be determined.

Structured interviews, such as the Disturbances of Attachment Interview (DAI) may be used to inquire about specific signs of the disorder (Smyke, Dumitrescu, & Zeanah, 2002; Zeanah et al., 2004; Zeanah, Smyke, Koga, Carlson, & Bucharest Early Intervention Project Core Group, 2005) and often are used to make the diagnosis. Standardized observational procedures that elicit the child's responses to familiar and unfamiliar caregivers in order to distinguish between the child's responses to putative attachment figures and to unfamiliar adults have been used in research and also may be useful in clinical settings (Boris et al., 2004; McLaughlin et al., 2010; Zeanah et al., 2005).

Interviews and observations should include questioning about the child having one or more adults from whom he or she seeks comfort, reassurance, nurturing, and protection, particularly in times of distress. In addition, failing to use the attachment figure for comfort, as occurs in the emotionally withdrawn/inhibited pattern, and exhibiting overly familiar behaviors with unfamiliar adults, as occurs in the indiscriminate/disinhibited pattern, should be identified.

The clinical examination provides an opportunity to observe and elicit attachment behaviors. The child's reaction on first meeting the interviewer (a stranger) can provide information about how a child references and/or seeks comfort from a caregiver in the context of a new person and setting. In addition, asking a parent to leave the room for a brief separation from the child can activate the child's attachment system and provide valuable information about how a child uses a parent upon reunion. Multiple observations and agreement between historical information and directly observed behaviors increase confidence in the diagnostic findings.

Historically, standardized observations of attachment behaviors were used to classify attachment but rarely to diagnose RAD. However, more recently, a clinical assessment of attachment involving a stranger, separations and reunions, and the introduction of a robot as a mildly distressing stimulus also has been used reliably to diagnosis attachment disorders in a clinical context (Boris et al., 2004; Shaffer, Huston, & Egeland, 2008). The use of standardized procedures provides the clinician the opportunity to observe children's patterns of attachment behaviors in a consistent manner, reducing the influence of other variables.

Epidemiology

While the exact incidence of RAD is unknown, it is thought to be relatively rare. Egger et al. (2006) found no cases of attachment disorders in a 307 subject study of 2- to 5-year-olds enriched for participants with high scores on the Child Behavioral Checklist recruited from a pediatric clinic. In a similarly designed study in Bucharest, Romania, of young children recruited from pediatric clinics, Gleason et al. (2011b) found no cases of RAD.

Rates of RAD in an at-risk sample of currently and formerly institutionalized children in Bucharest, Romania, were less than 5% both at 22 months and 54 months of age in one study (Gleason et al., 2011a) and too rare to assess longitudinally in another study of young children adopted out of institutions (O'Connor & Rutter, 2000). Studies of children placed into foster care due to child protective concerns show conflicting results as to diagnostic rates. A health information database review of all children placed into foster care in Utah in a four-year period suggested a 17% rate of attachment disorder, although this number reflects inclusion of DSED as well as adjustment disorders (Steele & Buchi, 2008). A study of 94 maltreated toddlers evaluated 3 months after placement in foster care in New Orleans found RAD rates of 35% using International Classification of Diseases (10th revision; ICD-10) criteria (18% withdrawn type only and 17% mixed withdrawn and disinhibited type) (Zeanah et al., 2004). Elevated rates may reflect the retrospective nature of the study or bias introduced by evaluators' knowledge of subjects' neglect history. Further research is necessary, especially among foster care populations, accounting for maltreatment history, age of symptom onset, and timing of the removal from the neglectful environment.

Comorbidity

Severe neglect that comes from early psychosocial deprivation leads to delays in cognition and language (Nelson et al., 2007), since the child may not have received adequate verbal stimulation or interaction during critical developmental periods. Growth parameters including height, weight, and head circumference can be diminished (Rutter, 1998), likely secondary to nutritional compromise. Though it is often immediately treatable, lingering effects can manifest in children's continued problems with food hoarding behavior, despite ample food availability (Parker & Forrest, 1993; Reber, 1996). One study of subjects raised in Romanian orphanages found an association between RAD and signs of depression (Gleason et al., 2011a), which may reflect the fact that both diagnoses can present with reduced positive affect.

Course

While the conditions that contribute to the development of RAD are present very early in a child's life, the diagnosis is not distinguishable until 9 months, when children are expected to form attachments to caregivers. Among children experiencing severe neglect, the behavioral features of RAD have been documented to persist to 12 years of age (Humphreys et al., 2017). Although elevated signs of RAD have been detected in children with histories of post-institutional rearing, it is unclear if any of these children reach the diagnostic threshold. Functional impairment in interpersonal relationships for children with RAD is well documented (Hodges & Tizard, 1989), manifested by decreased social competence appropriate for developmental age.

Differential Diagnosis

ASD shares several of the behavioral features seen in RAD. A child with ASD can manifest the same lack of positive affect and social reciprocity, as well as the developmental delays typically seen in RAD. Stereotypic rocking movements can be characteristic of either ASD or RAD (Smyke et al., 2002). A history of neglect required for the diagnosis of RAD would be the classic way to differentiate the two. Also, RAD lacks the repetitive rituals and restrictive interests that are typical of ASD. Individuals with ASD typically have developmental histories notable for stereotyped speech such as echolalia, persistent pronoun reversal, or scripted speech and frequently demonstrate ongoing problems with goal-oriented communication. In RAD, communication skills are comparable to the individual's developmental level. While a lack of attachment behaviors define RAD, a majority of studies of participants with ASD demonstrate attachment behaviors toward preferred caregivers, especially among subjects with higher cognitive capacity (Rutgers, Bakermans-Kranenburg, Ijzendoorn, & Berckelaer-Onnes, 2004).

While children with RAD typically have co-occurring language and cognitive delays, it must be distinguished from ID. Children with ID are not expected to manifest limited positive affect or reduced emotional responsiveness typically seen in RAD. Moreover, children with ID with a developmental age of at least 9 months are expected to exhibit selective attachment to caregivers.

Distinguishing RAD from depression and posttraumatic stress disorder among traumatized or neglected individuals can be difficult as each may present with blunted affect, social withdrawal, or emotional indifference. Seeking comfort when distressed will distinguish depressed and traumatized individuals from those with RAD as will the presence of overt intrusion symptoms (flashbacks, nightmares), increases in arousal or reactivity, or avoidance of reminders of trauma.

Etiology and Pathophysiology

Social/Environmental Factors

RAD shares a unique characteristic with other diagnoses within the trauma-and stressor-related disorders category within the DSM-5—the role of social and environmental factors in the etiology of the disorder. Institutionalized children or those in foster care experiencing isolation, limited stimulation, poor child/caregiver ratios, or neglect can develop attachment disorders (Bos et al., 2011). The severity of the adversity in a rearing environment is relevant. When two groups of institutionalized children were compared, the group with more consistent caregivers on the unit demonstrated fewer signs of attachment disorders (Smyke et al., 2002). A separate study found that a measure of "quality of caregiving" (meant to gauge the sensitivity/responsiveness of caregivers) was associated with signs of RAD in children who had grown up in institutions (Zeanah et al., 2005).

Children removed early from institutionalized care may have better outcomes than those removed later. For example, Smyke et al. (2010) showed infants removed from institutionalized care before 24 months of age developed more secure and more organized attachments at age 42 months than those removed after 24 months. Despite these findings, age of removal has less of an impact on the course of RAD than that of DSED. One study of institutionalized children found all subjects went on to have resolution of signs of RAD independent of age of adoption (Smyke et al., 2012).

Genetic Factors

Limited data are available concerning any genetic risk factors for RAD. In one study, Minnis et al. (2007) compared behaviors indicative of attachment disorder, such as inhibition and disinhibition, in monozygotic and dizygotic twins. Correlations of these behaviors between monozygotic twins were higher than those between dizygotic twins, supporting the idea of strong genetic influences. Additional research points to a genetic susceptibility for disorganized attachment in individuals with a particular dopamine D4 receptor (DRD4) polymorphism (Bakermans-Kranenburg & van Ijzendoorn, 2007). Still, this susceptibility only leads to an increased risk of disorganized attachment when combined with environmental factors.

Neurobiological Factors

Increasingly, research has demonstrated neurobiological effects of deprivation among institutionalized subjects. Magnetic resonance imaging (MRI) studies of institutionalized children have shown reductions in white matter connectivity in areas of the brain, including both the amygdala and prefrontal cortex, which are areas of higher cognition and emotion (Govindan, Behen, Helder, Makki, & Chugani, 2010). Other neurobiological differences demonstrated include reductions in grey and white matter volumes (Sheridan et al., 2012) and aberrant electrical activity (Marshall, Fox, & BEIP Core Group, 2004) that may normalize over time with subsequent adoption (Vanderwert et al., 2010).

These children also show lower overall levels of vasopressin, as well as lower levels of oxytocin after interactions with caregivers (Bos et al., 2011). These hormones are believed to contribute to prosocial behaviors. Providing more evidence for hormone disruptions, children adopted from institutionalized care show higher levels of cortisol when interacting with their new caregiver than with unfamiliar adults (Bos et al., 2011). While this line of evidence has not been studied directly in children with RAD, the available evidence from institutionalized children may point to new directions in research for other factors that play a role in attachment disorders.

Psychological Factors

While a diagnosis of RAD implies that a child endured adverse environmental conditions in early childhood, it is interesting that, even in this population, very few exposed children develop the disorder. One area of interest has been interactions between temperament, environmental factors, and caregiver behaviors. Temperament and attachment patterns have long been thought to be related to each other; for example, an infant's temperament may influence a parent's reaction to behaviors, thus influencing attachment (Zeanah et al., 2004). Additionally, the synergistic effects of negative temperaments when combined with adverse environmental situations may put a child at a higher risk of developing the disorder. Adverse effects also tend to negatively influence temperament, thus meaning that not only may a child with an irritable and negative affect temperament placed into foster care be prone to developing RAD but also these circumstances may worsen his temperament, increasing the likelihood of development of the disorder (Zeanah et al., 2004).

DISINHIBITED SOCIAL ENGAGEMENT DISORDER

Diagnostic Features

The essential diagnostic characteristic of this disorder is seen in children displaying socially and culturally inappropriate overly familiar social behavior with strangers. The child must be developmentally old enough and capable of forming selective attachments, at least 9 months of age. Children with DSED actively approach and interact with unfamiliar adults without verbal or physical reticence. They may also fail to check with an adult or caregiver when leaving and may even indiscriminately go with a stranger or unfamiliar adult, without hesitation. These uninhibited behaviors should not be better accounted for by attention deficit hyperactivity disorder (ADHD), impulsive type, or merely social extroversion. Finally, an environment in which the child was exposed to social neglect or deprivation where basic emotional needs were not met precedes the behaviors. Alternately, an environment in which the child experienced frequent caregiver changes (e.g., frequent foster care changes) or resided in an institution in which there was a high child to caregiver ratio, where basic emotional and social needs were not met, must have been present. The term "persistent" is used to specify when a child has exhibited symptoms of the disorder for longer than 12 months.

Assessment Issues

Much as in RAD, DSED is best assessed through interviews of adult caregivers about the child's typical behavior and direct observation of the child's behavior. Indiscriminate social behavior, which forms the essence of the disorder, may be assessed by comparing the child's behavior to a stranger and to a familiar caregiver, with subsequent questioning. A detailed history of the child's caregiving experiences is important in order to establish that deficiencies were sufficient to account for the child's social abnormalities. Therefore, details of the child's caregiving history, with attention to neglect, changes in primary caregiving relationships, or significant losses of primary caregivers should be determined.

An important confounding factor that can complicate assessment for DSED in the clinical interview is the presence or absence of selective attachments to a child's primary caregiver. Children with a clear diagnosis of DSED may have varying levels of attachment to a primary caregiver with some studies finding no attachment behaviors and some studies finding secure attachments (Zeanah & Gleason, 2015). Further research is required to understand how security of attachment to a parental figure might affect the development or course of DSED.

Structured interviews such as the Disturbances of Attachment Interview (Smyke et al., 2002, Zeanah et al., 2004, Zeanah et al., 2005) or the Preschool Age Psychiatric Assessment (Egger et al., 2006) may be used to inquire systematically about specific signs of the disorder and include diagnostic algorithms that assist with making the diagnosis. Several standardized observational procedures that allow the clinician to observe the child's social behaviors with unfamiliar adults have been studied, but only one has been used in clinical settings (Boris et al., 2004).

Epidemiology

While few studies assessing rates of the DSM-5 DSED diagnosis have been performed, research examining rates of the fourth edition of the *Diagnostic and Statistical Manual of Mental Disorders* disinhibited subtype of Reactive Attachment Disorder (RADd) are instructive. In a study of 2 to 5-year-old children recruited from pediatric clinics in Bucharest, Gleason et al. (2011b) found a weighted prevalence of 2% for RADd.

Disinhibited attachment disorder behaviors in 4- to 6-year-olds raised in institutions were seen in nearly 30% of children adopted between 24 and 42 months, in nearly 20% of children adopted between 6 and 24 months, and in nearly 5% of children adopted before 6 months (O'Connor et al., 2000). In this same adoptee population, by 11 years old, rates of severe RADd behaviors dropped to 9.9% with higher rates among those adopted after 6 months (Rutter, Colvert, et al., 2007).

A separate population of children institutionalized in Romanian orphanages was studied assessing for rates of attachment disorders over a 54-month period (Gleason et al., 2011a). In this study group, half of subjects were adopted between 12 and 31 months of age and others remained in orphanages. At the time of initial evaluation (average of 22 months), 30 months, 42 months, and 54 months, rates of RADd were 31.8%, 17.9%, 18% and 17.6%, respectively.

Pritchett, Rochat, Tomlinson, and Minnis (2013) studied youths in urban townships in South Africa and found a 12.5% incidence of attachment disorders. All the diagnosed youths were male and displayed the disinhibited symptoms of RAD. Minnis et al. (2013) conducted a large-scale study of an entire educational sector of a UK city, targeting high risk youths. All 1,600 of the students were screened for attachment disorders, followed by focused interviews. Those who screened in after the semistructured focused interview were subsequently evaluated face-to-face to confirm the diagnosis. Through this methodologically rigorous population-based sampling method, the authors determined that 1.4% (95% confidence interval 0.94–2.10) of children in their sample met diagnostic criteria for attachment disorders with RADd far outweighing the inhibited type. A study of 94 maltreated toddlers from one area of New Orleans evaluated 3 months after placement in foster care found rates of 22% of the ICD-10 diagnosis disinhibited attachment disorder (DAD) (5% disinhibited only and 17% mixed withdrawn and disinhibited type; Zeanah et al., 2004). A separate study assessed 60 children ages 6 to 11 years adopted at a mean age of 35 months in the UK following removal by child protective services (Kay et al., 2016). Rates of the ICD-10 diagnosis DAD were 49% possibly reflecting the late adoption age or the high number of care placements (mean of 3.1).

Finally, in a set of studies, Kay et al. (2012, 2016) examined the incidence of RAD among 158 individuals in looked-after care (LAC; the UK version of foster care) with a history of maltreatment but never institutionalized. Fifty-eight percent of individuals in the LAC group showed elevations (≥2 SD above low-risk sample mean) of Disinhibited Indiscriminate behavior; 52% of LAC group had elevations with the Attention Seeking behaviors constellation; and 56% had elevated Superficial Relationships scores. These scores are indicative of those at risk for developing RAD and DSED, previously not examined before.

Comorbidity

In DSED there have been consistent findings of associations with inattention and overactivity that may meet criteria for a separate diagnosis of ADHD. In a study of institutionalized Romanian adoptees, signs of DSED were associated with ADHD and more modestly associated with signs of disruptive behavior disorders by 54 months (Gleason et al., 2011). This study replicated similar associations found among studies of Romanian adoptees between the ages of 54 and 72 months (Rutter, Kreppner, et al., 2007).

This same study by Rutter, Kreppner, et al. (2007) found a significant minority of subjects (9.2%) who demonstrated "quasi-autism." These participants met criteria for autism on the Autism Diagnostic Interview but were differentiated from those with "true" autism by high rates of indiscriminant behavior (such as social approach), superior "spontaneity and flexibility of communication," and improvement in autism symptoms with adoption out of institutions. This finding is further complicated by the increased prevalence of cognitive and language delays known to be seen in populations who experienced severe neglect.

Course

While children may be neglected in the first year of life, the diagnosis of DSED is not made until the child is at least 9 months of age, after the developmental capacity to form selective attachment to caregivers is present. Prior to that age, it is developmentally expected that young children will show social engagement without discrimination. There is no evidence to date that neglect that begins after the age of 2 years is associated with the disorder (Wolkind, 1974). Like RAD, among children who remain in an insufficient rearing environment, there is evidence that signs of the disorder are stable over a period of years (Gleason et al., 2011a).

However, unlike RAD, signs of DSED can be resistant to change despite normalization of the caregiving environment. Among children adopted out of Romanian orphanages, some children continued to demonstrate signs of the disorder between ages 6 and 11 years (Rutter, Colvert, et al., 2007) and when assessed again at age 15 years old (Rutter et al., 2010). Among subjects who improved, the amount of improvement was sometimes modest and took at least 2 years after adoption to be identified. Sometimes signs of DSED were noted to be present even after developing secure attachments to adoptive caregivers (Chisholm, 1998).

Given the sometimes refractory nature of DSED, more is known about the functional impairment of this disorder throughout the child/adolescent life course. In toddlers, the disorder typically involves seeking physical closeness and lack of reticence with unfamiliar adults. In addition, affected children may exhibit separation protest from complete strangers after brief acquaintances. As children move into preschool years, they may display violation of social boundaries and attention-seeking behavior. Increasingly, they may display violation of boundaries with verbally intrusive and inappropriate questions. This over-familiarity with adults has been shown to shift to indiscriminate behavior with peers (Hodges & Tizard, 1989). Affected individuals are expected to have decreased social/emotional competence, peer relational problems, and higher rates of psychopathology (Rutter et al., 2010). These social deficits may be mediated in part by deficits in theory of mind and misattribution that have been found among those with this diagnosis (Kay & Green, 2016).

Differential Diagnosis

The social impulsivity seen in DSED is also a hallmark of several other disorders such as ADHD, Williams syndrome, and bipolar disorder, which can cause confusion between the several conditions. Despite this similarity, Gleason et al. (2011a) demonstrated the ability to differentiate DSED from ADHD. Children with ADHD demonstrate more prominent patterns of pervasive inattention or hyperactivity outside of social interactions. Williams syndrome is a genetic disorder in which affected individuals display many of the socially disinhibited behaviors associated with DSED. People with Williams syndrome can be distinguished by characteristic facial dysmorphology, cardiac and endocrine manifestations, and microdeletion within characteristic regions on chromosome 7 (Pober, 2010). Finally, social impulsivity seen in DSED must be distinguished from impulsive hyper-social behavior that can be seen in manic or hypomanic states. In bipolar disorder such impulsivity is expected to be episodic with periods that are distinguishable from a patient's previous functioning and associated with a constellation of associated mood changes (irritability, euphoria), grandiosity/flight of ideas, and decreased need for sleep.

Etiology and Pathophysiology

Social/Environmental Factors

Environmental factors play a central role in the development of DSED and in fact are considered necessary for the diagnosis of the disorder. Children growing up in neglectful environments have a much higher risk of developing DSED, and the length of time spent in the environment is correlated with symptom persistence. In a report about the Bucharest Early Intervention Project, children randomly assigned to foster care and placed before 24 months of age showed a reduction in signs of DSED by 42 months as compared to children with more prolonged institutionalization (Smyke et al., 2012), and the intervention effect was still evident at 12 years of age (Humphreys et al., 2017). The English and Romanian Adoptees (ERA) Study Team demonstrated similar time sensitivity with the lowest rates of DSED being seen in those adopted before 6 months (O'Connor et al., 2000). Similar to RAD, higher severity of neglect (as measured by consistency of caregivers) is linked to increased signs of DSED (Smyke et al., 2002). Pears et al. (2010) found signs of DSED were linked to the number of placement disruptions among children in foster care.

Despite similarities with RAD, symptoms of DSED may be less influenced by improvements in the quality of the caregiving environment after neglect is experienced. One study of children adopted out of Romanian orphanages found no relationship between caregiving quality and signs of DSED following placement. This finding seems supported by the fact that the ERA Study Team found subjects with persistent signs of DSED even by age 15 years. However, data in this area is mixed with at least one study showing reductions in indiscriminant behavior among subjects with more sensitive adoptive mothers (Van Den Dries, Juffer, van Ijzendoorn, Bakermans-Kranenburg, & Alink, 2012). It is unknown whether refractory signs of DSED are a function of the disorder or as yet unknown mediating qualities of the caregiving environment.

Genetic Factors

A preliminary study has explored genetic factors in children exposed to deprivation. Drury et al. (2012) showed that children who had the s/s genotype of the serotonin transporter gene variant (5HTTLPR) and the met66 allele of brain derived neurotropic factor (BDNF) showed the lowest levels of indiscriminate behavior among children in foster care but the highest levels among children remaining in institutions. These findings need to be replicated, but they illustrate the kind of approach to vulnerability factors that may lead to delineating individual differences in vulnerability to environmental risk.

Neurobiological Factors

There is an evolving body of research finding neurobiological factors linked to "indiscriminant friendliness" among study subjects who experienced the extremes of early neglect. One study of internationally adopted children found that participants with "stunted" growth had higher rates of disinhibited social behavior and higher evening cortisol levels (Johnson et al., 2011). This study implicates chronic stress (allosteric load) on the body as a mediating factor. Olsavsky et al. (2013) performed a functional MRI (fMRI) study of amygdala activation in response to presentation of mother versus stranger's faces in postinstitutionalized (PI) subjects. Among non-PI participants (controls) there were clear differences in patterns of amydala activation when comparing fMRI data upon viewing images of strangers versus images of their mothers' face. PI participants showed less discrimination in amygdala activation between strangers and mothers' faces, and this lack of variation in amygdala activation was associated with indiscriminant friendliness. Finally, Tarullo et al. (2011) have proposed a hypo-activation model of institutional rearing where PI and foster care children demonstrate associations between indiscriminant friendliness and EEG patterns suggesting decreased arousal states.

Rutter, Connor, and the ERA Study Team (2004) have theorized the existence of a sensitive period of developmental programming, wherein institutional deprivation during a key window of development may result in attachment disorders via neural damage. In support of this theory is the Rutter and colleagues' finding that disordered attachment behaviors were not associated with the consequences of malnutrition, cognitive age, or head circumference but were associated with institutional deprivation during the early developmental period. Therefore, deprivation itself is proposed to be the etiologic factor in behavior changes thought to have their roots in "biological programming."

Others have argued that extreme privation may disrupt the establishment of a foundation for neural networks to form in the brain, especially in the right hemisphere (Hardy, 2007). The right hemisphere is involved in affective experiences and is important for interpreting and conveying emotion. Healthy exchanges between infant and caregiver are proposed as key in this process. Therefore, a child in an abusive or neglectful environment during that sensitive period may not correctly develop the skills necessary for interpersonal relationships. Studies involving analyzing children institutionalized later in childhood or adolescence are needed to support these sensitive period theories in the development of disinhibited behavior.

Psychological Factors

Similar to RAD, certain temperaments may increase the risk of developing DSED when subjected to adverse environments, although this is quite challenging to study. A child with an exuberant temperament may be prone to making impulsive and spontaneous decisions, and, when put under the stresses of a neglectful early environment, this may develop into the disinhibited behaviors of DSED (Zeanah et al., 2004). Many studies have explored the relationship between externalizing disorders, specifically ADHD and the disinhibited behaviors associated with DSED. Gleason et al. (2011a) confirmed an association between disinhibited behavior and signs of ADHD in the sample of children in the Bucharest Early Intervention Program but still showed that these two disorders typically may not occur together. This may demonstrate an association between disinhibited behavior and poor social inhibitory control independent of an ADHD diagnosis.

TREATMENT FOR RAD AND DSED

The key intervention for these conditions is ensuring a caregiving environment that is sensitive, responsive, and likely to build a sense of security in the child (Boris, Zeanah, & Zeanah, C. H., & Work Group on Quality Issues, 2005). Currently there are no pharmacologic interventions for attachment disorders unless clinicians identify a separate comorbid condition such as ADHD. Among studies with subjects raised in institutions, the primary intervention is adoption into stable, safe, and emotionally available families. Studies of the quality of such adoptive families (as measured by the sensitivity and responsiveness of caregivers) have linked such measures to improvement in RAD but less robustly to DSED (Smyke et al., 2012). Such a finding may suggest a threshold effect of caregiving quality, wherein further enhancement does not further reduce signs of DSED. Therapeutic interventions that may hasten remission of signs of attachment disorders or treat refractory cases have been examined, but guidelines and effectiveness data is limited. Different psychotherapeutic approaches for children with attachment disorders are here described.

Psychoeducation of caregivers is, after ensuring safety of children, the first crucial step in helping families understand the context and proposed meaning behind disordered attachment behaviors. Such education may help caregivers who feel hurt or rejected by the absence or indiscriminant display of affection. Furthermore, this education can help guide caregivers in how to respond to their child. For instance, many clinicians advise that a child with RAD or DSED may need an overemphasized emotional response from parents in order to sufficiently establish new attachments and make the connection clear to the child (Lieberman, 2003). Restricting the child's contacts to family only, especially in the early months of placement, is often recommended for DSED, although no studies have evaluated this approach. Such restriction is thought to help the children learn to focus comfort and affection seeking to attachment figures.

Including the caregiver in therapy is important for treatment success. A study by Dozier, Stovall, Albud, and Bates (2001) found that maltreated children placed in foster care were more likely to develop secure attachments if their foster mothers were themselves securely attached. Manualized guidelines for treatments for working with families to foster caregiver sensitivity and emotional availability have been explored with promising results (Bernard et al., 2012) and should especially be considered in treatment refractory cases (Zeanah, Berlin, & Boris, 2011). Moreover, interventions that address the history of caregivers' own attachment styles and relationships may play a preventative role for infants at risk for developing attachment disorders (Cicchetti, Rogosch, & Toth, 2006). Infant–parent psychotherapy and child–parent psychotherapy can be used for the treatment of attachment disorders with modifications geared specifically for families dealing with these disorders.

Working individually with the caregivers or, when appropriate, children on specific strategies to manage maladaptive behaviors can also be helpful in strengthening the child's attachment (Boris et al., 2005). Interaction guidance therapy is a way to incorporate working with both child and caregiver and involves shaping positive behaviors through suggestion and positive reinforcement during interactions between the child and caregiver. Basic behavioral or cognitive behavioral therapy (CBT) may also be helpful in DSED to assist the child or teenager in learning socially appropriate behaviors. Research has implicated social cognitive abnormalities in this disorder, which may be particularly well addressed with CBT.

The presence of co-occurring RAD or DSED can reduce the effectiveness of trauma-focused therapies. A randomized controlled trial titled, "It's My Turn Now" targeted internalizing and externalizing disordered youth exposed to interparental violence within a Dutch sample. Results indicated that RAD and DSED negatively impacted recovery from trauma, such that treatment outcomes for both internalizing and externalizing disorders were slowed in individuals with RAD or DSED compared to individuals without the comorbidities. The authors hypothesized that youth with attachment disturbance lacked appropriate social engagement necessary to fully benefit from the therapy process, thereby reducing the therapy's potency (Overbeek, de Schipper, Lamers-Winkelman, & Schuengel, 2014).

A study by Dozier, Peloso, Lewis, Laurenceau, and Levine (2008) examined the Attachment and Biobehavioral Catch-up manualized intervention for children in foster care. To measure the efficacy of the program, cortisol levels were measured for the interventional group of foster children, a control group of foster children with no intervention program, and a control group of children never in foster care and not receiving any intervention. The intervention program combined the teaching of self-regulatory capabilities and focused on teaching parents how to be responsive to their child's emotions, along with attachment security. Cortisol levels of those children participating in the intervention were lower after the Strange Situation Test compared to the foster care control group. Even more surprising, cortisol levels from the control group that had never been in foster care did not statistically differ from those children in foster care receiving the intervention. Research such as this provides important insight into ways of treating children with attachment disorders.

SUMMARY

A small number of individuals from neglectful or abusive environments during critical developmental periods go on to display a variety of problematic behaviors as a result of their experiences. During these times of neglect and abuse, and sometimes even months and years afterward, they have difficulty regulating and managing their social relationships. Descriptions in the DSM-5 provide further refinement of what researchers have been describing for many years—though the etiology may be similar, there are important distinctions between children who go on to develop RAD and those developing the new diagnosis of DSED.

Despite the newer nosology, little is known about what constitutes efficacious care for these vulnerable children, opening up opportunities for valuable contributions to the treatment literature. Until treatment efficacy studies show the best form of therapy, practitioners are often left to rely on pragmatically designed symptom-focused treatment.

REFERENCES

Ainsworth, M. D. S, Blehar, M. C., Waters, E., & Wall, S. *Patterns of attachment: A psychological study of the strange situation*. Hillsdale, NJ: Erlbaum, 1978.

American Psychiatric Association. (1980). *Diagnostic and statistical manual of mental disorders* (3rd ed.). Washington, DC: American Psychiatric Assocation.

American Psychiatric Association. (2013). *Diagnostic and statistical manual of mental disorders* (5th ed.). Arlington, VA: American Psychiatric Publishing.

Bakermans-Kranenburg, M. J., & van Ijzendoorn, M. H. (2007). Research review: Genetic vulnerability or differential susceptibility in child development: The case of attachment. *Journal of Child Psychology & Psychiatry, 48*, 1160–1173.

Bernard, K., Dozier, M., Bick, J., Lewis-Morrarty, E., Lindheim, O., & Carlson, E. (2012). Enhancing attachment organization among maltreated children: Results of a randomized clinical trial. *Child Development, 83*(2), 623–636.

Boris, N. W., Hinshaw-Fuselier, S. S., Smyke, A. T., Scheeringa, M. S., Heller, S. S., & Zeanah, C. H. (2004). Comparing criteria for attachment disorders: Establishing reliability and validity in high-risk samples. *Journal of the American Academy of Child & Adolescent Psychiatry, 43*, 568–577.

Boris, N. W., Zeanah, C. H., & Work Group on Quality Issues. (2005). Practice parameter for the assessment and treatment of children and adolescents with reactive attachment disorder of infancy and early childhood. *Journal of the American Academy of Child & Adolescent Psychiatry, 44*, 1206–1219.

Bos, K., Zeanah, C. H., Fox, N. A., Drury, S. S., McLaughlin, K. A., & Nelson, C. A. (2011). Psychiatric outcomes in young children with a history of institutionalization. *Harvard Review of Psychiatry, 19*, 15–24.

Chisholm, K. (1998). A three-year follow-up of attachment and indiscriminant friendliness in children adopted from Romania orphanages. *Development and Psychopathology, 7*, 283–294.

Cicchetti, D., Rogosch, F. A., & Toth, S. L. (2006). Fostering secure attachments in infants in maltreating families through preventative interventions. *Development and Psychopathology, 18*, 623–645.

Dozier, M., Peloso, E., Lewis, E., Laurenceau, J. P., & Levine, S. (2008). Effects of an attachment-based intervention on the cortisol production of infants and toddlers in foster care. *Developmental Psychopathology, 20*, 845–859.

Dozier, M., Stovall, K. C., Albud, K. E., & Bates, B. (2001). Attachment for infants in foster care: The role of caregiver state of mind. *Child Development, 72*, 1467–1477.

Drury, S. S., Gleason, M. M., Theall, K. P., Smyke, A. T., Nelson, C. A., Fox, N. A., & Zeanah, C. H. (2012). Genetic sensitivity to the caregiving context: The influence of 5httlpr and BDNF val66met on indiscriminate social behavior. *Physiology and Behavior, 16*, 728–735.

Egger, H. L., Erkanli, A., Keeler, G., Potts, E., Walter, B. K., & Angold, A. (2006). Test-retest reliability of the preschool age psychiatric assessment (PAPA). *Journal of the American Academy of Child & Adolescent Psychiatry, 45*, 538–549.

Giltaij, H. P., Sterkenburg, P. S., & Schuengel, C. (2015). Psychiatric diagnostic screening of social maladaptive behaviour in children with mild intellectual disability: Differentiating disordered attachment and pervasive developmental disorder behaviour. *Journal of Intellectual Disability Research, 59*(2), 138–149. doi:10.1111/jir.12079

Gleason, M. M., Fox, N. A., Drury, S., Smyke, A., Egger, H. L., Nelson, C. A. III, Gregas, M. C., & Zeanah, C. H. (2011a). Validity of evidence-derived criteria for reactive attachment disorder: indiscriminately social/disinhibited and emotionally withdrawn/inhibited types. *Journal of the American Academy of Child and Adolescent Psychiatry, 50*, 216–231.

Gleason, M. M., Zamfirescu, A., Egger, H. L., Nelson, C. A. III, Fox, N. A., & Zeanah, C. H. (2011b). Epidemiology of psychiatric disorders in very young children in a Romanian pediatric setting. *European Journal of Child and Adolescent Psychiatry, 20*, 527–535.

Govindan, R. J., Behen, M. E., Helder, E., Makki, M. I., & Chugani, H. T. (2010). Altered water diffusivity in cortical association tracts in children with early deprivation identified with tract-based spatial statistics (TBSS). *Cerebral Cortex, 20*, 561–569.

Hardy, L. T. (2007). Attachment theory and reactive attachment disorder: Theoretical perspectives and treatment implications. *Journal of Child and Adolescent Psychiatric Nursing, 20*, 27–39.

Hodges, J., & Tizard, B. (1989). Social and family relationships of ex-institutional adolescents. *Journal of Child Psychology and Psychiatry, 30*, 77–97.

Humphreys, K. L., Nelson, C. A., Fox, N. A., & Zeanah, C. H. (2017). Signs of reactive attachment disorder and disinhibited social engagement disorder at age 12 years: Effects of institutional care history and high-quality foster care. *Development and Psychopathology, 29*(2), 675–684.

Johnson, A., Bruce, J., Tarullo, A. R., & Gunnar, M. R. (2011). Growth delay as an index of allostatic load in young children: Predictions to disinhibited social approach and diurnal cortisol activity. *Development and Psychopathology, 23*, 859–871.

Kay, C. L., & Green, J. (2016). Social cognitive deficits and biases in maltreated adolescents in UK out-of-home care: Relation to disinhibited attachment disorder and psychopathology. *Developmental Psychopathology, 28*(1), 73–83.

Kay, C. L., Green, J., & Sharma, K. (2016). Disinhibited attachment disorder in UK adopted children during middle childhood: Prevalence validity and possible developmental origin. *Journal of Abnormal Child Psychology, 44*(7), 1375–1386.

Lieberman, A. F. (2003). The treatment of attachment disorder in infancy and early childhood: Reflections from clinical intervention with later-adopted foster care children. *Attachment and Human Development, 5*, 279–282.

Main, M., & Solomon, J. (1990). Procedures for identifying infants as disorganized/disoriented during the Ainsworth Strange Situation. In M. T. Greenberg, D. Cicchetti, & E. M. Cummings (Eds.), *.Attachment in the preschool years: Theory, research, and intervention* (pp. 161–182). Chicago: University of Chicago Press.

Marshall, P. J., Fox, N. A., & BEIP Core Group. (2004). A comparison of the electroencephalogram between institutionalized and community children in Romania. *Journal of Cognitive Neuroscience, 16*(8), 1327–1338.

McLaughlin, K. A., Kubzansky, L. D., Dunn, E. C., Waldinger, R., Vaillant, G., & Koenen, K. C. (2010). Childhood social environment, emotional reactivity to stress, and mood and anxiety disorders across the life course. *Depression and Anxiety, 27*, 1087–1094.

Minnis, H., Macmillan, S., Pritchett, R., Young, D., Wallace, B., Butcher, J., . . . Gillberg, C. (2013). Prevalence of reactive attachment disorder in a deprived population. *British Journal of Psychiatry, 202*(5), 342–346. doi:10.1192/bjp.bp.112.114074

Minnis, H., Reekie, J., Young, D., O'Connor, T., Ronald, A., Gray, A., & Plomin, R. (2007). Genetic, environmental and gender influences on attachment disorder behaviours. *British Journal of Psychiatry, 190*, 490–495.

Nelson, C. A., Zeanah C. H., Fox, N. A., Marshall, P. J., Smyke, A. T., & Guthrie, D. (2007). Cognitive recovery in socially deprived young children: The Bucharest early intervention project. *Science, 318*, 1937–1940.

O'Connor, T. G., Rutter, M. R., Beckett, C., Keaveney, L. Kreppner, J. M., & ERA Study Team (2000). The effects of global severe privation on cognitive competence: Extension and longitudinal follow-up. *Child Development, 71*, 376–390.

O'Connor, T. G., & Rutter, M. (2000). Attachment disorder behavior following early severe deprivation: Extension and longitudinal follow-up. *Journal of the American Academy of Child and Adolescent Psychiatry, 39*, 703–712.

Olsavsky, A. K., Telzer, E. H., Shapiro, M., Humphreys, K. L. Flannery, J., Goof, B., & Tottenham, N. (2013). Indiscriminate amygdala response to mothers and strangers after early maternal deprivation. *Biological Psychiatry, 74*, 853–860.

Overbeek, M. M., de Schipper, J. C., Lamers-Winkelman, F., & Schuengel, C. (2014). Risk factors as moderators of recovery during and after interventions for children exposed to interparental violence. *American Journal of Orthopsychiatry, 84*(3), 295–306. doi:10.1037/ort0000007

Parker, K. C., & Forrest, D. (1993). Attachment disorder: An emerging concern for school counselors. *Elementary School Guidance and Counseling, 27*, 209–215.

Pears, K. C., Bruce, J., Fisher, P. A., & Kim, H. (2010). Indiscriminate friendliness in maltreated foster children. *Child Maltreatment, 15*, 64–75.

Pritchett, R., Rochat, T. J., Tomlinson, M., & Minnis, H. (2013). Risk factors for vulnerable youth in urban townships in South Africa: The potential contribution of reactive attachment disorder. *Vulnerable Children and Youth Studies, 8*(4), 310–320. doi:10.1080/17450128.2012.756569

Pober, B. R. (2010). Williams-Beuren syndrome. *New England Journal of Medicine, 362*(3), 239–252.

Reber, K. (1996). Children at risk for reactive attachment disorder: Assessment, diagnosis, and treatment. *Progress: Family Systems Research and Therapy, 5*, 83–98.

Rutgers, A. H., Bakermans-Kranenburg, M. J., Ijzendoorn, M. H., & Berckelaer-Onnes, I. A. (2004). Autism and attachment: A meta-analytic review. *Journal of Child Psychology and Psychiatry, 45*, 1123–1134.

Rutter, M. (1998). Developmental catch-up, and deficit, following adoption after severe global early privation. English and Romanian Adoptees (ERA) Study Team. *Journal of Child Psychology and Psychiatry, 39*(4), 465–476.

Rutter, M., O'Connor, T. G., & English and Romanian Adoptees (ERA) Study Team. (2004). Are there biological programming effects for psychological development? Findings from a study of Romanian adoptees. *Developmental Psychology, 40*, 81–94.

Rutter, M., Colvert, E., Kreppnes, J., Beckett, C., Castle, J., Groothues, C., . . . Sonuga-Barke, E. J. S. (2007). Early adolescent outcomes for institutionally deprived and non deprived adoptees. I: Disinhibited attachment. *Journal of Child Psychology and Psychiatry, 48*, 17–30.

Rutter, M., Kreppner, J., Croft, C., Murin, M., Colvert, E., Beckett, C., Castle, J., & Sonuga-Barke, E. (2007). Early adolescent outcomes for institutionally-deprived and nondeprived adoptees. III: Quasi-autism. *Journal of Child Psychology and Psychiatry, 48*, 1200–1207.

Rutter, M., Kreppner, J., & Sonuga-Barke, E. (2009). Emanuel Miller lecture: Attachment insecurity, disinhibited attachment, and attachment disorders: Where do research findings leave the concepts? *Journal of Child Psychology and Psychiatry*, *50*, 529–543.

Rutter, M., Sonuga-Barke, E. J., Beckett, C., Castle, J., Kreppnes, J., Kumsta, R., . . . Gunnar, M. R. (2010). Deprivation-specific psychological patterns: Effects of institutional deprivation. *Monographs of the Society for Research in Child Development*, *75*(1), Serial No. 295.

Shaffer, A., Huston, L., & Egeland, B. (2008). Identification of child maltreatment using prospective and self-report methodologies: A comparison of maltreatment incidence and relation to later psychopathology. *Child Abuse and Neglect*, *32*, 682–692.

Sheridan, M. A., Fox, N. A., Zeanah, C. H., McLaughlin, K. A., & Nelson, C. A. (2012). Variation in neural development as a result of exposure to institutionalization early in childhood. *Proceedings of the National Academy of Sciences*, *109*, 12927–12932.

Steele, J. S., & Buchi, K. F. (2008). Medical and mental health of children entering the Utah foster care system. *Pediatrics*, *122*, e703–e709.

Smyke, A. T., Dumitrescu, A., & Zeanah, C. H. (2002). Attachment disturbances in young children. I: The continuum of caretaking casualty. *Journal of the American Academy of Child & Adolescent Psychiatry*, *41*, 972–982.

Smyke, A. T., Zeanah, C. H., Fox, N. A., Nelson, C. A., & Guthrie, D. (2010). Placement in foster care enhances quality of attachment among young institutionalized children. *Child Development*, *81*(1), 212–223.

Smyke, A. T., Zeanah, C. H., Gleason, M. M., Drury, S. S., Fox, N. A., Nelson, C. A., & Guthrie, D. (2012). A randomized controlled trial comparing foster care and institutional care for children with signs of reactive attachment disorder. *American Journal of Psychiatry*, *169*, 508–514.

Tarullo, A. R., Garvin, M. C., & Gunnar, M. (2011). Atypical EEG power correlates with indiscriminately friendly behavior in internationally adopted children. *Developmental Psychology*, *47*, 417–431.

Tizard, B., & Rees, J. (1975). The effect of early institutional rearing on the behavior problems and affectional relationships of four-year-old children. *Journal of Child Psychology and Psychiatry*, *16*, 61–73.

Van Den Dries, L., Juffer, F., van Ijzendoorn, M. H., Bakermans-Kranenburg, M. J., & Alink, L. R. A. (2012). Infants' responsiveness, attachment, and indiscriminate friendliness after international adoption from institutions or foster care in China: Application of emotional availability scales to adoptive families. *Development and Psychopathology*, *24*, 49–64.

Vanderwert, R. E., Marshall, P. J., Nelson, C. A., Zeanah, C. H., & Fox, N. A. (2010). Timing of intervention affects brain electrical activity in children exposed to severe psychosocial neglect. *PLoS One*, *5*(7), 1–5.

Vervoort, E., De Schipper, J. C., Bosmans, G., & Verschueren, K. (2013). Screening symptoms of reactive attachment disorder: Evidence for measurement invariance and convergent validity. *International Journal of Methods in Psychiatric Research*, *22*(3), 256–265. doi:10.1002/mpr.1395

Vorria, P., Papaligoura, Z., Dunn, J., van Ijzendoorn, M., Steele, H., Kontopoulou, A., & Sarafidou, E. (2003). Early experiences and attachment relationships of Greek infants raised in residential group care. *Journal of Child Psychology and Psychiatry*, *44*, 1–14.

Wolkind, S. N. (1974). The components of "affectionless psychopathy" in institutionalized children. *Journal of Child Psychology and Psychiatry*, *15*, 215–20.

Zeanah, C. H., Berlin, L. J., & Boris, N. W. (2011). Practitioner review: Clinical applications of attachment theory and research for infants and young children. *Journal of Child Psychology and Psychiatry*, *52*, 819–833.

Zeanah, C., & Gleason, M. M. (2010). *Reactive attachment disorder: A review for DSM-V*. American Psychiatric Association, Arlington, VA: American Psychiatric Publishing.

Zeanah, C. H., & Gleason, M. M. (2015). Annual research review: Attachment disorders in early childhood—clinical presentation, causes, correlates and treatment. *Journal of Child Psychology and Psychiatry*, *56*(3), 207–222.

Zeanah, C. H., Scheeringa, M., Boris, N. W., Heller, S. S., Smyke, A. T., & Trapani, J. (2004). Reactive attachment disorder in maltreated toddlers. *Child Abuse and Neglect*, *28*, 877–888.

Zeanah, C. H., Smyke, A. T., Koga, S. F., Carlson, E., & Bucharest Early Intervention Project Core Group. (2005). Attachment in institutionalized and community children in Romania. *Child Development*, *76*, 1015–1028.

3

Posttraumatic Stress Disorder

FREDERICK J. STODDARD JR., DAVID M. BENEDEK,
MOHAMMED R. MILAD, AND ROBERT J. URSANO

INTRODUCTION

Posttraumatic stress disorder (PTSD) affects all ages across the globe and when chronic can bring persistent suffering and impaired function. Its diagnosis offers the opportunity for early intervention. PTSD is the subject of intensive research at every level—developmental, epidemiological, as well as from clinical to genetic/genomic, translational, neurobiological, neuropsychological, and psychological. Computational methods with "big data," statistical modeling, and machine learning are beginning to emerge and are likely to accelerate this research; handheld and wearable devices will soon make possible instant inputs and clinical integration as well as rapid applications of findings. The findings from research on PTSD are changing education and the ways clinicians practice, offering the hope for improved care of those experiencing traumatic stress. Those at particular risk for PTSD include children and adolescents, women, soldiers, refugees and survivors of genocide, sexual orientation minorities, racial and ethnic minorities, patients with burns, injuries and medical trauma, and victims of rape, violence, accidents, and disasters. PTSD is highly comorbid with neurodevelopmental, affective, anxiety conduct and substance use disorders (Kessler et al., 1995). PTSD has a neurobiological foundation (Pitman et al., 2012) and evidenced-based biopsychosocial treatments (Foa, Keane, & Friedman, 2008; Yehuda et al., 2015; Ross et al., 2016).

DSM-5 DIAGNOSTIC CRITERIA FOR PTSD

While many criteria are retained from the fourth edition of the Diagnostic and Statistical Manual of Mental Disorders (American Psychiatric Association, 2000), there are significant changes in the fifth edition (DSM-5) for PTSD, with greater clarity, explanation, and some modified and added criteria (American Psychiatric Association, 2013) (Table 3.1). The avoidance and numbing criterion was divided into two clusters, with emotional numbing no longer required to establish a diagnosis but included as a potential manifestation of the "negative alterations of cognition and mood" symptom cluster. Also, while acute and chronic PTSD are no longer distinguished as part of the diagnosis (it is a descriptor) in DSM-5, "delayed expression" is now specified if full diagnostic criteria are not met until 6 months after the traumatic event. In addition, "with dissociative symptoms" is now specified in persons who meet full diagnostic criteria and experience either persistent or recurrent symptoms of depersonalization of derealization (or both). Finally, modified criteria define "PTSD for children 6 years and younger" (Chapter 8) and its variants (i.e., with depersonalization, derealization, and/or delayed expression).

Changes from DSM-IV-TR

The move of PTSD into a new category, trauma- and stressor-related disorders, is one of the largest changes in DSM-5, from the fourth edition, text revision (DSM-IV-TR) (DSM-5, p. 812; Houston et. al., 2013) and reflects the expectation that there will be other trauma- and stressor- related disorders as the science of disorders mature. Since first named as a diagnosis in the third edition of the DSM (DSM-III), PTSD had been included within the category of anxiety disorders. Similar to other diagnoses in medicine, the reclassification of PTSD (along with acute stress disorder, adjustment disorder, and several child-specific disorders) into a new diagnostic class was based on recognition of a common etiology for these conditions. PTSD has similarities to anxiety disorders including *re-experiencing*, which occurs also in panic disorder; *avoidance*, also present in social phobia and obsessive-compulsive disorder; and *arousal*, also seen in panic disorder and generalized anxiety disorder. It also

TABLE 3.1. SUMMARY OF DSM-5 PTSD CRITERIA A-H AND SUBTYPES [FOR FULL CRITERIA, SEE DSM-5]

Criterion	Description	Example	Required	Difference from DSM-IV
Criterion A	Experiencing a traumatic event	Direct experiencing, in-person witnessing, learning someone close was exposed to a severe stressor	Direct: violent or accidental. Indirect: extreme exposure.	Criterion A2, reaction of fear, helplessness, or horror" dropped.
Criterion B	One or more intrusion symptoms associated with the trauma(s), beginning afterwards.	1) Recurrent memories; children > 6, posttraumatic play. 2) Recurrent dreams, nightmares 3) Dissociation, e.g. flashbacks. Children: play re-enactment 4) Severe distress at reminders. 5) Physiological reactions to reminders.	One or more.	No change
Criterion C	Avoidance of reminders	Avoidance of stimuli linked to the trauma: 1) Memories, thoughts, or feelings about the trauma. 2) External reminders	One or both.	This cluster is separated from Criterion D.
Criterion D	Negative alterations in cognitions and mood beginning or worsening after the trauma	1) Inability to recall the trauma, from dissociative amnesia, not head injury, alcohol or drugs. 2) Negative beliefs or expectations about oneself, others or the world. 3) Distorted cognitions about the trauma(s), blame for self or others. 4) Persistent negative emotional state e.g. fear, horror, anger, guilt, sadness, shame, confusion. 5) Markedly diminished interest in activities. 6) Feelings of detachment or estrangement from others. 7) Inability to experience positive emotions.	Two or more.	This cluster is separated from Criterion C.
Criterion E	Alterations in arousal and reactivity	1) Irritable behaviour and angry outbursts 2) Reckless or self-destructive behavior 3) Hypervigilance 4) Exaggerated startle response 5) Problems with concentration 6) Sleep disturbance	Two or more.	#2 is added.
Criterion F	Duration	Duration of the disturbance (Criteria B, C, D, and E) is more than 1 month."	Acute Stress Disorder is < 1 month.	No change

TABLE 3.1. CONTINUED

Criterion	Description	Example	Required	Difference from DSM-IV
Criterion G	Function	The disturbance causes clinically significant distress or impairment in social, occupational, or other functioning.	Impaired function required in one of these areas.	No change
Criterion H	Exclusion	Not attributable to the physiological effects of a substance or another medical condition.	Symptoms not from other medical causes.	This is a new addition.
Subtypes	Specifiers	*Preschool*: Criteria for children under 6.	4 symptoms required.	This is new.
		Dissociative: added if there are dissociative symptoms, either depersonalization or derealization.	Added symptoms.	This is new.
		Delayed expression: emergence of symptoms after a time they were not present or did not meet criteria.		No change from Delayed Onset.

has shared elements with affective disorders. For some patients, depressive symptoms are more significant in PTSD than anxiety symptoms. For this reason, persistent negative alterations in cognitions and mood were added to the DSM-5 criteria for PTSD (Friedman et al., 2011). Sleep disturbance, included within the "altered arousal/ reactivity" symptom cluster, is a core symptom, although perhaps not a hallmark in DSM-5. Germain (2013) advised that "the field is ripe for prospective and longitudinal studies in high risk groups to clarify how changes in sleep physiology and neurobiology contribute to increased risk of poor psychiatric outcomes" (p. 372). With further research, it will become clearer once the diagnostic algorithms for PTSD are further tested whether or not a more "parsimonious" structure or set of symptoms for PTSD exists (Armour, 2015), which very likely would include sleep disturbance.

Controversies

Controversies between several sectors within psychiatry and psychology prevented PTSD from becoming recognized as a formal diagnosis until DSM-III in 1980, and child variants were not added until the revision (DSM-III-R) several years later. Some controversies continue, or continue to strengthen the acceptance of its importance. *Is PTSD a real condition?* This question prevented its acceptance as a diagnostic category until DSM III, since it was not judged to meet the same nosological criteria for a "real" diagnosis, for instance, as depression, schizophrenia, character disorders, autism, or even neuroses. Methodical descriptive and nosological research demonstrated its validity leading to acceptance as a diagnosis and to advocacy for those who had experienced the effects of psychological trauma.

Biological Versus Psychological?

Some of the earliest theories of psychopathology diverged here. Organic causes of psychopathology were assumed to be the etiology of psychoses, and other conditions, by neurologists and psychiatrists with the goal being to find the offending organic cause, or the curative organic treatment.

Psychoanalytic Versus Biological?

On the other hand, psychoanalysis and many other psychological theories minimized biological factors, emphasizing psychological factors as causative such as early trauma, adverse relationships, and stressful life events. Depression, except for involutional melancholia, was largely considered a psychological disorder until antidepressants appeared. Also, for many years, psychotherapy was the primary treatment of schizophrenia until antipsychotic medications were discovered and proven effective.

False Memory Syndrome?

For children, the debate about "false memory syndrome" was fought, mainly resulting in broader acceptance of the validity of the diagnosis of PTSD and broader recognition of the prevalence in society of denial, avoidance, and minimization of the reality of posttraumatic memories and symptoms. In adults, that debate led to examples of individuals "using" this, like other, diagnoses for personal gain, such as inappropriate disability benefits. More common, however, are inappropriate denials of benefits to contain costs for those who have suffered terrible sequelae of trauma. The course of these controversies attest to the importance of the research on this diagnosis and treatment.

Case Example 1

A 14-year-old boy, Ashraf, was seen in pediatric consultation, with an Arabic interpreter, due to a question of recurrent pain and PTSD from burn wounds sustained from a bomb in his neighborhood four months earlier, requiring extensive acute surgical care and a recent right forearm amputation. He was somewhat sad but curious and engaged readily in drawing a self-portrait and playing catch with a football, and his mood lightened. Despite intense initial fear and reluctance, he eventually shared details of his intrusive memories of fearing his own death and recurrent nightmares of the bombing including fears for the lives of his best friend and his family. He explained that the pain medicine helped but didn't work long enough, leaving him with more fear of staff hurting him and with frightening dreams waking him from sleep. When asked if he was considering a prosthetic arm, he expressed hope about that and looked forward to one being fitted and using it once his wounds had healed more.

Comment: This adolescent boy, Ashraf, suffered severe injuries and has intrusive memory and avoidance/numbing and hyperarousal symptoms consistent with PTSD including recurrent nightmares (Ross et al., 1989; Stoddard et al., 1996) from exposure to the bombing and his near-death experience. This related also to the pain of amputation and his changed body image from his burn injuries (Stoddard & Saxe, 2001). He showed mild numbing, and his fearfulness and reluctance to speak were also new phobic and avoidance symptoms, not present pre-injury.

Note. For each illustrative case in this chapter, all names and case vignettes are fictitious. Any resemblance to actual individuals are coincidental.

In modern times, a number of authors have moved the study of trauma forward. Medical psychology sought to label the phenomena as associated with war with terms such as "soldier's heart" during the Civil War, "shell shock" in World War I, and "combat fatigue" in World War II, all of which were seen as stigmatizing for the soldier. After Boston's Cocoanut Grove Nightclub Fire in 1942 in which 492 people—many of them young—died, Stanley Cobb, Erich Lindemann, and Alexandra Adler presented the symptoms and treatments of the survivors with burn injuries whom they treated and their grieving families. These are basic to our knowledge of the symptoms, syndromes, and treatments of PTSD (Cobb & Lindemann, 1943; Adler, 1943, Lindemann, 1944). Robert Lifton describes posttraumatic symptoms in those who endured "brainwashing" in the Korean War (Lifton, 1963) and the horrors of atomic weapons and the suffering of survivors of Hiroshima (Lifton, 1968). Lenore Terr's (1979, 1991) clinical observations and study of the "Children of Chowchilla" who were kidnapped on a school bus, describing their posttraumatic persistent fears, reenactments in play and behaviors, and the lasting impacts of trauma in childhood was critical to our developmental understanding of PTSD. Judith Herman (1992), in *Trauma and Recovery: The Aftermath of Violence from Domestic Abuse to Political Terror*, was also ground-breaking in describing the trauma endured by women who are victims of rape and violence and their psychotherapeutic care. And Jonathan Shay's *Achilles in Vietnam: Combat Trauma and the Undoing of Character* (Shay, 1994) and *Odysseus in America: Combat Trauma and the Trials of Homecoming* (Shay, 2002) unforgettably link the symptoms of posttraumatic stress disorder of soldiers in Vietnam and on their return home to the heroic and tragic tales of Achilles and Odysseus. Art, music, drama and film, history, and literature portray traumatic stress and the symptoms which follow of distressing and intrusive memories, nightmares, irritability, hypervigilance, avoidance, emotional numbing, and posttraumatic re-enactments.

DEVELOPMENTAL EFFECTS OF TRAUMA AND STRESS

There are linkages of early life traumas (Dvir et al., 2014) and stressors and of PTSD (Morey et al., 2016), to the emergence of other psychopathological disorders throughout development (Pynoos et al., 1999; Carrion & Kletter, 2012; Cohen et al., 2017; Danese, 2017; Palmer & Raskind, 2016). However, the neurobiological mechanisms by which these changes occur over a lifetime are much less studied (DeBellis & Zisk, 2014). These observations are important for the minority of children exposed to traumatic events and their risk of subsequent psychopathology (Stoddard, 2014). The symptoms of most mental disorders and other medical illnesses can be increased by stressful life experiences (Bremner, 1999), including posttraumatic sleep disturbances (Stoddard et al., 1996). Of equal interest are how and why the majority of people exposed to severe stressors manifest resilience and do not develop PTSD or other psychopathology.

Injuries and illness at particular phases of life have differing impacts on biopsychosocial development from infancy to old age, with greater impact over the life span the earlier they occur and with most severe impacts tending to come from more severe injuries or illnesses. Trauma and stress symptoms associated with cardiovascular, infectious, autoimmune and other diseases, and surgery or traumatic injury have been associated with onset of illness, impaired or delayed healing, or extended lengths of stay, following medical and surgical illness (Stoddard, in press). A new groundbreaking translational study indicated how stress is associated with the mechanism of cardiovascular disease. Tawakol et al. (2017) found that emotional stress, as indicated by PET/CT brain scanning of amygdala activity, independently and robustly predicted cardiovascular disease events, mediated by increased bone marrow activity and arterial inflammation. They interpret their findings as biological evidence supporting preventive interventions to reduce stress and in turn cardiovascular disease.

There is additional evidence that preventing or reducing the trauma, stressors, or stress response, improve outcomes. These findings have major implications for innovative interventions throughout the life cycle to prevent or reduce the impacts of trauma and stress in the medical setting early in the treatment process. Known impacts of early life stress are impairments in learning, behavior, and both physical and mental well-being (Shonkoff & Garner, 2012), as well as psychiatric disorders as shown in Box 3.1.

> **BOX 3.1. DISORDERS IN LATER LIFE ASSOCIATED WITH CHILDHOOD STRESS AND TRAUMA**
>
> Learning Disabilities
> Attachment Disorders
> Depression
> Anxiety Disorders
> Borderline and other Personality Disorders
> Psychotic Disorders
> Substance Abuse Disorders
> Chronic Pain Syndromes
>
> *Danese & Lewis, 2017*

EPIDEMIOLOGY

While covered in detail in Chapter 7, some general points are addressed here. The methods of epidemiology are being applied to trauma- and stressor-related disorders with ever more powerful computing tools in order to study possible associations with adverse outcomes and to determine what interventions are possible or best. DSM-5 (p. 276) reports lifetime prevalence using DSM-IV criteria at age 75 years as 8.7%, with prevalence for US adults over 12 months as 3.5%. Lower rates of 0.5% to 1.0% are found in most other countries. Rates are up to one-third to one-half for survivors of rape, combat, captivity, and genocide.

Children and adolescents are at significant risk due to poverty, cognitive and emotional immaturity, dependency on parents and caretakers (National Academy of Sciences, 2016), and the potential lifelong negative and positive impacts of early trauma (Terr, 1979, 1991; Stoddard, 2014). Young children are at risk specifically due to "permanent changes in brain structure and function" from the burdens of toxic stress from "poverty, violence, maltreatment, exploitation and oppression" (Shonkoff & Garner, 2012; Shonkoff, 2017). DSM-5 includes new criteria for children under 6 years (Chapter 8). Specifically for children aged 6 to 18, a meta-analysis of psychological risk factors for PTSD found medium to large effect sizes for factors relating to the subjective experience of the stressor event and posttrauma low social support, peritraumatic fear, perceived life threat, social withdrawal, comorbid psychological problem, poor family functioning, distraction, and thought suppression (Trickey et al., 2012).

Adult risk factors for trauma and for PTSD are the most extensively studied. DSM-5 (p. 278) identifies pretraumatic risks such as prior exposure, temperament, and female gender; peritraumatic risks like greater trauma "dose" exposure, injury, or dissociation; and posttraumatic risks such as emergence of acute stress disorder and financial or trauma-related losses. Additional risks include age, education, IQ, race and ethnicity, sexual orientation, pretrauma psychopathology, prior trauma exposure, family psychiatric history, and neurobiological factors (Sayed et al., 2015). Childhood sexual and physical abuse are risk factors for PTSD as well as a wide range of medical, psychological, behavioral, and sexual disorders, including depression, anxiety, and substance abuse over the adult life course (Paolucci et al., 2001; Maniglio, 2009; Lindert et al., 2014). Women are at increased risk for PTSD (Chapter 15).

Analysis of data by Slopen et al. (2016) from the 2014–2015 National Survey of Children's Health revealed black, Hispanic, and particularly children *from lower income groups* were at highest risk of exposure to adverse childhood experiences or adversity (Box 3.2). Risks are, persistently, even higher for boys and men of color (Jones et al., 2012).

There is considerable interest in comorbidity of PTSD and drug use disorders, including possible overlap in their neurochemistry and neurocircuitry. In a national epidemiological study on alcohol and related conditions of 36,309 people, drug use disorders are highly correlated with PTSD and affective, anxiety, and personality disorders (Grant et al., 2016). A review of studies of opiate addiction indicates a very high rate of comorbidity with PTSD, in one study indicating 30% comorbidity (Fareed et al., 2013). A U.S. Veterans Administration study revealed rapidly increasing rates of coprescribing of opioids and benzodiazepines for 66,210 veterans with PTSD over an 11-year period (2003–2011). This pointed to a possible contribution of opioid prescribing for veterans with PTSD to the rise in opioid addiction (Hawkins et al., 2015).

The prevalence of PTSD among prisoners or those who have been to prison is little studied. A study of juveniles in detention in Chicago found nearly all had experienced one or more traumatic events, usually witnessing violence, and rates of PTSD of 11.2% in the prior year (Abram et al., 2004). A survey of 5,008 black American adults found a history of incarceration for 566, of whom 67 (12.59%) had a lifetime history of PTSD, compared to 333 (7.92%) of 4,109 with no incarceration (Anderson et al., 2016), while assessment of PTSD in a Latino prison population found 13.4% with PTSD and 11.6% with subthreshold PTSD for a total of 25% with significant PTSD symptoms (Caraballo et al., 2013). A review of 14 studies in Britain looked at affective and anxiety disorders and PTSD and found rates of either/both anxiety and depression of 30% to 75% (Leigh-Hunt & Perry, 2015). An estimate for prevalence of PTSD for those who are or were imprisoned, based on these studies, suggests a range of 12% to 25% with PTSD or significant symptoms and 30% to 75% if depression and other anxiety disorders are also assessed. A review of 14 studies found elderly prisoners at very high risk for multiple psychopathological disorders but, oddly, only 6% for PTSD (Di Lorito et al., 2017). It is not stated if these rates are lowered by psychotherapy or psychopharmacological treatment.

A meta-analysis of indigenous populations throughout the Americas found, compared to nonindigenous populations, these groups have greater PTSD and social phobia but lower rates of other anxiety and depressive disorders (Kisely et al., 2017). Immigrant groups also had significant but less risk. The injured and medically ill, both children and adults, experience greater risk due to their illness experience, medical-surgical trauma (e.g., pain, the injury or illness, or adverse effects of treatment), and life-threatening events (Stoddard et al., 2011, 2013).

Roberts et al. (2010, 2012) reported that sexual orientation minorities are at a 1.6 to 3.9 elevated risk of PTSD relative to a heterosexual comparison

BOX 3.2. ADVERSE CHILDHOOD EXPERIENCES

- Financial Hardship
- Parent Divorce/Separation or Death
- Parent History of Jail
- Domestic Violence
- Neighborhood Violence
- Household member with Mental Illness or Drug/Alcohol Problem
- Unfair Treatment due to Race/Ethnicity)

group. Elders (Chapter 9) may carry with them positive or negative psychological outcomes from traumatic event exposures while serving in the military when young (Palmer & Raskind, 2016). This is also true for women (Kaiser et al., 2017). Those who serve in the military are at increased risk, especially those in combat roles; women have increased risk related to sexual trauma as well (Ritchie, 2015). Much of the research on PTSD since Vietnam has come through the United States' and other nations' military medical services and the U.S. Veteran's Administration.

Regarding disaster survivors (Chapter 10), while no generalization can be made about PTSD rates, variables known to affect degree of traumatization include age, gender (F>M), prior trauma, exposure, proximity to the disaster, social supports, loss of family or friends, and injury or other illness. Survivors of genocide, as noted in Chapter 1, have high rates of traumatization and variable rates of PTSD related to factors including age, gender, social support, loss of family or friends, and injury or other illness. People with serious and persistent mental illness are also at risk for PTSD, either as a precursor or comorbidity and/or secondary to the onset of psychosis and hospitalization, and are the subjects of studies to treat it (Ruggeri et al., 2000; Mueser et al., 2010; Sin et al., 2015).

BOX 3.3. MODELS OF PTSD

Biological
- Physiological
- Neurochemical and Epigenetic
- Genetic
- Neuroendocrine

Psychological
- Developmental
- Phenomenological/Descriptive
- Cognitive
- Psychodynamic
- Neuropsychological/Circuitry

BIOLOGICAL MODELS OF PTSD

There is a progression of models for PTSD from psychological based only on symptoms to biological models related to physiological, endocrine, neurobiological, and most recently, genetic evidence of PTSD (Box 3.3). One of the first of the biological models were *physiological* studies of autonomic parameters, for example, skin conductance and heart rate, and facial muscle reactivity electromyography, which demonstrated increased physiological reactivity to external trauma-related stimuli and internal mental imagery of the event. "These findings have been interpreted within a framework of Pavlovian conditioning, in which the traumatic event serves as the unconditioned stimulus, the emotional response to it serves as the unconditioned response, trauma-related cues serve as conditioned stimuli, and the physiological reactions serve as conditioned responses" (Stoddard, Simon, & Pitman, 2015, p. 460). The underlying biological mechanisms of PTSD are becoming clearer and are based fundamentally on molecular, neurochemical, and cellular actions and brain circuitry (Pitman et al., 2012; McIntyre et al., 2012; Yehuda et al., 2015; Ross et al., 2017). Twin studies (Gilbertson et al., 2002; Stein et al., 2002) strengthened the evidence for genetic factors increasing susceptibility to PTSD (accounting for at least 30% of the susceptibility). Neurobiological discoveries have helped PTSD's biological foundations as a disease to be accepted broadly, not limited to subjective statements of the past or reported symptoms without a biological basis.

NEUROCHEMISTRY, NEUROBIOLOGY, AND GENETICS

The neurochemical (Chapter 14) and neurobiological (Chapter 15) mechanisms of PTSD are becoming better understood, although much of the research has focused on adult military members. PTSD symptoms appear to vary depending on cortical (e.g., prefrontal cortex) and subcortical (e.g., amygdala and hippocampus circuitry). Animal studies provide a model for understanding amygdala-based fear conditioning and endocrine responses governed by the hypothalamic-pituitary-adrenal axis and their roles in PTSD. However, these models lack the cortical areas similar to the human prefrontal cortex and cognitive capacity to control stress and modulate fear. These differences—along with the availability of new technologies—suggest the importance of studying individual human differences utilizing contemporary neurochemical and neuroimaging and other methods to study the pathophysiology of PTSD (Yehuda, 2015, p. 1; Ross et al., 2017).

The genetics and genomics of PTSD (Chapter 17) remain to be fully elucidated but there is some progress with the likelihood of several genes and epigenetic factors being relevant. There is evidence that genetic factors determine risk for exposure to trauma and for PTSD. Smoller (2015) writes that the findings support "moderately heritabilities for PTSD (in the range of 30–50%) and [for] high-risk trauma exposure (in the range of 30–60%) and that genetic influences on them are highly overlapping." New larger cohorts are being studied. In addition, a Veteran's Administration based postmortem brain bank for PTSD is now in process. This means that understanding of brain function at the cellular and circuit level are significantly advancing through functional genomics, with the availability of genetic tools to decipher neuronal diversity and function and model brain disorders in other species. The existence of a gene editing tool (Heidenreich & Zhang, 2016) suggests that genomic understanding and treatment of many diseases, including PTSD, may move more quickly.

New computational methods are also becoming available. With the utilization of neuroimaging tools and the acquisition of large amounts of psychometric and demographic data, the field is now beginning to consider the use of machine learning and computational modeling tools to integrate large data sets to better our understanding of the neurobiology of PTSD. There is also the thinking that these models may help inform the field of possible biological markers that can be used to diagnose and assess treatment outcomes. Additionally, symptom cluster analysis using "big data" analytic methods appear promising in clarifying whether it is a narrowly defined PTSD syndromal diagnosis or actually a dimensional disorder with variable expression across populations. Biomarkers (Daskalakis et al., 2010) are a major focus and several are promising, such as glucocorticoids (e.g., cortisol), the NR3C1 gene which encodes the glucocorticoid receptor, the FKBP5 gene and other stress-sensitive genes, peripheral blood mononuclear cell sensitivity to glucocorticoids, and "master regulators" related to inflammation being either transcription regulators or cytokine/growth factors (Box 3.4).

In addition, longer duration research, attempting to *stage* the course of biological variants of PTSD, offers an alternative approach to classify its different manifestations, its characteristics with structural and functional neuroimaging, and the relationships of stress hormones enhancing memory consolidation, and immunological/inflammatory factors influencing differing manifestations and trajectories over time and their responses to treatment (McFarlane et al., 2017). Neuroactive steroids, glucocorticoids, allopregnanolone and pregnanolone, 17 beta-estradiol, and GABAergic neuroactive steroids or agents which enhance their synthesis or degradation are candidates for clinical trials to investigate whether they aid memory extinction and extinction retention (Rasmusson et al., 2017). Genetic and epigenetic factors are under increasing scrutiny also as referred to above and in detail in Chapter 16.

BOX 3.4. POTENTIAL BIOMARKERS FOR PTSD IN THE BLOOD

1. Glucocorticoids (GC)
2. NRC31 gene for GC Receptor
3. FKBP5 and other genes sensitive to stress
4. Mononuclear cell sensitivity to GC
5. Master regulators of inflammation: transcription or cytokine/growth factors

Daskalakis et al., 2016

Case Example 2

A 23-year-old woman, Cindy, was seen on referral from her primary care physician for evaluation of emotional trauma and memory problems following a car accident two years earlier in which she was not physically injured. On examination she reported recurrent dreams of the accident, dissociative amnesia not present before for key aspects of the experience, tearfulness associated with remembering, trouble concentrating, and reluctance to drive after it occurred. She had prior panic symptoms qualifying as panic disorder as well, and these were increased on reexposure to the location of the accident and other reminders. When seen, she was six months pregnant with fears that her child might be affected by her PTSD symptoms and depression, which made her symptoms even more distressing as they were also impacting her relationship with her husband of one year.

Comment: This woman presents with some typical PTSD symptoms, and comorbid panic disorder, after a traumatic stressor, with her symptoms including recurrent involuntary dreams, dissociative amnesia, distress with reminders, persistent tendency to avoid driving, persistent and apparently exaggerated negative beliefs about her unborn child, and altered mood not present before the car accident.

PSYCHOLOGICAL MODELS OF PTSD

Several psychological models and factors inform the understanding of PTSD, differentiating psychological symptoms and treatments related to age, gender, culture, phase of the life cycle, resilience, and types of psychotherapy. The psychological models of traumatology include developmental, phenomenological, cognitive, psychodynamic, and neuropsychological. The first has already been addressed. Phenomenological psychology focuses on describing the observed phenomena rather than attributing causation. Cognitive psychology, the source of cognitive behavioral therapy (CBT), describes modes of thinking and increasing interfaces with neuropsychological knowledge from neurobiology and neuroimaging. Psychodynamic approaches began with the psychoanalytic theories of Freud and moved to ego psychology, object relations, self-psychology, and intersubjective models, each of which have distinct therapeutic approaches (Schottenbauer et al., 2008). Cognitive therapy and CBT are evidence-based and effective in relieving PTSD symptoms for over a month after traumatic exposure (Sin et al., 2015).

DIAGNOSTIC ASSESSMENT

Certain conditions or factors are necessary in order to interview people who have been exposed to a traumatic event. This requires skill and consideration for the specific trauma or stressor they have endured in order to foster a relationship, obtain their history, assess for possible posttraumatic stress symptomatology, make a diagnosis, and plan treatment together with the patient.

BUILDING A THERAPEUTIC ALLIANCE

The therapeutic alliance refers to the capacity to form a trusting relationship with the therapist based on the early maternal/child relationship (Zetzel, 1956). Elements of an alliance around diagnosis and therapy includes goals, tasks, and bonds. For effective therapy the patient and therapist must agree on common goals and on the therapeutic tasks to achieve them. In the course of working together on these, the bond of patient and therapist becomes a positive attachment of trust and confidence. Objective and empathic attentive listening and inquiry, with open-ended questions about the patient's psychiatric history including medical history, provides a basis for broadly understanding the origins of the patient's distress, experience over time, and his or her own explanation for the causes of the illness. The diagnostic process is of practical use in gathering information about the patient's strengths and vulnerabilities, capacity for self-expression, and the person's explanatory model for his or her problem or illness. This process, elicited with empathy for the patient's distress, facilitates gathering the symptoms he or she has and concluding what the diagnosis is, communicating understanding, and building a therapeutic alliance with the patient.

The process of building a trusting relationship with the patient has been and is subject to focused study which has confirmed the particular importance of the therapeutic alliance which is developmentally thought to be derived from the patient's early attachment style as a child and problems of early separation and loss, described by Bowlby (1964). Of core therapeutic elements or "the common factors" aiding healing through psychotherapy, the therapeutic alliance is very important (Frank, 1964). It was found to predict outcome in both psychotherapy and psychopharmacology treatments (Krupnick et al., 1996), and recently Milrod et al. (2014) identified its relevance as a trusting relationship between patient and therapist in the treatment of anxiety disorders. A further step in psychotherapeutic treatment is aiding patients in finding meaning in their experience(s), as the elements of their narrative histories begin to come together and they feel less anxious and uncertain as to what is happening to them. In describing the importance of this in listening to children, Anna Freud in 1964 spoke to students at Case Western Reserve Medical School about the child's experience of bodily illness, highlighting the reality of their pain and anxiety in causing them to express extreme fear and distress often in behavior (Freud, 1952).

There are significant differences in eliciting a history of trauma for different age groups, ethnicities, socioeconomic groups, females and males, types of trauma, and between those with single traumas versus multiple or complex traumas. For instance "meeting" the patient to optimize the opportunity for self-expression about psychologically traumatic experiences can entail play with a child (Meersand & Gilmore, 2018), which may include reenactments in play of their trauma termed "posttraumatic play" (Terr, 1981). Meeting the older patient includes other steps, such as explanation about what a diagnostic evaluation is with a very anxious patient, requesting an interpreter for a patient whose native language is different from one's own, learning whether or not a female patient is comfortable being interviewed by a man, or arranging a home visit for an elderly patient. Sharing a traumatic experience with a stranger can be unsettling and requires effort to help the patient feel more comfortable, the first step in building a therapeutic alliance.

Another element in establishing a trusting therapeutic alliance in relation to traumatic experiences occurs through empathic interest in the patient's bodily feelings related to and after the trauma especially whether or not the patient is experiencing current physical pain, and what its location, duration and severity is (Stoddard & Saxe, 2001). Further inquiry into pain, including emotional suffering, as exemplified by the technique of inquiry into bodily experience and memory associated with the trauma, as taught by Dr. Elvin Semrad, conveys both interest in their story of the trauma and therapeutic interest in relieving their suffering related to it (Van der Kolk, 1994). Dr. Semrad's central, intentionally provocative, serious question to patients was "where do you feel it in your body?" They responded in their own words with their narrative of the memories of their experience. This empathic approach led some patients to grieve, crying for the first time about the traumas they had been through.

ASSESSMENT CONSIDERATIONS IN CHILDREN

Diagnostic assessment varies for children under 6 years based on the new PTSD diagnostic criteria for that age group. School-age children or adolescents may need to play or talk about their latest video game before being able to share information about what they have endured (per American Psychiatric Association guideline and others). Some patients may choose not to speak about their traumatic event initially, requiring more than one session to establish trust and gentle encouragement, before elaborating about it. Shy, fearful, withdrawn, or medicated patients may have difficulty and may need specific direct questions if information about traumatic experiences are to be elicited.

Diagnostic Criteria

The DSM-5 recognizes that in addition to anxiety- and fear-based symptomatology, many individuals with PTSD have clinical characteristics which are more anhedonic and dysphoric, consistent with the high comorbidity of PTSD with depression, and also externalizing angry and aggressive or dissociative symptoms. In DSM-5, there are five clusters for *children over 6 years, adolescents*, and *adults*. They are "A-E" with varying numbers of required symptoms, and requirements E, F, and G also. "A" is exposure in one or more of four ways: to actual or threatened death, serious injury or sexual violence directly, witnessing, learning about it occurring to a close family member or friend, or repeated and extreme exposure to aversive details of the events. "B" is presence of at least one of five intrusion symptoms beginning after the traumatic event, including distressing memories, distressing dreams, dissociative reactions, intense distress at exposure to internal or external cues, or marked physiological reactions to reminders. "C" are at least one of two persistent avoidance symptoms, including avoidance of or efforts to avoid distressing memories, thoughts, or feelings about or closely associated with the event, or avoidance of or efforts to avoid external reminders that arouse distressing memories, thoughts, or feelings about or closely associated with the traumatic event(s). "D" are at least two or more of seven negative alterations in cognitions and mood associated with the traumatic event(s), including inability to remember (typically dissociative amnesia not due to head injury or substances); persistent negative beliefs or expectations about oneself or the world; persistent distorted cognitions about the cause or consequences of the traumatic event(s) leading the individual to blame self or others; persistent negative emotions such as fear, horror, anger, guilt, or shame; markedly diminished interest in significant activities; feelings of estrangement or detachment from others; or persistent inability to experience positive emotions; and at least two of six marked alterations in arousal or reactivity associated with the traumatic event(s): irritability or angry outbursts, reckless and self-destructive behavior, hypervigilance, exaggerated startle response, problems concentrating, or sleep disturbances such as difficulty falling or staying asleep or restless sleep. Therefore, the minimum number of required symptoms is a total of seven symptoms, including at least one from each cluster, in order to make a diagnosis of PTSD. Arriving at a diagnosis only occurs after eliciting responses regarding the required symptom criteria which is normally elicited directly but can be done over time, or using a symptom and criterion checklist, or by asking a relative or caregiver in the case of a child or elder under the care of a family member or caregiver. "F" specifies that the duration must be at least one month. "G" specifies that the disturbance causes clinically significant distress or impairment in social, occupational, or other important areas (e.g., school) functioning. "H" specifies that the disturbance is not attributable to the physiological effects of a substance including drugs and medications or to another medical illness.

ASSESSMENT INSTRUMENTS

The clinical interview remains the "gold standard" for the assessment of PTSD for several reasons: (a) an interview allows for a detailed explanation of the nature of the traumatic stressor or stressors, (b) an interactive process allows for the best understanding of confusing symptoms (the ability to distinguish or articulate the difference between intrusive recollections and flashbacks), and (c) the clinical interview allows for the progressive elaboration of symptoms in a manner sensitive to the emotional needs of the patient at the time of assessment.

However, several clinician-administered and self-report instruments can be used to obtain diagnostic information in the aftermath of traumatic exposure. The most widely used instruments are listed in Box 3.5.

Several of these instruments were developed originally for DSM-IV but have since been adapted for and used extensively in clinical and research environments to quantify diagnostic criteria and measure DSM-5 PTSD symptom severity. The PTSD module of the Structured Clinical Interview for DSM-IV (SCID-IV) used open-ended questions about traumatic exposure (supplemented with examples) as well as questions about each of the 17 symptoms of PTSD, duration of disturbance, and functional impairment (First et al., 1995). The PTSD module SCID for DSM 5 has been developed in a similar format asking open-ended questions about each of the 20 symptoms of DSM-5 PTSD and is presently being validated. The most commonly used PTSD measure in research prior to the transition to DSM-5 was the Clinician-Administered PTSD scale (CAPS), which asked the patient about the frequency and severity of each symptom rating each on a scale of 1 to 4 yielding a total score of between zero and 136. A minimum score of 50 was used as an entry criterion for PTSD research (Blake et al., 1990). The CAPS has been revised to reflect the new diagnostic criteria, and new scoring and threshold scores have been developed allowing a clinician to assess severity (mild, moderate, severe) as well current (past month and/or past week) as well as lifetime diagnosis (Weathers, et al. 2013). The PTSD Checklist for DSM-5 is a self-report measure that can be completed by patients. It takes approximately 5 to 10 minutes to complete, and results are easily interpreted by clinicians according to a variety of scoring rules (Weathers, et al., 2013). Such a report can be used to assess symptom severity at initial presentation and to track symptoms as treatment progresses.

Regardless of the interview techniques or instruments used to quantify symptoms, it is important to note that the DSM-5 specifies that the diagnosis should better explain the symptoms (e.g., why symptoms represent PTSD, a trauma- and stressor-related disorder), than a depressive, anxiety, or dissociative disorder or a substance use disorder or other general medical condition.

BOX 3.5. INSTRUMENTS USED IN THE ASSESSMENT AND DIAGNOSIS OF PTSD

- The Structured Clinical Interview for DSM 5 (SCID-5)
- The Clinician-Administered PTSD Scale (CAPS)
- The Davidson Trauma Scale (DTS)
- The Impact of Events Scale Revised (IES-R)
- The Life Events Checklist for DSM-5 (LEC-5)
- The PTSD Checklist for DSM-5 (PCL-5)

TREATMENT CONSIDERATIONS

At the conclusion of the diagnostic evaluation, the final step is to discuss with the patient the presence (or absence) of the PTSD diagnosis, the prognosis, and then to engage in a discussion about whether and when to proceed with treatment. The pla nning, designing, and carrying out the course of treatment will often differ for patients in special populations, with different trauma experiences, medical histories, family or cultural characteristics, or resources and social supports. It is important to listen and observe the patient's response to learning the presence or absence of the diagnosis of PTSD since it can be experienced in varying ways such as being upsetting, confirmatory, alien, supportive, or stigmatizing. For some patients, anxiety, language difficulty, cultural barriers, a general mistrust of clinicians, or other factors may interfere with their understanding of either this or an alternative diagnosis as potentially helpful to them. They may require simpler explanation, or explanations responding to their questions, before the meaning of the diagnosis and what may help becomes clear.

Case Example 3

Mr. Smith is a 46-year-old electrician, on disability, who sustained 50% total body surface area burns at work one year before, requiring acute trauma surgeries and many plastic and reconstructive procedures for his injuries and extensive scars. His surgeon referred him for evaluation of PTSD and depression since his injury. Despite pride in having overcome rehabilitation challenges, he presented with feelings of intense distress about his sexual attractiveness, sexual functioning, and marriage, due to his scars although he had no genital injury. He avoided sex due to these preoccupations but could function sexually, had persistent negative emotional states with depressive mood, angry feelings, and difficulty having loving feelings toward his wife, who was angry too. He felt estranged from her and had altered arousal with angry outbursts and insomnia but no nightmares. His PTSD, and comorbid adjustment disorder with depression, improved over three years of CBT, couples therapy, and paroxetine for both PTSD and depression. He was unable to return to work.

Comment: Mr. Smith presents with mixed, somewhat atypical PTSD symptoms fulfilling DSM-5 criteria, after a 50% burn and scarring, extensive painful surgical care and rehabilitation, with sequelae including distress at living with reminders of his injuries and his wife's reactions to them, distress with reminders of his scarring in his sexual relationship, a persistent tendency to avoid sex, new persistent and severe feelings of anger, and anger outbursts toward his wife, feelings of estrangement from and difficulty experiencing loving feelings towards her, and negative mood. These were not present before his burn injury. His impairments in both social and occupational functioning, and despite moderate alcohol use, no substances or other medical condition explained his PTSD symptoms. His long-term evidence-based psychotherapeutic and psychopharmacological treatments effectively helped to reduce his symptoms and improve his marital relationship.

TREATMENT

Psychotherapies

These include psychodynamic (generally for complicated and chronic PTSD), CBT, eye-movement desensitization and relaxation (EMDR), and others. CBT treatment interventions—including exposure and cognitive processing treatments—are the most evidence supported and are based on cognitive psychology and the idea that traumatic experience results in fear memories and overgeneralized response to reminders of the traumatic experience. Behavior therapy focuses on identifying and extinguishing maladaptive behavioral responses to triggers or cues of the fear memory. CBT is thus targeted to neurocircuitry involved in thoughts and behaviors, or areas of the brain or circuits devoted to particular functions such as autonomic responsivity, emotional regulation, and executive functioning (Bisson & Andrew, 2007; Bisson et al., 2007; Foa et al., 2008). Clinical trials have also demonstrated the efficacy of EMDR in PTSD—although subsequent dismantling studies have suggested that the eye-movement component of this exposure-based cognitive therapy is unnecessary (Benedek et al., 2009).

Somatic and/or Pharmacotherapy

A range of medications and other somatic approaches to the treatment of PTSD have been evaluated in clinical trials in the last quarter-century. These are presented in detail in later chapters. Importantly, pharmacotherapies for PTSD presently considered "first-line" on the basis of evidence from randomized controlled trials include selective serotonin-reuptake inhibitors, serotonin-norepinephrine reuptake inhibitors, and—with regard to associated sleep disturbance and nightmares—alpha-1 antagonists (Capehart, 2017). Neurostimulation techniques including vagus nerve stimulation, transcranial magnetic stimulation, and deep brain stimulation are currently being explored, as are alternative approaches such animal-assisted therapy, yoga, meditation, and acupuncture—although thus far only the latter has demonstrated efficacy in well-designed clinical trials.

A range of treatment guidelines for trauma therapies are available for adults and children and are further discussed in Section IV. The most recent ones are based on critical review of evidence from randomized controlled clinical trials, and these universally describe exposure-based cognitive therapy including prolonged exposure or cognitive processing therapy as first-line treatment for adults with PTSD. Several, but not all published guidelines suggest that medications (i.e., from those medication classes noted earlier) should be also considered as first line approaches. Available evidence suggests pharmacotherapy is not as effective as CBT in combat-related PTSD (Benedek et al. 2009). The extent to which practice parameters or guidelines are used differs depending on the system of care to which patients have access, from extensive use to none (which is surprisingly common). Treatment guidelines do not define the standard of care but are increasingly available online or in handheld treatment decision-facilitating applications. Research is currently examining the extent to which these clinical decision support tools and applications actually improve clinical outcomes. To the extent that these do prove beneficial, they must anticipate the incorporation of new evidence for medications, complementary and alternative approaches, and new psychotherapies currently being explored.

PRACTICE PARAMETERS

Selected practice parameters or treatment guidelines for PTSD are as follows.

For Adults

American Psychological Association (2017) Clinical Practice Guideline for the Treatment of PTSD. Retrieved from http://www.apa.org/ptsd-guideline/ptsd.pdf on 01/21/2018.

Bandelow et al. World Federation of Societies of Biological Psychiatry (WFSBP) guidelines for the pharmacological treatment of anxiety, obsessive-compulsive and post-traumatic stress disorders: first revision. *The World Journal of Biological Psychiatry*. 2008;9(4):248–312.

Foa et al. *Effective treatments for PTSD: Practice guidelines from the International Society for Traumatic Stress Studies* (2nd ed.). New York: Guilford; 2009.

National Collaborating Centre for Mental Health. The management of posttraumatic stress disorder in primary and secondary care. National Institute for Clinical Excellence Guidelines (NICE), UK, 2005. (Last updated 2016; in development [GID-NG10013]; expected date 2018)

Stein et al. WCA recommendations for the long-term treatment of posttraumatic stress disorder. *CNS Spectrums*. 2003 Aug; 8(8) Suppl. 1: 31–39.

Ursano et al. *American Psychiatric Association practice guidelines for the treatment of patients with acute stress disorder and posttraumatic stress disorder*. Washington, DC: American Psychiatric Association; 2004.

Department of Veterans Affairs and Department of Defense. *VA/DoD clinical practice guideline for management of post-traumatic stress and acute stress disorder* 2017. Retrieved from https://www.healthquality.va.gov/guidelines/MH/ptsd/VADoDPTSDCPGFinal012418.pdf.

For Children

Cohen JA, Bukstein O, Walter H, et al. Practice parameters for the assessment and treatment of children and adolescents with posttraumatic stress disorder. *Journal of the American Academy of Child and Adolescent Psychiatry*. 2010;49:414–430.

SUMMARY AND CONCLUSIONS

Posttraumatic stress disorder was a new diagnosis in the DSM III in 1980, while the condition was recognized long before its acceptance as a formal diagnosis. The process of diagnostic assessment for PTSD requires steps to assist the patient in relating as comfortably as possible in the process: empathy for the patient's experience of having endured one or more traumatic events, attention to eliciting and/or observing the presence or absence of PTSD symptoms which make up the criteria for diagnosis, a willingness to acknowledge what is not known, and awareness that the sharing of traumatic events may evolve over time as the patient's comfort increases. The diagnostic criteria for posttraumatic stress disorder have been significantly modified in DSM-5 from DSM-IV, and PTSD is now placed in a new class "trauma and stressor-related disorders." Changes from DSM-IV include the elimination of the A2 criterion which required a subjective reaction of "fear, helplessness or horror" to the traumatic event, and the addition of the "persistent negative alterations in cognitions and mood" symptom cluster. There is a subcategory of "PTSD for children 6 years and younger"(Chapter 8), and specifiers for three variants: with depersonalization, derealization, and delayed expression.

Epidemiological studies reveal both resilience after traumatic events in most of those exposed to severe traumatic events and significant rates of PTSD in a significant minority. Risk factors are important determinants of individual vulnerability for adult PTSD, with early life trauma, toxic stress such as abuse, neglect, or poverty being significant predictors. The prevalence of PTSD varies with different degrees of exposure and different populations with high rates for those exposed to combat or rape and lower rates for those who endure other abuse, disasters, and injuries. Knowledge of the biological foundations of PTSD continues to increase with new findings in epidemiology, neurochemistry, genetics, neurobiology, and neuroimaging and across the life cycle. Current research directions seem likely to further improve knowledge about PTSD or help to resolve existing diagnostic and therapeutic challenges. As knowledge of the neurobiology of PTSD expands, so too will treatment options. There is great need throughout the world to reduce early life toxic stressors leading to PTSD and other adverse outcomes. Thus the prevention of PTSD remains an unmet need but a very worthwhile goal.

REFERENCES

Abram KM, Teplin LA, Charles DR, Longworth SL, McClelland GM, Dulcan MK. Posttraumatic stress disorder and trauma in youth in juvenile detention. *Arch Gen Psychiatry.* 2004 Apr;61(4):403–410.

Adler, A. Neuropsychiatric complications in victims of Boston's cocoanut grove disaster. *JAMA.* 1943;123(17):1098–1101. doi:10.1001/jama.1943.02840520014004

Anderson RE, Geier TJ, Cahill SP. Epidemiological associations between posttraumatic stress disorder and incarceration in the National Survey of American Life. *Crim Behav Ment Health.* 2016 Apr;26(2):110–123. doi:10.1002/cbm.1951. PMID:25732512

American Psychiatric Association. *Diagnostic and statistical manual of mental disorders,* 4th ed., text rev. Washington, DC: American Psychiatric Association, 2000.

American Psychiatric Association. *Diagnostic and statistical manual of mental disorders,* 5th ed. Arlington, VA: American Psychiatric Association, 2013.

Armour C. The underlying dimensionality of PTSD in the diagnostic and statistical manual of mental disorders: where are we going? *Eur J Psychotraumatology.* 2015;6:28074.

Benedek DM, Friedman MJ, Zatzick D, Ursano RJ. *Guideline watch: Practice guideline for the treatment of patients with acute stress disorder and posttraumatic stress disorder.* Arlington, VA: American Psychiatric Press; 2009.

Bisson J, Andrew M. Psychological treatments of post-traumatic stress disorder (PTSD). *Cochrane Database Syst Rev.* 2007;3:CD003388.

Bisson JI, Ehlers A, Matthews R, et al. Psychological treatments for chronic post-traumatic stress disorder: Systematic review and meta-analysis. *Br J Psychiatry.* 2007;190:97–104.

Bremner JD. Does stress damage the brain? *Biol Psychiatry.* 1999;45:797–805.

Capehart B. Psychopharmacology of PTSD. Paper presented at MGH Psychiatry Academy, March 20, 2017.

Caraballo JN, Pérez-Pedrogo C, Albizu-García CE. Assessing post-traumatic stress symptoms in a Latino prison population. *Int J Prison Health.* 2013;9(4):196–207. doi:10.1108/IJPH-02-2013-0004

Carrion VG, Kletter H. Posttraumatic stress disorder: Shifting towards a developmental framework. *Child Adolesc Psychiatric Clin N Am.* 2012;21:573–591. http://dx.doi.org/10.1016/j.chc.2012.05.004

Cobb S, Lindemann E. Neuropsychiatric observations. *Ann Surg.* 1953;117(6):814–824.

Cohen JR, Suvarna V, Menon RC, et al. The distal consequences of physical and emotional neglect in emerging adults: A person-centered, multi-wave, longitudinal study. *Child Abuse Neglect.* 2017;63:151–161 http://dx.doi.org/10.1016/j.chiabu.2016.11.030

Danese A, Moffitt TE, Arseneault L, et al. The origins of cognitive deficits in victimized children: Implications for neuroscientists and clinicians. *Am J Psychiatry.* 2017;174:349–361; doi:10.1176/appiajp201616030333

Davidson JT, Book SW, Colket JT, et al. (1997). Assessment of a new self-rating scale of post-traumatic stress disorder. *Psychological Medicine.* 1997;27:153–160.

Dvir Y, Julian D, Ford JD, Hill M, Frazier JA. Childhood maltreatment, emotional dysregulation, and psychiatric comorbidities. *Harv Rev Psychiatry.* 2014;22(3):149–161. doi:10.1097/HRP.0000000000000014\

Daskalakis NP, Cohen H, Nievergelt CM, Baker DG, Buxbaum JD, Russo SJ, Yehuda R. New translational perspectives for blood-based biomarkers of PTSD: From glucocorticoid to immune mediators of stress susceptibility. *Exp Neurol.* 284:133–140.

DeBellis MD, Zisk A. The biological effects of childhood trauma. *Child Adolesc Psychiatric Clin*

N Am. 2014;23(2):185–222. http://dx.doi.org/10.1016/j.chc.2014.01.002

Di Lorito C, Völlm B, Dening T. Psychiatric disorders among older prisoners: A systematic review and comparison study against older people in the community. *Aging Ment Health.* 2017 Feb 7:1–10. doi:10.1080/13607863.2017.1286453

Fareed A, Eilender P, Haber M, Bremner J, Whitfield N, Drexler K. Comorbid posttraumatic stress disorder and opiate addiction: A literature review. *J Addict Dis.* 2013;32(2):168–179. doi:10.1080/10550887.2013.795467

First MB, Spitzer RL, Gibbon M, Williams JB. *Structured Clinical Interview for DSM-IV Axis I disorders—Patient Edition* (SCID I/P Version 2). New York: Biometrics Research Department, New York State Psychiatric Institute; 1995.

Foa EB, Keane TM, Friedman MJ, Cohen JA. *Effective treatments for PTSD: Practice guidelines from the international society for traumatic stress studies*, 2nd ed. New York: Guilford; 2008.

Frank, JS. *Persuasion and healing: A comparative study of psychotherapy.* New York: Schocken; 1964.

Freud A. The role of bodily illness in the mental life of children. *Psychoanalytic Study Child.* 1952;7(1):69–81. doi:10.1080/00797308.1952.11823153

Friedman MJ, Resick PA, Bryant RA, Strain J, Horowitz M, Spiegel D. Classification of trauma- and stressor-related disorders in DSM-5. *Depress Anxiety.* 2011;28(9):737–749. doi:10:1002/da.20845

Germain A. Sleep disturbance and the hallmark of PTSD: Where are we now? *Am J Psychiatry.* 2013;170:372–382.

Gilbertson MW, Shenton ME, Ciszewski A, et al. Smaller hippocampal volume predicts pathologic vulnerability to psychological trauma. *Nat Neurosci.* 2002;5:1242–1247.

Grant BF, Saha TD, Ruan WJ, et al. Epidemiology of DSM-5 drug use disorder: Results from the National Epidemiologic Survey on Alcohol and Related Conditions-III. *JAMA Psychiatry.* 2016 Jan;73(1):39–47. doi:10.1001/jamapsychiatry.2015.2132.PMID:26580136

Hawkins EJ, Malte CA, Grossbard JR, Saxon AJ. Prevalence and trends of concurrent opioid analgesic and benzodiazepine use among Veterans Affairs patients with post traumatic stress disorder, 2003–2011. *Pain Med.* 2015 Oct;16(10):1943–1954. doi:10.1111/pme.12787

Heidenreich M, Zhang, F. Applications of CRISPR-Cas systems in neuroscience. *Nat Rev Neurosci.* 2016 Jan;17(1):36–44. doi:10.1038/nrn.2015.2

Herman J. *Trauma and recovery: The aftermath of violence—from domestic abuse to political terror.* New York: Basic Books; 1992.

Houston AA, Webb-Murphy J, Delaney E. (2013). *From DSM-IV-R to DSM-5: Changes in posttraumatic stress disorder.* COSC Research Facilitation. Retrieved from www.nccosc.navy.mil

Institute of Medicine. *Treatment of posttraumatic stress disorder: An assessment of the evidence.* Washington, DC: National Academies Press; 2008.

Jones DJ, Crump AD, Lloyd JJ. Health disparities in boys and men of color. Editorial. *Am J Pub Health.* 2012;102(2):S170–S172.

Kaiser AP, Wang J, Davison EH, Park CL, Stellman, JM. Stressful and positive experiences of women who served in Vietnam. *J Women Aging.* 2017;29(1):26–38. doi:10.1080/08952841.2015.1019812

Kessler RC, Sonnega A, Bromet E, Hughes M, Nelson, CB. Posttraumatic stress disorder in the National Comorbidity Survey. *Arch Gen Psychiatry.* 1995;52:1048–1060.

Kisely S, Alichniewics KK, Black E, Siskind D, Spurling G, Toombs M. The prevalence of depression and anxiety disorders in indigenous people of the Americas: A systematic review and metanalysis. *J Psych Res.* 2017;84:137–212. http://dx.doi.org/10.1016/j.jpsychires.2016.09.032 0022-3956/

Krupnick JL, Sotsky SM, Simmens S, Moyer J, Elkin I, Watkins J, Pilkonis PA. The role of the therapeutic alliance in psychotherapy and pharmacotherapy outcome: Findings in the National Institute of Mental Health Treatment of Depression Collaborative Research Program. *J Consult Clin Psychol.* 1996;64(3):532–539.

Leigh-Hunt N, Perry A. A systematic review of interventions for anxiety, depression, and PTSD in adult offenders. *Int J Offender Ther Comp Criminol.* 2015 Jun;59(7):701–725. doi:10.1177/0306624X13519241. Review. PMID: 24441030

Lifton RJ. *Thought reform and the psychology of totalism.* New York: W. W. Norton; 1963.

Lifton RJ. *Death in life: Survivors of Hiroshima.* New York: Random House; 1968.

Lindemann E. Symptomatology and management of acute grief. *Am J Psychiatry.* 1944;101(2):141–148. doi:10.1176/ajp.101.2.141

Lindert J, von Ehrenstein OS, Grashow R, Gal G, Braehler E, Weisskopf MG. Sexual and physical abuse in childhood is associated with depression and anxiety over the life course: Systematic review and meta-analysis. *Int J Public Health.* 2014;59:359–372. doi:10.1007/s00038-013-0519-5

Maniglio R. The impact of child sexual abuse on health: A systematic review of reviews. *Clin Psychol Rev.* 2009;29:647–657.

McFarlane AC, Lawrence-Wood E, Van Hooff M, et. al. The need to take a staging approach to the biological mechanisms of PTSD and its treatment.

Curr Psychiatry Rep. 2017;19:10. doi:10.1007/s11920-017-0761-2

McIntyre CK, McGaugh JL, Williams CL, et al. Interacting brain systems modulate memory consolidation. *Neurosci Biobehav Rev*. 2012;36:1750–1762.

Meersand P, Gilmore KJ. Play therapy: a psychodynamic primer for the treatment of young children. Arlington, VA: American Psychiatric Association Publishing, 2018.

Milrod B, Markowitz JC, Gerber AJ, Cyranowski J, Altemus M, Shapiro T, Hofer M, Glatt C. Childhood separation anxiety and the pathogenesis and treatment of adult anxiety. *Am J Psychiatry*. 2014 Jan;171(1):34–43. doi:10.1176/appi.ajp.2013.13060781

Morey RA, Haswell CC, Hooper SR, De Bellis MD. Amygdala, hippocampus, and ventral medial prefrontal cortex volumes differ in maltreated youth with and without chronic posttraumatic stress disorder. *Neuropsychopharmacology*. 2016;41:791–801.

Mueser KT, Lu W, Rosenberg SD, Wolfe R. The trauma of psychosis: Posttraumatic stress disorder and recent onset psychosis. *Schizophr Res*. 2010;116:217–227.

National Academy of Sciences, Engineering, and Medicine. *Parenting matters: Supporting parents of children ages 0–8*. Washington, DC: National Academies Press; 2016.

Palmer BW, Raskind MA. Posttraumatic stress disorder and aging. *Am J Geriatr Psychiatry*. 2016 Mar;24(3):177. http://dx.doi.org/10.1016/j.jagp.2016.01.133

Paolucci EO, Genuis ML, Violato C. A meta-analysis of the published research on the effects of child sexual abuse. *J Psychology*. 2001;135(1):17–36.

Pitman RK, Rasmusson AM, Koenen KC, et al. Biological studies of post-traumatic stress disorder. *Nat Rev Neurosci*. 2012;13:769–787.

Pynoos RS, Steinberg AM, Piacentini JC. A developmental psychopathology model of childhood traumatic stress and intersection with anxiety disorders. Review article. *Biol Psychiatry*. 1999 Dec 1;46(11):1542–1554.

Rasmusson AM, Marx CE, Pineles SL, Locci A, Scioli-Salter ER, Nillni YI, Liang JJ, Graziano P. Neuroactive steroids and PTSD treatment. *Neurosci Lett*. 2017;649:156–163. doi:http://dx.doi.org/doi:10.1016/j.neulet.2017.01.054

Ritchie EC, Bell MR, Gallaway MS, et al. Female soldiers and post-traumatic stress disorder. In: EC Ritchie and AL Naclerio, Eds. *Women at war*, 22–33. New York: Oxford University. Press; 2015.

Roberts AL, Austin BS, Corliss HL, Vandermorris AK, Koenen KC. Pervasive trauma exposure among U.S. sexual orientation minority adults and risk of posttraumatic stress disorder. *Am J Public Health*. 2010;100(12):2433–2441.

Roberts AL, Rosario M, Corliss HL, Koenen KD, Austin SB. Elevated risk of posttraumatic stress in sexual minority youths: Mediation by childhood abuse and gender nonconformity. *Am J Public Health*. 2012;102(8):1587–1593.

Ross DA, Arbuckle MR, Travis MJ, Dwyer JB, van Schalkwyk GI, Ressler KJ. An integrated neuroscience perspective on formulation and treatment planning for posttraumatic stress disorder: An educational review. *JAMA Psychiatry*. 2017;74(4):407–415. doi:10.1001/jamapsychiatry.2016.3325. PMID:28273291

Ross RJ, Ball WA, Sullivan KA, Caroff SN. Sleep disturbance as the hallmark of posttraumatic stress disorder. *Am J Psychiatry*. 1989;146:697–707.

Ruggeri M, Leese M, Thornicroft G, Bisofti G, Tansella M. Definition and prevalence of severe and persistent mental illness. *Br J Psychiatry*. 2000;177:149–155.

Sayed S, Iacoviello BM, Charney DS. Risk factors for the development of psychopathology following trauma. *Current Psychiatry Rep*. 2015;17(70). doi:10.1007/s11920-015-0612-y

Shay J. *Achilles in Vietnam: Combat trauma and the undoing of character*. New York: Scribner; 1994.

Shay J. *Odysseus in America: Combat trauma and the trials of homecoming*. New York: Scribner; 2002.

Schottenbauer MA, Glass CR, Arnkoff DB, Gray SH. Contributions of psychodynamic approaches to treatment of PTSD and trauma: A review of the empirical treatment and psychopathology literature. *Psychiatry*. 2008;71(1):13–34.

Shonkoff J. Expanding the evidence base to drive more productive early childhood investment. *Lancet* 2017;389:14–16. http://dx.doi.org/10.1016/S0140-6736(16)31702-0

Shonkoff J, Garner AS. Technical report: The lifelong effects of early childhood adversity and toxic stress. *Pediatrics*. 2012;129:e232–e246. www.pediatrics.org/cgi/doi/10.1542/peds.2011-2663 doi:10.1542/peds.2011-2663

Sin J, Spain D, Furuta M, Murrells T, Norman I. Psychological interventions for post-traumatic stress disorder (PTSD) in people with severe mental illness. *Cochrane Database Sys Rev*. 2015;1. doi:10.1002/14651858.CD011464

Slopen N, Shonkoff JP, Albert MA, Yoshikawa H, Jacobs A, Stoltz R, Williams DR. Racial disparities in child adversity in the U.S.: Interactions with family immigration history and income. *Am J Prev Med*. 2016;50(1):47–56.

Smoller JW. The genetics of stress-related disorders: PTSD, depression, and anxiety disorders. *Neuropsychopharm Rev*. 2016;41:297–319. doi:10.1038/npp.2015.266

Stein MB, Jang KL, Taylor S, et al. Genetic and environmental influences on trauma exposure and posttraumatic stress disorder symptoms: A twin study. *Am J Psychiatry*. 2002;159:1675–1681.

Stoddard FJ. Outcomes of traumatic exposure. *Child Adolesc Psychiatric Clin N Am.* 2014;23(2):243–256.

Stoddard FJ, Chedekel DS, Shakun L. Dreams in burned children. In: D. Barrett, Ed. *Trauma and dreams*, 25–45. Cambridge, MA: Harvard University Press; 1996.

Stoddard FJ. Wound healing and depression. In: J Strain, Ed. *Depression as a systemic illness.* New York: Oxford University Press, in press.

Stoddard FJ, Saxe GN. Ten-year research review of physical injuries. *J Am Acad Child Adolesc Psychiatry.* 2001;40(10):1128–1145.

Stoddard FJ, Sheridan RL, Martyn JAJ, Czarnik JE, Deal VT. Pain management. In: EC Ritchie, Ed. *Combat and operational behavioral health*, 339–358. (Textbooks of Military Medicine). Washington, DC: Department of the Army, Office of the Surgeon General, Borden Institute; 2011.

Stoddard FJ, Sheridan R, Martyn J, Selter L, Greenberg, DB. General surgery: Basic principles. In: BS Fogel, DB Greenberg, Eds. *Psychiatric care of the medical patient*, 3rd ed., 1367–1388. New York: Oxford University Press; 2015.

Tawakol A, Ishai A, Takx RA, Figueroa AL, Ali A, Kaiser Y, Truong QA, Solomon CJ, Calcagno C, Mani V, Tang CY, Mulder WJ, Murrough JW, Hoffmann U, Nahrendorf M, Shin LM, Fayad ZA, Pitman RK. Relation between resting amygdalar activity and cardiovascular events: a longitudinal and cohort study. *Lancet.* 2017;389:834–845.

Terr LC. Children of Chowchilla: A study of psychic trauma. *Psychoanal Study Child.* 1979;34:547–623.

Terr LC. "Forbidden games": Post-traumatic child's play. *J Am Acad Child Psychiatry.* 1981;20:740–759.

Terr LC: Childhood traumas: An outline and overview. *Am J Psychiatry.* 1991;148:10–20.

Trickey D, Siddaway AP, Meiser-Stedman R, Serpell L, Field AP, Wilson MA, Reagan LP. A meta-analysis of risk factors for post-traumatic stress disorder in children and adolescents. *Clin Psychol Rev.* 2012;32:122–138.

van der Kolk, BA. The body keeps the score: Memory and the evolving psychobiology of posttraumatic stress. *Harv Rev Psychiatry.* 1994 Jan-Feb;1(5):253–265.

Weathers FW, Litz BT, Keane TM, Palmieri PA, Marx BP, Schnurr PP. *The PTSD Checklist for DSM-5 (PCL-5)*, 2013. Retrieved from www.ptsd.va.gov

Yehuda R, Hoge CW, McFarlane AC, et al. Post-traumatic stress disorder. *Nature Rev/Dis Primers.* 2015; Oct 1(8):1–22. doi:10.1038/nrdp.2015.57

Zetzel, ER. Current concepts of transference. *Int J Psychoanal.* 1956;37(4–5):369–376.

ADDITIONAL RESOURCES

Chang JC, Yen AM, Chen HH, Chen SL, Chiu SY, Fann JC, Lee CS. Comorbid diseases as risk factors for incident posttraumatic stress disorder (PTSD) in a large community cohort (KCIS no.PSY4). *Sci Rep.* 2017 Jan 27;7:41276. doi:10.1038/srep41276

Cohen JA, Scheeringa MS. Post-traumatic stress disorder diagnosis in children: Challenges and promises. *Dialogues Clin Neurosci.* 2009;11:91–99.

Danese A, Lewis SJ. Psychoneuroimmunology of early-life stress: The hidden wounds of childhood trauma? *Neuropsychopharmacology.* 2017 Jan;42(1):99–114. doi:10.1038/npp.2016.198. PMID:27629365

Davydow DS, Gifford JM, Desai SV, et al. Posttraumatic stress disorder in general intensive care unit survivors: A systematic review. *Gen Hosp Psychiatry.* 2008;30:421–434.

Elhai JD, Palmieri PA. The factor structure of posttraumatic stress disorder: A literature update, critique of methodology, and agenda for future research. *J Anxiety Disord.* 2011;25(6):849–854. doi:10:1016/j.janxdis. 2011.04/007

Editorial. Special issue: New perspectives in PTSD. *Exp Neurol.* 2016;284:115–118. http://dx.doi.org/10.1016/j.expneurol.2016.09.011

Eilender P, Haber M, Bremner J, Whitfield N, Drexler K. Comorbid posttraumatic stress disorder and opiate addiction: A literature review. *J Addict Dis.* 2013;32(2):168–179. doi:10.1080/10550887.2013.795467

Lehrner A, Yehuda R. Biomarkers of PTSD: Military applications and considerations. *Eur J Psychotraumatol.* 2014;5:1–11.

Schmeltzer SN, Herman JH, Sah R. Neuropeptide Y(NPY) and posttraumatic stress disorder (PTSD): A translational update. *Exp Neurol.* 2016;284:196–210 http://dx.doi.org/10.1016/j.expneurol.2016.06.020

Slopen S, McLaughlin KA, Shonkoff JP. Interventions to improve cortisol regulation in children: A systematic review. *Pediatrics.* 2014;133:312–326. doi:10.1542/peds.2013-1632

Stoddard FJ Jr, Simon MN, Pitman RK. Trauma- and stressor-related disorders. In LR Yudofsky, Ed. *American Psychiatric Publishing textbook of psychiatry: DSM-5 edition*, 6th ed., 455–498. Washington, DC: American Psychiatric Press; 2014.

Strawn JR, Keeshin BR, DelBello MP, Geracioti TD, Putnam FW. Psychopharmacological treatment of posttraumatic stress disorder in children and adolescents: A review. *J Clin Psychiatry.* 2010;71:932–941.

Yehuda R. Post-traumatic stress disorder. *N Engl J Med.* 2002;346:108–114.

4

Acute Stress Disorder

RICHARD A. BRYANT

Acute stress disorder (ASD) was introduced as a new diagnosis in 1994 in the fourth edition of the *Diagnostic and Statistical Manual of Mental Disorders* (DSM-IV; American Psychiatric Association, 1994). This diagnosis has led to much new research into the nature of acute psychological reactions to trauma, as well considerable developments in how acute traumatic stress is assessed and treated. This chapter reviews the current diagnostic criteria, the nature of trajectories of traumatic stress responses, known mechanisms of ASD, and prevailing assessment and treatment procedures.

BACKGROUND TO THE ASD DIAGNOSIS

There has been a long-standing tradition in the diagnosis of posttraumatic stress disorder (PTSD) to limit the diagnosis to severe reactions that persist for at least one month after trauma exposure. Prior to the development of DSM-IV, there was concern that this approach limited access to health care in the United States because in the absence of a formal diagnosis, accessing health care could be problematic. Accordingly, it was proposed in the development of DSM-IV that a diagnosis was needed that would fill this diagnostic gap and that by identifying people who are more severely distressed there would be a formal means of facilitating access to health care.

There was a second goal of the new ASD diagnosis, which was to identify acutely traumatized people who would be most likely to subsequently develop PTSD. This was noted at the time as an important step forward because numerous studies had indicated that whereas many people display acute distress in the initial days after trauma exposure, most of these people will not progress to develop PTSD (Bryant, 2003). Accordingly, a major challenge for early intervention for people after trauma has been to disentangle those people in the acute phase who have a transient stress response from those displaying the early signs of a chronic course of PTSD. It was proposed that ASD would provide a solution, at least to some degree, to this problem (Koopman, Classen, Cardeña, & Spiegel, 1995).

In DSM-IV the ASD diagnosis required that the individual needed to be exposed to a traumatic event in which there was actual or threatened death or serious injury and they experienced fear, helplessness, or horror. Four additional symptom clusters needed to be satisfied. Three of these clusters were similar to the PTSD criteria, insofar as the person needed to exhibit one or more re-experiencing symptoms, marked avoidance of stimuli that remind the individual of the trauma, and marked anxiety or arousal symptoms. These symptoms also had to cause significant distress or impairment and last for a minimum of two days and a maximum of four weeks. The distinctive symptom cluster of ASD involved dissociative symptoms which required at least three of the following dissociative symptoms: (a) a subjective sense of numbing, detachment, or absence of emotional responsiveness; (b) reduced awareness of surroundings; (c) derealization; (d) depersonalization; and (e) dissociative amnesia. The historical roots of this emphasis on dissociation in ASD can be traced to the work of Janet in the early 20th century (Janet, 1907), who proposed that some trauma survivors respond to traumatic experiences by splitting awareness of their distressed state from consciousness. Janet posited that this reaction placed demands on one's psychological resources, which led to subsequent psychopathological states. This perspective became popular in the years prior to DSM-IV, and this led to the notion that dissociative symptoms in the aftermath of trauma were pivotal in moderating subsequent PTSD (van der Kolk & van der Hart, 1989). Accordingly, it was proposed that dissociative responses to the trauma in the acute phase resulted in limited access to trauma memories, which would limit processing of emotional experiences and lead to ongoing PTSD (Spiegel, Koopman, & Classen, 1994). Supporting this idea was early evidence that dissociation in the acute phase was associated with subsequent PTSD (Cardeña & Spiegel, 1993; Holen, 1993), and which has been replicated numerous times (Ehlers, Mayou, & Bryant, 1998; Murray, Ehlers, & Mayou, 2002).

CRITICISMS OF THE ASD DIAGNOSIS

There were numerous criticisms of the ASD diagnosis when it appeared. First, there was criticism that DSM-IV allowed dissociative symptoms to occur during the trauma *or* during its aftermath. The ambiguity over the time frame of dissociative responses was problematic because dissociative reactions that occur during a trauma may actually limit encoding of the traumatic experience and in this sense may be protective (Horowitz, 1997), whereas dissociative responses that persist may limit access to encoded trauma memories and their affect and contribute to posttraumatic stress symptoms. In this sense it is worth noting that most dissociative reactions after trauma abate with time (Davidson, Kudler, Saunders, & Smith, 1990). Further, persistent dissociative responses are linked to both acute (Panasetis & Bryant, 2003) and chronic (Briere, Scott, & Weathers, 2005) posttraumatic reactions. This pattern is underscored by evidence that factor-analytic studies demonstrates two subscales of the major measure of acute dissociation, the Peritraumatic Dissociative Experiences Questionnaire (Marmar, Weiss, & Metzler, 1997); one subscale involved reduced awareness and is not strongly correlated with symptoms of psychopathology (e.g., those which may cause clinically significant distress or result in social or occupational dysfunction), whereas the Derealization/Depersonalization subscale is (Brooks et al., 2009).

ASD AND PTSD

As noted, one of the goals of the ASD diagnosis was to identify recently trauma-exposed individuals who would subsequently develop PTSD. Following the introduction of the ASD diagnosis in DSM-IV, a series of longitudinal studies were conducted that assessed ASD in the initial month after trauma exposure and subsequently assessed for PTSD. A review of 22 published longitudinal studies highlights the major findings from these studies (Bryant, 2011). First, across most studies most trauma survivors with ASD subsequently met criteria for PTSD. That is, the ASD diagnosis performed well in that most people with the disorder did not remit but continued to have longer-term PTSD. However, the sensitivity in predicting PTSD was poor. That is, most trauma survivors who eventually developed PTSD did not meet the criteria for ASD initially. Several studies that assessed subsyndromal ASD, which typically required meeting three of the four ASD symptom clusters (but not dissociation), found that the sensitivity in predicting PTSD was better if one used subsyndromal ASD; however, even these studies found only very modest sensitivity in predicting PTSD (Bryant, Creamer, O'Donnell, Silove, & McFarlane, 2008a; Harvey & Bryant, 1998b, 1999d).

Several studies have focused on the relationship between ASD and PTSD in children. An interesting pattern emerges in studies that address the predictive capacity of ASD in children. The five child studies that have assessed ASD and PTSD longitudinally (Bryant, Salmon, Sinclair, & Davidson, 2007; Dalgleish et al., 2008; Ji, Xiaowei, Chuanlin, & Wei, 2010; Kassam-Adams & Winston, 2004; Meiser-Stedman, Yule, Smith, Glucksman, & Dalgleish, 2005) suggest that ASD is an even weaker predictor of PTSD in children than adults. The significant majority of children who develop PTSD after trauma do not display ASD initially, and this may be attributed to the poor understanding of dissociative responses in children after trauma.

TRAJECTORIES OF POSTTRAUMATIC STRESS

Understanding ASD requires appreciation of the trajectories of posttraumatic stress responses. In earlier conceptualizations of traumatic stress, most work converged on the notion that whereas acute stress responses were more common in the acute phase, there was a trend for adaptation by most people in a way that only a minority experienced chronic PTSD (Galea et al., 2003; Riggs, Rothbaum, & Foa, 1995). In contrast, there is now awareness that the course of traumatic stress is not linear. For example, in one longitudinal study of traumatically injured patients who were assessed in the hospital and again 3, 12, and 24 months later, it was found that the rate of PTSD remained fairly constant over time—but approximately half of people who had PTSD, or even subsyndromal PTSD, at any time point had a different status at the next assessment (Bryant, O'Donnell, Creamer, McFarlane, & Silove, 2013). This highlights the dynamic nature of PTSD status over time, and this appears to be strongly influenced by ongoing stressors after the trauma.

One of the newer developments in this area in recent years has been recognition of the limiting factor of diagnostic categories because one only needs to alter one symptom and persons who previously met diagnostic criteria shift from being a "case" to being a "non-case" (see later discussion of incidence). More sophisticated statistical approaches have mapped trajectories by using latent growth mixture modeling, which permits distinct groups to be identified in way that individual variation over time. Rather than assuming that all people follow the same path, it permits different trajectories to be mapped. Different investigations have robustly noted (a) a resilient class that consistently shows few PTSD symptoms, (b) a recovery class with initial distress then gradual remission, (c) a delayed reaction class with initial low symptom levels but increased symptoms over time, and (d) a chronic distress class with consistently high PTSD levels. Most of these studies indicate that approximately three-quarters of trauma survivors enjoying minimal distress across time. It is impressive that these patterns have been observed in survivors of traumatic injury (Bryant, et al., 2015), SARS infection (Bonanno et al., 2008), women diagnosed with breast cancer (Lam et al., 2010), disaster (Pietrzak, Van Ness, Fried, Galea, & Norris, 2013), disaster and terrorist attacks (Norris, Tracy, & Galea, 2009), and military personnel deployed to the Middle East (Bonanno et al., 2012). These studies indicate that how a person adapts following trauma cannot be accurately assessed in the acute phase because the longer status of an individual will change over time (except for the majority of people who will remain consistently resilient).

ASD IN DSM-5

The evidence reviewed above was important in laying the foundation for changes in the ASD diagnosis in the fifth edition of the DSM (DSM-5; American Psychiatric Association, 2013). On the basis of the ASD having poor predictive capacity, one of the most important changes in DSM-5 was that the ASD diagnosis was no longer intended to predict subsequent PTSD (Bryant, Friedman, Spiegel, Ursano, & Strain, 2011). The emphasis of the diagnosis was shifted solely to identifying people who are experiencing severe stress reactions and may require mental health assistance.

There were numerous other changes made in DSM-5. In DSM-IV the diagnosis of ASD required satisfaction of four different symptom clusters. Whereas several factor analytic studies of ASD symptoms have supported the DSM-IV conceptualization of the four factors (Brooks et al., 2008; Cardeña, Koopman, Classen, Waelde, & Spiegel, 2000; Wang et al., 2000), others have found that the four-factor structure does not accommodate ASD responses (Armour, Elklit, & Shevlin, 2013; Bryant, Moulds, & Guthrie, 2000). As a result, in DSM-5 the diagnosis of ASD was restructured such that it did not require specific symptom clusters to be present. Instead, it was decided that a minimum of 9 out of a possible 14 symptoms should be present. This was deemed to reflect people who suffered severe stress reactions that may warrant mental health intervention. Other changes were introduced in the wake of increasing evidence. The number of dissociative symptoms were reduced from the five to two: (a) reduced awareness of one's surroundings was deleted on the grounds that it pertained predominantly to responses occurring during the trauma, (b) symptoms of derealization and depersonalization were combined into a single item because of the documented overlap between these two responses (Harvey & Bryant, 1999c); and (c) dissociative amnesia was retained. There was also a minor shift in the time frame of when ASD can be diagnosed. There is evidence that many people who will experience stress reactions in the initial days after trauma will subsequently report fewer reactions in the following weeks (Solomon, Laor, & McFarlane, 1996), and so the change was extended from two to three days.

INCIDENCE OF ASD

In contrast to most psychiatric disorders, there is an absence of epidemiological studies of ASD. Because it is not a chronic disorder, it is unusual for population studies to index this disorder in the context of traumatic events that occurred in the previous month. Hence, knowledge of the incidence of ASD is restricted to studies that are conducted on trauma-exposed populations within one month of exposure. These studies have led to quite varied rates of ASD. For example, ASD has been reported following motor vehicle accidents (13% to 21%; Harvey & Bryant, 1998b), mild traumatic brain injury (14%; Harvey & Bryant, 1998a), assault (16% to 19%; Brewin, Andrews, Rose, & Kirk, 1999; Harvey & Bryant, 1999b), burns (10%; Harvey & Bryant, 1999b), industrial accidents (6%; Harvey & Bryant, 1999b), and witnessing a mass shooting (33%; Classen, Koopman, Hales, & Spiegel, 1998). It is worth noting that these studies employed the DSM-IV criteria for ASD diagnosis, and there is limited evidence regarding the incidence of ASD using the DSM-5 criteria. Using DSM-5 criteria, ASD has been noted in 10% of bank robbery victims (Armour & Hansen, 2015) and 14% of traumatic injury patients (Bryant et al., 2015); however, further studies are needed to establish a robust evidence base of the incidence of ASD using the DSM-5 definition.

BIOLOGICAL MODELS OF ASD

Arguably the major model of acute traumatic stress involves biological processes. This perspective typically involves fear conditioning models, which posit that psychological trauma triggers noradrenergic and glucocorticoid activation, which fosters consolidation of trauma memories. Fear conditioning models propose that the fear experienced at the time of trauma causes strong associative conditioning between the fear and many stimuli associated with the trauma and that when one is confronted with trauma reminders, conditioned responses are triggered; these responses may include re-experiencing symptoms, such as intrusive memories and physiological reactivity (Pitman, 1989). In support of this model is much evidence that psychophysiological reactivity is activated in PTSD patients when exposed to trauma reminders (Blanchard, Kolb, Gerardi, Ryan, & Pallmeyer, 1986; Orr, Pitman, Lasko, & Herz, 1993). It is proposed that most people adapt to a traumatic experience by virtue of extinction learning, in which trauma survivors are exposed to trauma reminders without any harmful consequences and thereby new learning occurs that the previously conditioned reminders now signal safety (Milad, Rauch, Pitman, & Quirk, 2006). In this sense, PTSD can be regarded as an example of failed extinction learning (Myers & Davis, 2007).

Consistent with fear conditioning models, studies have examined resting heart rate immediately after trauma exposure because sympathetic arousal may reflect the level of fear conditioning. These studies have noted that higher resting heart rates in adults and children in the days after trauma exposure predict subsequent PTSD (Bryant, Creamer, O'Donnell, Silove, & McFarlane, 2008b; Shalev et al., 1998). This pattern is also reflected in the finding that elevated respiration rate in the first 48 hours predicts PTSD (Bryant et al., 2008b). More direct support for the process of fear conditioning is a finding that phasic increases in heart rate in response to trauma reminders are a stronger predictor of PTSD than resting state heart rate (O'Donnell, Creamer, Elliott, & Bryant, 2007). It is also worth noting that nearly all people with ASD reported having panic symptoms during the trauma, and most of these persist in the weeks after the event (Nixon & Bryant, 2003).

We have noted that only a minority of people develop PTSD, and there is evidence that one of the key risk factors for PTSD is if they are predisposed to enhanced conditioning or impaired extinction before the trauma exposure. For example, one study assessed newly recruited firefighters, who at the time of assessment were in class-based training and had not commenced active duty, on conditioning paradigms. This study found that recruits' skin conductance and eyeblink startle reactions in response to startling tones predicted their level of acute stress symptoms within a month of subsequently being exposed to a traumatic event as a fire-fighter (Guthrie & Bryant, 2005). This observation may suggest that the tendency to be reactive to stressors increases vulnerability to fear conditioning. In a more direct study of conditioning, this study also assessed extinction learning on an experimental task before trauma exposure and found that the level of PTSD two years after commencing firefighting duties was predicted by impoverished extinction learning as a recruit (Guthrie & Bryant, 2006). This finding has been replicated in both first responders and military personnel who were assessed prior to exposure to traumatic events (Lommen, Engelhard, Sijbrandij, van den Hout, & Hermans, 2013; Orr et al., 2012). These findings strongly indicate that individual differences in extinction learning are pivotal in the risk for PTSD.

COGNITIVE MODELS OF ASD

The other influential model focuses on cognitive mechanisms. This model proposes that traumatic stress is moderated by (a) the manner in which the trauma is encoded in memory and (b) excessively negative appraisals about the traumatic experience and the aftermath (Ehlers & Clark, 2000). In terms of appraisals, cognitive models posit that trauma response is influenced by how the survivor interprets trauma experiences, especially regarding one's role in the trauma, one's vulnerability for future harm, and one's worth as a person. Specifically, the appraisals of vulnerability (e.g., "I can never feel safe again"), one's role in the trauma (e.g., "the attack was my fault"), or one's worth (e.g., "I am a terrible mother for not coping better") can contribute substantially to the acute and chronic stress response.

Much evidence supports this model, with people with chronic PTSD displaying distorted appraisals (Dunmore, Clark, & Ehlers, 1997; Ehlers et al., 1998; Ehlers & Steil, 1995). In terms of acute stress, people with ASD exaggerate both the probability of negative events happening to them and also the severity of how adverse those events would be (Smith & Bryant, 2000; Warda & Bryant, 1998). Further, negative appraisals in the acute phase are predictive of later PTSD (Dunmore, Clark, & Ehlers, 2001; Engelhard, van den Hout, Arntz, & McNally, 2002; Murray et al., 2002; Wikman, Molloy, Randall, & Steptoe, 2011). Relatedly, cognitive styles that are characterized by ruminating after a traumatic event are also predictive of later PTSD (Ehlers, Mayou, & Bryant, 2003; Kleim et al., 2007; Mayou et al., 2002).

Cognitive models also emphasize the importance of how memories are encoded and consolidated. The strong arousal at the time of trauma purportedly results in details of the trauma being encoded in a predominantly sensory (and often visual) manner. That is, a motor vehicle accident survivor may have recurring images of the grill of the truck he smashed into but have patchy recall of other events as they occurred. According to this model, this form of encoding ("data-driven processing") leads to fragmented memories of the trauma that foster a sense of "nowness" in which person re-experiences the memory as if it is still in the present. Consistent with this perspective, data-driven processing has been associated with intrusive memories and PTSD (Ehring, Ehlers, & Glucksman, 2008; Halligan, Clark, & Ehlers, 2002; Halligan et al., 2002). Moreover, data-driven processing in the acute phase is linked with heart rate increase in response to trauma-related stimuli (Ehlers et al., 2010). Similarly, children with ASD report more sensory-laden memories of their trauma, which in turn mediates the relationship between perceived threat of a trauma and severity of ASD (Meiser-Stedman, Dalgleish, Smith, Yule, & Glucksman, 2007). Also people with ASD have fragmented memories (Harvey & Bryant, 1999a), which accords with the proposal that acute stress is associated with memory disorganization.

ASSESSMENT OF ASD

Several assessment instruments have been introduced to index ASD symptoms. The Acute Stress Disorder Interview (ASDI) was initially developed based on the DSM-IV items (Bryant, Harvey, Dang, & Sackville, 1998). Comprising 19 dichotomously scored items based on the DSM-IV dissociative (5 items), reexperiencing (4 items), avoidance (4 items), and arousal (6 items) symptoms. It possesses good internal consistency (r = .90), test–retest reliability (r = .88), sensitivity (91%), and specificity (93%) relative to independent clinician diagnosis of ASD, based on DSM-IV criteria (Bryant et al., 1998). Following the changes to the ASD diagnosis in DSM-5, the interview has modified to match the DSM-5 criteria (Bryant, 2016); however, this recent adaptation has not yet been subjected to psychometric evaluation.

In terms of self-report measures, the first measure developed was the Stanford Acute Stress Reaction Questionnaire (SASRQ; Cardeña, Classen, & Spiegel, 1991). The more recent version of the SASRQ is a 30-item self-report inventory that encompasses each of the DSM-IV ASD symptoms (Cardeña, Koopman, Classen, Waelde, & Spiegel, 2000). The other major self-report measure is the Acute Stress Disorder Scale (ASDS), which is based on the same items and wording as the ASDI. Each item is scored on a 5-point scale to index symptom severity (Bryant et al., 2000). Test–retest reliability between two to seven days was strong (r = 0.94). Predictive ability of the ASDS has been reported using a cut-off score of 56 on the ASDS, predicting 91% of those who developed PTSD and 93% of those who did not. The ASDS has also been updated to incorporate DSM-5 changes (Bryant, 2016), although it has yet to be validated.

It is also worth noting that other measures have been developed to assess acute trauma reactions. Depression is a very common posttraumatic stress response (Bryant et al., 2010; Shalev et al., 1998), and so one scale was developed to screen acutely traumatized individuals for depression and posttraumatic stress. The Posttraumatic Adjustment Scale (PAS; O'Donnell et al., 2008) comprises 10 items that are each scored on a 5-point scale. In terms of predicting subsequent PTSD 12 months after trauma, the PAS-P has been shown to have strong sensitivity (.82) and specificity (.84) but modest positive predictive power (.28). In terms of predicting subsequent depression, the PAS-D had a sensitivity of .72 and a specificity of .74, positive predictive power of .30 (O'Donnell et al., 2008).

TREATING ASD

Psychotherapy Approaches

Similar to the status of treatment of PTSD, the evidence indicates that the treatment of choice for ASD is trauma-focused cognitive behavior therapy (CBT). Treatment guidelines around the world recommend this approach for the treatment of ASD and prevention of PTSD (Foa, Keane, Friedman, & Cohen, 2009; National Clinical Institute of Excellence, 2005). This therapy typically begins with education about psychological trauma and then focuses on anxiety management, exposure therapy, and cognitive restructuring. Education intends to normalize the trauma response, explains basic mechanisms for ASD symptoms, and discusses how core symptoms will be treated during therapy. Anxiety management techniques intend to reduce arousal through breathing retraining, relaxation skills, and self-talk. Arguably the most central technique of CBT is exposure therapy, which can involve both imaginal and in vivo exposure. Imaginal exposure (also called prolonged exposure) directs patients to "relive" their trauma for prolonged periods (often for at least 30 minutes; Foa, 2011). This involves people providing a detailed narrative of their experience with the goal of accessing emotional engagement and relevant details. This technique is often combined with in vivo exposure, which involves graded exposure to stimuli that causes distress (the patient initially remains in proximity to mildly distressing trauma reminders) and then repeating this exercise with increasingly distressing scenarios situations. Most programs also include cognitive restructuring, which teaches patients to identify and evaluate the evidence for negative automatic thoughts and develop more realistic appraisals of these factors.

The Evidence for Psychotherapy Approaches

A series of trials have now been conducted that have evaluated trauma-focused CBT in rigorous randomized studies. The initial study, focused on trauma survivors who met criteria for ASD, were randomly allocated to either CBT or supportive counseling (SC; Bryant, Harvey, Dang, Sackville, & Basten, 1998). The CBT program included education about posttraumatic reactions, relaxation training, cognitive restructuring, and imaginal and in vivo exposure that was conducted in five 1.5-hour weekly individual therapy sessions. The SC condition included trauma education and more general problem-solving skills training that occurred at the same frequency as CBT. At six months follow-up, there were fewer participants in the CBT group (20%) who met diagnostic criteria for PTSD compared to SC participants (67%). This pattern has been replicated across a series of subsequent studies that each showed that brief CBT led to lower rates of subsequent PTSD relative to supportive counseling (Bryant, Moulds, Guthrie, & Nixon, 2003, 2005; Bryant, Moulds, & Nixon, 2003; Bryant, Sackville, Dang, Moulds, & Guthrie, 1999). A major issue that often confronts clinicians is the extent to which therapy should focus on exposure versus cognitive restructuring. To address the issue of the relative benefits of exposure and cognitive restructuring, one study randomized trauma survivors to either five weekly sessions of (a) imaginal and in vivo exposure, (b) cognitive restructuring, or (c) assessment only (Bryant et al., 2008); this study found that patients who received exposure therapy had lower levels of PTSD, depression, and anxiety than those in the other conditions, indicating that emotional processing of trauma memories should be included in treatment if optimal clinical gains are to be achieved.

Other early intervention studies have not focused on individuals who meet ASD criteria but have focused on individuals with elevated levels of posttraumatic stress in the acute phase. A very large trial randomized 242 patients admitted to an emergency department and who met criteria for either full or subsyndromal ASD to either prolonged exposure, cognitive restructuring, wait-list (who were then randomized to exposure or cognitive restructuring after 12 weeks), escitalopram (selective serotonin reuptake inhibitors [SSRI]), or placebo (Shalev et al., 2012). Nine months after treatment, PTSD rates were comparable across exposure (21%) and restructuring (22%) conditions, relative to the much higher rates in the SSRI (42%) and placebo (47%) conditions. Significantly, there were no longer-term differences between those who received the early or later provision of CBT. This outcome is consistent with the observation that effect sizes found in most CBT treatments of ASD or early PTSD are comparable to effect sizes of CBT for chronic PTSD (Foa et al., 2009). Other controlled trials have applied CBT to patients with acute PTSD, with both positive and negative results (Bisson, Shepherd, Joy, Probert, & Newcombe, 2004; Sijbrandij et al., 2007). Reflecting the overall evidence, a meta-analysis of four studies of CBT for ASD relative to supportive counseling reported the relative risk for a PTSD diagnosis was (0.36; 95% confidence interval 0.17–0.78; Kornør et al., 2008). A larger meta-analysis including studies with patients meeting criteria for ASD or acute PTSD came to a similar conclusion (Roberts, Kitchiner, Kenardy, & Bisson, 2009).

Pharmacological Approaches

In contrast to the evidence on psychotherapeutic approaches, there is a paucity of evidence for pharmacological interventions. In the previously reviewed Jerusalem study that randomized patients to either prolonged exposure, cognitive restructuring, wait-list (who were then randomized to exposure or cognitive restructuring after 12 weeks), escitalopram (SSRI), or placebo (Shalev et al., 2012), nine months after treatment, rates of PTSD in exposure (21%) and restructuring (22%) conditions were lower than rates in the SSRI (42%) and placebo (47%) conditions. Another study of ASD patients also found no greater benefit of escitalopram relative to placebo (Suliman et al., 2015). In terms of pharmacological interventions with children, one randomized trial reported that seven days of treatment with imipramine was more effective in treating symptoms of ASD in 25 child and adolescent burns victims than chloral hydrate (Robert, Blakeney, Villarreal, Rosenberg, & Meyer, 1999), although another study with burnt children found no effect for imipramine (Robert et al., 2008). Several small and uncontrolled trials have used benzodiazepines to address the acute anxiety, agitation, or sleep problems that commonly occur in the immediate aftermath of trauma exposure, with mixed results suggesting that benzodiazepines can reduce stress symptoms (Gelpin, Bonne, Peri, & Brandes, 1996; Mellman, Byers, & Augenstein, 1998); it should be noted, however, that persistent use may lead to exacerbation of PTSD symptoms.

Another line of research has attempted to reduce PTSD symptoms by reducing noradrenergic response in the acute phase through administration of beta-blockers in the initial days of trauma exposure. Using propranolol within the initial days after trauma, there has been evidence of reduced PTSD symptoms in an uncontrolled trial (Vaiva et al., 2003), evidence of reduced fear-conditioned response in a controlled study (Pitman et al., 2002), and negative findings in other controlled studies (Hoge et al., 2012; Stein, Kerridge, Dimsdale, & Hoyt, 2007). Overall, a meta-analysis of available evidence suggests propranolol is not a secondary prevention strategy to reduce PTSD (Argolo, Cavalcanti-Ribeiro, Netto, & Quarantini, 2015).

Although no randomized controlled trials have been conducted, there is reason to believe that morphine in the acute phase after trauma may reduce later PTSD. Morphine can serve to reduce noradrenergic release, and animal work indicates that morphine injections into the amygdala impairs acquisition of fear conditioning (Clark, Jovic, Ornellas, & Weller, 1972) and impairs memory for fear conditioning (McNally & Westbrook, 2003). Several studies have demonstrated that greater morphine dose in the initial days after trauma exposure is associated with reduced subsequent PTSD in both adults (Bryant, Creamer, O'Donnell, Silove, & McFarlane, 2009; Holbrook, Galarneau, Dye, Quinn, & Dougherty, 2010) and children (Nixon et al., 2010; Saxe et al., 2001). It is important to note that none of these studies represent controlled trials, and so one needs to be cautious about interpreting any causal relationship.

SUMMARY

Over the past 20 years the field of acute traumatic stress has grown enormously. Much has been learned about the course of traumatic stress responses, the mechanisms underpinning ASD, and the means by which PTSD can be limited by focusing early interventions on people with full or subsyndromal levels of ASD. It is now recognized that the nature and course of traumatic stress responses are more complex than was initially thought, and accordingly the confidence we have in predicting PTSD from acute reactions is now more modest than it used to be. Trajectory analyses suggest that we have better capacity to identify people who are likely to follow a resilient course and will not require mental health assistance than identifying people who will need assistance. This suggests that agencies may have more success in conducting surveillance of those who are not resilient and providing treatment to these individuals when they require it, rather than expecting to be able to identify PTSD individuals on the basis of acute responses.

REFERENCES

American Psychiatric Association. (1994). *Diagnostic and Statistical Manual of Mental Disorders* (4th ed.). Washington, DC: American Psychiatric Association.

American Psychiatric Association.(2013). *Diagnostic and Statistical Manual for Mental Disorders* (5th ed.). Washington, DC: American Psychiatric Association.

Argolo, F. C., Cavalcanti-Ribeiro, P., Netto, L. R., & Quarantini, L. C. (2015). Prevention of posttraumatic stress disorder with propranolol: A meta-analytic review. *Journal of Psychosomatic Research*, *79*, 89–93.

Armour, C., Elklit, A., & Shevlin, M. (2013). The latent structure of acute stress disorder. *Psychological Trauma, 5*, 18–25.

Armour, C., & Hansen, M. (2015). Assessing DSM-5 latent subtypes of acute stress disorder dissociative or intrusive? *Psychiatry Research, 225*, 476–483.

Bisson, J. I., Shepherd, J. P., Joy, D., Probert, R., & Newcombe, R. G. (2004). Early cognitive-behavioural therapy for post-traumatic stress symptoms after physical injury: Randomised controlled trial. *British Journal of Psychiatry, 184*, 63–69.

Blanchard, E. B., Kolb, L. C., Gerardi, R. J., Ryan, P., & Pallmeyer, T. P. (1986). Cardiac response to relevant stimuli as an adjunctive tool for diagnosing post-traumatic stress disorder in Vietnam veterans. *Behavior Therapy, 17*(5), 592–606.

Bonanno, G. A., Ho, S. M., Chan, J. C., Kwong, R. S., Cheung, C. K., Wong, C. P., & Wong, V. C. (2008). Psychological resilience and dysfunction among hospitalized survivors of the SARS epidemic in Hong Kong: A latent class approach. *Health Psychology, 27*(5), 659–667.

Bonanno, G. A., Mancini, A. D., Horton, J. L., Powell, T. M., Leardmann, C. A., Boyko, E. J., et al. (2012). Trajectories of trauma symptoms and resilience in deployed U.S. military service members: Prospective cohort study. *British Journal of Psychiatry, 200*(4), 317–323.

Brewin, C. R., Andrews, B., Rose, S., & Kirk, M. (1999). Acute stress disorder and posttraumatic stress disorder in victims of violent crime. *American Journal of Psychiatry, 156*(3), 360–366.

Briere, J., Scott, C., & Weathers, F. (2005). Peritraumatic and persistent dissociation in the presumed etiology of PTSD. *American Journal of Psychiatry, 162*(12), 2295–2301.

Brooks, R., Bryant, R. A., Silove, D., Creamer, M., O'Donnell, M., McFarlane, A. C., & Marmar, C. R. (2009). The latent structure of the Peritraumatic Dissociative Experiences Questionnaire. *Journal of Traumatic Stress, 22*(2), 153–157.

Brooks, R., Silove, D., Bryant, R., O'Donnell, M., Creamer, M., & McFarlane, A. (2008). A confirmatory factor analysis of the Acute Stress Disorder Interview. *Journal of Traumatic Stress, 21*(3), 352–355.

Bryant, R. A. (2003). Early predictors of posttraumatic stress disorder. *Biological Psychiatry, 53*(9), 789–795.

Bryant, R. A. (2011). Acute stress disorder as a predictor of posttraumatic stress disorder: A systematic review. *Journal of Clinical Psychiatry, 72*, 233–239.

Bryant, R. A. (2016). *Acute stress disorder: What it is and how to treat it.* New York: Guilford.

Bryant, R. A., Creamer, M., O'Donnell, M. L., Silove, D., & McFarlane, A. C. (2008a). A multisite study of the capacity of acute stress disorder diagnosis to predict posttraumatic stress disorder. *Journal of Clinical Psychiatry, 69*(6), 923–929.

Bryant, R. A., Creamer, M., O'Donnell, M., Silove, D., & McFarlane, A. C. (2008b). A multisite study of initial respiration rate and heart rate as predictors of posttraumatic stress disorder. *Journal of Clinical Psychiatry, 69*(11), 1694–1701.

Bryant, R. A., Creamer, M., O'Donnell, M., Silove, D., Clark, C. R., & McFarlane, A. C. (2010). The psychiatric sequelae of traumatic injury. *American Journal of Psychiatry, 167*, 312–320.

Bryant, R. A., Creamer, M., O'Donnell, M., Silove, D., & McFarlane, A. C. (2009). A study of the protective function of acute morphine administration on subsequent posttraumatic stress disorder. *Biological Psychiatry, 65*, 438–440.

Bryant, R. A., Creamer, M., O'Donnell, M., Silove, D., McFarlane, A. C., & Forbes, D. (2015). A comparison of the capacity of DSM-IV and DSM-5 acute stress disorder definitions to predict posttraumatic stress disorder and related disorders. *Journal of Clinical Psychiatry, 76*, 391–397.

Bryant, R. A., Friedman, M. J., Spiegel, D., Ursano, R., & Strain, J. (2011). A review of acute stress disorder in DSM-5. *Depression and Anxiety, 28*(9), 802–817.

Bryant, R. A., Harvey, A. G., Dang, S. T., & Sackville, T. (1998). Assessing acute stress disorder: Psychometric properties of a structured clinical interview. *Psychological Assessment, 10*(3), 215–220.

Bryant, R. A., Harvey, A. G., Dang, S. T., Sackville, T., & Basten, C. (1998). Treatment of acute stress disorder: A comparison of cognitive-behavioral therapy and supportive counseling. *Journal of Consulting and Clinical Psychology, 66*(5), 862–866.

Bryant, R. A., Mastrodomenico, J., Felmingham, K. L., Hopwood, S., Kenny, L., Kandris, E., et al. (2008). Treatment of acute stress disorder: A randomized controlled trial. *Archives of General Psychiatry, 65*(6), 659–667.

Bryant, R. A., Moulds, M. L., & Guthrie, R. M. (2000). Acute Stress Disorder Scale: A self-report measure of acute stress disorder. *Psychological Assessment, 12*(1), 61–68.

Bryant, R. A., Moulds, M., Guthrie, R., & Nixon, R. D. (2003). Treating acute stress disorder following mild traumatic brain injury. *American Journal of Psychiatry, 160*(3), 585–587.

Bryant, R. A., Moulds, M. L., Guthrie, R. M., & Nixon, R. D. V. (2005). The additive benefit of hypnosis and cognitive-behavioral therapy in treating acute stress disorder. *Journal of Consulting and Clinical Psychology, 73*(2), 334–340.

Bryant, R. A., Moulds, M. L., & Nixon, R. V. (2003). Cognitive behaviour therapy of acute stress disorder: A four-year follow-up. *Behaviour Research and Therapy, 41*(4), 489–494.

Bryant, R. A., Nickerson, A., Creamer, M., O'Donnell, M., Forbes, D., Galatzer-Levy, I., McFarlane, A. C., & Silove, D. (2015). The trajectory of posttraumatic stress following traumatic injury: A six-year follow-up. *British Journal of Psychiatry, 206*, 417–423.

Bryant, R. A., O'Donnell, M., Creamer, M., McFarlane, A. C., & Silove, D. (2013). A multi-site analysis of the fluctuating course of posttraumatic stress disorder. *JAMA: Psychiatry, 70*, 839–846.

Bryant, R. A., Sackville, T., Dang, S. T., Moulds, M., & Guthrie, R. (1999). Treating acute stress disorder: An evaluation of cognitive behavior therapy and supporting counselling techniques. *American Journal of Psychiatry, 156*(11), 1780–1786.

Bryant, R. A., Salmon, K., Sinclair, E., & Davidson, P. (2007). The relationship between acute stress disorder and posttraumatic stress disorder in injured children. *Journal of Traumatic Stress, 20*(6), 1075–1079.

Cardeña, E., Classen, C., & Spiegel, D. (1991). *Stanford Acute Stress Reaction Questionnaire.* Stanford, CA: Stanford University Medical School.

Cardeña, E., Koopman, C., Classen, C., Waelde, L. C., & Spiegel, D. (2000). Psychometric properties of the Stanford Acute Stress Reaction Questionnaire (SASRQ): A valid and reliable measure of acute stress. *Journal of Traumatic Stress, 13*(4), 719–734.

Cardeña, E., & Spiegel, D. (1993). Dissociative reactions to the San Francisco Bay Area earthquake of 1989. *American Journal of Psychiatry, 150*(3), 474–478.

Clark, A. G., Jovic, R., Ornellas, M. R., & Weller, M. (1972). Brain microsomal protein kinase in the chronically morphinized rat. *Biochemical Pharmacology, 21*, 1989–1990.

Classen, C., Koopman, C., Hales, R., & Spiegel, D. (1998). Acute stress disorder as a predictor of posttraumatic stress symptoms. *American Journal of Psychiatry, 155*(5), 620–624.

Dalgleish, T., Meiser-Stedman, R., Kassam-Adams, N., Ehlers, A., Winston, F., Smith, P., et al. (2008). Predictive validity of acute stress disorder in children and adolescents. *British Journal of Psychiatry, 192*(5), 392–393.

Davidson, J., Kudler, H. S., Saunders, W. B., & Smith, R. D. (1990). Symptom and comorbidity patterns in World War II and Vietnam veterans with posttraumatic stress disorder. *Comprehensive Psychiatry, 31*(2), 162–170.

Dunmore, E., Clark, D. M., & Ehlers, A. (1997). Cognitive factors in persistent versus recovered post-traumatic stress disorder after physical or sexual assault: A pilot study. *Behavioural and Cognitive Psychotherapy, 25*(2), 147–159.

Dunmore, E., Clark, D. M., & Ehlers, A. (2001). A prospective investigation of the role of cognitive factors in persistent posttraumatic stress disorder (PTSD) after physical or sexual assault. *Behaviour Research and Therapy, 39*(9), 1063–1084.

Ehlers, A., & Clark, D. M. (2000). A cognitive model of posttraumatic stress disorder. *Behaviour Research and Therapy, 38*(4), 319–345.

Ehlers, A., Mayou, R. A., & Bryant, B. (1998). Psychological predictors of chronic posttraumatic stress disorder after motor vehicle accidents. *Journal of Abnormal Psychology, 107*(3), 508–519.

Ehlers, A., Mayou, R. A., & Bryant, B. (2003). Cognitive predictors of posttraumatic stress disorder in children: Results of a prospective longitudinal study. *Behaviour Research and Therapy, 41*(1), 1–10.

Ehlers, A., & Steil, R. (1995). Maintenance of intrusive memories in posttraumatic stress disorder: A cognitive approach. *Behavioural and Cognitive Psychotherapy, 23*(3), 217–249.

Ehlers, A., Suendermann, O., Boellinghaus, I., Vossbeck-Elsebusch, A., Gamer, M., Briddon, E., et al. (2010). Heart rate responses to standardized trauma-related pictures in acute posttraumatic stress disorder. *International Journal of Psychophysiologyl, 78*(1), 27–34.

Ehring, T., Ehlers, A., & Glucksman, E. (2008). Do cognitive models help in predicting the severity of posttraumatic stress disorder, phobia, and depression after motor vehicle accidents? A prospective longitudinal study. *Journal of Consulting and Clinical Psychology, 76*(2), 219–230.

Engelhard, I. M., van den Hout, M. A., Arntz, A., & McNally, R. J. (2002). A longitudinal study of "intrusion-based reasoning" and posttraumatic stress disorder after exposure to a train disaster. *Behaviour Research and Therapy, 40*(12), 1415–1424.

Foa, E. B. (2011). Prolonged exposure therapy: Past, present, and future. *Depression and Anxiety, 28*(12), 1043–1047.

Foa, E. B., Keane, T. M., Friedman, M. J., & Cohen, J. A. (Eds.). (2009). *Effective treatments for PTSD: Practice guidelines from the International Society of Traumatic Stress Studies* (2nd ed.). New York: Guilford.

Galea, S., Vlahov, D., Resnick, H., Ahern, J., Susser, E., Gold, J., et al. (2003). Trends of probable posttraumatic stress disorder in New York City after the September 11 terrorist attacks. *American Journal of Epidemiology, 158*(6), 514–524.

Gelpin, E., Bonne, O., Peri, T., & Brandes, D. (1996). Treatment of recent trauma survivors with benzodiazepines: A prospective study. *Journal of Clinical Psychiatry, 57*, 390–394.

Guthrie, R. M., & Bryant, R. A. (2005). Auditory startle response in firefighters before and after trauma exposure. *American Journal of Psychiatry, 162*(2), 283–290.

Guthrie, R. M., & Bryant, R. A. (2006). Extinction learning before trauma and subsequent posttraumatic stress. *Psychosomatic Medicine, 68*(2), 307–311.

Halligan, S. L., Clark, D. M., & Ehlers, A. (2002). Cognitive processing, memory, and the development of PTSD symptoms: Two experimental analogue studies. *Journal of Behavior Therapy and& Experimental Psychiatry, 33*(2), 73–89.

Harvey, A. G., & Bryant, R. A. (1998a). Acute stress disorder after mild traumatic brain injury. *Journal of Nervous and Mental Disease, 186*(6), 333–337.

Harvey, A. G., & Bryant, R. A. (1998b). The relationship between acute stress disorder and posttraumatic stress disorder: A prospective evaluation of motor vehicle accident survivors. *Journal of Consulting and Clinical Psychology, 66*(3), 507–512.

Harvey, A. G., & Bryant, R. A. (1999a). A qualitative investigation of the organization of traumatic memories. *British Journal of Clinical Psychology, 38*, 401–405.

Harvey, A. G., & Bryant, R. A. (1999b). Acute stress disorder across trauma populations. *Journal of Nervous and Mental Disease, 187*(7), 443–446.

Harvey, A. G., & Bryant, R. A. (1999c). Dissociative symptoms in acute stress disorder. *Journal of Traumatic Stress, 12*(4), 673–680.

Harvey, A. G., & Bryant, R. A. (1999d). The relationship between acute stress disorder and posttraumatic stress disorder: A 2-year prospective evaluation. *Journal of Consulting and Clinical Psychology, 67*(6), 985–988.

Hoge, E. A., Worthington, J. J., Nagurney, J. T., Chang, Y., Kay, E. B., Feterowski, C. M., et al. (2012). Effect of acute posttrauma propranolol on PTSD outcome and physiological responses during script-driven imagery. *CNS Neuroscience & Therapeutics, 18*, 21–27.

Holbrook, T. L., Galarneau, M. R., Dye, J. L., Quinn, K., & Dougherty, A. L. (2010). Morphine use after combat injury in Iraq and post-traumatic stress disorder. *New England Journal of Medicine, 362*, 110–117.

Holen, A. (1993). The North Sea oil rig disaster. In J. P. Wilson & B. Raphael (Eds.), *International handbook of traumatic stress syndromes* (pp. 471–478). New York: Plenum.

Horowitz, M. J. (1997). *Stress response syndromes: PTSD, grief, and adjustment disorders* (3rd ed.). Northvale, NJ: Jason Aronson.

Janet, P. (1907). *The major symptoms of hysteria*. New York: Macmillan.

Ji, L., Xiaowei, Z., Chuanlin, W., & Wei, L. (2010). Investigation of posttraumatic stress disorder in children after animal-induced injury in China. *Pediatrics, 126*(2), e320–e324.

Kassam-Adams, N., & Winston, F. K. (2004). Predicting child PTSD: The relationship between acute stress disorder and PTSD in injured children. *Journal of the American Academy of Child & Adolescent Psychiatry, 43*(4), 403–411.

Kleim, B., Ehlers, A., & Glucksman, E. (2007). Early predictors of chronic post-traumatic stress disorder in assault survivors. *Psychological Medicine, 37*(10), 1457–1467.

Koopman, C., Classen, C., Cardeña, E., & Spiegel, D. (1995). When disaster strikes, acute stress disorder may follow. *Journal of Traumatic Stress, 8*(1), 29–46.

Kornør, H., Winje, D., Ekeberg, Ø., Weisaeth, L., Kirkehei, I., Johansen, K., & Steiro, A. (2008). Early trauma-focused cognitive-behavioural therapy to prevent chronic post-traumatic stress disorder and related symptoms: A systematic review and meta-analysis. *BMC Psychiatry, 8*, 81.

Lam, W. W., Bonanno, G. A., Mancini, A. D., Ho, S., Chan, M., Hung, W. K., et al. (2010). Trajectories of psychological distress among Chinese women diagnosed with breast cancer. *Psychooncology, 19*(10), 1044–1051.

Lommen, M. J., Engelhard, I. M., Sijbrandij, M., van den Hout, M. A., & Hermans, D. (2013). Pre-trauma individual differences in extinction learning predict posttraumatic stress. *Behaviour Research and Therapy, 51*(2), 63–67.

Marmar, C. R., Weiss, D. S., & Metzler, T. J. (1997). The Peritraumatic Dissociative Experiences Questionnaire. In J. P. Wilson & T. M. Keane (Eds.), *Assessing psychological trauma And PTSD* (pp. 412–428). New York: Guilford.

Mayou, R. A., Ehlers, A., & Bryant, B. (2002). Posttraumatic stress disorder after motor vehicle accidents: 3-year follow-up of a prospective longitudinal study. *Behaviour Research & Therapy, 40*(6), 665–675.

McNally, G. P., & Westbrook, R. F. (2003). Opioid receptors regulate the extinction of Pavlovian fear conditioning. *Behavioral Neuroscience, 117*, 1292–1301.

Meiser-Stedman, R., Dalgleish, T., Smith, P., Yule, W., & Glucksman, E. (2007). Diagnostic, demographic, memory quality, and cognitive variables associated with acute stress disorder in children and adolescents. *Journal of Abnormal Psychology, 116*(1), 65–79.

Meiser-Stedman, R., Yule, W., Smith, P., Glucksman, E., & Dalgleish, T. (2005). Acute stress disorder and posttraumatic stress disorder in children and adolescents involved in assaults or motor vehicle accidents. *American Journal of Psychiatry, 162*(7), 1381–1383.

Mellman, T. A., Byers, P. M., & Augenstein, J. S. (1998). Pilot evaluation of hypnotic medication during acute traumatic stress response. *Journal of Traumatic Stress, 11*, 563–569.

Milad, M. R., Rauch, S. L., Pitman, R. K., & Quirk, G. J. (2006). Fear extinction in rats: Implications for human brain imaging and anxiety disorders. *Biological Psychology, 73*(1), 61–71.

Murray, J., Ehlers, A., & Mayou, R. A. (2002a). Dissociation and post-traumatic stress disorder: Two prospective studies of road traffic accident survivors. *British Journal of Psychiatry, 180*, 363–368.

Murray, J., Ehlers, A., & Mayou, R. A. (2002b). Dissociation and post-traumatic stress disorder: Two prospective studies of road traffic accident survivors. *British Journal of Psychiatry, 180*, 363–368.

Myers, K. M., & Davis, M. (2007). Mechanisms of fear extinction. *Molecular Psychiatry, 12*(2), 120–150.

National Institute of Clinical Excellence. (2005). *The management of PTSD in adults and children in primary and secondary care*. Wiltshire, UK: Cromwell Press.

Nixon, R. D., & Bryant, R. A. (2003). Peritraumatic and persistent panic attacks in acute stress disorder. *Behaviour Research and Therapy, 41*(10), 1237–1242.

Nixon, R. D., Nehmy, T. J., Ellis, A. A., Ball, S. A., Menne, A., & McKinnon, A. C. (2010). Predictors of posttraumatic stress in children following injury: The influence of appraisals, heart rate, and morphine use. *Behaviour Research and Therapy, 48*, 810–815.

Norris, F. H., Tracy, M., & Galea, S. (2009). Looking for resilience: Understanding the longitudinal trajectories of responses to stress. *Social Science and Medicine, 68*(12), 2190–2198.

O'Donnell, M. L., Creamer, M., Elliott, P., & Bryant, R. (2007). Tonic and phasic heart rate as predictors of posttraumatic stress disorder. *Psychosomatic Medicine, 69*, 256–261.

O'Donnell, M. L., Creamer, M. C., Parslow, R., Elliott, P., Holmes, A. C., Ellen, S., et al. (2008). A predictive screening index for posttraumatic stress disorder and depression following traumatic injury. *Journal of Consulting and Clinical Psychology, 76*(6), 923–932.

Orr, S. P., Lasko, N. B., Macklin, M. L., Pineles, S. L., Chang, Y., & Pitman, R. K. (2012). Predicting post-trauma stress symptoms from pre-trauma psychophysiologic reactivity, personality traits and measures of psychopathology. *Biology of Mood and Anxiety Disorders, 2*(1), 8.

Orr, S. P., Pitman, R. K., Lasko, N. B., & Herz, L. R. (1993). Psychophysiological assessment of posttraumatic stress disorder imagery in World War II and Korean combat veterans. *Journal of Abnormal Psychology, 102*(1), 152–159.

Panasetis, P., & Bryant, R. A. (2003). Peritraumatic versus persistent dissociation in acute stress disorder. *Journal of Traumatic Stress, 16*(6), 563–566.

Pietrzak, R. H., Van Ness, P. H., Fried, T. R., Galea, S., & Norris, F. H. (2013). Trajectories of posttraumatic stress symptomatology in older persons affected by a large-magnitude disaster. *Journal of Psychiatric Research, 47*, 520–526.

Pitman, R. K. (1989). Post-traumatic stress disorder, hormones, and memory. *Biological Psychiatry, 26*(3), 221–223.

Pitman, R. K., Sanders, K. M., Zusman, R. M., Healy, A. R., Cheema, F., Lasko, N. B., et al. (2002). Pilot study of secondary prevention of posttraumatic stress disorder with propranolol. *Biological Psychiatry, 51*, 189–192.

Riggs, D. S., Rothbaum, B. O., & Foa, E. B. (1995). A prospective examination of symptoms of posttraumatic stress disorder in victims of nonsexual assault. *Journal of Interpersonal Violence, 10*(2), 201–214.

Robert, R., Blakeney, P. E., Villarreal, C., Rosenberg, L., & Meyer, W. J. III. (1999). Imipramine treatment in pediatric burn patients with symptoms of acute stress disorder: A pilot study. *Journal of the American Academy of Child & Adolescent Psychiatry, 38*(7), 873–882.

Robert, R., Tcheung, W. J., Rosenberg, L., Rosenberg, M., Mitchell, C., Villarreal, C., et al. (2008). Treating thermally injured children suffering symptoms of acute stress with imipramine and fluoxetine: A randomized, double-blind study. *Burns, 34*, 919–928.

Roberts, N. P., Kitchiner, N. J., Kenardy, J., & Bisson, J. I. (2009). Systematic review and meta-analysis of multiple-session early interventions following traumatic events. *American Journal of Psychiatry, 166*(3), 293–301.

Saxe, G., Stoddard, F., Courtney, D., Cunningham, K., Chawla, N., Sheridan, R., et al. (2001). Relationship between acute morphine and the course of PTSD in children with burns. *Journal of the American Academy of Child & Adolescent Psychiatry, 40*, 915–921.

Shalev, A. Y., Ankri, Y., Israeli-Shalev, Y., Peleg, T., Adessky, R., & Freedman, S. (2012). Prevention of posttraumatic stress disorder by early treatment: Results from the Jerusalem Trauma Outreach and Prevention Study. *Archives of General Psychiatry*, *69*(2), 166–176.

Shalev, A. Y., Freedman, A., Peri, T., Brandes, D., Sahara, T., Orr, S., & Pitman, R. K. (1998). Prospective study of posttraumatic stress disorder and depression following trauma. *American Journal of Psychiatry*, *155*(5), 630–637.

Shalev, A. Y., Sahar, T., Freedman, S., Peri, T., Glick, N., Brandes, D., et al. (1998). A prospective study of heart rate response following trauma and the subsequent development of posttraumatic stress disorder. *Archives of General Psychiatry*, *55*(6), 553–559.

Sijbrandij, M., Olff, M., Reitsma, J. B., Carlier, I. V. E., de Vries, M. H., & Gersons, B. P. R. (2007). Treatment of acute posttraumatic stress disorder with brief cognitive behavioral therapy: A randomized controlled trial. *American Journal of Psychiatry*, *164*(1), 82–90.

Smith, K., & Bryant, R. A. (2000). The generality of cognitive bias in acute stress disorder. *Behaviour Research and Therapy*, *38*(7), 709–715.

Solomon, S., Laor, N., & McFarlane, A. (1996). Acute posttraumatic reactions in soldiers and civilians. In B. A. Van der Kolk, A. C. McFarlane, & L. Weisaeth (Eds.), *Traumatic stress: The effects of overwhelming experience on mind, body and society* (pp. 102–114). New York: Guilford.

Spiegel, D., Koopman, C., & Classen, C. (1994). Acute stress disorder and dissociation. *Australian Journal of Clinical and Experimental Hypnosis*, *22*(1), 11–23.

Stein, M. B., Kerridge, C., Dimsdale, J. E., & Hoyt, D. B. (2007). Pharmacotherapy to prevent PTSD: Results from a randomized controlled proof-of-concept trial in physically injured patients. *Journal of Traumatic Stress*, *20*, 923–932.

Suliman, S., Seedat, S., Pingo, J., Sutherland, T., Zohar, J., & Stein, D. J. (2015). Escitalopram in the prevention of posttraumatic stress disorder: A pilot randomized controlled trial. *BMC Psychiatry*, *15*, 24.

Vaiva, G., Ducrocq, F., Jezequel, K., Averland, B., Lestavel, P., Brunet, A., et al. (2003). Immediate treatment with propranolol decreases posttraumatic stress disorder two months after trauma. *Biological Psychiatry*, *54*, 947–949.

van der Kolk, B., & van der Hart, O. (1989). Pierre Janet and the breakdown of adaptation in psychological trauma. *American Journal of Psychiatry*, *146*(12), 1530–1537.

Wang, X., Gao, L., Shinfuku, N., Zhang, H., Zhao, C., & Shen, Y. (2000). Longitudinal study of earthquake-related PTSD in a randomly selected community sample in north China. *American Journal of Psychiatry*, *157*(8), 1260–1266.

Warda, G., & Bryant, R. A. (1998). Cognitive bias in acute stress disorder. *Behaviour Research and Therapy*, *36*(12), 1177–1183.

Wikman, A., Molloy, G. J., Randall, G., & Steptoe, A. (2011). Cognitive predictors of posttraumatic stress symptoms six months following acute coronary syndrome. *Psychology & Health*, *26*(8), 974–988.

5

Adjustment Disorder

ALLISON M. B. WEBB, SHANNON C. FORD, AND PATCHO N. SANTIAGO

INTRODUCTION

Adjustment disorder is a psychiatric diagnosis that has undergone numerous iterations within the *Diagnostic and Statistical Manual of Mental Health Disorders* (DSM). It is characterized by an immediate or almost immediate maladaptive or pathologic psychological response to a stressor. When the stressor is removed, there is the expectation that the patient returns to his or her previous level of functioning within six months. The diagnosis is not made if the patient's symptoms are better explained by another major psychiatric diagnosis. Historically, this relegated adjustment disorder to a subsyndromal status, despite evidence of its severity and serious impact on the lives of patients.[1] This chapter provides an overview of its historical development, diagnostic criteria with a discussion regarding potential controversies, epidemiology, neurobiology, and other differential diagnostic and treatment considerations, closing with the presentation of a case illustrating application of the criteria and clinical characteristics of adjustment disorder.

HISTORICAL DEVELOPMENT OF ADJUSTMENT DISORDER IN THE DSM

The concept of a pathologic and transient reaction to a life-stressor is not new, although it was not always identified as adjustment disorder. This diagnosis was initially described in the first edition of the (DSM-I)[2] as acute versus chronic brain syndrome, thought to potentially be due to problems with "cerebral tissue function" or a "transient situational personality disorder." Psychiatrists surmised that the patient's character had an acute transient change in response to a stressful situation. In patients who could adapt, the symptoms would resolve when the stress diminished. In DSM-I, these disorders were separated from an "adult situation reaction," which was a "superficial maladjustment to a difficult situation or to newly experienced environmental factors" and manifested by "anxiety, alcoholism, asthenia, poor efficiency, low morale, and unconventional behaviors."[2]

In 1968 the second edition of the DSM (DSM-II)[3] labeled these disorders "transient situational disturbances" with subcategories classifying an "adjustment reaction" into a life stage: infancy, childhood, or adulthood. The "disturbance" was an "acute reaction to overwhelming emotional stress." Two key diagnostic elements were developed that persisted in future editions. First, the stress reaction could be of any severity. Second, the symptoms could not be attributed to an underlying mental disorder. The expectation (consistent in all DSM editions) was that the symptoms would completely resolve with the elimination of the stressor. This assumption did not entirely hold up in studies performed on the predictive value of the diagnosis, however. A study by Andreasen et al. (1982) found that after a five-year follow up of patients diagnosed with transient situational disturbances, only 44% of adolescents compared with 71% of adults were well at follow-up with resolution of their symptoms.[4] The authors suggested that these data might indicate the diagnosis had poor predictive validity and describe a heterogeneous group of patients.

Adjustment disorder was incorporated into International Classification of Diseases (ICD), ninth revision, in 1978, and the third edition of the DSM (DSM-III)[5] in 1980. It was placed in its own separate category, and this description became the basis for subsequent DSM editions. Defined as a "maladaptive reaction to an identifiable psychosocial stressor or stressors," the symptoms had to disrupt normal functioning, occur within the first three months of the stressor being present, and resolve within six months of the stressor being removed. The subjective level of distress experienced does not have to correlate to the severity of the stressor. The subtypes were based on predominant symptom presentation: anxious, depressed, disturbance of conduct, mixed disturbance of emotions and conduct, physical complaints (in the revised third edition of the DSM), withdrawal, work (or academic) inhibition, and not otherwise specified. The diagnosis is not made if there is a pattern of overreaction across multiple events or the exacerbation of a previous psychiatric diagnosis.

The tenth revision of the ICD (ICD-10) was published in 1992, two years prior to the fourth edition of the DSM (DSM-IV). This update categorized adjustment disorder under "Reaction to Severe Stress and Adjustment Disorders" and required symptoms to present within one month of the stressor; if the stressor persisted beyond six months, the diagnosis was changed to prolonged depressive reaction. The DSM-IV[6] changes published in 1994 kept adjustment disorders in a separate diagnostic category and recharacterized the stressors, subtypes, and timeline based on epidemiological evidence.[6] In one outpatient study, over one-third of patients had their stressor present for over one year,[7] and to include this and similar findings, the DSM-IV added two specifiers: acute (stressor duration of less than six months) and chronic (stressor or its effects have a duration greater than six months). Both ICD-10 and DSM-IV continued the requirement that symptoms could not persist for more than six months after the termination of the stressor. DSM-IV removed the subtypes of adjustment disorder with work or academic inhibition, with withdrawal, and with mixed emotional features due to the low prevalence of these categories.[8] There was, however, ongoing debate as to what defined a pathologic response to a stressor, as opposed to experiencing a normal response.[9] ICD-10 does not require clinical significance in the severity of symptom presentation, though difficulty in performing daily routine is mentioned. The lack of specificity has caused variance in the diagnosis and limited research in the field.[10]

DSM-5: RATIONALE FOR AND IMPLICATIONS OF A NEW DIAGNOSTIC CLASS

The fifth edition of the DSM (DSM-5) moved the independent category of adjustment disorders to the "Trauma and Stressor-Related Disorders" (TSRD) diagnostic class, similar to the ICD 10 classification; this was the most significant change made from DSM-IV.[11] Like many changes, this sparked discussion. Proponents noted that adjustment disorder, acute stress disorder, and posttraumatic stress disorder (PTSD) are the only psychiatric diagnoses that rely on the presences of an external event, which is a common, unifying theme for the new section.[12] It was also felt that moving to a new category would help overcome challenges in researching and operationalizing the diagnosis.[13] Concern did exist that more data regarding the diagnosis needed to be acquired before moving it to the TSRD diagnostic class.[14] Einsle et al. proposed that any stressful event, whether traumatic or not, would contribute to formation of intrusive symptoms and avoidance behavior.[15] They, and others, proposed that adjustment disorders occur along a spectrum of syndromes with acute stress disorder and PTSD.[16] The final decision to move the class was based on an improved understanding about the response to trauma and that stressors cause multiple emotional and behavioral responses, not just anxiety.[16] Also, adjustment disorder can be used as a diagnosis when the full criteria are not met or the stressor severity does not meet the required threshold for acute stress disorder or PTSD.

The TSRD diagnostic class has created a spectrum to describe abnormal responses to stress, and symptoms range from adjustment disorder to PTSD.[12] Consistent symptoms among these syndromes is avoidance behavior and intrusion symptoms.[17] The adjustment disorder diagnosis remains highly informed by clinical judgment rather than a set of well-defined criteria, contributing to, and caused by, the lack of empirical evidence available.[12] Proposed criteria in the eleventh revision of the ICD for adjustment disorder are part of the effort to make the criteria more specific and consistent in its application. The diagnosis maintains its place under "Disorders Specifically Associated with Stress" with more specific criteria, described as "preoccupation with the stressor or its consequences, including excessive worry, recurrent and distressing thoughts about the stressor, or constant rumination about its implications, as well as by failure to adapt to the stressor that causes significant impairment in personal, family, social, educational, occupational or other important areas of functioning."[18–20]

The DSM-5 diagnostic criteria retained the ability to describe a temporary emotional state in a way that could be less stigmatizing than other mental disorders, or to be utilized as a provisional diagnosis while continuing to see how the course of illness plays out, though there is ongoing concern that experiencing a normal response to stress could be diagnosed as a mental disorder.[13,21]

Adjustment disorders represent clinically significant distress between normal responses and major psychiatric diagnoses.[22] It cannot be diagnosed if the symptoms can be better explained by a major psychiatric diagnosis; however, it can be diagnosed concurrently if another diagnosis is comorbid. There is utility in having a more moderate diagnosis and patients with the diagnosis do portend a better clinical outcome than their counterparts with major mood disorders.[23] Some note that the diagnosis also provides an opportunity to finance treatment for patients who would benefit but who might not meet the criteria for a full blown psychiatric disorder,[14] and there is diagnostic "sensitivity" such that it is able to pick up patients that require psychiatric care. This sensitivity may come at the expense of specificity, making it more difficult for operationalized study of outcomes and rigorous research.[13] Despite the lack of interrater reliability, the diagnosis has validity and is seen in both the outpatient and inpatient settings.[10] While it has a very positive prognosis, it can cause significant disability, to include an increased risk of suicide.

Despite these forces at work, the features and criteria of the diagnosis have remained similar to previous editions of the DSM. Authors note this is largely due to the lack of empirical evidence on adjustment disorder.[12] The subtypes in the DSM-5 are adjustment disorder with depressed mood, anxiety, mixed anxiety and depressed mood, disturbance of conduct, mixed disturbance of emotions and conduct, and unspecified. Adjustment disorders can also be acute (less than six months' duration) and persistent (or chronic, greater than six months' duration).

The criticisms and controversies surrounding this diagnosis do not stop there. Most notable is the view that adjustment disorder is a subsyndromal, wastebasket, or marginal diagnosis that does not communicate the degree of clinically significant dysfunction and suffering a patient may experience. Others argue that there is no clear separation between adjustment disorder and normal adaptive reactions, making normal human reaction pathologic.[24] A 1987 study by Fabrega et al. found that patients diagnosed with adjustment disorder were indeed "less ill" than patients diagnosed with a specific disease using metrics such as frequency of symptoms and levels of adaptive functioning at time of evaluation and during the previous year.[25] However, both this study and another in 1995 endorsed that patients with adjustment disorder were much closer to those with identifiable psychiatric diagnoses than well patients.[23,25] Strain et al specifically stated in a 1993 article that "in DSM-III . . . the adjustment disorders were intended to provide . . . a diagnosis that is not a full blown disorder."[8] However, these patients are not without suffering. A small study[26] found that individuals with adjustment disorder demonstrated higher interdaily mood variability or affective reactivity than those with major depressive disorders or normal controls. This controversy has led to the conceptualization of adjustment disorders in three possible ways, supported by different authors: that adjustment disorder is in fact its own specific disorder, that it is a subthreshold clinical syndrome, or that it is a precursor to more severe disorders.[4,23]

Many argue that because adjustment disorders have a poor boundary to one side with normal stress response and to the other with full-blown disorder, more stringent criteria would make this diagnosis less difficult to study.[12]

EPIDEMIOLOGY

Despite the diagnosis being recognizable in some form throughout all versions of the DSM, it does remain a poorly identified disorder.[27] Adjustment disorder is the seventh most prevalent diagnostic class used in mental health treatment,[28,29] but the larger psychiatric epidemiology studies such as the Epidemiological Catchment Area study[30] or the National Comorbidity Study[31] and its replication[32] did not include adjustment disorder as part of their evaluations. Efforts have been made to assess the prevalence, which varies based on patient location. The Outcome of Depression International Network study looked at the subtype of adjustment disorder with depressed mood and found 0.9% of the general population meet the criteria for an adjustment disorder if clinically significant impairment is a qualifier and 1.4% of the general population if that is not a factor.[22] Another study showed the prevalence of adjustment disorder in primary care settings was found to be 2.94%, though physicians did not detect all cases.[33] In the consult-liaison setting of inpatient medical-surgical wards, the prevalence increased to approximately 21%.[34,35] Estimates suggest about 1% of the general population, 1.5% of emergency department patients, 5% to 21% of consult-liaison hospitalized patient referrals, and up to 9% to 36% of psychiatric patients have an adjustment disorder.[35-40] Though sometimes in an inpatient psychiatric setting, this diagnosis can be useful initially, as one study found that 40% of inpatient psychiatric hospitalizations with an admission diagnosis of adjustment disorder had a different diagnosis upon discharge.[41] Women are diagnosed twice as often as men, though this gender variance does not occur in children or adolescents.[24]

The discrepancy between prevalence in various studies has sometimes been attributed to differences in diagnosis made based on structured interviews (discussed later) versus when a clinical evaluation leads to the diagnosis.[42] In structured interviews, patients are more often diagnosed with depression as opposed to adjustment disorder. Of those who are given the diagnosis of adjustment disorder in structured clinical interviews, 45% are still prescribed an antidepressant.[27] Researchers hypothesize this is due to the increased presence of antidepressants, which allow clinicians to prescribe more liberally and thus influencing their clinical diagnosis associated with the prescribed medication,[1] as it has been observed the frequency of an adjustment disorder is declining while the diagnosis of depression is increasing.[43]

The prevalence of adjustment disorders comorbid with organic mental disorders was estimated in a consult-liaison setting to be 7%; personality disorder was 15%, and psychoactive substance abuse disorder was 7%.[37] Comorbid suicidality is also common, though a wide range is reported of 2.7% to 50% of patients with suicidal ideation or self-injurious behavior having these thoughts secondary to an adjustment disorder.[44-46]

COMORBIDITY AND SUICIDAL IDEATION AND ADJUSTMENT DISORDER

Adjustment disorders may advance into a major mental disorder,[4] and comorbid substance use disorders are common[41] while some patients may be experiencing adjustment disorders in the context of a personality disorder.[47] One study found that of inpatient hospitalization for adjustment disorder and suicidal ideation, 67% were also diagnosed with borderline personality disorder or antisocial personality disorder.[48] Another found that 27% of adolescents being treated for adjustment disorder (but without suicidal ideation) in an outpatient setting frequently suffered from alcohol misuse, but the rate went up to 41% in those with suicidal ideation.[49]

In the discussions between DSM-III and DSM-IV regarding subtypes of adjustment disorder, scholars debated the utility of a subtype of adjustment disorder with suicidal behavior in reaction to a stressor.[8] Suicidal ideation is a relatively frequent occurrence in patients with adjustment disorder; up to 25% of adolescents[49] and 60% of adults[48] with adjustment disorder have suicidal behavior. Underscoring the significance of adjustment disorders, a study by Runeson reported that in patients diagnosed with adjustment disorder, there was a one-month interval between initial diagnosis and emergence of suicidal ideation compared with a 3-month interval in depression, a 30-month interval in personality disorder, and a 47-month interval in patients with schizophrenia.[50] For adults in India, adjustment disorder was found in one study to be the most common diagnosis of those dying by suicide.[51] The presence of suicidal ideation in adjustment disorder should alert clinicians to the significance of distress that patients with this diagnosis can have, and they should remember that it can appear quickly in those who may not initially report it.

THE NEUROBIOLOGY OF ADJUSTMENT DISORDER

Little is known about the biological basis of adjustment disorder. One prospective study by Kumano et al. examined regional brain metabolism using PET in patients diagnosed with cancer.[52] The patients' neuro-metabolisms were analyzed prior to development of adjustment disorder. Those patients who developed adjustment disorder had baseline decreased glucose metabolism in the right medial frontal gyrus and increased glucose metabolism in the left caudate and subcallosal gyrus and right posterior cingulate and anterior cingulate. This study showed a possibility that risk for development of adjustment disorder could be predicted with neuroimaging. Another study by Rocco et al. analyzed cortisol levels as a possible biomarker for the diagnosis of adjustment disorder.[53] They found that patients who developed adjustment disorder after experiencing a mugging had lower levels of morning cortisol but normal dexamethasone suppression tests. This finding may also help clinicians distinguish between adjustment disorder and major depression. However, examining the neurophysiology of the hypothalamic-pituitary-adrenocortical axis in patients with adjustment disorder after suicide attempt found similar biological markers compared to those with major depression, rather than any unique indicators.[54] Certainly, understanding and characterizing a biological basis for adjustment disorder is an area for future research and development.

DISTINGUISHING DEPRESSION FROM ADJUSTMENT DISORDER WITH DEPRESSED MOOD

The most common diagnostic overlap is that between adjustment disorder with depressed mood and major depression. Historically, a diagnosis of "reactive depression" served as a theoretical precursor to adjustment disorder with depressed mood. While the diagnosis of reactive depression allowed clinicians diagnostic flexibility and the ability to recognize pathologic response to a stressor, it also caused considerable diagnostic confusion,[21] and reactive depression was replaced by adjustment disorder with depressed mood.

In many studies, adjustment disorder with depressed mood has significant overlap with depression. One study by Despland et al. showed that 83% of patients diagnosed with depression also have experienced major life events. (Of course, 100% of those diagnosed with adjustment disorder had recent life events given the diagnostic requirement to have a stressor.)[23] Baumeister et al. emphasize that while patients with both diagnoses might experience similar life events, the clinician should focus on whether or not the life stressor caused the psychiatric disorder directly.[21] Further, they also summarize that "no study has identified specific distinguishing symptoms" between adjustment disorder and major depression.[21]

ASSESSMENT INSTRUMENTS FOR ADJUSTMENT DISORDER

There were no standardized instruments for adjustment disorder, limiting its rigorous study. However, the Diagnostic Interview Adjustment Disorder is a new instrument connecting a stressor to distress and impairment.[55] In addition, three full-length structured interviews, the Schedule for Clinical Assessment in Neuropsychiatry,[56] the Structured Clinical Interview (SCID) for DSM-IV,[57] and the SCID for DSM-5[58] include sections on adjustment disorder. However, issues arise with structured interviews that limit diagnosis of adjustment disorder.[57,58] The SCID instructs interviewers that the diagnosis cannot be made if criteria for other disorders are met as specified in the DSM-IV and DSM-5 criteria. Using these interviews, clinically depressive symptoms in response to a stressor qualify as a major depressive episode if the symptoms are severe and persist for longer than two weeks. In a study of psychiatric outpatients, 36% of those seen were clinically diagnosed with adjustment disorder, but this changed to only 11% when the SCID was applied.[37] Thus, once a major depressive episode is diagnosed, adjustment disorder is excluded. Since adjustment disorder criteria meet a lower threshold than major mood and anxiety disorders, the more severe diagnosis being made may risk inappropriate treatment.[1] Other structured interviews do not include adjustment disorder.[34] In comparisons, the diagnosis is made more often during an unstructured than a structured clinical diagnostic interview.[12]

Einsle et al. created a validated questionnaire to screen for adjustment disorder.[15] It was based on the theory that adjustment disorder is a stress-response syndrome,[17] had good construct validity, and supported inclusion of adjustment disorder within this DSM-5 category of TSRD.

TREATMENT FOR ADJUSTMENT DISORDER

Adjustment disorders are typically treated with supportive interventions, both psychotherapeutic and psychopharmacological, and external, such as, when possible, removing or reducing the stressor. Since removing a stressor often is not feasible, the primary task in treating adjustment disorder becomes helping patients manage the extremes of their response to the severity of the stressor itself.[34] Supportive psychotherapy,[59] psychodynamic psychotherapy,[60,61] cognitive behavioral therapy,[62–65] interpersonal psychotherapy,[66,67] group therapy,[68] and psychological first aid[69] have potential benefit in treating adjustment disorder. In psychotherapy, identifying how the patient understands and responds to stress, and translating those emotions into words, allows for improved tolerance and response to the stressor.

Arends and colleagues, in a 2012 Cochrane database review, conducted a systematic review of treatment interventions for employees experiencing adjustment disorders and their effectiveness at returning employees to work.[70] The authors found 10 psychotherapy treatment interventions (five cognitive therapy and five problem-solving therapy) and a combined treatment of psychotherapy and relaxation techniques but no psychopharmacologic treatment programs of sufficient quality to include in their review. While there were no improvements in return to work full-time in the treatments groups in general, a small effect was found for return to part-time work occurring 17 days faster on average for the problem-solving therapy treatment groups when compared to controls. While the evidence was of low to moderate quality because of the small number of participants in a small number of studies, the review underscores the importance of further examination of what treatments may be effective for adjustment disorder.

The Cochrane database identifies two randomized control trials for the treatment of adjustment disorders, one a cognitive-behavioral intervention for employees with a goal of developing coping skills in a group of employees and the other an occupational intervention using mirror therapy treatment for patients experiencing depressive symptoms after a myocardial infarction. The first study's intervention occurred in three stages similar to stress inoculation training, where participants first sought to understand a loss of control that they were experiencing, then identify problem-solving strategies for their sources of stress, and finally implement those strategies in their lives.[65] The second study also had three phases: (1) the body block, to increase attentiveness to physical cues and understanding of health and disease models; (2) the cognitive block, to examine modes of thinking, and improve self-esteem; and (3) the integration block, to accept and adapt to the disease.[71] Both treatments emphasized phases that provide specific goals to be achieved and an examination of both the roadblocks to achieving those goals and how to overcome them. Any psychotherapeutic treatment for adjustment disorder may incorporate the identification of adaptive skills to be learned, with encouragement and reinforcement as those skills replace maladaptive behaviors in daily living and direction in anticipation of setbacks that might promote a return of old habits.[72]

Other specific psychotherapies have been investigated for their efficacy in the treatment of adjustment disorders. Brief psychotherapy may be effective in the treatment of minor depressive episodes[59] and has been a mainstay of treatment of adjustment disorder, presumably because therapy is often time-limited and ends with resolution of a stressor. Thus treatment frequently focuses on reducing or avoiding the stressor, or reducing the emotional reaction to the stressor, and a therapist can help a patient identify the significance and implication of stressful life events and from there serve as a springboard to thinking through a more balanced evaluation of their circumstances to reduce a stressor's affective power. Similarly, interpersonal psychotherapy's (IPT) focus on one of the four problem areas of bereavement, interpersonal role disputes, role transitions, or interpersonal deficits makes it well suited to treating adjustment disorders, which frequently stem from such contexts. For example, Markowitz and colleagues have employed IPT in the treatment of HIV-positive individuals struggling with tremendous upheaval in their lives.[73,74] Other studies looking at patients dealing with medical conditions have similarly found success in improving mood symptoms and reducing impairment with support groups.[75–77]

In contrast to the psychotherapies, there is controversy about use of medication, compared to psychotherapy alone, though many psychiatrists prescribe antidepressant medications such as the selective serotonin reuptake inhibitors for adjustment disorder like they would depressive disorders.[78] Despite little data from randomized control trials for these diagnoses, there is still a known response to antidepressants and anxiolytics in patients with depression and anxiety, and medication should be considered especially if the patient remains symptomatic after three months of psychotherapy.[79,80] While clinicians may need to frequently infer the possible treatment of adjustment disorder in heterogeneous study populations, research on medications for the treatment of adjustment disorder specifically may be gaining some traction. In 2015, Stein examined the treatment of adjustment disorder with anxiety using etifoxine versus alprazolam, finding that the former was effective, though subjects taking the latter showed continued improvement after four weeks,[81]which is consistent with the efficacy of benzodiazepines for anxiety.[81] Nevertheless, caution is encouraged since adjustment disorder may signal the onset of a more severe disorder. At the same time, as Andreasen and colleagues found, despite some of the data on an increased risk of suicide, after five years most adults (71%) and many adolescents (44%) were doing well after experiencing and adjustment disorder, though risk factors for poor outcomes include chronicity and behavioral disturbances.[4] Still, adjustment disorder is generally less disabling long term than other major mental disorders, and there remains the probability of a good outcome relative to other mental disorders, especially after the resolution of the triggering stressor.[47]

Case Illustration

Here we use a case to further outline points to consider for this diagnosis.

An 18-year-old, active-duty, female sailor in the US Navy presented to the emergency department of a military hospital for evaluation of suicidal ideation. Before enlisting, she described herself as an academically minded student with goals of having a successful Navy career and gaining a debt-free education through her service. She was in good health with no history of psychiatric illness, suicidal ideation, or symptoms of past depressive episodes. She had no family history of mental disorder, but her mother had recent diagnoses of worsening hypertension and diabetes. However, within days of starting Navy basic training, she became distressed with worry and anxiety related to training, and she found it difficult to make friends. Despite being an A and B student in high school, when she took the Armed Services Vocational Aptitude Battery, a placement entrance exam, she scored so poorly that she entered the Navy as an "undesignated seaman" where, in her own words, "all I do is chip paint." She had hoped to become a hospital corpsman, or medic, which she could use as a springboard to entering a health care profession. After completing basic training, she presented to her first duty station on an amphibious assault ship to perform maintenance such as painting, like other sailors. She soon began to experience daily progressive worry, low mood, and crying spells. She had less than five hours of interrupted sleep per night and lost weight. Ultimately, every time she had to report for work, she began to have suicidal thoughts, without a plan or intent. When she told a peer that she would rather "just never wake up in the morning ever again" and "rather die than report to duty," it was reported to her commanding officer, and she was referred for psychiatric evaluation. She said, "the Navy has made me miserable," but "I would not be unhappy if I had been assigned a better job." Many of her emotions were lessened or absent on days when she did not have to present to work, and she continued to enjoy her leisure activities. The patient's commanding officer was confounded by her reaction to these stressors.

Comment: This case illustrates many of the diagnostic criteria and features of adjustment disorders. The predominant feature, criterion A, is the presence and emergence of these emotional and behavioral symptoms in relation to acute occupational and situational stressors. The patient had a number of life changes surrounding her joining the Navy. She had left an ailing mother who was her main social support and reason for not committing suicide. She had moved across the country for her first duty station, leaving any other supports she had. She felt betrayed by the Navy who had promised her a successful career of progression and education, only to find that her entrance scores were too low to be guaranteed the job she wanted. The patient's symptoms occurred almost immediately after the onset of basic training; she had anxiety, worry, and low mood. She denied having these symptoms prior to leaving home. The temporal development of these symptoms with the stressors fulfills and illustrates criterion A for adjustment disorder.

The patient's symptoms were clinically significant both in the marked distress that they caused her and her degree of impairment. This illustrates criterion B. The stressor does not meet criteria for acute stress disorder or PTSD because it was not a trauma that included threatened death, serious injury, or sexual violation. There was a discrepancy in the degree of the stressor as portrayed by the patient and observed by her commanding officer. She described stress related to the "meaninglessness" of her position and her perceived inability to understand how to prepare for retaking her entrance exam. Her command reported that she was mostly performing orientation duties such a completing paperwork and had only "chipped paint" for fewer than four hours in a single eight-hour shift. They also reported they had prepared a clear study plan for her and that the exam is not onerous in terms of content. Her psychiatric team also felt that her distress was disproportionate to the actual stressors, further fulfilling criterion B for the diagnosis of adjustment disorder.

She was diagnosed with adjustment disorder with mixed anxiety and depressed mood. She presented with notable symptoms of low mood, tearfulness, hopelessness, worry, and nervousness. To meet the criteria of adjustment disorder, the patient's disturbance cannot meet criteria for another mental disorder, as stated in criterion C. She displayed some characteristics of major depressive disorder and generalized anxiety disorder, which were on the differential for this patient. Those symptoms consistent with major depressive disorder included depressed mood, weight loss, insomnia, feelings of worthlessness, and indecisiveness, but her depressed mood and loss of interest were fleeting. When she was not faced with presenting to work or making decisions regarding her future, her symptoms lessened and were manageable, and she found enjoyment in activities she liked. She appeared more overwhelmed than depressed on interviews and in her interactions with others. All of these factors supported a diagnosis of adjustment disorder over a major depressive episode. The final criterion is resolution of symptoms after the stressor terminates. She stabilized on the inpatient ward and returned to her unit, where she was able to retake the entrance exam and improve her score. She was reassigned to a new position that she enjoyed, and her symptoms resolved within three months of being moved to a different department.

This case illustrates both the diagnostic criteria of the disorder as well as the character of one type of patient with adjustment disorder. In her case, her suffering is recognized and a medical system followed her longitudinally to help resolve her illness throughout its course.

CONCLUSION

Adjustment disorder is a useful clinical diagnosis that can identify patients with clinical distress due to stressors, yet do not meet criteria for other TSRDs or an affective disorder. It is not necessarily mild but can be self-limiting and resolve without intensive treatment. The diagnosis remains loosely defined and requires more subjective clinical interpretation than other diagnoses. One future direction may be driven by the National Institute of Mental Health's introduction of the Research Domain Criteria (RDoC). Cuthbert and Insel describe "the seven pillars" of differences between the RDoC and the constructs behind the DSM, leading to one possible end where adjustment disorders may be studied not as an afterthought but as rigorously as its more famous diagnostic relative, PTSD.[82] Adjustment disorders represent a significant public health concern in terms of morbidity and disability. A significant risk of suicidal ideation and suicide is associated with them. Clinicians are wise to treat patients with adjustment disorders with the same energy and concern as those experiencing other mental disorders.

REFERENCES

1. Casey P, Bailey S. Adjustment disorders: the state of the art. *World Psychiatry.* 2011;10(1):11–18.
2. *Diagnostic and statistical manual of mental disorders.* 1st ed. Washington, DC: American Psychiatric Association; 1952.
3. *Diagnostic and statistical manual of mental disorders.* 2nd ed. Washington, DC: American Psychiatric Assocation; 1968.
4. Andreasen NC, Hoenk PR. The predictive value of adjustment disorders: a follow-up study. *The American Journal of Psychiatry.* 1982;139(5):584–590.
5. *Diagnostic and statistical manual of mental disorders.* 3rd ed. Washington, DC: American Psychiatric Association; 1987.
6. *Diagnostic and statistical manual of mental disorders.* 4th ed. Washington, DC: American Psychiatric Association; 1994.
7. Andreasen NC, Wasek P. Adjustment disorders in adolescents and adults. *Archives of General Psychiatry.* 1980;37(10):1166–1170.
8. Strain JJ, Newcorn J, Wolf D, Fulop G, Davis W. Considering changes in adjustment disorder. *Hospital & Community Psychiatry.* 1993;44(1):13–15.
9. Wakefield JC. Diagnosing DSM-IV—Part I: DSM-IV and the concept of disorder. *Behaviour Research and Therapy.* 1997;35(7):633–649.
10. Patra BN, Sarkar S. Adjustment disorder: current diagnostic status. *Indian Journal of Psychological Medicine.* 2013;35(1):4–9.
11. American Psychiatric Association, American Psychiatric Association, Force DSMT. *Diagnostic and statistical manual of mental disorders: DSM-5.* Washington, DC: American Psychiatric Association; 2013.
12. Strain JJ, Friedman MJ. Considering adjustment disorders as stress response syndromes for DSM-5. *Depression and Anxiety.* 2011;28(9):818–823.
13. Baumeister H, Kufner K. It is time to adjust the adjustment disorder category. *Current Opinion in Psychiatry.* 2009;22(4):409–412.
14. Laugharne J, van der Watt G, Janca A. It is too early for adjusting the adjustment disorder category. *Current Opinion in Psychiatry.* 2009;22(1):50–54.
15. Einsle F, Kollner V, Dannemann S, Maercker A. Development and validation of a self-report for the assessment of adjustment disorders. *Psychology, Health & Medicine.* 2010;15(5):584–595.
16. Friedman MJ, Resick PA, Bryant RA, Strain J, Horowitz M, Spiegel D. Classification of trauma and stressor-related disorders in DSM-5. *Depression and Anxiety.* 2011;28(9):737–749.
17. Maercker A, Einsle F, Kollner V. Adjustment disorders as stress response syndromes: a new diagnostic concept and its exploration in a medical sample. *Psychopathology.* 2007;40(3):135–146.
18. ICD-11 Beta Draft (Mortality and Morbidity Statistics), 6B33 Adjustment disorder. (n.d.). Retrieved from http://apps.who.int/classifications/icd11/browse/l-m/en - / http%3a%2f%2fid.who.int%2ficd%2fentity%2f264310751).
19. Maercker A, Brewin CR, Bryant RA, et al. Diagnosis and classification of disorders specifically associated with stress: proposals for ICD-11. *World Psychiatry.* 2013;12(3):198–206.
20. Maercker A, Brewin CR, Bryant RA, et al. Proposals for mental disorders specifically associated with stress in the International Classification of Diseases-11. *Lancet.* 2013;381(9878):1683–1685.
21. Baumeister H, Maercker A, Casey P. Adjustment disorder with depressed mood: a critique of its

DSM-IV and ICD-10 conceptualisations and recommendations for the future. *Psychopathology.* 2009;42(3):139–147.
22. Dowrick C, Casey P, Dalgard O, et al. Outcomes of Depression International Network (ODIN). Background, methods and field trials. ODIN Group. *British Journal of Psychiatry.* 1998;172:359–363.
23. Despland JN, Monod L, Ferrero F. Clinical relevance of adjustment disorder in DSM-III-4 and DSM-IV. *Comprehensive Psychiatry.* 1995;36(6):454–460.
24. Casey P, Dowrick C, Wilkinson G. Adjustment disorders: fault line in the psychiatric glossary. *British Journal of Psychiatry.* 2001;179:479–481.
25. Fabrega H Jr, Mezzich JE, Mezzich AC. Adjustment disorder as a marginal or transitional illness category in DSM-III. *Archives of General Psychiatry.* 1987;44(6):567–572.
26. Hall DP, Benedek DM. Adjustment disorder criteria. *Hospital & Community Psychiatry.* 1993;44(6):592.
27. Fernández A, Mendive JM, Salvador-Carulla L, et al. Adjustment disorders in primary care: prevalence, recognition and use of services. *British Journal of Psychiatry.* 2012;201:137–142.
28. Reed GM, Roberts MC, Keeley J, et al. Mental health professionals' natural taxonomies of mental disorders: implications for the clinical utility of the ICD-11 and the DSM-5. *Journal of Clinical Psychology.* 2013;69(12):1191–1212.
29. Evans SC, Reed GM, Roberts MC, et al. Psychologists' perspectives on the diagnostic classification of mental disorders: results from the WHO-IUPsyS Global Survey. *International Journal of Psychology.* 2013;48(3):177–193.
30. Myers JK, Weissman MM, Tischler GL, et al. Six-month prevalence of psychiatric disorders in three communities 1980 to 1982. *Archives of General Psychiatry.* 1984;41(10):959–967.
31. Kessler RC, Sonnega A, Bromet E, Hughes M, Nelson CB. Posttraumatic stress disorder in the National Comorbidity Survey. *Archives of General Psychiatry.* 1995;52(12):1048–1060.
32. Druss BG, Wang PS, Sampson NA, et al. Understanding mental health treatment in persons without mental diagnoses: results from the National Comorbidity Survey Replication. *Archives of General Psychiatry.* 2007;64(10):1196–1203.
33. Fernandez A, Mendive JM, Salvador-Carulla L, et al. Adjustment disorders in primary care: prevalence, recognition and use of services. *British Journal of Psychiatry.* 2012;201:137–142.
34. Strain JJ, Diefenbacher A. The adjustment disorders: the conundrums of the diagnoses. *Comprehensive Psychiatry.* 2008;49(2):121–130.
35. Popkin MK, Callies AL, Colon EA, Stiebel V. Adjustment disorders in medically ill inpatients referred for consultation in a university hospital. *Psychosomatics.* 1990;31(4):410–414.
36. Koran LM, Sheline Y, Imai K, et al. Medical disorders among patients admitted to a public-sector psychiatric inpatient unit. *Psychiatric Services.* 2002;53(12):1623–1625.
37. Shear MK, Greeno C, Kang J, et al. Diagnosis of nonpsychotic patients in community clinics. *American Journal of Psychiatry.* 2000;157(4):581–587.
38. Strain JJ, Smith GC, Hammer JS, et al. Adjustment disorder: a multisite study of its utilization and interventions in the consultation-liaison psychiatry setting. *General Hospital Psychiatry.* 1998;20(3):139–149.
39. Jones R, Yates WR, Williams S, Zhou M, Hardman L. Outcome for adjustment disorder with depressed mood: comparison with other mood disorders. *Journal of Affective Disorders.* 1999;55(1):55–61.
40. Kuhn M, Ehlert U, Rumpf HJ, Backhaus J, Hohagen F, Broocks A. Onset and maintenance of psychiatric disorders after serious accidents. *European Archives of Psychiatry and Clinical Neuroscience.* 2006;256(8):497–503.
41. Greenberg WM, Rosenfeld DN, Ortega EA. Adjustment disorder as an admission diagnosis. *American Journal of Psychiatry.* 1995;152(3):459–461.
42. Casey P, Doherty A. Adjustment disorder: implications for ICD-11 and DSM-5. *British Journal of Psychiatry.* 2012;201:90–92.
43. Diefenbacher A, Strain JJ. Consultation-liaison psychiatry: stability and change over a 10-year-period. *General Hospital Psychiatry.* 2002;24(4):249–256.
44. Haw C, Hawton K, Houston K, Townsend E. Psychiatric and personality disorders in deliberate self-harm patients. *British Journal of Psychiatry.* 2001;178(1):48–54.
45. Schnyder U, Valach L. Suicide attempters in a psychiatric emergency room population. *General Hospital Psychiatry.* 1997;19(2):119–129.
46. Gupta B, Trzepacz PT. Serious overdosers admitted to a general hospital: comparison with nonoverdose self-injuries and medically ill patients with suicidal ideation. *General Hospital Psychiatry.* 1997;19(3):209–215.
47. Looney JG, Gunderson EK. Transient situational disturbances: course and outcome. *American Journal of Psychiatry.* 1978;135(6):660–663.
48. Kryzhanovskaya L, Canterbury R. Suicidal behavior in patients with adjustment disorders. *Crisis.* 2001;22(3):125–131.

49. Pelkonen M, Marttunen M, Henriksson M, Lonnqvist J. Suicidality in adjustment disorder—clinical characteristics of adolescent outpatients. *European Child & Adolescent Psychiatry.* 2005;14(3):174–180.
50. Runeson BS, Beskow J, Waern M. The suicidal process in suicides among young people. *Acta Psychiatrica Scandinavica.* 1996;93(1):35–42.
51. Manoranjitham SD, Rajkumar AP, Thangadurai P, Prasad J, Jayakaran R, Jacob KS. Risk factors for suicide in rural south India. *British Journal of Psychiatry.* 2010;196(1):26–30.
52. Kumano H, Ida I, Oshima A, et al. Brain metabolic changes associated with predispotion to onset of major depressive disorder and adjustment disorder in cancer patients—a preliminary PET study. *Journal of Psychiatric Research.* 2007;41(7):591–599.
53. Rocco A, Martocchia A, Frugoni P, et al. Inverse correlation between morning plasma cortisol levels and MMPI psychasthenia and depression scale scores in victims of mobbing with adjustment disorders. *Neuroendocrinology Letters.* 2007;28(5):610–613.
54. Lindqvist D, Traskman-Bendz L, Vang F. Suicidal intent and the HPA-axis characteristics of suicide attempters with major depressive disorder and adjustment disorders. *Archives of Suicide Research.* 2008;12(3):197–207.
55. Cornelius LR, Brouwer S, de Boer MR, Groothoff JW, van der Klink JJ. Development and validation of the Diagnostic Interview Adjustment Disorder (DIAD). *International Journal of Methods in Psychiatric Research.* 2014;23(2):192–207.
56. Wing JK, Babor T, Brugha T, et al. SCAN: Schedules for Clinical Assessment in Neuropsychiatry. *Archives of General Psychiatry.* 1990;47(6):589–593.
57. First MB, Gibbon M, Williams JBW. *Structured Clinical Interview for DSM-IV Axis I Disorders, Clinician Version* (SCID-CV). Washington, DC: American Psychiatric Press; 1996.
58. First MB WJ, Karg RS, Spitzer RL. *Structured Clinical Interview for DSM-5—Research Version* (SCID-5 for DSM-5, Research Version; SCID-5-RV). Arlington, VA: American Psychiatric Association Publishing; 2015.
59. Maina G, Forner F, Bogetto F. Randomized controlled trial comparing brief dynamic and supportive therapy with waiting list condition in minor depressive disorders. *Psychotherapy and Psychosomatics.* 2005;74(1):43–50.
60. Subic-Wrana C, Greenberg LS, Lane RD, Michal M, Wiltink J, Beutel ME. Affective change in psychodynamic psychotherapy: Theoretical models and clinical approaches to changing emotions. *Zeitschrift fur Psychosomatische Medizin und Psychotherapie.* 2016;62(3):207–223.
61. Kramer U, Pascual-Leone A, Despland JN, de Roten Y. One minute of grief: emotional processing in short-term dynamic psychotherapy for adjustment disorder. *Journal of Consulting and Clinical Psychology.* 2015;83(1):187–198.
62. Craig A, Hancock K, Dickson H. Improving the long-term adjustment of spinal cord injured persons. *Spinal Cord.* 1999;37(5):345–350.
63. Kavitha C, Rangan U, Nirmalan PK. Quality of life and marital adjustment after cognitive behavioural therapy and behavioural marital therapy in couples with anxiety disorders. *Journal of Clinical and Diagnostic Research.* 2014;8(8):Wc01-04.
64. Skruibis P, Eimontas J, Dovydaitiene M, Mazulyte E, Zelviene P, Kazlauskas E. Internet-based modular program BADI for adjustment disorder: protocol of a randomized controlled trial. *BMC Psychiatry.* 2016;16:264.
65. van der Klink JJ, Blonk RW, Schene AH, van Dijk FJ. Reducing long term sickness absence by an activating intervention in adjustment disorders: a cluster randomised controlled design. *Occupational and Environmental Medicine.* 2003;60(6):429–437.
66. Neugebauer R, Kline J, Bleiberg K, et al. Preliminary open trial of interpersonal counseling for subsyndromal depression following miscarriage. *Depression and Anxiety.* 2007;24(3):219–222.
67. Neugebauer R, Kline J, Markowitz JC, et al. Pilot randomized controlled trial of interpersonal counseling for subsyndromal depression following miscarriage. *Journal of Clinical Psychiatry.* 2006;67(8):1299–1304.
68. Sundquist J, Lilja A, Palmer K, et al. Mindfulness group therapy in primary care patients with depression, anxiety and stress and adjustment disorders: randomised controlled trial. *British Journal of Psychiatry.* 2015;206(2):128–135.
69. True PK, Benway MW. Treatment of stress reaction prior to combat using the "BICEPS" model. *Military Medicine.* 1992;157(7):380–381.
70. Arends I, Bruinvels DJ, Rebergen DS, et al. Interventions to facilitate return to work in adults with adjustment disorders. *Cochrane Database of Systematic Reviews.* 2012;12:Cd006389.
71. Gonzalez-Jaimes EI, Turnbull-Plaza B. Selection of psychotherapeutic treatment for adjustment disorder with depressive mood due to acute myocardial infarction. *Archives of Medical Research.* 2003;34(4):298–304.
72. Beitman BD, Manring J. *Textbook of psychotherapeutic treatments.* Arlington, VA: American Psychiatric Publishing; 2009.

73. Markowitz JC, Klerman GL, Perry SW. Interpersonal psychotherapy of depressed HIV-positive outpatients. *Hospital & Community Psychiatry.* 1992;43(9):885–890.
74. Markowitz JC, Kocsis JH, Fishman B, et al. Treatment of depressive symptoms in human immunodeficiency virus-positive patients. *Archives of General Psychiatry.* 1998;55(5):452–457.
75. Spiegel D. Mind matters in cancer survival. *Psycho-oncology.* 2012;21(6):588–593.
76. Goodwin PJ. Support groups in advanced breast cancer. *Cancer.* 2005;104(11 Suppl):2596–2601.
77. Akechi T, Okuyama T, Onishi J, Morita T, Furukawa TA. Psychotherapy for depression among incurable cancer patients. *Cochrane Database of Systematic Reviews.* 2008(2):Cd005537.
78. Olfson M, Marcus SC, Pincus HA, Zito JM, Thompson JW, Zarin DA. Antidepressant prescribing practices of outpatient psychiatrists. *Archives of General Psychiatry.* 1998;55(4):310–316.
79. Simon GE, Rossom RC, Beck A, et al. Antidepressants are not overprescribed for mild depression. *Journal of Clinical Psychiatry.* 2015;76(12):1627–1632.
80. Stewart JW, Quitkin FM, Klein DF. The pharmacotherapy of minor depression. *American Journal of Psychotherapy.* 1992;46(1):23–36.
81. Stein DJ. Etifoxine versus alprazolam for the treatment of adjustment disorder with anxiety: a randomized controlled trial. *Advances in Therapy.* 2015;32(1):57–68.
82. Cuthbert BN, Insel TR. Toward the future of psychiatric diagnosis: the seven pillars of RDoC. *BMC Medicine.* 2013;11:126.

6

Persistent Complex Bereavement Disorder

MEREDITH E. CHARNEY,* SARAH WIEMAN, NICOLE LEBLANC, AND NAOMI SIMON

INTRODUCTION

Grief is an intensely painful but natural and normal psychological response following the death of a loved one. Although there is no uniform pattern for adapting to loss, for the majority of people, acute grief naturally evolves over time into a more integrated, less painful form of grief in a way that is healthy and adaptive; this enables return to a satisfying life without the deceased. However, a growing literature has shown that complications can arise such that the natural recovery from acute grief stalls and grief becomes persistently intense and debilitating. This condition has been termed "traumatic grief" (Cohen, Mannarino, & Staron, 2006; Kaplow, Layne, Pynoos, Cohen, & Lieberman, 2012), "prolonged grief" (Prigerson et al., 2009; Bryant et al., 2014), and "complicated grief" (Shear et al., 2011) in the literature. In the fifth edition of the *Diagnostic and Statistical Manual of Mental Disorders* (DSM-5), the term "persistent complex bereavement disorder" (PCBD; p. 289) is used to describe this impairing grief reaction and is included as a subtype of "Other Specified Trauma- and Stressor-Related Disorder" (309.89 [F 43.8]). DSM-5 indicates the need for additional research to determine the best diagnostic criteria prior to its acceptance as a formal DSM diagnosis. Despite the need to finalize the diagnostic criteria, there is a wealth of evidence for complicated grief as an identifiable, independent condition and a debilitating syndrome that is comprised of symptoms that interfere with adaptation and re-engagement in life after bereavement (Horowitz et al., 1997; Langner & Maercker, 2005; Prigerson et al., 2009; Shear et al., 2011; Simon et al., 2007; Simon et al., 2011). Further, several randomized controlled trials have supported the efficacy of targeted psychotherapies for individuals with complicated grief (Bryant et al., 2014; Kersting, Brahler, Glaesmer, & Wagner, 2011; Shear, Frank, Houck, & Reynolds, 2005; Shear et al., 2016; Shear et al., 2014). Because of its simplicity and the substantial prior clinical literature using the term, this chapter uses the term "complicated grief" (CG). This chapter describes the etiology, diagnostic and clinical features, differential diagnosis, epidemiology, pathophysiology, assessment, and treatment of CG.

ETIOLOGY

Loss of an Attachment Relationship

The theory of attachment as proposed by Bowlby (1978) suggests that humans have a biological instinct to seek out secure attachments with other people. A securely attached relationship provides a secure base from which one can explore and try new things, as well as a source of comfort and safety during periods of stress by

* Corresponding author: Massachusetts General Hospital Director of Psychotherapy and Training, MGH Center for Anxiety & Traumatic Stress Disorders Staff Psychologist, Red Sox Foundation and Massachusetts General Hospital Home Base Program One Bowdoin Square, 6th Floor Boston, MA 02114. Phone: 617-724-1037. Fax: 617-643-0730. Email: mecharney@partners.org

being available, sensitive, and responsive (Shear & Shair, 2005). In adulthood, people form these reciprocal relationships with the ones they love, as each person offers the other a sense of belonging and support. Mental representations of secure relationships develop based on both explicit and implicit memory (Shear, 2010). One's explicit memory uses the factual and narrative history of the relationship to predict how the person will act in the future. One's implicit memory creates intuitive knowledge about the loved one.

When a loved one dies, the secure relationship is lost. Explicit memory easily assimilates to this new information; however, implicit memory requires repeated physical and imaginal experiences to adjust the mental representation and learned predictions (rules) about the person and the attachment relationship (Shear, 2010). Directly following a loss, explicit and implicit memories are at odds. When there is a mismatch between narrative experience and implicit, intuitive predictions or expectations about the relationship, people tend to disregard the experience instead of changing these predictions or expectations (Shear, 2010). This creates a sense of disbelief about the death. With separation in a close relationship, the attachment system is activated if reunion is possible. In acute grief, before the loss is integrated into the implicit, mental representation of the relationship, yearning and emotional pain are heightened as the attachment system is activated attempting to seek reunion. There is a sense of internal disorganization, leading to symptoms such as disrupted sleep, attention, and concentration; physiological or emotional dysregulation; and difficulty with habitual tasks (Shear, 2010). During the normal grieving process, the mental representation of the attachment relationship eventually changes to incorporate the loss of the loved one. In CG, this mental representation of the person and the attachment relationship does not fully incorporate the loss. Instead, patients experience a persistent feeling of traumatic loss as they feel continued discord between their explicit memory of the loss and implicit representation of the loved one and their attachment relationship. This is hypothesized to contribute to the prolonged, intense, and distressing nature of grief in those with CG.

DIAGNOSTIC AND CLINICAL FEATURES

Signs and Symptoms

Grief is characterized by particular thoughts (e.g., preoccupation with the deceased), emotions (e.g., yearning), behaviors (e.g., behavioral deactivation), and physiological reactions (e.g., disturbed sleep; Shear et al., 2007). For most individuals, grief lessens in frequency and intensity over time (Bonanno et al., 2002). However a subset experience complicating reactions (e.g., maladaptive beliefs, excessive avoidance) that stall recovery and prolong grief. Prolonged and severe grief symptoms, coupled with these complicating features, comprise the CG syndrome.

Cognitive

Intrusive thoughts of the deceased are common in CG (Meert et al., 2011). Intrusions may include positive memories of the deceased, memories of the death, images of the deceased's last moments, and distressing images of the future (Boelen & Huntjens, 2008). Maladaptive beliefs may also occur in CG, including negative views of the self (e.g., "I'm worthless"), life (e.g., "life is meaningless"), and the future (e.g., "the future is bleak"), as well as catastrophic interpretations of grief symptoms (e.g., "I'm going crazy"; Boelen, van den Bout, & van den Hout, 2006). These beliefs are considered maladaptive because they generate negative emotions and interfere with coping behaviors (Boelen, van den Bout, et al., 2006).

Individuals with CG may also engage in grief-related rumination (Meert et al., 2011), which includes repetitive negative thinking about the loss and loss-related emotions (Eisma et al., 2015). Grief-related rumination may regard the injustice of the loss, ways the death could have been prevented, and/or difficulties with adjustment post-loss (Eisma et al., 2015). Individuals with CG also often report difficulty thinking about or planning for the future (Cozza et al., 2016). Experimental research indicates that individuals with CG have an impaired ability to imagine specific future events without the deceased, which may contribute to this sense of hopelessness (Robinaugh & McNally, 2013). Repetitive thoughts about reunion with the deceased also occur; these are described in the following sections.

Emotional

Yearning, pining, or longing for the deceased is a common emotional symptom of CG (Meert et al., 2011). The subjective experience of yearning is an intense, appetitive desire for reunion with the deceased (Robinaugh et al., 2016). Among those with CG, self-reported yearning is correlated with neural activation in the nucleus accumbens, which is a region associated with reward processing (O'Connor et al., 2008). Individuals with CG also often report sadness and emotional pain (Cozza et al., 2016). These pangs of emotional pain have been hypothesized to be analogous to the negative affective experience that accompanies physical injuries (Eisenberger, 2015; MacDonald & Leary, 2005). This hypothesis is supported by data indicating that grief reminders trigger activation in the dorsal anterior cingulate cortex, which is a region that is active during physical pain processing (Kersting, Ohrmann, et al., 2009; O'Connor et al., 2008). Emotional pain is especially important to assess clinically, as it predicts both suicidal thoughts and behaviors among bereaved individuals (Robinaugh, 2017).

Loneliness is another common symptom of CG (Meert et al., 2011). Loneliness serves as an emotional signal that one's social supports are absent or unavailable (Cacioppo, Grippo, London, Goossens, & Cacioppo, 2015). Loss can trigger loneliness if the deceased was a primary source of emotional or instrumental support for the bereaved, and may be exacerbated by maladaptive beliefs (e.g., "no one understands what I'm going through"). Individuals with CG may also experience bitterness or anger related to the loss (Meert et al., 2011). Shock, disbelief, and emotional numbness are also common (Meert et al., 2011). Shock and disbelief sometimes manifest as a feeling of "unrealness" about the loss, which is described as the subjective sense that the deceased could return at any moment (Boelen, 2010). Finally, individuals with CG may report survivor guilt for being alive while their loved one has died, or they may feel guilt for some aspect of the death (Shear et al., 2007).

Behavioral

Excessive avoidance is a hallmark symptom of CG (Meert et al., 2011). Individuals with CG engage in avoidance to limit distressing emotions such as yearning and emotional pain (Shear et al., 2007). While an ability to both approach and avoid the intensity of the loss can be adaptive in normal grief, when used inflexibly or excessively avoidance is thought to prevent acceptance of the loss and stall recovery (Shear et al., 2007). Those with CG might avoid reminders of the deceased (e.g., people, places, and activities), the loss (e.g., the deceased's doctor, the final resting place), or death/illness (e.g., sick relatives, funerals; Shear et al., 2007). Grief-related avoidance predicts functional impairment earlier and beyond CG symptom severity, as it restricts individuals' behavior and limits opportunities for positive emotions (Shear et al., 2007).

Individuals with CG may also demonstrate excessive proximity seeking of reminders of the deceased as part of a desire for reunion (Meert et al., 2011). They might linger over pictures/scrapbooks, wear the deceased's clothing, or spend a great deal of time in rooms or other places associated with the deceased. The pathological nature of proximity seeking is equivocal (for conflicting results, see Boelen, Stroebe, Schut, & Zijerveld, 2006; Field, Holen, & Horowitz, 1999). An important distinction may be the function of the behavior (i.e., maintaining a connection to the deceased vs. avoiding acknowledging the reality of the loss), as well as the degree to which excessive proximity seeking interferes with other, adaptive behaviors that enable engagement in life without the deceased.

Behavioral deactivation is also observed among many individuals with CG (Monk, Houck, & Shear, 2006). In one study, individuals with the disorder were less likely to engage in a variety of daily activities (e.g., socializing, eating meals, going outside, exercising, and doing work/housework) than control participants (Monk et al., 2006). They were also significantly more likely to report napping and snacking (Monk et al., 2006). Individuals with CG experience disrupted daily rhythms, which can contribute to behavioral deactivation and reduced opportunities for positive reinforcement. Finally, individuals with CG are at increased risk for suicidal thoughts and behaviors. In one treatment-seeking sample, 65% of bereaved individuals reported suicidal ideation, 29% reported indirect suicidal behavior (e.g., not taking medicines), and 9% reported a previous suicide attempt (Szanto et al., 2006). In this sample, suicidal behavior was predicted by CG symptom severity (Szanto et al., 2006).

Physiological

Individuals with CG also report physiological symptoms that contribute to distress and impairment. Sleep quality is typically poor, especially among patients with comorbid depression (Germain, Caroff, Buysse, & Shear, 2005; Hinton, Field, Nickerson, Bryant, & Simon, 2013; Maytal et al., 2007; Milic et al., 2017) or bipolar disorder (Maytal et al., 2007). Dreams of the dead may also be prominent, particularly in some cultures (Hinton, Field, Nickerson, Bryant, & Simon, 2013). Physiological distress is also common in response to reminders of the deceased and the loss. In one study, 40% of patients with CG reported a least one full or limited symptom grief-related panic attack within the past week (Bui, Horenstein, et al., 2015). The majority of patients who experienced grief-related panic attacks found them distressing and reported anticipatory anxiety about having more attacks (Bui, Horenstein, et al., 2015). More research is needed to understand the physiological underpinnings of CG.

Diagnostic Criteria

Grief experts have argued for the inclusion of a persistent maladaptive grief in the DSM for years, citing research indicating that it is a distinct syndrome, observed across cultures, that causes distress and impairment and demonstrates response to targeted treatment (Bryant, 2012; Hinton et al., 2013; Maytal et al., 2007; Meert et al., 2011; Milic et al., 2017). Ultimately the disorder was included in the DSM-5 as a subtype of "Other Specified Trauma- and Stressor-Related Disorder" as well as in the appendix section "Conditions for Further Study," with the name "Persistent Complex Bereavement Disorder" (CG) and proposed diagnostic criteria as follows (American Psychiatric Association, 2013):

A: Death of a loved one

B: Separation distress, experienced more days than not for at least 12 months since the loss (defined by at least one of the following):
- Persistent yearning/longing
- Intense sorrow and emotional pain
- Preoccupation with the deceased
- Preoccupation with the circumstances of the death

C: Associated symptoms, experienced more days than not for at least 12 months since the loss (defined by at least six of the following):
- Difficulty accepting the death
- Disbelief/emotional numbness
- Difficulty with positive reminiscing
- Bitterness or anger
- Maladaptive appraisals (e.g., self-blame)
- Excessive avoidance
- A desire to die
- Difficulty trusting others
- Feeling alone or detached
- Feeling life is meaningless or empty
- Identity confusion
- Loss of interest

D: Clinically significant distress/impairment

E: The response is inconsistent with the person's cultural, religious, or age norms.

The DSM-5 PCBD criteria have received some criticism. One issue is that empirical data were not available regarding the performance of the PCBD criteria prior to their publication (Wakefield, 2013), and prior research had examined alternate criteria sets. Findings reported by both Cozza et al. (2016) and Mauro et al. (2017) derived from different large, diverse clinical and community samples that compared CG, prolonged grief, and PCBD suggest that the PCBD criteria fail to capture a significant proportion of individuals with clinically significant grief and find that CG criteria best identifies individuals with clinically significant, impairing grief. Cozza et al. (2016) suggest that the PCBD criteria miss clinically significant cases because they require too many symptoms under Criterion C and that the criteria could be improved by reducing the required number of associated symptoms to one. Another unresolved question is the appropriate timeframe for diagnosing PCBD. The DSM-5 PCBD criteria require that an individual be bereaved for at least 12 months before he or she can receive a diagnosis. In contrast, criteria sets for CG (Meert et al., 2011; Shear et al., 2011; Simon et al., 2011) and prolonged grief (Prigerson et al., 2009) both proposed and provide support that a diagnosis should be made after six months. Debate regarding the optimal criteria will likely continue as proposals are considered for the 11th revision of the International Classification of Diseases (due in 2018) and DSM-5.1. Until consensus is reached, a score of $\geq$ 30 on the Inventory of Complicated Grief (ICG; Prigerson et al., 1995) alongside clinical assessment of distress, impairment, time course, and differential diagnosis can most simply be used in practice as a proxy for the diagnosis. Further, a five-item Brief Grief Questionnaire screening tool is available (see later discussion: Ito et al., 2012; Shear, Jackson, Essock, Donahue, & Felton, 2006).

Comorbidity

The symptoms of CG can be reliably distinguished from those of other mental disorders (Boelen & van den Bout, 2005). Nevertheless, psychiatric comorbidity is common among individuals with CG and should be carefully assessed (Simon et al., 2007). In one study, 75% of primary CG patients met criteria for at least one comorbid mood or anxiety disorder: 25% had one comorbidity, 31% had two comorbidities, 14% had three comorbidities, and 6% had four or more comorbidities (Simon et al., 2007). The most common co-occurring disorder was major depressive disorder (MDD; 55%), followed by posttraumatic stress disorder (PTSD; 49%), and generalized anxiety disorders (18%; Simon et al., 2007). Most comorbid disorders had an age of onset prior to CG, which suggests that pre-existing mood and anxiety disorders increase risk for CG. Further, the presence of a comorbid disorder predicted greater CG symptom severity, greater sleep disruption, and more severe work and social impairment in this sample.

CG is likely underrecognized in psychiatric settings. The little available data suggest that rates of comorbid CG in psychiatric samples are high. For example, one study identified elevated rates of CG among those with primary anxiety disorders (Marques et al., 2013). Rates of comorbid CG are also elevated among those with primary unipolar and bipolar mood disorders (Kersting, Kroker, et al., 2009; Simon et al., 2005; Sung et al., 2011). Mood and anxiety disorder patients with comorbid CG have lower quality of life, greater functional impairment, and higher rates of lifetime suicide attempts (Marques et al., 2013; Simon et al., 2005). Identification and diagnosis of comorbid CG in psychiatric samples is clinically important.

DIFFERENTIAL DIAGNOSIS

The differential diagnoses for CG include normative grief, major depression, and PTSD. Complicated grief is a distinct disorder; however, as noted, major depression and PTSD are often comorbid in bereaved adults (Simon et al. 2007). However, studies such as those by Simon and colleagues have found that a proportion of those with CG have no comorbid conditions.

CG versus Normative Grief

Experiencing intense grief in the early months following the loss of a loved one is typical and to be expected. Most bereaved adults experience intense acute grief in the months following a loss, and it tends to be characterized by symptoms including yearning, sorrow, intrusive thoughts of the deceased, and emptiness. For most bereaved individuals, the intense acute grief diminishes within 6 to 12 months following the death (Bonanno et al., 2002; Prigerson & Jacobs, 2001; Prigerson et al., 1999) and those individuals are able to accept the reality of the loss, find meaning in life, and establish/reestablish life goals, activities, and relationships. It is common for those with normative grief to experience surges in grief symptoms from time to time. Anniversaries, holidays, or other stressors can temporarily increase grief and distress. However, these reactions tend to be time limited and eventually subside. In contrast, for those with CG, symptoms are more intense and unrelenting. People get stuck in the acute grief phase of grieving and are unable to meaningfully move forward and heal. No significant reduction in symptoms is seen in the expected 6- to 12-month post-loss time period, and acute grief symptoms can persist for years if untreated.

CG versus Depression

There are overlapping symptoms between major depression and CG including sadness, crying, social withdrawal, sleep disturbance, and suicidality (Shear et al., 2011; Shear et al., 2005). However, the experience of these symptoms occurs for different reasons for depression and CG. In depression, sadness and tearfulness is generalized and all-encompassing and not related to something specific. In CG, sadness and tearfulness is related to the loss of a loved one and missing a loved one and tends to not be generalized. In depression, the social isolation is more generalized and anhedonia is present. In CG, social isolation is specific to the loss and related to avoiding painful reminders of the deceased. In addition, there are symptoms of CG that are unique to bereavement/grief and not found in individuals with depression. This includes intense yearning or preoccupation with the deceased, wishes to be reunited with the deceased, proximity seeking related to the deceased, emotional distress specifically related to the loss, and avoidance of painful reminders related to the deceased.

CG versus PTSD

In addition, there is overlap, but also factors that distinguish, between PTSD and CG. This is particularly the case when the death has been violent, sudden, and/or accidental. Both CG and PTSD can include a sense of shock, intrusive images of the death, avoidance related to the death, feeling distant from others, sleep difficulties, and poor concentration (Shear et al., 2011; Shear et al. 2005). However, CG and PTSD are also distinct in several important ways. First, the predominant emotion in PTSD is fear; in CG, the predominant emotions are longing and sadness (Shear et al., 2011; Shear et al., 2005). In addition, the nature of intrusive thoughts and avoidance are different for PTSD and CG. In PTSD, intrusive thoughts and memories are associated with the traumatic event itself resulting in a prolonged sense of threat (Brewin & Holmes, 2003). Intrusive thoughts in CG are focused on thoughts of the deceased and the circumstances of the death (Prigerson et al., 1999). Avoidance in PTSD is related to reducing perceptions of threat. Avoidance in CG is related to avoid painful reminders, sadness related to the loss, as well as the permanence of the loss. Finally, there are symptoms of CG that are not typically observed in PTSD, including intense yearning for the deceased and proximity seeking to the reminders.

EPIDEMIOLOGY

Prevalence and Risk Factors

The lack of finalized, standardly accepted criteria for the diagnosis of CG poses a challenge for determining the prevalence of CG in the general population. The results of a representative population-based survey ($N = 2520$) showed that the prevalence of CG in the general sample was 3.7%, while the prevalence for CG in the bereaved subsample was 6.7% (Kersting et al., 2011). Many different risk factors including the loss of a child, spouse, or family member; pre-existing psychological disorders; high attachment to and dependence on the deceased; general negative cognitions; and the lack of meaning-making or preparedness surrounding the death have each been associated with CG. Demographic risk factors for CG include being female, older age (>61), and lower socioeconomic status (Kersting et al., 2011).

As might be expected, the nature of the relationship to the deceased plays a role in grief, and several studies support that having a close, familial relationship to the deceased is a risk factor for developing CG. For instance, a study examining parents who had lost a child estimated the prevalence of CG among this population to be as high as 60% (Meert et al., 2011), while the prevalence of CG amongst bereaved spouses ranges from 10% to 20% (Lobb et al., 2010; Meert et al., 2010). In a study by Mitchell, Kim, Prigerson, and Mortimer-Stephens (2004), suicide survivors who were family members of the deceased experienced significantly more severe symptoms of CG compared to suicide survivors that were in-laws, friends, or co-workers of the deceased. In this sample, 43% of the variance in CG scores was explained by the relationship to the deceased.

Furthermore, the prevalence of CG is higher in individuals who have a mood disorder, as has been demonstrated for both bipolar disorder and major depression (Simon et al., 2005; Sung et al., 2011). Adversities during childhood also increase one's risk for developing CG. Higher CG prevalence has been reported for bereaved adults who experienced abuse, the death of a parent, and separation anxiety as a child (Silverman, Johnson, & Prigerson, 2001; Vanderwerker, Jacobs, Parkes, & Prigerson, 2006).

In addition, both secure and insecure attachments styles are related to the development of CG (Bonanno et al., 2002; Van Doorn, Kasl, Beery, Jacobs, & Prigerson, 1998). von Doorn and colleagues found that both an insecure attachment style and a secure, supportive spouse were independently associated with CG. Caregivers may be another group at risk, and CG has been shown to be elevated in caregivers who feel they lack social support following the loss of a loved one (Schulz, Boerner, Shear, Zhang, & Gitlin, 2006).

Cognitive conceptualizations such as negative cognitions and resistance to change may also contribute to risk for CG. Global negative beliefs, negative worldviews, and avoidance of emotional problems have all been linked to increased possibility for CG development (Boelen, van den Bout, & van den Hout, 2003a, 2003b). Additionally, bereaved individuals who are generally averse to lifestyle change are at higher risk of developing CG (Beery et al., 1997). How one makes sense of the loss is another contributing factor. In a study on parents who had lost their child, the inability to conceptualize the loss posed the greatest risk for developing CG (Keesee, Currier, & Neimeyer, 2008). Neimeyer, Baldwin, and Gillies (2006) have also demonstrated an interaction between this sense-making and ongoing attachment to the deceased; continuing one's bond to the deceased after the death was predictive of higher levels of CG if the person was unable to make sense of that loss.

Lastly, the nature of the death, which includes many elements, is also an important contributor to the development of CG. Sudden, unexpected, or violent losses may bring additional challenges for the bereaved to cope with (Kristensen, Weisaeth, & Heir, 2012; Nakajima, Ito, Shirai, & Konishi, 2012; Tal et al., 2017). A small body of literature has suggested that sudden and violent deaths may be associated with higher rates of CG amongst the bereaved, ranging from 12% to as high as 78% in one report, though rates have varied widely and more research is clearly needed (Kristensen et al., 2012; Nakajima et al., 2012). Suicide-related CG can be especially challenging, with recent data suggesting even greater occurrence of self-blame as well as impaired work and social functioning compared to those with CG due to other types of losses (Tal et al., 2017). These types of losses can also result in a range of other conditions, most notably PTSD and MDD, which may in turn complicate the usual adaptations to loss and increase risk for CG. Prior research has also suggested feeling unprepared for the death is associated with CG (Barry, Kasl, & Prigerson, 2002). In contrast, a study by Vanderwerker and Prigerson (2004) found that participants who felt they prepared in advance for the loss and also had a good support system had lower CG prevalence.

PATHOPHYSIOLOGY

Neurobiology

Although the pathogenesis of CG has yet to be determined, one study used functional magnetic resonance imaging and found that CG has unique neurobiological correlates compared to acute grief (O'Connor et al., 2008). These findings suggest that CG is neurobiologically different than the natural grieving process. O'Connor and colleagues examined the neural activity of 23 women who had lost a female family member to breast cancer in the past 18 months. The women were exposed to pictures and word composites to remind them of the death. Compared to those without CG (n = 12), those with CG (n = 11) showed higher neural activation in the nucleus accumbens, a brain region associated with reward. This heightened reward activation when reminded of the deceased may hinder adjustment to the loss (O'Connor et al., 2008). Additional neuroimaging studies have suggested potential roles for disrupted prefrontal processing during emotion processing (Arizmendi, Kaszniak, & O'Connor, 2016), as well as potential differences in cognitive function and whole brain volume compared to normal grief (Saavedra Perez et al., 2015). Although immune activation and cortisol responses have been hypothesized in CG, consistent with CG as a stress response disorder, minimal biomarker data is available to support these hypotheses, although one recent study of bereaved older adults did find lower morning and diurnal cortisol in those with complicated versus normal grief (O'Connor, 2012; Saavedra Perez et al., 2017; Simon, 2012). Although there is much to learn from prior grief, attachment, and stress-related condition studies that may be relevant, more research is needed to elucidate the underlying biology associated with CG.

ASSESSMENT

Screening

Routine screening for CG in psychiatric settings could increase recognition of the disorder and allow for more timely access to treatment. The Brief Grief Questionnaire (BGQ) is a five-item instrument designed for this purpose (Shear, Jackson, Essock, Donahue, & Felton, 2006). The BGQ has good internal consistency (Nakajima et al., 2012; Shear et al., 2006) and captures a cluster of grief-related symptoms that are distinct from general psychological distress (Nakajima et al., 2012). Scores ≥ 8 on the BGQ indicate probable CG, and scores between 5 and 7 indicate subthreshold CG (Shear et al., 2006). Fujisawa et al. (2010) used the BGQ to screen for CG in a representative, bereaved sample and found that 2.4% had probable CG and 22.7% had subthreshold CG. In contrast, Shear et al. (2006) identified 23% with probable CG and 21% with subthreshold CG among individuals who had lost a loved one in the 9/11 attacks.

Clinical Evaluation

Clinical evaluation of patients with possible CG should include a diagnostic assessment for current and lifetime psychiatric disorders, suicide risk, medical history, mental status examination, and treatment history. The Structured Clinical Interview for DSM-5 (SCID-5; First, Williams, Karg, & Spitzer, 2015), or similar structured assessment, can help facilitate information gathering.

However, CG symptoms are not directly assessed via standard psychiatric assessments such as the SCID-5. Clinicians must therefore inquire separately about the circumstances of the loss as well as the severity and intensity of CG symptoms. The Structured Clinical Interview for

Complicated Grief (SCI-CG; Bui, Mauro, et al., 2015) is a clinician-administered assessment that can be used to obtain the information necessary to diagnosis CG. The SCI-CG includes questions about loss-related variables (e.g., patient's relationship to the deceased, date and cause of death) as well as 31 questions about the presence versus absence of specific CG symptoms (Bui, Mauro, et al., 2015). The SCI-CG has excellent psychometric properties including excellent interrater reliability, good test–retest reliability, and good convergent validity with other CG symptom measures (Bui, Mauro, et al., 2015). The majority of clinicians who use the SCI-CG find it easy to use and helpful in understanding their patients' symptoms (Bui, Mauro, et al., 2015).

Self-Report

Self-report measures of CG symptom severity and clinical features are available for research and clinical use. The ICG (Prigerson et al., 1995) is the most widely-used self-report measure of CG symptom severity. To complete the ICG, patients rate the frequency of 19 CG symptoms on a 5-point Likert scale, ranging from 0 (*never*) to 4 (*always*). The ICG has excellent internal consistency and demonstrates good convergent validity with other grief symptom measures (Prigerson et al., 1995). A cut-off score of >25 identified the top 20% of the sample and could be used to diagnosis CG (Prigerson et al., 1995). Grief researchers later proposed a cut-off score of ≥ 30 as the diagnostic threshold (Meert et al., 2011).

Researchers have also developed self-report scales to assess specific clusters of CG symptoms. The Yearning in Situations of Loss Scale (YSL; O'Connor & Sussman, 2014) is a 21-item self-report measure of yearning, as well as the thoughts and behaviors that typically accompany yearning. The YSL has demonstrated excellent internal consistency in a treatment-seeking sample (Robinaugh et al., 2016). The Grief Related Avoidance Questionnaire (GRAQ; Shear et al., 2007) is a 15-item self-report measure that assesses specific grief-related avoidance behaviors. The GRAQ has excellent internal consistency in a treatment seeking sample and predicts decrements in work and social functioning, above and beyond CG symptom severity (Shear et al., 2007). The Typical Beliefs Questionnaire (TBQ; Skritskaya et al., 2017) is a 25-item measure of common, maladaptive, grief-related cognitions. The TBQ has excellent internal consistently in a treatment-seeking sample and demonstrates sensitivity to change with treatment (Skritskaya et al., 2017). Finally, the Grief Cognitions Questionnaire (GCQ; Boelen & Lensvelt-Mulders, 2005) is a 38-item self-report measure that also assesses common maladaptive cognitions among those with CG. The GCQ has demonstrated excellent internal consistency (Boelen & Lensvelt-Mulders, 2005). These self-report measures can assist with the rapid identification of problematic thoughts and behaviors to target in treatment.

TREATMENT

Complicated Grief Therapy

For the majority of bereaved individuals, treatment is unnecessary. Over time, a natural recovery process occurs and individuals are able to continue on with their lives unassisted. However, for bereaved individuals who meet criteria for CG, an empirically supportive psychotherapy is available. Complicated grief therapy (CGT) is a 16-session manualized weekly treatment designed to specifically target symptoms of CG. CGT integrates an attachment model and cognitive-behavioral therapy (CBT) components and focuses on both grief and restoration strategies designed to assist in the natural recovery process following loss (Shear, 2010; Stroebe & Schut, 1999). Grief strategies include revisiting the memory of the death as well as exposure to painful reminders of the deceased that have previously been avoided. These strategies increase tolerance of the distress associated with these memories and reminders and help the patient make peace with a painful reality and accept the finality of the death. The restoration strategies target goals and aspirations for the short and long term to help the patient envision a life without the deceased that allows for joy and satisfaction. Restoration also includes increasing pleasurable and rewarding activities.

Numerous randomized controlled trials support the effectiveness of CGT for treatment of CG (Shear et al., 2005; Shear et al., 2016; Shear et al., 2014). In a randomized controlled trial examining the efficacy of CGT compared to interpersonal therapy (N = 83), Shear and colleagues (2005) found that participants randomly assigned to CGT showed a significantly higher response rate and a significantly faster time to response compared to those receiving interpersonal therapy. A second study by Shear and colleagues (2014) examined the efficacy of CGT compared to interpersonal therapy in a population of older adults (N = 151) (a population vulnerable to CG). Researchers found that twice as many people responded to CGT compared to interpersonal therapy. Furthermore, CGT led to greater symptom reduction, greater change in illness severity, and greater rate of improvement in impairments related to CG (Shear et al., 2014).

CGT has also been shown to be more efficacious than the antidepressant citalopram in treating CG symptoms (Shear et al., 2016). In a study examining CGT verses citalopram, participants (n = 395) received either citalopram (n = 101), placebo (n = 99), CGT with citalopram (n = 99), or CGT with placebo (n = 96). Results revealed that the addition of citalopram did not significantly improve CGT outcome such that the response rate of CGT + placebo versus CGT +citalopram was not significantly different and that the majority improved in both treatment conditions. In addition, suicidal ideation was substantially more improved among participants receiving CGT than among those who did not. However, CGT with the addition of citalopram showed a greater decrease in depressive symptoms compared to CGT+ placebo. Therefore, if a patient is experiencing co-occurring depressive symptoms, supplementing therapy with citalopram could be a beneficial option.

Cognitive-Behavioral Therapy

There is emerging evidence that CBT adapted to target grief that specifically includes an exposure component may be efficacious in treating CG. Bryant and colleagues (2014) examined if a group CBT for grief supplemented with four individual sessions of exposure therapy (reliving the experience of the death of their loved one) was more effective than group CBT supplemented with four individual sessions of supportive. The patients who received the exposure therapy showed greater reductions in CG symptoms, depression, negative appraisals, and functional impairment. These results suggests that exposure sessions that focus on the death help reduce grief symptoms (Bryant et al., 2014).

Pharmacotherapy for CG

Research on the effectiveness of pharmacotherapy to treat CG is emerging. Several studies suggest that antidepressants can relieve depressive symptoms that are related to bereavement; however, the effect on grief severity appears to be less robust (Reynolds et al., 1999; Shear et al., 2016; Zisook, Shuchter, Pedrelli, Sable, & Deaciuc, 2001; Zygmont et al., 1998). For instance, in a sample of bereaved individuals with major depression treated with bupropion, Zisook and colleagues (2001) found a significant response in reducing depression; grief severity decreased but the effect was not as strong. Other research suggests the use of antidepressants in enhancing outcomes for individuals in CGT. In an examination of naturalistic data on combining antidepressants with CGT, Simon et al. (2008) found that those who remained on antidepressants were less likely to drop out of CGT. In addition, Simon and colleagues found that those in CGT who were concurrently on antidepressants showed a higher response rate compared to those who were not receiving concomitant antidepressant medication. However, as noted, antidepressant effects were not robust when compared to CGT alone or in combination with CGT (Shear et al., 2016), and more research is needed to determine whether other medication approaches may be effective or not.

SUMMARY

Grief is a natural reaction following the loss of a loved one. A subset of bereaved individuals are unable to progress beyond the acute grief period and go on to develop CG. CG is a distinct and debilitating condition with a growing literature supporting its existence, its optimal diagnostic criteria, as well as effective treatments. It is currently described in DSM-5 as "persistent complex bereavement disorder" and classified as a subtype of "Other Specified Trauma- and Stressor-Related Disorder" (309.89 [F 43.8]) within the trauma- and stressor-related disorders category, yet there is a growing weight of evidence supporting CG as a diagnosis. Complicated grief is clearly distinct from depression and anxiety, causes significant distress and impaired functioning, is associated with negative outcomes including elevated suicide risk, and responds to targeted treatment. Further research will continue to enhance our understanding of the causes, psychological and biological correlates, and most effective treatment approaches for this patient population.

REFERENCES

American Psychiatric Association. *Diagnostic and Statistical Manual of Mental Disorders*,

5th ed. Arlington, VA: American Psychiatric Publishing, 2013.

Arizmendi, B., Kaszniak, A. W., & O'Connor, M. F. (2016). Disrupted prefrontal activity during emotion processing in complicated grief: An fMRI investigation. *Neuroimage, 124*(Pt A), 968–976. doi:10.1016/j.neuroimage.2015.09.054

Barry, L. C., Kasl, S. V., & Prigerson, H. G. (2002). Psychiatric disorders among bereaved persons: The role of perceived circumstances of death and preparedness for death. *American Journal of Geriatric Psychiatry, 10*(4), 447–457.

Beery, L. C., Prigerson, H. G., Bierhals, A. J., Santucci, L. M., Newsom, J. T., Maclejewski, P. K., . . . Reynolds, Charles F. (1997). Traumatic grief, depression and caregiving in elderly spouses of the terminally ill. *OMEGA-Journal of Death and Dying, 35*(3), 261–279.

Boelen, P. (2010). A sense of "unrealness" about the death of a loved-one: An exploratory study of its role in emotional complications among bereaved individuals. *Applied Cognitive Psychology, 24*, 238–251. doi:10.1002/acp.1557

Boelen, P. A., van den Bout, J., & van den Hout, M. A. (2003a). The role of cognitive variables in psychological functioning after the death of a first degree relative. *Behaviour Research and Therapy, 41*(10), 1123–1136.

Boelen, P. A., van den Bout, J., & van den Hout, M. A. (2003b). The role of negative interpretations of grief reactions in emotional problems after bereavement. *Journal of Behavior Therapy and Experimental Psychiatry, 34*(3–4), 225–238. doi:10.1016/j.jbtep.2003.08.001

Boelen, P., & Huntjens, R. J. C. (2008). Intrusive images in grief: An exploratory study. *Clinical Psychology and Psychotherapy, 15*(4), 217–226. doi:10.1002/cpp.568

Boelen, P., & Lensvelt-Mulders, G. J. L. M. (2005). Psychometric properties of the Grief Cognitions Questionnaire. *Journal of Psychopathology and Behavioral Assessment, 27*(4), 291–303. doi:10.1007/s10862-005-2409-5

Boelen, P., Stroebe, M., Schut, H. A. W., & Zijerveld, A. M. (2006). Continuing bonds and grief: A prospective analysis. *Death Studies, 30*, 767–776. doi:10.1080/07481180600852936

Boelen, P., & van den Bout, J. (2005). Complicated grief, depression, and anxiety as distinct postloss syndromes: A confirmatory factor analysis study. *American Journal of Psychiatry, 162*, 2175–2177. doi:10.1176/appi.ajp.162.11.2175

Boelen, P., van den Bout, J., & van den Hout, M. (2006). Negative cognitions and avoidance in emotional problems after bereavement: A prospective study. *Behaviour Research and Therapy, 44*, 1657–1672. doi:10.1016/j.brat.2005.12.006

Bonanno, G. A., Wortman, C. B., Lehman, D. R., Tweed, R. G., Haring, M., Sonnega, J., . . . Nesse, R. M. (2002). Resilience to loss and chronic grief: A prospective study from preloss to 18-months postloss. *Journal of Personality and Social Psychology, 83*(5), 1150–1164.

Bowlby, J. (1978). Attachment theory and its therapeutic implications. *Adolescent Psychiatry, 6*, 5–33.

Brewin, C. R., & Holmes, E. A. (2003). Psychological theories of posttraumatic stress disorder. *Clinical Psychology Review, 23*(3), 339–376.

Bryant, R. A. (2012). Grief as a psychiatric disorder. *The British Journal of Psychiatry, 201*, 9–10. doi:10.1192/bjp.bp.111.102889

Bryant, R. A., Kenny, L., Joscelyne, A., Rawson, N., Maccallum, F., Cahill, C., . . . Nickerson, A. (2014). Treating prolonged grief disorder: A randomized clinical trial. *JAMA Psychiatry, 71*(12), 1332–1339. doi:10.1001/jamapsychiatry.2014.1600

Bui, E., Horenstein, A., Shah, R., Skritskaya, N., Mauro, C., Wang, P. S., . . . Simon, N. (2015). Grief-related panic symptoms in complicated grief. *Journal of Affective Disorders, 170*, 213–216. doi:10.1016/j.jad.2014.08.028

Bui, E., Mauro, C., Robinaugh, D. J., Skritskaya, N., Wang, Y., Gribbin, C., . . . Shear, M. K. (2015). The structured clinical interview for complicated grief: Reliability, validity, and exploratory factor analysis. *Depression and Anxiety, 32*, 485–492. doi:10.1002/da.22385

Cacioppo, S., Grippo, A. J., London, S., Goossens, L., & Cacioppo, J. T. (2015). Loneliness: Clinical import and interventions. *Perspective on Psychological Science, 10*(2), 238–249. doi:10.1177/1745691615570616

Cohen, J. A., Mannarino, A. P., & Staron, V. R. (2006). A pilot study of modified cognitive-behavioral therapy for childhood traumatic grief (CBT-CTG). *Journal of the American Academy of Child and Adolescent Psychiatry, 45*(12), 1465–1473. doi:10.1097/01.chi.0000237705.43260.2c

Cozza, S. J., Fisher, J. E., Mauro, C., Zhou, J., Ortiz, C. D., Skritskaya, N. A., . . . Shear, M. K. (2016). Performance of DSM-5 persistent complex bereavement disorder criteria in a community sample of bereaved family members. *American Journal of Psychiatry, 173*, 919–929. doi:10.1176/appi.ajp.2016.15111442

Eisenberger, N. I. (2015). Social pain and the brain: Controversies, questions, and where to go from here. *Annual Review of Psychology, 66*, 601–629. doi:10.1146/annurev-psych-010213-115146

Eisma, M. C., Schut, H., Stroebe, M., Boelen, P., van den Bout, J., & Stroebe, W. (2015). Adaptive and maladaptive rumination after the loss: A three-wave longitudinal study. *British Journal of Clinical Psychology, 54*(2), 163–180. doi:10.1111/bjc.12067

Field, N. P., Holen, A., & Horowitz, M. J. (1999). The relation of continuing attachment to adjustment in conjugal bereavement. *Journal of Consulting and Clinical Psychology, 67*(2), 212–218. doi:10.1037/0022-006X.67.2.212

First, M. B., Williams, J. B. W., Karg, R. S., & Spitzer, R. L. (2015). *Structured Clinical Interview for DSM-5 Disorders, Clinician Version* (SCID-5-CV). Arlington, VA: American Psychiatric Association.

Fujisawa, D., Miyashita, M., Nakajima, S., Ito, M., Kato, M., & Kim, Y. (2010). Prevalence and determinants of complicated grief in general population. *Journal of Affective Disorders, 127*, 352–358. doi:10.1016/j.jad.2010.06.008

Germain, A., Caroff, K., Buysse, D. J., & Shear, M. K. (2005). Sleep quality in complicated grief. *Journal of Traumatic Stress, 18*(4), 343–346. doi:10.1002/jts.20035

Hinton, D. E., Field, N. P., Nickerson, A., Bryant, R. A., & Simon, N. (2013). Dreams of the dead among Cambodian refugees: Frequency, phenomenology, and relationship to complicated grief and posttraumatic stress disorder. *Death Studies, 37*(8), 750–767. doi:10.1080/07481187.2012.692457

Horowitz, M. J., Siegel, B., Holen, A., Bonanno, G. A., Milbrath, C., & Stinson, C. H. (1997). Diagnostic criteria for complicated grief disorder. *American Journal of Psychiatry, 154*(7), 904–910. doi:10.1176/ajp.154.7.904

Ito, M., Nakajima, S., Fujisawa, D., Miyashita, M., Kim, Y., Shear, M. K., . . . Wall, M. M. (2012). Brief measure for screening complicated grief: reliability and discriminant validity. *PLoS One, 7*(2), e31209. doi:10.1371/journal.pone.0031209

Kaplow, J. B., Layne, C. M., Pynoos, R. S., Cohen, J. A., & Lieberman, A. (2012). DSM-V diagnostic criteria for bereavement-related disorders in children and adolescents: Developmental considerations. *Psychiatry, 75*(3), 243–266. doi:10.1521/psyc.2012.75.3.243

Keesee, N. J., Currier, J. M., & Neimeyer, R. A. (2008). Predictors of grief following the death of one's child: The contribution of finding meaning. *Journal of Clinical Psychology, 64*(10), 1145–1163. doi:10.1002/jclp.20502

Kersting, A., Brahler, E., Glaesmer, H., & Wagner, B. (2011). Prevalence of complicated grief in a representative population-based sample. *Journal of Affective Disorders, 131*(1–3), 339–343. doi:10.1016/j.jad.2010.11.032

Kersting, A., Kroker, K., Horstmann, J., Ohrmann, P., Baune, B. T., Arolt, V., & Suslow, T. (2009). Complicated grief in patients with unipolar depression. *Journal of Affective Disorders, 118*, 201–204. doi:10.1016/j.jad.2009.01.033

Kersting, A., Ohrmann, P., Pedersen, A., Kroker, K., Samberg, D., Bauer, J., . . . Suslow, T. (2009). Neural activation underlying acute grief in women after the loss of an unborn child. *American Journal of Psychiatry, 166*, 1402–1410. doi:10.1176/appi.ajp.2009.08121875

Kristensen, P., Weisaeth, L., & Heir, T. (2012). Bereavement and mental health after sudden and violent losses: a review. *Psychiatry, 75*(1), 76–97. doi:10.1521/psyc.2012.75.1.76

Langner, R., & Maercker, A. (2005). Complicated grief as a stress response disorder: Evaluating diagnostic criteria in a German sample. *Journal of Psychosomatic Research, 58*(3), 235–242. doi:10.1016/j.jpsychores.2004.09.012

Lobb, E. A., Kristjanson, L. J., Aoun, S. M., Monterosso, L., Halkett, G. K., & Davies, A. (2010). Predictors of complicated grief: A systematic review of empirical studies. *Death Studies, 34*(8), 673–698. doi:10.1080/07481187.2010.496686

MacDonald, G., & Leary, M. R. (2005). Why does social exclusion hurt? The relationship between social and physical pain. *Psychological Bulletin, 131*(2), 202–223. doi:10.1037/0033-2909.131.2.202

Marques, L., Bui, E., LeBlanc, N. J., Porter, E., Robinaugh, D. J., Dryman, M. T., . . . Simon, N. (2013). Complicated grief symptoms in anxiety disorders: Prevalence and associated impairment. *Depression and Anxiety, 30*, 1211–1216. doi:10.1002/da.22093

Mauro, C., Shear, M. K., Reynolds, C., Simon, N., Zisook, S., Skritskaya, N., . . . Glickman, K. (2017). Performance characteristics and clinical utility of diagnostic criteria proposals in bereaved treatment-seeking patients. *Psychological Medicine, 47*(4), 608–615. doi: 10.1017/S0033291716002749

Maytal, G., Zalta, A. K., Thompson, E., Chow, C. W., Perlman, C., Ostacher, M. J., . . . Simon, N. M. (2007). Complicated grief and impaired sleep in patients with bipolar disorder. *Bipolar Disorder, 9*(8), 913–917. doi:10.1111/j.1399-5618.2007.00446.x

Meert, K. L., Shear, K., Newth, C. J., Harrison, R., Berger, J., Zimmerman, J., . . . Human Development Collaborative Pediatric Critical Care Research Network. (2011). Follow-up study of complicated grief among parents eighteen months after a child's death in the pediatric intensive care unit.

Journal of Palliative Medicine, *14*(2), 207–214. doi:10.1089/jpm.2010.0291

Meert, K. L., Donaldson, A. E., Newth, C. J. L., Harrison, R., Berger, J., Zimmerman, J., . . . Willson, D. F. (2010). Complicated grief and associated risk factors among parents following a child's death in the pediatric intensive care unit. *Archives of Pediatrics & Adolescent Medicine*, *164*(11), 1045–1051.

Milic, J., Saavedra Perez, H., Zuurbier, L. A., Boelen, P. A., Rietjens, J. A., Hofman, A., & Tiemeier, H. (2017). The longitudinal and cross-sectional associations of grief and complicated grief with sleep quality in older adults. *Behavioral Sleep Medicine*. Advance online publication. doi:10.1080/15402002.2016.1276016

Mitchell, A. M., Kim, Y., Prigerson, H. G., & Mortimer-Stephens, M. (2004). Complicated grief in survivors of suicide. *Crisis*, *25*(1), 12–18. doi:10.1027/0227-5910.25.1.12

Monk, T., Houck, P., & Shear, M. K. (2006). The daily life of complicated grief patients—What gets missed, what gets added? *Death Studies*, *30*, 77–85. doi:10.1080/07481180500348860

Nakajima, S., Ito, M., Shirai, A., & Konishi, T. (2012). Complicated grief in those bereaved by violent death: The effects of post-traumatic stress disorder on complicated grief. *Dialogues in Clinical Neuroscience*, *14*(2), 210–214.

Neimeyer, R. A., Baldwin, S. A., & Gillies, J. (2006). Continuing bonds and reconstructing meaning: Mitigating complications in bereavement. *Death Studies*, *30*(8), 715–738. doi:10.1080/07481180600848322

O'Connor, M. F. (2012). Immunological and neuroimaging biomarkers of complicated grief. *Dialogues in Clinical Neuroscience*, *14*(2), 141–148.

O'Connor, M. F., Wellisch, D. K., Stanton, A. L., Eisenberger, N. I., Irwin, M. R., & Lieberman, M. D. (2008). Craving love? Enduring grief activates brain's reward center. *Neuroimage*, *42*(2), 969–972. doi:10.1016/j.neuroimage.2008.04.256

O'Connor, M., & Sussman, T. J. (2014). Developing the yearning in situations of loss scale: Convergent and discriminant validity for bereavement, romantic break-up, and homesickness. *Death Studies*, *38*(7), 450–458. doi:10.1080/07481187.2013.782928

Prigerson, H. G., Horowitz, M. J., Jacobs, S. C., Parkes, C. M., Aslan, M., Goodkin, K., . . . Maciejewski, P. K. (2009). Prolonged grief disorder: Psychometric validation of criteria proposed for DSM-V and ICD-11. *PLoS Medicine*, *6*(8), e1000121. doi:10.1371/journal.pmed.1000121

Prigerson, H. G., & Jacobs, S. C. (2001). Perspectives on care at the close of life. Caring for bereaved patients: "All the doctors just suddenly go." *JAMA*, *286*(11), 1369–1376.

Prigerson, H. G., Maciejewski, P. K., Reynolds, C., Bierhals, A. J., Newsom, J. T., Fasicza, A., . . . Miller, M. (1995). Inventory of Complicated Grief: A scale to measure maladaptive symptoms of loss. *Psychiatry Research*, *59*, 65–79. doi:10.1016/0165-1781(95)02757-2

Prigerson, H. G., Shear, M. K., Jacobs, S. C., Reynolds, C. F., 3rd, Maciejewski, P. K., Davidson, J. R., . . . Zisook, S. (1999). Consensus criteria for traumatic grief. A preliminary empirical test. *British Journal of Psychiatry*, *174*, 67–73.

Reynolds, C. F. 3rd, Miller, M. D., Pasternak, R. E., Frank, E., Perel, J. M., Cornes, C., . . . Kupfer, D. J. (1999). Treatment of bereavement-related major depressive episodes in later life: A controlled study of acute and continuation treatment with nortriptyline and interpersonal psychotherapy. *American Journal of Psychiatry*, *156*(2), 202–208. doi:10.1176/ajp.156.2.202

Robinaugh, D. J. (2017). *Psychological pain and its relation to complicated grief, depression, and suicidal thoughts and behaviors in bereaved adults.* Paper presented at the Anxiety and Depression Association of American Annual Conference, San Francisco, CA.

Robinaugh, D. J., Mauro, C., Bui, E., Stone, L., Shah, R., Wang, Y., . . . Simon, N. M. (2016). Yearning and its measurement in complicated grief. *Journal of Loss and Trauma*, *21*(5), 410–420. doi:10.1080/15325024.2015.1110447

Robinaugh, D. J., & McNally, R. J. (2013). Remembering the past and envisioning the future in bereaved adults with and without complicated grief. *Clinical Psychological Science*, *1*(3), 290–300. doi:10.1177/2167702613476027

Saavedra Perez, H. C., Direk, N., Milic, J., Ikram, M. A., Hofman, A., & Tiemeier, H. (2017). The impact of complicated grief on diurnal cortisol levels two years after loss: A population-based study. *Psychosomatic Medicine*, *79*(4), 426–433. doi:10.1097/PSY.0000000000000422

Saavedra Perez, H. C., Ikram, M. A., Direk, N., Prigerson, H. G., Freak-Poli, R., Verhaaren, B. F., . . . Tiemeier, H. (2015). Cognition, structural brain changes and complicated grief. A population-based study. *Psychological Medicine*, *45*(7), 1389–1399. doi:10.1017/S0033291714002499

Schulz, R., Boerner, K., Shear, K., Zhang, S., & Gitlin, L. N. (2006). Predictors of complicated grief among dementia caregivers: A prospective study of bereavement. *The American Journal of Geriatric Psychiatry*, *14*(8), 650–658.

Shear, K., Frank, E., Houck, P. R., & Reynolds, C. F. 3rd. (2005). Treatment of complicated grief: A randomized controlled trial. *JAMA*, *293*(21), 2601–2608. doi:10.1001/jama.293.21.2601

Shear, K. M., Jackson, C. T., Essock, S. M., Donahue, S. A., & Felton, C. J. (2006). Screening for complicated grief among Project Liberty service recipients 18 months after September 11, 2001. *Psychiatric Services*, *57*(9), 1291–1297. doi:10.1176/appi.ps.57.9.1291

Shear, K., & Shair, H. (2005). Attachment, loss, and complicated grief. *Developmental Psychobiology*, *47*(3), 253–267. doi:10.1002/dev.20091

Shear, M. K. (2010). Complicated grief treatment: The theory, practice and outcomes. *Bereavement Care*, *29*(3), 10–14. doi:10.1080/02682621.2010.522373

Shear, M. K., Monk, T., Houck, P., Melhem, N., Frank, E., Reynolds, C. F., & Sillowash, R. (2007). An attachment-based model of complicated grief including the role of avoidance. *European Archives of Psychiatry and Clinical Neuroscience*, *257*(8), 453–461. doi:10.1007/s00406-007-0745-z

Shear, M. K., Reynolds, C. F., 3rd, Simon, N. M., Zisook, S., Wang, Y., Mauro, C., . . . Skritskaya, N. (2016). Optimizing treatment of complicated grief: A randomized clinical trial. *JAMA Psychiatry*, *73*(7), 685–694. doi:10.1001/jamapsychiatry.2016.0892

Shear, M. K., Simon, N., Wall, M., Zisook, S., Neimeyer, R., Duan, N., . . . Keshaviah, A. (2011). Complicated grief and related bereavement issues for DSM-5. *Depression and Anxiety*, *28*(2), 103–117. doi:10.1002/da.20780

Shear, M. K., Wang, Y., Skritskaya, N., Duan, N., Mauro, C., & Ghesquiere, A. (2014). Treatment of complicated grief in elderly persons: A randomized clinical trial. *JAMA Psychiatry*, *71*(11), 1287–1295. doi:10.1001/jamapsychiatry.2014.1242

Silverman, G. K., Johnson, J. G., & Prigerson, H. G. (2001). Preliminary explorations of the effects of prior trauma and loss on risk for psychiatric disorders in recently widowed people. *Israel Journal of Psychiatry and Related Sciences*, *38*(3–4), 202–215.

Simon, N. M. (2012). Is complicated grief a post-loss stress disorder? *Depression and Anxiety*, *29*(7), 541–544. doi:10.1002/da.21979

Simon, N. M., Pollack, M. H., Fischmann, D., Perlman, C., Muriel, A. C., Moore, C. W., . . . Shear, M. K. (2005). Complicated grief and its correlates in patients with bipolar disorder. *Journal of Clinical Psychiatry*, *66*(9), 1105–1110. doi:10.4088/JCP.v66n0903

Simon, N. M., Shear, K. M., Thompson, E. H., Zalta, A. K., Perlman, C., Reynolds, C. F., . . . Silowash, R. (2007). The prevalence and correlates of psychiatric comorbidity in individuals with complicated grief. *Comprehensive Psychiatry*, *48*(5), 395–399. doi:10.1016/j.comppsych.2007.05.002

Simon, N. M., Wall, M. M., Keshaviah, A., Dryman, M. T., LeBlanc, N. J., & Shear, M. K. (2011). Informing the symptom profile of complicated grief. *Depression and Anxiety*, *28*(2), 118–126. doi:10.1002/da.20775

Skritskaya, N., Mauro, C., Olonoff, M., Qiu, X., Duncan, S., Wang, Y., . . . Shear, M. K. (2017). Measuring maladaptive cognitions in complicated grief: Introducing the Typical Beliefs Questionnaire. *The American Journal of Geriatric Psychiatry*, *25*(5), 541–550. doi:10.1016/j.jagp.2016.09.003

Stroebe, M., & Schut, H. (1999). The dual process model of coping with bereavement: Rationale and description. *Death Studies*, *23*(3), 197–224. doi:10.1080/074811899201046

Sung, S. C., Dryman, M. T., Marks, E., Shear, M. K., Ghesquiere, A., Fava, M., & Simon, N. M. (2011). Complicated grief among individuals with major depression: Prevalence, comorbidity, and associated features. *Journal of Affective Disorders*, *134*(1–3), 453–458. doi:10.1016/j.jad.2011.05.017

Szanto, K., Shear, M. K., Houck, P., Reynolds, C., Frank, E., Caroff, K., & Silowash, R. (2006). Indirect self-destrutive behavior and overt suicidality in patients with complicated grief. *Journal of Clinical Psychiatry*, *67*(2), 233–239. doi:\10.4088/JCP.v67n0209

Tal, I., Mauro, C., Reynolds, C. F. 3rd, Shear, M. K., Simon, N., Lebowitz, B., . . . Zisook, S. (2017). Complicated grief after suicide bereavement and other causes of death. *Death Studies*, *41*(5), 267–275. doi: 10.1080/07481187.2016.1265028

Van Doorn, C., Kasl, S. V., Beery, L. C., Jacobs, S. C., & Prigerson, H. G. (1998). The influence of marital quality and attachment styles on traumatic grief and depressive symptoms. *The Journal of Nervous and Mental Disease*, *186*(9), 566–573.

Vanderwerker, L. C., Jacobs, S. C., Parkes, C. M., & Prigerson, H. G. (2006). An exploration of associations between separation anxiety in childhood and complicated grief in later life. *Journal of Nervous and Mental Disease*, *194*(2), 121–123. doi:10.1097/01.nmd.0000198146.28182.d5

Vanderwerker, L. C., & Prigerson, H. G. (2004). Social support and technological connectedness as protective factors in bereavement. *Journal of Loss and Trauma*, *9*(1), 45–57.

Wakefield, J. C. (2013). DSM-5 grief scorecard: Assessment and outcomes of proposals to pathologize grief. *World Psychiatry*, *12*(2), 171–173.

Zisook, S., Shuchter, S. R., Pedrelli, P., Sable, J., & Deaciuc, S. C. (2001). Bupropion sustained release for bereavement: Results of an open trial. *Journal of Clinical Psychiatry*, *62*(4), 227–230.

Zygmont, M., Prigerson, H. G., Houck, P. R., Miller, M. D., Shear, M. K., Jacobs, S., & Reynolds, C. F. 3rd. (1998). A post hoc comparison of paroxetine and nortriptyline for symptoms of traumatic grief. *Journal of Clinical Psychiatry*, *59*(5), 241–245.

7

Epidemiology of Trauma- and Stressor-Related Disorders

DAVID M. BENEDEK

INTRODUCTION

Clinical epidemiology describes the distribution of disease—and those factors correlated with the presence of disease—with regard to rates of prevalence, incidence and associated risk, or protective factors.

For trauma and stressor-related disorders (TSRD), risk factors include—by definition—the various traumatic exposures (or stressors) that precipitate illness but also a variety of demographic, socioeconomic, genetic, and environmental factors. Thus epidemiologic study characterizing risk may help identify measures targeted to reducing specific types of risk as well areas of inquiry during history taking or clinical evaluation to aid early detection or to assess ongoing treatment for TSRD.

Epidemiologic study at the turn of this century provided evidence of the prevalence, longitudinal course, and risk factors associated with posttraumatic stress disorder (PTSD) and helped to clarify the connection between exposure to trauma and symptom onset and progression (McFarlane, 2004). Historically, the symptoms of PTSD were attributed to causes ranging from the whims of the gods, innate character deficits, to the blast effects from exploding ordinance. However, support for the existence of PTSD as a constellation of symptoms correlating with traumatic exposures has been consistently derived from large population-based studies that administered mental health diagnostic interviews to a random sample of households in the United States (e.g., Kessler et al., 1995; Kessler et al., 2005) as well as Australia (Creamer et al., 2001) and Europe (Darves-Bornoz et al., 2008) and replicated most recently through a series of studies derived from the World Mental Health (WMH) surveys—in South Africa, Japan, and European nations (Atwoli et al., 2015).

Epidemiologic research has also demonstrated that PTSD is underdiagnosed in medical settings. Magruder and colleagues (2005) reported that less than half of patients with a diagnosis of PTSD established by epidemiologic surveillance had a diagnosis of PTSD in their medical records. This disconnect between having and being diagnosed with illness is important because untreated PTSD is associated with impairments in multiple domains of life, (Davidson et al., 2004), high rates of physical and medical comorbidity (Kessler et al. 1995; Stein et al., 2000; Magruder et al., 2005; Kessler et al., 2005), and increased health service utilization (Schnurr et al., 2000; Stein et al., 2000; Deykin et al., 2001). Since traumatized individuals are more likely to present to primary care than to specialty mental health settings (Kimerling et al., 1994), knowledge of the epidemiology of disease entities help clinicians and policymakers direct attention to all appropriate environments of care.

Complicating any review of the epidemiology of TSRD is the fact that diagnostic criteria defining these disorders have evolved in the past 30 years. Recent changes to definition of "caseness" for PTSD and acute stress disorder (ASD) have altered the extent to which previous studies may be generalized to reflect the current rates. For example, today's definition of PTSD in the fifth edition of the *Diagnostic and Statistical Manual of Mental Disorders* (DSM-5; American Psychiatric Association [APA], 2013) requires presence of symptoms of negative alterations in mood and cognition not necessary in the fourth edition, text revision of the DSM (DSM-IV-TR; APA, 2000). On the other hand, the immediate reaction to traumatic exposure involving fear or horror necessary was to establish the diagnosis of PTSD in the fourth edition of the DSM (DSM-IV; APA, 1994) while this requirement is eliminated in the DSM-5. Even the definition of what constitutes a necessarily traumatic exposure has been broadened to include learning of such experience in others close to the patient or vicarious repeated exposure to the details of another's trauma.

With these limitations in mind, this chapter begins with a review of the epidemiology of traumatic exposure, that is, what is known about the prevalence of traumatic experience in the general population and other more specific subpopulations, and then highlights the epidemiology of the specific DSM-5 TSRD that may be diagnosed in adults: PTSD, ASD, and adjustment disorder. (Note: Chapter 2 of this volume includes a discussion of the epidemiology of reactive attachment disorder and disinhibited social engagement disorder; Chapter 8 highlights the epidemiology of PTSD in children; and Chapter 6 includes a discussion of the epidemiology of persistent complex bereavement disorder which is included in DSM-5 as an area for further study.) Most epidemiologic studies of TSRD have been based on pre-DSM-5 diagnostic definitions. But these studies must inform current clinical practice until new data emerges. In addition, much more attention has been devoted to the epidemiology of PTSD than to ASD—and even less has been devoted to the epidemiology of adjustment disorder, or its specific subtypes. After highlighting the results of epidemiologic studies to date, the chapter concludes with a discussion of areas for further inquiry.

EPIDEMIOLOGY OF PTSD

In the DSM-5, PTSD symptoms are divided into four categories of symptom criteria: intrusion, avoidance, negative alternations in cognitions and mood, and hyperarousal. These symptoms must not be due to the effects of a substance or another medical condition, must be present for at least a month, and must cause clinically significant distress or impairment. Most importantly, the diagnosis may only be made when a patient has experienced "exposure to actual or threatened death, serious injury or sexual violence," via direct personal experience, witnessing the event(s) as it occurred to others, leaning of the violent or accidental death of a close friend or family member, or (as may be the case with first responders collecting human remains or police officers repeatedly exposed to the details of child abuse) experiencing repeated or extreme exposure to details of such events as they occurred in others (APA, 2013). Thus traumatic exposure is listed as "Criterion A" for the diagnosis of PTSD and for ASD and may also be the basis for establishing a diagnosis for adjustment disorder. Hence, any discussion of the epidemiology of TSRD should begin with a description of what is known about such exposures.

EPIDEMIOLOGY OF TRAUMATIC EXPOSURES

The majority of adults are exposed to a traumatic event (or events) in their lifetime, with women generally reporting fewer exposures than men in the United States and internationally. In the United States' general population, rates of exposure to one or more traumas range from 39% (Breslau et al., 1991) to as high as 90% (Breslau et al., 1998). Ten percent of men and 6% of women report being exposed to at least four events (Kessler et al., 1995). In Switzerland, exposure to potentially traumatic events was 28% (Hepp et al., 2006); in Australia, rates of exposure were 49.5% (women) and 64.6% (men; Creamer et al., 2001). The South African Stress and Health Survey reported a lifetime traumatic event prevalence rate of 73.8% (Atwoli et al. 2013), whereas rates in Europe and Japan ranged from 54% to 64% (Darves-Bonoz et al., 2008; Kawakami et al., 2014; de Vries and Olff, 2009). Differences in prevalence reflect historical, cultural, and political factors that vary across regions including varying rates of civil conflict, state-sanctioned political violence or discrimination, exposure to international combat, or natural or technological disasters. For example, physical violence and witnessing trauma occurring to another contributed the largest portion of all lifetime traumatic events in South Africa, whereas accidents and unexpected death of a loved one were the largest contributors in Europe (Atwoli et al., 2015). In the WMH surveys, certain sociodemographic characteristics were associated with *reduced* risk of traumatic event exposure including low education in Spain and Italy and low income in Northern Ireland. Unemployment *increased* risk of exposure in Spain and Northern Ireland (Atwoli et al., 2015).

Across nations other subpopulations such as combat troops are at particularly high risk of exposure. For example, Hoge et al. (2004) reported that 95% of US Army and Marine service members who served in the Iraq war and 84% of Army service members who served in Afghanistan were exposed to combat. Likewise, disaster workers or populations living in regions prone to natural disasters may be repeatedly exposed to traumatic events.

Although a reaction to traumatic exposure involving intense fear, helplessness, or horror

(Criterion A2) was necessary to the DSM-IV diagnosis of PTSD (APA, 2000) this requirement was eliminated in the DSM-5. This change resulted from epidemiologic findings suggesting that the inclusion of A2 only marginally attenuated the prevalence of PTSD, as compared to the absence of including A2 in the diagnosis (Weathers et al., 2007) and that the relationship between traumatic exposure, immediate reaction, and subsequent PTSD was further complicated by degree of preparedness for exposure in emergency and military personnel (Adler et al., 2008). Interview data from 202 military service members with combat-related traumatic experience revealed that 80% of the sample did not endorse A2 as written in DSM-IV-TR. However, members with and without this criterion A2 reaction reported similar rates of re-experiencing symptoms, hyperarousal symptoms, referral for treatment follow-up, and functional impairment. In the United States, epidemiologic surveillance has not occurred since the elimination of this diagnostic requirement from the DSM.

EPIDEMIOLOGY OF PTSD AFTER TRAUMA EXPOSURE

Despite the very high rates of traumatic exposure in the general population, relatively few people develop PTSD as defined by meeting sufficient threshold symptom criteria described by various evolutions of the DSM or the International Classification of Diseases. Using the third edition, revised version of the DSM (DSM-III-R) criteria for PTSD (APA, 1987), Breslau et al. (1991) reported a lifetime prevalence of 11% (31% of respondents exposed to trauma) in women and 6% (14% of trauma exposed) in men. Although men were more likely to experience trauma, Kessler et al. (1995) reported a lifetime prevalence of 7.8%, with women more than twice as likely to meet full diagnostic criteria (10.4%) compared to men (5%). In the United States, Kessler et al.'s (1999) 12-month prevalence was 3.9% and more recently was 3.5% with approximately one-third of the cases being serious, moderate, and mild severity as determined by functional status and self-injury risk factors (Kessler et al., 2005). While large US epidemiologic studies asked participants to identify the worst traumatic event ever experienced and assess for PTSD in relation to that event, the more recent WMH surveys assessed for PTSD in relation to both the worst lifetime traumatic event and a random event selected from a respondent's other life time traumas, and sample weights were then applied to create an accurate distribution of traumatic events in the sample population (Atwoli et al., 2013). Lifetime prevalence using this methodology ranged from 1.3% in Japan to 8.8% in Northern Ireland with other European nations and South Africa reporting a prevalence of approximately 2.3% (Atwoli et al., 2015).

Various studies have identified relationships between characteristics of the traumatic event (e.g., type, severity, frequency) and the development of PTSD. Kessler et al. (1995) reported the conditional risk of PTSD by trauma type in a US sample (see Table 7.1). In men, rape and combat exposure in a war was associated with the highest risk of developing PTSD, 65% and 39%, respectively. Being threatened with a weapon or being physically attacked was associated with the lowest risk (1% and 2%, respectively). In women, rape (46%) and being threatened with a weapon (33%)

TABLE 7.1. RELATION OF TRAUMATIC EXPOSURE TO PTSD IN THE NATIONAL COMORBIDITY SURVEY

Traumatic Event Type	Rate			
	Men		Women	
	Exposure	PTSD	Exposure	PTSD
Any trauma	61%	8%	51%	20%
Multiple traumas	35%	—	25%	—
Accidents	25%	6%	14%	9%
Threatened with weapon	19%	2%	7%	33%
Natural disaster with fire	19%	4%	15%	6%
Trauma experienced by close friend/relative	11%	4%	12%	10%
Physical attack	11%	2%	7%	21%
Combat	6%	39%	—	—
Physical abuse	3%	22%	5%	49%
Molestation/sexual abuse	3%	12%	12%	27%
Neglect	2%	24%	3%	20%
Rape	1%	65%	9%	46%
Other	2%	13%	>1%	33%

Note: PTSD = posttraumatic stress disorder.
Adapted from Kessler RC, et al.: Posttraumatic stress disorder in the National Comorbidity Survey. *Arch Gen Psychiatry* 52:1048–1060, 1995.

was associated with the highest risk, while exposure to a natural disaster (5%) was the lowest. Kessler et al. argued that, in general, interpersonal violence, more so than other traumas, is associated with the highest risk of PTSD development. In 2004, Hoge and colleagues reported rates of PTSD (determined by a self-report screening checklist) in combat-exposed troops ranged from 4% to 20%.

Kessler (2000) and McNally (2003) summarized findings from several other international studies (including refugees and children exposed to war trauma) and concluded that the conditional risk of PTSD is substantially higher among people exposed to horrific ongoing traumas in developing countries. In the WMH studies, conditional risk for developing PTSD was highest for witnessing traumatic events in South Africa (attributed to high rates of political or criminal violence occurring in public places) while exposure to sexual and physical violence was associated with the highest conditional risk in Europe and Japan (Atwoli et al., 2015). While unexpected death of a loved one was also associated with a high conditional risk in some European nations, the WMH surveys did not ascertain whether such deaths were either "violent or accidental" as required in the DSM-5 definition of PTSD.

Consistent with scope and intentionality of the trauma, rates of PTSD following natural disasters are lower than from technological (e.g., mining accident) or manmade disaster (e.g. religious uprising; Neria et al., 2008). There is a relationship between proximity to disaster site and rates of PTSD, such that victims of a natural disaster with direct exposure have the highest rates, followed by rescue workers, with the general population having the lowest rates (see Table 7.2). Similarly, factors like degree of physical injury, risk to life, fatalities, and severity of property destruction are important to consider and are predictive of high rates of PTSD (Neria et al., 2008).

SYMPTOM ONSET AND SUBTYPES

While PTSD may be diagnosed 30 days after traumatic exposure, a subpopulation of patients experience delayed onset of symptoms (i.e., onset occurring six months or later following exposure to traumatic event; APA, 2000). In DSM-5, "delayed onset" is replaced by the term "with delayed expression" as a specifier if the full criteria are not met until six months after the event, the same duration as in DSM-IV. In a sample of Vietnam veterans (Schnurr et al., 2003), symptom onset occurred 1.34 years after entry into Vietnam, with 40% of their sample reporting that symptoms first occurred 2 or more years after entering Vietnam. McFarlane (2004) discussed delayed onset PTSD and presented findings from several studies using civilian and veteran populations. Interestingly, some people experienced latency periods of decades. Grieger et al. (2006) reported that the majority (78.8%) of soldiers hospitalized as a result of injuries on the battlefield who reported PTSD and depression symptoms at 7 months reported no symptoms at 1-month following hospitalization. Other researchers reported an increase in prevalence from 7.6% at 3 months to 10% at 12 months post-injury, with nearly half of all 12-month cases being delayed onset (Carty et al., 2006).

The DSM-5 also allows for the specification of a dissociative subtype of PTSD, for patients who meet full criteria for PTSD and also exhibit marked symptoms of derealization and/or depersonalization (DSM-5). In 2005, Waelde and colleagues examined the structure of dissociation (as defined by amnesia, depersonalization, and absorption) in Vietnam veterans and found that 32% of those with PTSD could be classified as belonging to a dissociative group. Wolf, Miller, et al. (2012) subsequently used latent profile analysis of items indexing PTSD and dissociative symptom severity (as defined by depersonalization, derealization, and reduction in awareness) and demonstrated that about 12% of Vietnam veterans with PTSD scored uniquely high on symptoms of derealization and depersonalization and that this group was also associated with higher severity of flashbacks and a higher level of exposure to childhood and adult sexual assault. This pattern was replicated in additional male and female veteran and military PTSD samples with approximately 15% of the male sample and 30% of the female sample were assigned to the dissociative class (Wolf, Lunney, et al., 2012). In the same year, latent profile analysis of a civilian sample revealed that approximately 25% of the sample could be classified as belonging to a dissociative subgroup (Steuwe et al., 2012). Finally, Stein and colleagues (2013) demonstrated the dissociative subtype in a sample of over 25,000 individuals from 16 different countries and found that approximately 14% of the sample could be assigned to a dissociative group, demonstrating cross-cultural and cross-national generalizability of the dissociative subtype.

TABLE 7.2. PREVALENCE OF PTSD IN DISASTER VICTIMS AND RESPONDERS

Cohort and Event	Prevalence
Volunteers & Mental Health Workers* after Buffalo Creek Dam collapse	44% and 38%*
Firefighter responses to Australian bushfires	32%, 27%, 30%
Police responders to Hurricane Katrina	19%
Refugees who resettled in Western countries	3%-50%
Terrorist attacks (general review including responders and victims)	28%
New York City residents after 9/11 attacks	8%-20%
9/11 disaster workers and volunteers in New York City	8%-22.5% (9 studies)

Note: PTSD = posttraumatic stress disorder.
Adapted from Freed MC, et al.: Epidemiology. In: *Clinical Manual for the Management of PTSD*. Edited by DM Benedek and GH Wynn. Arlington, VA: American Psychiatric Publishing, 2009.

SYMPTOM TRAJECTORY

PTSD may resolve spontaneously or with treatment but is a chronic condition for many patients (Magruder et al., 2005). In Vietnam veterans, average symptom duration was 18.5 years, with 92.5% of veterans experiencing symptoms for more than 5 years, and 40.2% of veterans reporting a duration of 20 or more years (Schnurr et al., 2003). Kessler et al. (1995) found that 60% of patients with PTSD reached spontaneous remission in 72 months, but type of trauma affected time to remission (see chapter 18 of this volume for a more detailed discussion of factors influencing duration and severity of symptoms). Even with treatment, approximately one-third of respondents did not remit at 120 months (Kessler et al., 1995), suggesting that these treatment-refractory persons may experience lifelong symptoms. In the US Burden of Disease Study, Michaud et al., (2006) estimated PTSD to last on, average, four years for males and five years for females. In the WMH studies, exposure to sexual and physical violence were associated with the longest duration of symptoms in Europe, whereas the witnessing of violence was associated with the longest duration of symptoms in South Africa (Atwoli et al., 2015). Research also suggests that risk and resilience factors present pre-exposure, during the trauma, or after traumatic events can impact the severity and trajectory of PTSD (see Table 7.3). These factors include historical and family characteristics of the exposed individual (ethnicity, gender), characteristics of the event (e.g., frequency and duration and intensity of exposure), and environmental factors including social support, family history of mental illness, degree of injury, and subsequent financial or life stress. (Friedman, 2006; Hoge et al., 2004; Institute of Medicine, 2006; Kessler, 2000).

CORRELATES OF PTSD

In 2006 Keane et al. (2006) described three categories of PTSD correlates: (a) individual-specific pre-existing correlates include sex, age, race, mental health history, marital status, and prior traumas; (b) event-specific correlates, or aspects such as trauma severity, frequency, duration, intentionality, perceived threat, and the individual's emotional response; and (c) posttrauma factors such as social support. Other posttrauma factors in the literature include financial difficulties, social stressors (Galea et al., 2008), negative appraisals of the trauma and actions of others, avoidance coping, and hypervigilant safety behaviors (Brewin, 2008). These correlates have demonstrated varying degrees of predictive value in the development and maintenance of PTSD (Keane et al. 2006). Studies have identified different correlates and risk factors in different populations. While cross-cultural variation in the measurement or reporting of such factors may explain some discrepant findings amongst studies of different cohorts, disagreement exists about the relevance of many of these variables.

The idea that peritraumatic dissociation at the time of exposure is a risk factor for PTSD was important in the initial diagnostic conceptualization of ASD (see later discussion). However, more recent findings (van der Velden et al., 2008) suggest there is limited utility for peritraumatic dissociation as a predictor of PTSD symptom development. Other correlates following major physical trauma include chronic illness, blaming others, an unsettled compensation claim, unemployment, and use of a lawyer (Harris et al., 2008). In intensive care unit survivors (Davydow et al., 2008) prior psychopathology, greater benzodiazepine administration, and distressing memories about the intensive care unit were associated with a postinjury PTSD diagnosis.

Research clearly shows that PTSD frequently co-occurs with other mental disorders (Kessler et al., 1995; Magruder et al., 2005). However, those other mental disorders may be a

TABLE 7.3. FACTORS THAT MODIFY RISK AND TRAJECTORY OF PTSD

Pre-existing/Individual Factors	Event/Immediate Response Factors	Posttrauma Factors
Mental health history	Trauma type, severity, and proximity to event (more severe, manmade, and violent with the highest risk)	Perceived lack of social support
Gender (female)		Subsequent life stress (e.g., financial loss or injury or death of loved one)
Personality (external locus of control)	Perceived life threat	Stigma or other barriers to care
Socioeconomic status (lower, in most studies)	Peritraumatic dissociation	Community-level supports
Education level (lower)	Negative cognitions about self and world	Chronic pain/injury
Race (minority status)	Previous physical injury	
Previous traumatic exposure (cumulatively increases risk)		
Family psychiatric history		
Age (children and elderly at higher risk)		
Underlying medical conditions		
Poor social support		

Note: PTSD = posttraumatic stress disorder.

determinant, a consequence, or both. Research has demonstrated that pre-existing mental health conditions such as depression, anxiety disorders, substance use disorders, and conduct disorders (Breslau, 2002) increase the likelihood of PTSD development. For example, Koenen et al. (2008) reported in a longitudinal sample that 100% of those diagnosed with PTSD in the past year, and 94% of those with lifetime PTSD, met criteria for another mental disorder between the ages of 11 and 21 years old. The authors reported the odds (adjusted odds ratio) of having had a mental disorder by age 15 were 5.5 times greater for participants who developed PTSD when compared to those who experienced a trauma but did not develop PTSD. These findings suggest that a prior mental health history is a likely determinant of PTSD.

Studies also suggest that mental disorders (i.e., beyond those defined as TSRD) may also be a *consequence* of traumatic exposure. Copeland et al. (2007) followed cohorts of children for four to seven years to assess traumatic exposure and pre- and posttrauma mental health functioning. They demonstrated that children exposed to trauma had nearly two times the rates of mental health disorders than those not exposed. They also found that higher rates of posttraumatic stress. Although most of their sample did not meet full criteria for PTSD, subthreshold symptoms were also associated with higher rates of mental health diagnoses. These results were mediated by the number of trauma exposures, as number of exposures greater than one were associated with poorer functioning. Further statistical modeling demonstrated that age, prior anxiety, and previous trauma exposure were important determinants of trauma response in the next year. Other studies have also demonstrated that both combat veterans and civilian patients with traumatic exposures and PTSD are at increased risk for substance use disorders and in particular opioid dependence (Fareed et al., 2013).

The relationship between PTSD and suicide risk is complex. Some studies have shown that suicide risk is higher among those who experienced trauma due to the symptoms of PTSD (Ferrada-Noli et al., 1998; Amir et al., 1999; Fontana & Rosenheck, 1999; Thompson et al., 1999). Others suggest that higher risk for suicidal ideation and attempts in trauma-exposed populations may stem from comorbid psychiatric conditions (Fontana & Rosenheck, 1995). Still others suggest this risk remains elevated after controlling for other mental disorders and physical conditions (Sareen et al., 2005; Sareen et al., 2007). Research in Vietnam combat veterans with PTSD has suggested that combat-related guilt elevates the risk of suicidal ideation and suicide attempts (Hendin & Haas, 1991). Recent studies in veterans of operations in Iraq and Afghanistan suggest increased risk for suicidal ideation in veterans with PTSD (Jakupcak et al., 2009). While the dramatic increase in suicide rate in veterans of these conflicts has been the subject of considerable investigation, studies suggest multiple risk factors beyond trauma exposure or combat-related PTSD contribute to this increase (Rozanov & Carli, 2012).

The effects of trauma exposure appear to be cumulative, especially in women, such that exposures sensitize individuals to the effects of subsequent traumas, even if those subsequent events are of lesser magnitude (Breslau et al., 2007). As briefly reviewed by Keane et al. (2006), one explanation of the sensitization hypothesis is based in biology. That is, if normal stress hormones are activated over long periods (like during repeated exposures) brain physiology may be altered.

EPIDEMIOLOGY OF ACUTE STRESS DISORDER

Prior to the publication of the DSM-IV, diagnosis of severe posttraumatic mental illness was reserved for syndromes persisting for a minimum of one month. The diagnosis of ASD (for which symptoms are present from 2 to 30 days after traumatic exposure) was proposed in recognition of the ideas that relatively transient symptoms may still result in significant impairment, and that formal diagnostic "label" might also facilitate access to treatment for persons exhibiting clinically significant distress or impairment during this early post-exposure window. In DSM-IV, the diagnosis of ASD required the presence of at least three dissociative symptoms during the trauma or its aftermath (APA, 1994). Earlier studies suggested that proposed criteria (in particular, peritraumatic dissociation) would facilitate treatment by identifying persons at highest risk for the development of the more protracted symptoms of PTSD (Koopman et al., 1995). Longitudinal studies subsequently demonstrated that most persons meeting diagnostic criteria for ASD did indeed subsequently develop PTSD but also demonstrated that most persons with PTSD did *not* initially meet criteria for ASD (Bryant, 2011). Even after eliminating the requirement for dissociative symptoms, longitudinal studies demonstrated that most persons with PTSD did not first meet criteria for even this "subsyndromal" form of ASD. As a result, the predictive utility of the ASD diagnosis as initially proposed was called into question (van der Velden et al., 2008; Bryant et al., 2008, Harvey & Bryant 1998a, 1998b; Bryant, 2011). As it became evident that severe early symptoms did not adequately predict subsequent PTSD, other studies demonstrated that the course of PTSD itself was not linear. In a longitudinal study of physically injured patients requiring hospitalization, assessed at point of injury (hospitalization), 3, 12, and 24 months, incidence of PTSD remained relatively constant, but approximately half the persons meeting criteria for PTSD at one time point had a different status at the next (Bryant et al., 2013). This dynamic trajectory of PTSD symptoms across time was previously demonstrated in a cohort of battle injured service members at one hospitalization, 3, 6, and 12 months following injury (Grieger et al., 2006), casting further doubt on the notion that any observed initial response could predict symptom development. Therefore, a refocus in DSM-5 on best identifying those in acute distress rather than predicting PTSD led to a definition no longer requiring the presence of dissociative symptoms or symptoms from each PTSD specific cluster (i.e., paralleling PTSD) but instead requiring the presence of at least 9 of 14 symptoms (Bryant, 2013).

Prevalence of ASD

The fact that ASD is a transient disorder means its incidence is not assessed for in large-scale population studies such as the epidemiologic catchment area study of 1995, its replications, or in international surveys such as the WMH surveys. Estimates of the prevalence of ASD are limited to studies of trauma-exposed populations within one month of traumatic exposure. Given that ASD was introduced in DSM-IV in 1994 (American Psychiatric Association, 1994) and redefined in 2013, the majority of studies utilized DSM-IV criteria have used the earlier criteria. For example, using DSM-IV criteria rates of ASD following various types of trauma have been reported following motor vehicle accidents (13%–21%; Harvey & Bryant, 1998a, 1998b), after mild traumatic brain injury (14%; Harvey & Bryant, 1998b), after assault (16%–19%; Harvey & Bryant, 1999; Brewin et al., 1999), after burns (10%; Harvey & Bryant, 1998b), after witnessing a mass shooting (33%; Classen et al., 1998), and after industrial accidents (6%; Creamer & Manning, 1998; Harvey & Bryant, 1999). Using DSM-5 criteria, incidence of ASD has been reported in 10% of bank robbery victims (Armour & Hansen, 2015) and 14% of traumatic injury patients (Bryant et al., 2015). Clearly further studies are necessary to establish the incidence of ASD across traumatic other traumatic exposures and amongst specific subpopulations. Cross-national study has demonstrated that trauma exposure itself has significant downstream effects on physical health independent of PTSD (Scott et al., 2013). However, the extent to which presence of ASD (or any of its specific symptoms or symptom combinations) predicts this burden has not yet been explored.

EPIDEMIOLOGY OF ADJUSTMENT DISORDER

As with ASD, the larger epidemiologic surveillance efforts such as the Epidemiologic Catchment Area study (Bourdon et al., 1992), the National Comorbidity Study (Kessler et al., 1995), and its replication (Kessler et al., 2005) did not assess for or report the incidence or prevalence of adjustment disorders, nor have most recently conducted international surveys of mental health. One notable exception is the European Outcomes of Depression International Network study, which reported a prevalence rate of 0.5% using DSM-IV criteria (Ayuso-Mateos et al., 2001). However, this effort restricted adjustment disorder to the depressed mood subtype only (Ayuso-Mateos, et al., 2001; Casey et al., 2006). While efforts have been made to characterize the prevalence in specific subpopulations, these have been generally restricted to mental health care-seeking populations or those receiving medical care for non-psychiatric reasons. Studies have also been limited by either methodological approach such as chart review (Fabrega et al., 1987) or verbal autopsy review (Manoranjitham et al., 2010).

Within the United States it has been estimated that between 9% and 36% of patients seeking care in public-sector psychiatry receive a diagnosis of adjustment disorder (Koran et al., 2003). Roughly one-third of patients emergently evaluated for threats of self-harm receive an adjustment disorder diagnosis (Shear et al., 2000).

Studies of the prevalence of adjustment disorder in hospitalized patients referred to consult-liaison services has ranged from 11.5% to 21.5% (Snyder & Strain, 1989; Popkin et al., 1990). In an analysis of 1,039 consecutive referrals with seven teaching hospitals in the United States, Canada, and Australia, adjustment disorder was diagnosed in 12% of the patients, was the sole psychiatric diagnosis in 7.8%, and had been considered as a "rule out" diagnosis in an additional 10.6% (Strain et al., 1998). More recently, a meta-analysis of cancer patients based on 27 articles reported a pooled adjustment disorder prevalence rate of 19% (Mitchell et al., 2011).

To date there has been only one study of the prevalence of adjustment disorder in the aftermath of serious injury in adults (e.g., traumatic event meeting DSM-5 diagnostic criterion A for ASD or PTSD). In this multisite study, 826 injury patients were assessed during hospitalization and at 3 and 12 months for the presence of mood disorders, anxiety, and substance use disorders. Structured clinical interviews were used to assess diagnosis, severity or symptoms, and quality of life. The prevalence of adjustment disorder was 19% at 3 months and 16% at 12 months.

In subsequent analyses, participants with adjustment disorder reported worse outcomes relative to those with no psychiatric diagnosis but better outcomes compared with those diagnosed with other psychiatric disorders including depression and PTSD or depression (O'Donnell et al., 2016). While this study supported the inclusion of adjustment disorder as a response to criterion A trauma distinct from ASD or PTSD, persons meeting the diagnosis here did not clearly segregate into the mood, anxiety, conduct, or mixed subtypes specified in the DSM-5. Epidemiologic studies exploring the prevalence of subtypes described in DSM-5 in response to criterion A traumas other than physical injury requiring hospitalization or to less severe stressors as permitted by the diagnostic definition have not been conducted.

CONCLUSION

Persons with TSRD present for care in all health care arenas. Social and occupational burden seems to declare itself in areas not obviously linked to the specific symptoms defining these disorders. For a variety of reasons many sufferers do not seek care and go undiagnosed (Milliken et al., 2007). In a review, Seedat et al. (2006) reported that patients with PTSD have more impairments in quality of life than general public patients with other chronic physical conditions (e.g., diabetes, multiple sclerosis) or patients with anxiety disorders. PTSD ranks second only to depression in terms of the quality of life decrements associated with mental disorders. Regardless of the diagnostic definition or label applied, the burden of traumatic exposure has been quantified in social and occupational dysfunction beyond that represented by symptom expression (Schnurr et al., 2006; Magruder et al., 2005). In returning service members who fought in Iraq and Afghanistan, returnees reported a four-fold increase in concerns about interpersonal conflict (Milliken et al., 2007), had higher rates of attrition from the military (Hoge et al.,

2006), and reported a higher number of sick call visits, greater somatic complaints, lower ratings of general health, more physical symptoms, and more missed workdays (Hoge et al., 2007) than those without PTSD. In community (Zvolensky et al., 2008) and military/veteran samples (Smith et al., 2008), PTSD was associated with increased risks of smoking, even during a self-guided quit attempt (Zvolensky et al., 2008). PTSD is also associated with educational failure, work impairment (an estimated $3 billion loss in productivity in the United States), unemployment, and marital instability (Kessler, 2000). It is associated with increased mortality (Boscarino, 2008). Freed et al. (2009) summarized the preference-based metrics (a special class of health-related quality of life measures used in cost-effectiveness and disease burden analyses) for PTSD, and found the decrements associated with PTSD are comparable to those of major depression. When combined with measures of disease pervasiveness (e.g., incidence) and persistence (e.g., course of illness) PTSD ranks within the top 20 most burdensome diseases in the United States (Michaud et al., 2006).

Among the TSRD, the distribution of PTSD and its determinants have been by the far the most thoroughly characterized. Epidemiologic studies have shed light on the correlates and consequences of PTSD. It is clear that the effects ascribed to PTSD are observable across international, educational, and socioeconomic boundaries, and the burden of this illness extends far beyond distress that might be anticipated by the symptoms that define it. The transient nature of ASD and adjustment disorders suggests that the burden placed on sufferers, their families, and their communities must be less than that of PTSD. However, recent study has suggested that trauma exposure has effects on long-term health independent of PTSD effects (Scott et al., 2013). While the effects of stress on general health have also been described, a diverse range of stressors qualifying as those that might precipitate an adjustment disorder and the presumption that more transient TSRDs result in comparatively little morbidity or disease burden have contributed to a lack of attention to their epidemiology. Studies clarifying disease trajectory, correlates, and consequences have generally not been conducted for ASD or adjustment disorder. Hence the true burden of these conditions in terms of their associated comorbidity, impact on course of other chronic medical conditions, and quality of life of those whom they afflict has yet to be determined.

REFERENCES

Adler AB, Wright KM, Bliese PD, et al.: A2 diagnostic criterion for combat-related posttraumatic stress disorder. *J Trauma Stress* 21:301–308, 2008.

American Psychiatric Association: Diagnostic and Statistical Manual of Mental Disorders (3rd ed., text revision). Washington, DC: American Psychiatric Association, 1987.

American Psychiatric Association: *Diagnostic and statistical manual of mental disorders* (4th ed.). Washington, DC: American Psychiatric Association, 1994.

American Psychiatric Association. (2013). *Diagnostic and statistical manual of mental disorders* (5th ed.). Arlington, VA: American Psychiatric Publishing.

American Psychiatric Association: *Diagnostic and statistical manual of mental disorders* (4th ed., text revision). Washington, DC: American Psychiatric Association, 2000.

American Psychiatric Association: *Diagnostic and statistical manual of mental disorders* (5th ed.). Washington, DC: American Psychiatric Association, 2013.

Amir M, Kaplan Z, Efroni R, Kotler M: Suicide risk and coping styles in posttraumatic stress disorder patients. *Psychotherapy Psychosomatics* 68: 76–81, 1999. doi:10.1159/000012316

Armour C, Hansen M: Assessing DSM-5 latent subtypes of acute stress disorder dissociative or intrusive? *Psychiatry Research* 225:476–483, 2015.

Atwoli L, Stein DJ, Koenen KC, et al.: Epidemiology of posttraumatic stress disorder: prevalence, correlates and consequences. *Current Opin Psychiatry* 28(4):307–311, 2015.

Atwoli L, Stein DJ, Williams DR, et al.: Trauma and posttraumatic stress disorder in South Africa: Analysis from the South African Stress and Health Study. *BMC Psychiatry* 13:182, 2013.

Ayuso-Mateos J, Vazquez-Barquero J, Dowrick C, et al.: Depressive disorders in Europe: Prevalence figures from the ODIN study 2001. *Br J Psychiatry*179:308–316, 2001.

Boscarino JA: Psychobiologic predictors of disease mortality after psychological trauma: Implications for research and clinical surveillance. *J Nerv Ment Dis* 196:100–107, 2008.

Bourdon KH, Rae Locke BZ: Estimating the prevalence of mental disorders in U.S. adults from the Epidemiologic Catchment Area Survey. *Public Health* 107(6):663–668, 1992.

Breslau N, Davis GC, Andreski P, et al.: Traumatic events and posttraumatic stress disorder in an urban population of young adults. *Arch Gen Psychiatry* 48:216–222, 1991.

Breslau N: Epidemiologic studies of trauma, posttraumatic stress disorder, and other psychiatric disorders. *Can J Psychiatry* 47:923–929, 2002.

Breslau N, Anthony JC: Gender differences in the sensitivity to posttraumatic stress disorder: An epidemiological study of urban young adults. *J Abnorm Psychol* 116:607–611, 2007.

Breslau N, Kessler RC: The stressor criterion in DSM-IV posttraumatic stress disorder: An empirical investigation. *Biol Psychiatry* 50:699–704, 2001.

Breslau N, Kessler RC, Chilcoat HD, et al.: Trauma and posttraumatic stress disorder in the community: The 1996 Detroit Area Survey of Trauma. *Arch Gen Psychiatry* 55:626–632, 1998.

Brewin CR: What is it that a neurobiological model of PTSD must explain? *Prog Brain Res* 167:217–228, 2008.

Brewin CR, Andrews B, Rose S, Kirk M: Acute stress disorder and posttraumatic stress disorder in victims of violent crime. *Am J Psychiatry* 156:360, 1999.

Bryant RA, Creamer M, O'Donnell ML, Silove D, McFarlane AC: A multisite study of the capacity of acute stress disorder diagnosis to predict posttraumatic stress disorder. *J Clin Psychiatry* 69(6):923–929, 2008a.

Bryant RA, Friedman MJ, Spiegel D, et al.: A review of acute stress disorder in DSM-5. *Depress Anxiety* 28:802–817, 2011.

Bryant RA, O'Donnell M, Creamer M, McFarlane AC, Silove D: A multi-site analysis of the fluctuating course of posttraumatic stress disorder. *JAMA Psychiatry* 70:839–846, 2013.

Bryant RA, Creamer M, O'Donnell M, Silove D, McFarlane AC, Forbes D: A comparison of the capacity of DSM-IV and DSM-5 acute stress disorder definitions to predict posttraumatic stress disorder and related disorders. *J Clin Psychiatry* 76:391–397, 2015.

Carty J, O'Donnell ML, Creamer M: Delayed-onset PTSD: A prospective study of injury survivors. *J Affect Disord* 90:257–261, 2006.

Casey P, Maracy M, Kelly BD, et al.: Can adjustment disorder and depressive episode be distinguished? Results from ODIN. *J Affect Disord* 92:291–297, 2006.

Classen C, Koopman C, Hales R, Spiegel D: Acute stress disorder as a predictor of posttraumatic stress symptoms. *Am J Psychiatry* 155(5):620–624, 1998.

Copeland WE, Keeler G, Angold A, et al.: Traumatic events and posttraumatic stress in childhood. *Arch Gen Psychiatry* 64:577–584, 2007.

Creamer M, Burgess P, McFarlane AC: Post-traumatic stress disorder: Findings from the Australian National Survey of Mental Health and Well-being. *Psychol Med* 31:1237–1247, 2001.

Creamer M, Manning C: Acute Stress Disorder Following an Industrial Accident. *Australian Psychologist* 33:125–29, 1998.

Darves-Bornoz JM, Alonso J, de Girolamo G, de Graaf R, Haro JM, Kovess-Masfety V, Lepine JP, Nachbaur G, Negre-Pages L, Vilagut G. Main traumatic events in Europe: PTSD in the European study of the epidemiology of mental disorders survey. *J Trauma Stress* 21(5):455–62, 2008.

Davidson JR, Stein DJ, Shalev AY, et al.: Posttraumatic stress disorder: Acquisition, recognition, course, and treatment. *J Neuropsychiatry Clin Neurosci* 16:135–147, 2004.

Davydow DS, Gifford JM, Desai SV, et al.: Posttraumatic stress disorder in general intensive care unit survivors: A systematic review. *Gen Hosp Psychiatry* 30:421–434, 2008.

de Vries GJ, Olff M: The lifetime prevalence of traumatic events and posttraumatic stress disorder in the Netherlands. *J Trauma Stress* 22:259–267, 2009.

Deykin EY, Keane TM, Kaloupek D, et al.: Posttraumatic stress disorder and the use of health services. *Psychosom Med* 63:835–841, 2001.

Fabrega H Jr, Mezzich JE, Mezzich AC: Adjustment disorder as a marginal or transitional illness category in DSM-III. *Arch Gen Psychiatry* 44:567–572, 1987.

Fareed A, Eilender P, Habner M, et al.: Comorbid posttraumatic stress disorder and opiate addiction: A literature review. *J Addict Dis* 32(2):169–179, 2013.

Ferrada-Noli M, Asberg M, Ormstad K, Lundin T, Sundbom E: Suicidal behavior after severe trauma. Part 1: PTSD diagnoses, psychiatric comorbidity and assessment of suicidal behavior. *J Trauma Stress* 11:103–112, 1998.

Fontana A, Rosenheck R: Attempted suicide among Vietnam veterans: A model of etiology in a community sample. *Am J Psychiatry* 152:102–109, 1995.

Freed MC, Goldberg RK, Gore KL, et al.: Estimating the disease burden of combat-related posttraumatic stress disorder in United States veterans and military servicemembers. In *Handbook of Disease Burdens and Quality of Life Measures*. Edited by VR Preedy, RR Watson. New York: Springer-Verlag, 2009.

Friedman MJ: Posttraumatic stress disorder among military returnees from Afghanistan and Iraq. *Am J Psychiatry* 163:586–593, 2006.

Galea S, Tracy M, Norris F, et al.: Financial and social circumstances and the incidence and course of PTSD in Mississippi during the first two years after Hurricane Katrina. *J Trauma Stress* 21:357–368, 2008.

Grieger TA, Cozza SJ, Ursano RJ, et al.: Posttraumatic stress disorder and depression in battle-injured soldiers. *Am J Psychiatry* 163:1777–1783, 2006.

Harris IA, Young JM, Rae H, et al.: Predictors of posttraumatic stress disorder following major trauma. *ANZ J Surg* 78:583–587, 2008.

Havey AG, Bryant RA. The relationship between acute stress disorder and posttraumatic stress disorder: A prospective evaluation of motor vehicle accident survivors. *J Consult Clin Psychol* 66:507, 1998a.

Harvey AG, Bryant RA. Acute stress disorder after mild traumatic brain injury. *J Nerv Ment Dis* 186:333, 1998b.

Harvey AG, Bryant RA. Acute disorder across trauma populations. *J Nerv Ment Dis* 187:443, 1999.

Hendin H, Haas AP: Suicide and guilt as manifestations of PTSD in Vietnam combat veterans. *Am J Psychiatry* 148:586–591, 1991.

Hepp U, Gamma A, Milos G, et al.: Prevalence of exposure to potentially traumatic events and PTSD. The Zurich Cohort Study. *Eur Arch Psychiatry Clin Neurosci* 256:151–158, 2006.

Hoge CW, Auchterlonie JL, Milliken CS: Mental health problems, use of mental health services, and attrition from military service after returning from deployment to Iraq or Afghanistan. *JAMA* 295:1023–1032, 2006.

Hoge CW, Castro CA, Messer SC, et al.: Combat duty in Iraq and Afghanistan, mental health problems, and barriers to care. *N Engl J Med* 351:13–22, 2004.

Hoge CW, Terhakopian A, Castro CA, et al.: Association of posttraumatic stress disorder with somatic symptoms, health care visits, and absenteeism among Iraq war veterans. *Am J Psychiatry* 164:150–153, 2007.

Institute of Medicine, Subcommittee on Posttraumatic Stress Disorder of the Committee of Gulf War and Health: *Posttraumatic stress disorder: Diagnosis and assessment.* Washington, DC: National Academies Press, 2006.

Jakupcak M, Cook J, Imel Z, Rosenheck R, McFall M. PTSD as a risk factor for suicidal ideation in Iraq and Afghanistan war veterans. *J Trauma Stress* 22:303–306, 2009. doi:10.1002/jts.20423

Kawakami N, Tsuchiya M, Umeda M, Koenen KC, Kessler RC: Trauma and posttraumatic stress disorder in Japan: results from the World Mental Health Japan Survey. *J Psychiatr Res* 53:157–65, 2014.

Keane TM, Marshall AD, Taft CT: Posttraumatic stress disorder: Etiology, epidemiology, and treatment outcome. *Ann Rev Clin Psychol* 2:161–97, 2006.

Kessler RC: Posttraumatic stress disorder: The burden to the individual and to society. *J Clin Psychiatry* 61(Suppl. 5):4–12; discussion 13–14, 2000.

Kessler RC, Chiu WT, Demler O, et al.: Prevalence, severity, and comorbidity of 12-month DSM-IV disorders in the National Comorbidity Survey Replication. *Arch Gen Psychiatry* 62:617–627, 2005.

Kessler RC, Sonnega A, Bromet E, et al.: Posttraumatic stress disorder in the National Comorbidity Survey. *Arch Gen Psychiatry* 52:1048–1060, 1995.

Kessler RC, Sonnega A, Bromet E, et al.: Epidemiological risk factors for trauma and PTSD. In: *Risk factors for posttraumatic stress disorder.* Edited by R Yehuda. Washington, DC: American Psychiatric Press, 1999, pp. 23–60.

Kimerling R, Calhoun KS: Somatic symptoms, social support, and treatment seeking among. sexual assault victims. *J Consult Clin Psychol* 62:333–340, 1994.

Koenen KC, Moffitt TE, Caspi A, et al.: The developmental mental-disorder histories of adults with posttraumatic stress disorder: A prospective longitudinal birth cohort study. *J Abnorm Psychol* 117:460–466, 2008.

Koopman C, Classen C, Cardeña E, Spiegel D. When disaster strikes, acute stress disorder may follow. *J Trauma Stress* 8(1):29–46, 1995.

Koran LM, Sheline Y, Imai K: Medical disorders among patients admitted to a public sector psychiatric inpatient unit. *Psychiatr Serv* 53:1623–1625, 2003.

Magruder KM, Frueh BC, Knapp RG, et al.: Prevalence of posttraumatic stress disorder in Veterans Affairs primary care clinics. *Gen Hosp Psychiatry* 27:169–179, 2005.

Manoranjitham SD, Rajkumar AP, Thangadurai P, et al.: Risk factors for suicide in rural south India. *Br J Psychiatry* 196:26–30, 2010.

McFarlane A: The contribution of epidemiology to the study of traumatic stress. *Soc Psychiatry Psychiatr Epidemiol* 39:874–882, 2004.

McNally RJ: Progress and controversy in the study of posttraumatic stress disorder. *Ann Rev Psychol* 54:229–252, 2003.

Michaud CM, McKenna MT, Begg S, et al.: The burden of disease and injury in the United States 1996. *Popul Health Metr* 4:11, 2006.

Milliken CS, Auchterlonie JL, Hoge CW: Longitudinal assessment of mental health problems among active and reserve component soldiers returning from the Iraq war. *JAMA* 298:2141–2148, 2007.

Mitchell AJ, Chan M, Bhatti H, et al.: Prevalence of depression, anxiety, and adjustment disorder in oncological, haematological, and palliative-care settings: A meta-analysis of 94 interview-based studies. *Lancet Oncol* 12:160–174, 2011.

Neria Y, Nandi A, Galea S: Post-traumatic stress disorder following disasters: A systematic review. *Psychol Med* 38:467–480, 2008.

O'Donnell ML, Alkemade N, Creamer M, McFarlane AC, Silove D, Bryant RA, Felmingham K, Steel Z, Forbes D(1). A Longitudinal Study of Adjustment Disorder After Trauma Exposure. *Am J Psychiatry* 173(12):1231–1238, 2016.

Popkin MK, Callies AL, Colón EA, et al.: Adjustment disorders in medically ill inpatients referred for consultation in a university hospital. *Psychosomatics* 31:410–414, 1990.

Rozanov V, Carli V: Suicide among war veterans. *Int J Environ Res Public Health* 9(7):2504–2519, 2012.

Sareen J, Cox BJ, Stein MB, Afifi TO, Fleet C, Asmundson GJG: Physical and mental comorbidity, disability, and suicidal behavior associated with posttraumatic stress disorder in a large community sample. *Psychosom Med* 69:242–248, 2007.

Sareen J, Houlahan T, Cox B, Asmundson GJG: Anxiety disorders associated with suicidal ideation and suicide attempts in the National Comorbidity Survey. *J Nerv Ment Dis* 193:450–454, 2005.

Schnurr PP, Friedman MJ, Sengupta A, et al.: PTSD and utilization of medical treatment services among male Vietnam veterans. *J Nerv Ment Dis* 188:496–504, 2000.

Schnurr PP, Hayes AF, Lunney CA, et al.: Longitudinal analysis of the relationship between symptoms and quality of life in veterans treated for posttraumatic stress disorder. *J Consult Clin Psychol* 74:707–713, 2006.

Schnurr PP, Lunney CA, Sengupta A, et al.: A descriptive analysis of PTSD chronicity in Vietnam veterans. *J Trauma Stress* 16:545–553, 2003.

Scott KM, Koenen KC, Aguilar-Gaxiola S, et al.: Associations between lifetime traumatic events and subsequent chronic physical conditions: A cross-national, cross-sectional study. *PLoS One* 8e80573, 2013.

Seedat S, Lochner C, Vythilingum B, et al.: Disability and quality of life in post-traumatic stress disorder: Impact of drug treatment. *Pharmacoeconomics* 24:989–998, 2006.

Shear KM, Greeno C, Kang J: Diagnosis of nonpsychotic patients in community clinics. *Am J Psychiatry* 157:581–587, 2000.

Smith TC, Ryan MA, Wingard DL, et al.: New onset and persistent symptoms of post-traumatic stress disorder self reported after deployment and combat exposures: Prospective population based US military cohort study. *BMJ* 336:366–371, 2008.

Snyder S, Strain JJ: Differentiation of major depression and adjustment disorder with depressed mood in the medical setting. *General Hospital Psychiatry* 12:159–65, 1989.

Stein DJ, Koenen KC, Friedman MJ, Hill E, McLaughlin KA, Petukhova M, et al.: Dissociation in posttraumatic stress disorder: Evidence from the World Mental Health Surveys. *Biol Psychiatry*, 73:302–312, 2013.

Stein MB, McQuaid JR, Pedrelli P, et al.: Posttraumatic stress disorder in the primary care medical setting. *Gen Hosp Psychiatry* 22:261–269, 2000.

Steuwe C, Lanius RA, Frewen PA. Evidence for a dissociative subtype of PTSD by latent profile and confirmatory factor analyses in a civilian sample. *Depress Anxiety* 29:689–700, 2012.

Strain JJ, Newcorn J, Mezzich J, et al: *Adjustment disorder: the McArthur reanalysis. In DSM-IV source book* (Vol. 4, pp. 404–24). American Psychiatric Association, Washington, DC, 1998.

Thompson ME, Kaslow NJ, Kingree JB, Puett R, Thompson NJ, Meadows L: Partner abuse and posttraumatic stress disorder as risk factors for suicide attempts in a sample of low-income, inner-city women. *J Trauma Stress* 12:59–72, 1999. doi:10.1023/A:1024742215337

van der Velden PG, Wittmann L: The independent predictive value of peritraumatic dissociation for PTSD symptomatology after type I trauma: A systematic review of prospective studies. *Clin Psychol Rev* 28:1009–1020, 2008.

Waelde LC, Silvern L, Fairbank JA. A taxometric investigation of dissociation in Vietnam veterans. *J Trauma Stress* 18:359–369, 2005.

Weathers FW, Keane TM: The Criterion A problem revisited: Controversies and challenges in defining and measuring psychological trauma. *J Trauma Stress* West 20:107–121, 2007.

Wolf EJ, Lunney CA, Miller MW, Resick PA, Friedman MJ, Schnurr PP: The dissociative subtype of PTSD: A replication and extension. *Depress Anxiety* 29:679–688, 2012.

Wolf EJ, Miller MW, Reardon AF, Ryabchenko KA, Castillo D, Freund R: A latent class analysis of dissociation and posttraumatic stress disorder: Evidence for a dissociative subtype. *Arch Gen Psychiatry* 69:698–705, 2012.

Zvolensky MJ, Gibson LE, Vujanovic AA, et al.: Impact of posttraumatic stress disorder on early smoking lapse and relapse during a self-guided quit attempt among community-recruited daily smokers. *Nicotine Tob Res* 10:1415–1427, 2008.

8

PTSD in Children 6 Years and Younger

ALEXANDRA C. DE YOUNG AND MICHAEL S. SCHEERINGA

Young children are a high-risk population for exposure to traumatic events. Similar to older children and adults, young children are also at risk of developing trauma- and stressor-related disorders following trauma exposure, which in the fifth edition of the *Diagnostic and Statistical Manual of Mental Disorders* (DSM-5) includes the new subtype "posttraumatic stress disorder for children 6 years and younger," which is a major advance. Early childhood is associated with both a unique set of vulnerabilities that may put young children at risk of poor outcomes and rapid maturational growth that may enhance resilience. Because of the known detrimental short- and long-term effects of trauma across health outcomes, and variables enhancing resilience, the early and accurate assessment and treatment of posttrauma reactions is critical. However, the assessment and treatment of posttraumatic stress reactions can be challenging, particularly in very young children. This is an overview of the new DSM-5 subtype and what is known about posttraumatic stress disorder during early childhood. It outlines issues that complicate the accurate assessment of trauma-related problems in young children and describes and reviews the new DSM-5 category, instruments currently available, and the evidence for different treatment options.

THE BACKGROUND OF INCLUSION OF PTSD FOR CHILDREN 6 YEARS AND YOUNGER IN DSM-5

In response to concerns raised about the sensitivity of the criteria for children under age 6 years in the fourth edition of the DSM (DSM-IV), the age-related subtype of posttraumatic stress disorder (PTSD) for preschool children, "posttraumatic stress disorder children 6 years and younger" was proposed and published in the DSM-5 (American Psychiatric Association, 2013). Posttraumatic stress disorder for children 6 years and younger is the first developmental subtype of an existing disorder and represents a significant step for the DSM taxonomy. It is based on empirical validation of the PTSD alternative algorithm (PTSD-AA; Scheeringa, Zeanah, Drell, & Larrieu, 1995). Developmental modifications were incorporated in the PTSD-AA in all three of the main clusters of PTSD symptoms—intrusion/re-experiencing, avoidance/numbing, and increased arousal.

Intrusion/Re-experiencing Cluster

The change to the re-experiencing cluster was a relatively minor change in wording to increase face validity and, thereby, improve symptom detection. The old symptom of "recurrent and intrusive distressing recollections of the event" required three conditions to be counted; the symptom had to be (a) recurrent, (b) intrusive, and (c) distressing. Research showed empirically that very young children did not always manifest distress with their intrusive, unwanted thoughts. Some children were neutral or "over bright." Distressed reactions are common, but parents also commonly reported no affect or what appeared to be excitement.

Avoidance and Negative Alterations in Cognitions and Mood Clusters

Because many of the avoidance and negative cognition symptoms are highly internalized phenomena, the most significant changes in the criteria for preschool children are in this section. The major change was to require only one symptom in either the avoidance symptoms or negative alterations in cognitions and mood, instead of the DSM-IV threshold of three symptoms. The number of these symptoms that are possible to detect is simply fewer compared to adults. The symptoms of "loss of interests," "restricted range of affect," "detachment from loved ones," and "avoidance of thoughts or feelings related to the trauma" manifest in young children but are consistently ranked as some of the least frequent among the PTSD symptoms. The symptoms of "sense of a foreshortened future" and "inability to recall an important aspect of the event" were deleted because of the developmental challenges in manifesting and/or detecting them.

The wordings of two symptoms were modified to enhance face validity and symptom detection. Diminished interest in significant activities may manifest as constricted play. Feelings of detachment or estrangement may be manifest more behaviorally as social withdrawal.

Increased Arousal Cluster

Being the most behavioral and observable types of symptoms, few changes were needed for these problems. The symptoms "irritability or outbursts of anger" was modified to include "extreme temper tantrums" to enhance face validity.

Validation of PTSD Criteria for Young Children

Much evidence supports the criterion, convergent, discriminant, and predictive validities of the PTSD criteria for young children (reviewed in Scheeringa, Zeanah, & Cohen, 2011). Research using different trauma populations supported the developmental sensitivity and validity of this developmental subtype for PTSD in the DSM-5 (De Young, Kenardy, & Cobham, 2011; Gigengack, van Meijel, Alisic, & Lindauer, 2015; Scheeringa, Myers, Putnam, & Zeanah, 2012; Stoddard et al., 2017). Perhaps most convincingly, even when the threshold for the avoidance and numbing criterion was lowered from three symptoms to one symptom, cases that were diagnosed were still highly symptomatic, with means of 6 to 10 symptoms across different studies. Marked functional impairment across a range of domains has also been documented. Prospective longitudinal studies have also documented the longer-term stability of diagnoses and impairment over time.

The DSM-5 adopted the PTSD-AA criteria because of the rigorous and replicated studies of diagnostic validation (Scheeringa, Zeanah, et al., 2011), but the DSM-5 also included some additional changes. The additions in the DSM-5 criteria that were not examined in the studies on the PTSD-AA criteria included changes to the wording of the restricted range of affect symptom to limit it to only positive emotions (as opposed to positive or negative emotions) and the addition of a new symptom (i.e., "increased frequency of negative emotional states").

ASSESSING TRAUMA-RELATED SYMPTOMS DURING EARLY CHILDHOOD

Very young children typically fall within the highest risk category for exposure to sexual and physical abuse, unintentional injury, and witnessing domestic violence (U.S. Department of Health and Services, 2009). Additionally, due to the unique developmental factors associated with early childhood (e.g., rapid rate of neurobiological development, limited emotion regulation skills, importance of a protective attachment relationship), the risk of adverse psychological and physiological consequences may be greater.

There is growing recognition, including the addition of this subtype of PTSD to DSM-5, that young children develop PTSD or posttraumatic stress reactions following trauma exposure at rates equivalent or even higher than older children and adults (De Young et al., 2011; Meiser-Stedman, Smith, Glucksman, Yule, & Dalgleish, 2008; Scheeringa, Wright, Hunt, & Zeanah, 2006; Scheeringa & Zeanah, 2008; Scheeringa, Zeanah, Myers, & Putnam, 2003). A number of developmental issues create challenges for assessment of traumatic reactions in very young children. Some of the difficulties related to recognition of PTSD in young children are illustrated in the following case.

Case Example
Tammy and the Ice Cream Truck

During the summer months, an ice cream truck would drive slowly around Tammy's neighborhood, playing the familiar ice cream truck music over the loudspeaker. Tammy, six years old, tried to race out of the house as usual to stop the truck, her mother close behind. The ice cream truck stopped opposite their house across the street. After the exciting moments of trying to decide which ice cream to choose, her mother purchased a chocolate-covered vanilla ice cream ice cream bar, and they started back toward their house.

They could not see the car coming down the street because their view was blocked by the truck. Tammy's eyes were on her ice cream bar and her mother, though she was holding Tammy's hand, was a step behind. As she stepped out from behind the truck, the car struck; Tammy instinctively ducked and went underneath the car, which dragged her for about 30 feet. Miraculously, no bones were broken, and she suffered only cuts and extensive bruises.

At a pediatric check-up one month later, it appeared that Tammy was physically fine with no major scars. The pediatrician told them she was enormously lucky and would be fine. The mother, however, told the pediatrician that now the girl refused to cross their street anywhere. The mother asked the pediatrician, "Should I be worried?" To which the pediatrician replied that she did not need to worry, hoping to comfort her, and that being scared of crossing a street after an accident like this was normal.

The mother was not so sure, so after waiting another six months she finally brought Tammy to a mental health clinic. The clinician told her that very young children did not really develop PTSD and to just give it some more time.

The mother knew in her gut that something was not right, so she brought Tammy to another clinic, this time to see one of the authors (MS), where a standardized assessment for PTSD was conducted. The mother described how Tammy would place two dolls on the sidewalk in front of their house, making sure that they were holding hands. Then Tammy would get on her bicycle, and, starting about 50 feet away from the dolls, ride as fast as she could toward the dolls, always running over the smaller of the two dolls. She would do this repeatedly until her mother distracted her. Tammy also had seven other symptoms of PTSD and met full diagnostic criteria for the disorder.

WHAT IS KNOWN ABOUT PTSD DURING EARLY CHILDHOOD

Historical Background of Assessment of PTSD

Due both to their limited language development and the common misconception that all young children are resilient to the effects of trauma, there has been skepticism about the existence of PTSD in this age group. Strong empirical evidence from multiple studies, however, has demonstrated that young children develop PTSD. Young children present with many of the same PTSD symptoms as older children and adults (i.e. re-experiencing, avoidance, and hyperarousal). However, the research also indicates that PTSD manifests differently across different stages of child development (Salmon & Bryant, 2002; Scheeringa, 2011).

Epidemiology

Exposure to life-threatening traumatic events is common in young children. The youngest children are more likely to be maltreated compared to older children. Of all substantiated maltreatment reports in the United States in 2011, 27% were younger than 3 years and 20% were 3 to 5 years, for a total of 314,910 victims (U.S. Department of Health and Services, 2012). The National Violence Against Women Survey (Tjaden & Thoennes, 1998) estimated that 1.9 million women in the United States are assaulted each year, and the majority of those are witnessed by young children. The rate of death due to accidental injuries is twice as high in 1- to 4-year-old children (8.6 per 100,000) compared to 5- to 14-year-old children (4.0 per 100,000; Hoyert & Xu, 2012). Young children also experience burns, especially scalds (Glass, Nejad, Fricchione, & Stoddard, in press), dog attacks (Gaensbauer, 1995), frightening medical procedures (De Young, Kenardy, Cobham, & Kimble, 2012), and disasters (Scheeringa & Zeanah, 2008), and they frequently witness community violence (Taylor, Zuckerman, Harik, & Groves, 1992) and war (Laor et al., 1996). Generalizing these figures to the world's population, 30 million children younger than 6 years old annually exposed to psychological trauma may be a conservative estimate.

Few epidemiological studies have looked at lifetime prevalence rates of PTSD in the general preschool population. Two studies in pediatric primary care samples reported prevalence rates of 0.6% (Egger & Angold, 2006) and 0.1% (Lavigne et al., 1996). However, it is not clear how thoroughly interviewers in those studies probed about traumatic events and internalized PTSD symptoms, which can impact detection rates (Cohen & Scheeringa, 2009; Scheeringa, 2011).

Studies that utilized developmentally sensitive PTSD criteria with young children exposed to single-event traumas have reported prevalence rates of 6.5% to 29% for acute stress reactions in the first month after a motor vehicle accident (MVA; Meiser-Stedman et al., 2008) or burn injury (Stoddard et al., 2006). PTSD rates vary from 3%- to 5% within the first two months following a variety of injury types (e.g., burns, gun shots, MVA, sports injuries; De Young et al., 2012; Scheeringa et al., 2006; Stoddard et al., 2017), 10% six months post-MVA (Meiser-Stedman et al., 2008) or burn (De Young et al., 2012), 25% six months after a gas explosion in Japan (Ohmi et al., 2002), and 13.2% on average 15 months after a burn injury (Graf, Schiestl, & Landolt, 2011). Studies investigating the impact of mass trauma have documented PTSD-AA prevalence rates ranging from 17% 9 to 12 months post 9/11 (DeVoe, Bannon, & Klein, 2006), 31% following direct exposure to terrorism in Israel (Cohen & Gadassi, 2009), 21% to 37.8% in children exposed to war-related trauma (Feldman & Vengrober, 2011; Kaufman-Shriqui et al., 2013) and up to 50% 6 months to 2.5 years following Hurricane Katrina (Scheeringa & Zeanah, 2008). The rates of PTSD following a variety of events (mostly witnessing or being subject to interpersonal violence range from 26% in non-help-seeking community samples (Levendosky, Huth-Bocks, Semel, & Shapiro, 2002; Scheeringa et al., 2003) to 60% to 69% in clinic samples (Scheeringa, Peebles, Cook, & Zeanah, 2001; Scheeringa et al., 1995). If the DSM-IV criteria alone had been adopted in these studies, the PTSD prevalence rates would have been substantially lower (Table 8.1).

Clinical Course and Long-Term Outcomes

The majority of children and adolescents are resilient or experience only transient distress following trauma exposure. Areas of great interest are identifying just what protective factors support resilient adaptation and how to enhance them in young children (De Young et al., 2012). However, prospective longitudinal studies with preschool children who experienced an accidental trauma (MVA or burn) have shown that 10% did not experience any reduction in trauma symptoms, retaining a PTSD diagnosis 6 months post-accident (De Young et al., 2012; Meiser-Stedman et al., 2008). Equally concerning, Scheeringa, Zeanah, Myers, and Putnam (2005) found significant stability of PTSD symptoms over a two-year period in a sample of 62 children (1 to 6 years) with mixed traumatic experiences. Analyses demonstrated the PTSD symptoms did not remit over time or from community treatment. Additionally, 74% of children continued to have functional impairment even when they did not meet full PTSD criteria at the two-year assessment. Contrary to widely held beliefs, these findings indicate that PTSD in young children is not a normative reaction that children simply "grow out of" (Cohen & Scheeringa, 2009). Rather, it appears that, if left untreated, trauma during early childhood can follow a chronic and unremitting course in a clinically significant proportion of children.

Developmental Issues

The assessment of PTSD is relatively more difficult compared to other disorders and in young children is further complicated by the developmental considerations unique to early childhood. First, PTSD is one of the only disorders that require an etiological component. Therefore memory of the event is required for the development of PTSD. Research indicates that even very young children are able to encode and remember traumatic events up to several years later (Howe, Toth, & Cicchetti, 2006). Children are developing nonverbal memory capacities through infancy, spotty verbal memory emerges around 18 months of age, and autobiographical narrative skills emerge around 36 months and then become increasingly sophisticated (Fivush, 1998). However, prior knowledge and language skills can influence the amount and nature of information that enters and is encoded in memory as well as what the very young child is able to report to others (Salmon & Bryant, 2002). Limited verbal skills in infants and toddlers further complicate the assessment as parents may not be aware of the child's exposure to a traumatic event. In some cases young children may only be able to communicate trauma through behaviors or play. Additionally, due to their developmental capacities, a young child's perception of threat and danger may be different compared to adults. Thus adults may underestimate the impact a potentially traumatic event has had on their child. Further, as traumatic memories are unpleasant, children will often avoid talking about them. Multiple factors therefore contribute to the difficulty in accurately determining if a child has been exposed to a traumatic event.

Second, there are currently 18 possible PTSD symptoms in the DSM-5 criteria. At least nine of these symptoms are highly internalized symptoms (e.g., avoidance of internalized reminders, intrusive recollections). Parents are typically poor at identifying internalizing symptoms, and this is particularly the case for young children who are preverbal or have limited language skills (Scheeringa et al., 2003). Additionally, PTSD symptoms manifest differently at different developmental stages (Scheeringa, 2011). For example, young children often present with temper tantrums or aggressive behavior after a trauma. Whilst these symptoms are common and normal in children of this age, parents may mistakenly assume that these changes are due to the "terrible twos" rather than potential trauma signs that need to be monitored and assessed. Interviewers also need to be aware of developmental differences in symptom presentation (e.g., intrusive symptoms manifest in many preschool children as play reenactments; young children are less likely to present with avoidance symptoms). Given that assessments during early childhood often rely

TABLE 8.1. PREVALENCE OF PSYCHOLOGICAL DISORDERS AND COMORBIDITY IN YOUNG TRAUMATIZED CHILDREN

Author and Year	Trauma	*N*	Age	Assessment Time and Measure	Findings
			Interpersonal		
Scheeringa and Zeanah (1995)	Witnessed IPV, sexual and physical abuse	12	18–48 mths	Ax: 0–14 mths Semistructured interview	PTSD-AA: 69%[a] vs DSM-IV: 13%
Scheeringa et al. (2001)	Witnessed IPV, sexual and physical abuse	15	13–47 mths	Ax: 0–22 mths (M = 6.6 mths) PTSD-SSIORIYC	PTSD-AA: 60% [a] vs DSM-IV: 20%
Scheeringa et al. (2003)	MVA, accidental injury, abuse, witnessed IPV, cancer	62	20 mths–6 yrs	Ax: 2–52 mths (M = 11.3 mths) PTSD-SSIORIYC, DISC-IV	PTSD-AA: 26% vs DSM-IV: 0% Comorbidity: SAD = 63%; MDD = 6%; ADHD = 38%; ODD = 75%
Scheeringa et al. (2005)	Same sample as above	T2: 47 T3: 35	20 mths–6 yrs	Ax: 1 and 2 yrs post T1 Ax. DISC-V	T2: PTSD-AA: 23.4% vs DSM-IV: 2.1% T3: PTSD-AA: 22.9% vs DSM-IV: 11.4%
Levendosky et al. (2002)	DV	39	3–5 yrs	Most recent event of DV occurred within 1 yr of ax. PTSD-PAC checklist	PTSD-AA: 26% [a] vs DSM-IV: 3%
Scheeringa et al. (2012)	Witnessed IPV, accidental injury, abuse, Hurricane Katrina	284	3–6 yrs	Ax: not reported PAPA	PTSD-AA: 45% vs DSM-IV: 13% vs DSM-5: 44%
			Terrorism/War		
DeVoe et al. (2006)	September 11 Terrorist Attack	180	0–5 yrs	Ax: 9–12 mths PTSD-SSIORIYC	PTSD-AA: 17%.
E. Cohen and Gadassi (2009)	Exposed to terrorist events in Israel	29	3.57.5 yrs	Ax: not reported PTSDSSIORIYC	PTSD-AA: 31% vs DSM-IV: 2%
Feldman and Vengrober (2011)	Exposed to war-related trauma	148	1.5–5 yrs	Ax: not reported Clinical interview	PTSD-DC:0-3R: 37.8%
Kaufman-Shriqui et al. (2013)	Missile attacks during Gaza War	167	4–6.5 yrs	Ax: within 1st month after cessation of hostilities. Modified CPSS	PTSD-AA: 21%.
Natural Disaster					
Scheeringa and Zeanah (2008)	Hurricane Katrina	70	3–6 yrs	Ax: 6 mths-2–5 yrs PAPA	PTSD-AA: 50% vs DSM-IV: 15.7%. Comorbidity: ODD = 61%; MDD = 43%; ADHD = 33%; SAD = 21%.

(*continued*)

TABLE 8.1. CONTINUED

Author and Year	Trauma	*N*	Age	Assessment Time and Measure	Findings
			Single-Event		
Ohmi et al. (2002)	Gas explosion	32	32–73 mths	Ax: 6 mths CPTSD-RI modified	PTSD-AA: 25% [a] vs DSM-IV: 0%.
Scheeringa et al. (2006)	Injury (e.g. from MVA, gun shots, sporting, burns)	21	0–6 yrs	Ax: 2 mths PTSDSSI	PTSD-AA: 14.3% vs DSM-IV: 4.8%.
Meiser-Stedman et al. (2008)	MVA	62	2–6 yrs	Ax: 2–4 wks and 6 mths PTSD-SSIORIYC, ADIS-P	2–4 wks: PTSD-AA[b]: 6.5% vs ASD: 1.7% 6 mths: PTSD-AA: 10% vs DSM-IV: 1.7%
Stoddard et al. (2006)	Accidental burns	52	12–48 mths	Ax: within 1 mth PTSD-SSIORIYC	PTSD-AA[b] = 29%
De Young et al. (2012)	Accidental burns	130	1–6 yrs	Ax: 4–6 wks and 6 mths DIPA	4-6 wks: PTSD-AA & PTSD-DSM-V: 25% vs DSM-IV: 5%; 6 mths: PTSD-AA & PTSD-DSM-V: 10% vs DSM-IV: 0% Comorbidity: SAD = 39%; MDD = 0%; ADHD = 39%; ODD = 77%
Graf et al. (2011)	Accidental burns	76	12–49 mths	Ax: Avg 15 mths PTSD-SSIORIYC	PTSD-AA: 13.2% vs DSM-IV: 1.3%

Note: ADHD = attention deficit hyperactivity disorder; ADIS-P = Anxiety Disorder Interview Schedule—Parent version; Ax = assessment time points post-trauma; CPSS = Child PTSD Symptom Scale; CPTSD-RI = Child Post-Traumatic Stress Disorder Reaction Index, modified based on PTSD-AA; DC:0-3R = diagnostic classification of mental health and developmental disorders of infancy and early childhood; DISC-IV = Diagnostic Interview Schedule for Children, Version 4; DIPA = Diagnostic Infant Preschool Assessment; DV = domestic violence; DSM-IV = *Diagnostic and Statistical Manual of Mental Disorders*, 4th ed; IPV = interpersonal violence; MDD; major depressive disorder; mths = months; MVA = motor vehicle accident; ODD = oppositional defiant disorder; PAPA = Preschool Age Psychiatric Assessment; PTSD = posttraumatic stress disorder; PTSD-AA = alternative posttraumatic stress disorder algorithm; PTSD-PAC: measure of PTSD symptoms in preschool children developed specifically for study and not inclusive of all symptoms; PTSD-SSIORIYC = PTSD Semi-Structured Interview & Observational Record for Infants & Young Children; SAD = separation anxiety disorder; T2 = Time 2; T3 = Time 3; yrs = years.

[a]Original PTSD-AA that only required one symptom from each cluster. [b]Used PTSD-AA to assess for acute stress reactions within the first month.

solely on parent report, it is much harder to accurately identify trauma symptoms in infants and preschoolers.

Finally, the impact of trauma during early childhood should include an assessment of the parent–child relationship. Young children have limited emotional self-regulation capacities, and it is developmentally appropriate to rely on caregivers for assistance with emotion regulation, particularly during times of distress. If parents are suffering from depression or PTSD following traumas, they may be impaired in their ability to detect and respond effectively to their children's emotional needs. Imprudent parents may allow their children to be repeatedly exposed to traumatic incidents and/or reminders of past traumatic events, thereby triggering new fear and distress responses. In addition, anxious parents may directly influence their children's exposure to traumatic reminders (e.g., by allowing avoidance) and may thereby impede their children's recovery. Finally, parental reports of their children's distress may be influenced by their own distress levels. It is therefore important to understand the relationship between child and parent distress during a trauma assessment.

ETIOLOGY

Neurobiology of PTSD in Early Childhood

The modest heritability of PTSD in families appears well established, although attempts to identify the specific genes involved have encountered inconsistent results and failed replication studies (Koenen et al., 2011). Studies have focused on genes that regulate dopamine and serotonin neurotransmitters, as well as genes involved in the regulation of the hypothalamic-pituitary-adrenal (HPA) axis. Very few of these studies have examined very young children (Amstadter, Nugent, & Koenen, 2009; Drury, Brett, Henry, & Scheeringa, 2013; Drury, Theall, Keats, & Scheeringa, 2009).

Alterations of the stress response systems, including the HPA axis and the autonomic nervous system, have been demonstrated in children with abuse histories or PTSD (Gunnar & Fisher, 2006; Scheeringa, Zeanah, Myers, & Putnam, 2004). The direction of findings, however, has been inconsistent, perhaps due to the complex interaction of these stress response systems and differences across development. One of the greatest challenges for research into the etiology of PTSD is the ability to differentiate pre-existing differences in neurobiology and consequences of exposure to trauma and the psychological sequelae.

Volumetric differences in the amygdala, hippocampus, cerebellum, and prefrontal cortex have been associated with PTSD in adults, but these have not been consistently reported in children and adolescents (Choi, Jeong, Rohan, Polcari, & Teicher, 2009). No known studies have examined structural brain differences in very young children, and no studies have imaged brains of children prior to traumatic events to determine a causal pathway for any structural differences.

Psychosocial Factors

Multiple factors are likely to contribute to the development of PTSD including underlying neurobiological differences as well as differences in the posttraumatic environment. Although female gender, a history of child abuse/neglect, and limited perceived social support have been identified as risk factors for the development of PTSD in adults, research into the etiology of PTSD, specifically in infants, toddlers, and preschoolers, is scarce. Emerging research with young children has yielded inconsistent findings on age (Feldman & Vengrober, 2011; Scheeringa et al., 2006; Scheeringa & Zeanah, 1995; Scheeringa et al., 2005) and gender (Graham-Bermann & Levendosky, 1997; Green et al., 1991; Scheeringa & Zeanah, 1995, 2008; Scheeringa et al., 2003) as predictors of outcomes. One study of preschool children ages 1 to 5 years indicated that closer proximity to the traumatic event (bombing) increased the prevalence of avoidance symptoms but not other symptoms (Feldman & Vengrober, 2011). Premorbid emotional and behavioral difficulties and larger burn size have been associated with more PTSD symptoms in young burn victims (De Young, Hendrikz, Kenardy, Cobham, & Kimble, 2014; Graf et al., 2011; Stoddard et al., 2017).

One highly relevant component to a young child's environment, particularly in times of distress or trauma exposure, is the caregiving relationship. Given the reliance of young children on their caregiver, it is not surprising that another predictor of PTSD in young children is witnessing a threat to a primary caregiver (Scheeringa et al., 2006; Scheeringa & Zeanah, 1995). Additionally, a growing number of studies have documented a significant relationship between parent distress and child PTSD symptoms (De Young et al., 2011; Hall et al., 2006). The following models have been proposed to explain the significant association between child and parent distress following trauma: (a) parenting models (i.e., traumatized parents are impaired in their ability to provide emotional support and effective parenting practices), (b) bidirectional models (i.e., trauma affects both the child and parent and each person's symptomatology exacerbates that of the other), and (c) shared genetic vulnerability models (Scheeringa, 2009).

While it has been generally believed that parenting models with unidirectional effects from parents to children are of most importance (Feldman & Vengrober, 2011), other evidence challenges this notion. Scheeringa, Myers, Putnam, and Zeanah (2015) followed a cohort of 1- to 6-year-old children who had all been exposed to trauma over two years and measured maternal sensitivity in a variety of ways. They found that higher maternal sensitivity, not lower, was a significant mediator that predicted higher levels of children's PTSD symptoms over time. The authors speculated that children impacted their parents more than parents impacted children.

KNOWN CORRELATES, ASSOCIATED PROBLEMS, AND COMORBIDITIES

Research has identified several additional symptoms that are common in young traumatized children but are not critical for a PTSD diagnosis (De Young et al., 2011; Scheeringa et al., 2003). These symptoms include increased separation anxiety, new onset of fears not related to trauma (e.g., the dark, going to the bathroom alone), new aggressive and oppositional behavior, and regression in developmental skills (e.g., verbal skills, dressing skills, and toileting).

Consistent with older children and adults, comorbidity with PTSD is also common in young children (Table 8.1). Recent research has reported that PTSD was comorbid with at least one other disorder 73% to 89% of the time in preschool children exposed to Hurricane Katrina (Scheeringa & Zeanah, 2008) or burn injury (De Young et al., 2012). Separation anxiety disorder and oppositional defiant disorder (ODD) are the most common co-occurring conditions (De Young et al., 2012; Scheeringa & Zeanah, 2008; Scheeringa et al., 2003). Studies with preschool children have also shown that new onset disorders following a natural disaster or burn injury did not occur without the presence of posttraumatic stress symptoms (PTSS; De Young et al., 2012; Scheeringa & Zeanah, 2008). These findings suggest that a PTSD syndrome may be the core posttrauma response.

Young children are often first noticed by adults as having something wrong with them due to associated problem behavior rather than due to the internalized PTSD symptoms. The high rates of comorbidity with PTSD provide further support for concerns that children who exhibit high emotion and deregulated behavior may receive a number of erroneous primary diagnoses such as attention-deficit/hyperactivity disorder (ADHD) and ODD instead of PTSD following trauma (Scheeringa & Zeanah, 2008). Given that it is particularly difficult to accurately identify internalized PTSD symptoms in young children (e.g., avoidance of thoughts), there is a substantial risk of targeting the more easily observable behavioral symptoms for treatment without understanding the concurrent underlying PTSD symptomatology (Scheeringa & Zeanah, 2008). These findings have important implications for the assessment and treatment of PTSD and comorbid conditions, particularly in young children, and clearly highlight the importance of screening for trauma and traumatic stress symptoms in children who present with disruptive behavioral problems.

BEST PRACTICES IN ASSESSMENT FOR PTSD DURING EARLY CHILDHOOD

Next we provide an overview of the measures that are available to assess for trauma-related symptoms in very young children. Whilst there has been an emergence in assessment measures for this age group in recent years, there are important issues that need to be noted with the available measures. None of the measures have undergone rigorous and replicated systematic evaluations. Different types of measures are best for different purposes, so, as with all psychiatric syndromes, there is no single best assessment measure for all purposes. Additionally, due to the limited cognitive and verbal capacities of young children, all the measures rely on parent self-report. This is therefore associated with limitations inherent with parent report (i.e., underreporting of internalizing symptoms, bias due to own distress or guilt). The measures chosen for review and included in Table 8.2 are based on the following criteria: (a) they provide a measure of traumatic stress reactions, (b) psychometric properties have been published in at least one research study, and (c) the measure has been used with children under the age of 6 years. The measures are reviewed in the categories of trauma exposure checklists, diagnostic interviews, and parent-report questionnaires.

TABLE 8.2. SUMMARY OF ASSESSMENT MEASURES

Measure	Age Range	General Information / Purpose	Administration/Length/Scoring	Psychometric Properties
		Diagnostic Interviews		
Diagnostic Infant and Preschool Assessment (DIPA; Scheeringa & Haslett, 2010)	1–6 years	• Assesses psychopathology in childhood (13 DSM-IV Axis-I disorders) • Provides PTSD diagnosis? Yes, DSM-V and PTSD-AA criteria • Other information: Used in clinical and research settings • Costs? No	• Format: Semi-structured interview • Administered by: Clinician • Conducted with: Primary caregiver • Length of administration: 517 Questions PTSD module: 63 Questions • Requirements: Clinical or research training	• Reliability: TR: PTSD-AA ICC α=.87–.98; PTSD-AA κ= .56–1.00 • Validity: CONC w/CBCL PTSD Scale: Continuous: r=.15–.24 for PTSD-AA; Categorical: κ =.48 for PTSD-AA-RA, κ=.12 for PTSD-AA-Clinician
Preschool Age Psychiatric Assessment (PAPA; Egger, et al., 2006)	2–5 years	• Assesses for broad range of psychological disorders including PTSD • Provides PTSD diagnosis? Yes, DSM-IV, DC:0-3R and RDC-PA • Other information: Spanish, Romanian and Norwegian translations	• Format: Structured interview • Administered by: Clinician • Conducted with: Primary caregiver • Length of administration: Avg 100 mins • Requirements: Graduate, training and supervision	• Reliability: TR: PTSD ICC α= 0.56; PTSD κ=0.73
		Questionnaires		
The Trauma Symptom Checklist for Young Children (TSCYC; Briere, 2005)	3–12 years	• Assesses posttraumatic symptoms and comorbid difficulties • Provides PTSD diagnosis? No • Other information: • 9 subscales: 4 PTSD-related, Sexual Concerns, Anxiety, Depression, Dissociation, and Anger/Aggression • Contains two rater validity scales • Costs? Yes • Spanish and Swedish translations	• Format: Observer-report questionnaire • Items: 90 items rated on a 4-point scale • Completed by: Primary caregiver • Length: 15 mins (+8 mins to score) • Scoring: Norms based on sex and age (3–4, 5–9, 10–12) • Manual available? Yes • Requirements: Graduate training	• Reliability: IC: α=.55-.94 • Validity: Clinical scales associated with sexual abuse, physical abuse, and witnessing domestic violence Posttraumatic Stress Total Scale: SPEC = .957; SENS = .545

TABLE 8.2. CONTINUED

Measure	Age Range	General Information / Purpose	Administration/Length/Scoring	Psychometric Properties
Pediatric Emotional Distress Scale (PEDS) (Saylor et al., 1999)	2–10 years	• Assesses trauma related symptoms • Provides PTSD diagnosis? No • Other information: Yields a total distress score and three sub-scale scores: Anxious/ Withdrawn, Fearful and Acting Out • Costs? No	• Format: Observer-report questionnaire • Items: 17 general behavior items; 4 trauma-specific items on a 4-point scale • Completed by: Primary caregiver • Length: 7 mins (+4 mins to score) • Requirements: Psychologist	• Reliability: IC: α=.84–.85; IRR = .65; TR = .56 • Validity: CONC: PEDS Tot w/ ECBI $r = .62$, $p <.0001$ DISC: Differentiates between trauma-exposed and non-trauma exposed children
Pediatric Emotional Distress Scale Early Screener (PEDS-ES) (Kramer, Hertli & Landolt, 2013)	2–6 years	• Early screening tool for PTSD • Provides PTSD diagnosis? No • Other information: Cutoff score of 8 is recommended. • Costs? No	• Format: Observer-report questionnaire • Items: 17 general behavior items; 4 trauma-specific items on a 4-point scale • Completed by: Primary caregiver • Length: 7 mins (+4 mins to score) • Requirements: Psychologist	• Reliability: IC: α=.76. • Validity: SENS = .85; SPEC= .64; PPV = .41; NPV = .93.
PTSD Symptoms in Preschool Children (PTSD-PAC) (Levendosky et al., 2002)	3–5 years	• Assesses posttraumatic symptoms • Provides PTSD diagnosis? No • Costs? No	• Format: Observer-report questionnaire • Items: 18 items, yes/no format • Completed by: Primary caregiver • Length:10 minutes (+5 mins to score) • Manual available? No • Requirements: Interpretation requires psychologist and familiarity with the DSM-IV criteria	• Reliability: IC: α = .79
Preschool Posttraumatic Stress Symptoms Inventory (PPSSI) (Graham-Bermann et al., 2008).	3–5 years	• Assesses posttraumatic symptoms • Provides PTSD diagnosis? No • Costs? No	• Format: Observer-report questionnaire • Items: 17 items, 3-point scale • Completed by: Primary caregiver • Manual available? No	• Reliability: IC: α = .86 • Validity: CONV w/ CBCL PTSD scale $r = .24$, $p <.01$.

Note: CBCL = Child Behavior Checklist; CONC = concurrent validity; CONV = convergent validity; DSM-IV = *Diagnostic and Statistical Manual of Mental Disorders*, 4th ed; DISC = discriminant validity; Dx = diagnosis; DC:0-3R = diagnostic classification of mental health and developmental disorders of infancy and early childhood; IC = internal consistency; ICC = intraclass correlation statistic; IRR = interrater reliability; NPV = negative predictive value; PPV = positive predictive value; PTSD = posttraumatic stress disorder; PTSD-AA = alternative posttraumatic stress disorder algorithm; PTSD-RI = PTSD-Reaction Index; *rs* = Pearson *rs*; RA = research Assistant; RDC-PA = Research Diagnostic Classification System—Preschool Age; SENS = sensitivity; SPEC = specificity; TR = test–retest reliability; w/ = with.

Trauma Exposure Checklists

There are several parent-report trauma exposure checklists or interviews available to screen for a history of exposure to traumatic events (e.g., accidents, abuse, witnessing violence, terrorism, natural disasters). There is one known measure available that just screens for the presence of trauma exposure, the Traumatic Events Screening Inventory–Parent Report Revised (TESI-PRR; Ippen et al., 2002). This is a 24-item version of the original TESI and was revised to be more developmentally sensitive to the traumatic experiences that young children may experience. The Diagnostic Infant Preschool Assessment (DIPA; Scheeringa & Haslett, 2010) and Preschool Age Psychiatric Assessment (Egger et al., 2006) both include a screen for traumatic events as the first part of the interview assessment of PTSD symptoms. An advantage of using the Traumatic Life Events checklist in the DIPA is that it asks about the presence of 12 types of traumatic events and obtains information on first and last dates of trauma exposure and the frequency of occurrence. It then asks about the worst event for the child and follows into the assessment of the child's specific reactions to the event/s.

Diagnostic Interviews

Given the challenges of PTSD assessment in early childhood, structured or semi-structured diagnostic parent report interviews are the most reliable and valid method for assessing trauma-related symptoms in young children (Scheeringa et al., 2001). (See Table 8.2.)

The DIPA (Scheeringa & Haslett, 2010) is a semi-structured diagnostic interview that is conducted with the primary caregiver of children aged between 1 and 6 years of age. The PTSD module was developed from, and meant to replace the Posttraumatic Stress Disorder Semi-Structured Interview and Observational Record for Infants and Young Children (Scheeringa & Zeanah, 1994). The PTSD module screens for exposure to 12 potentially traumatic events, assesses for symptoms commonly seen in young traumatized children, and provides a measure of functional impairment and distress associated with the overall symptoms. The DIPA is the only interview for PTSD that has been tested in a clinical sample, showing acceptable test–retest reliability and construct validation (Scheeringa & Haslett, 2010). A new version of the DIPA with Likert-style ratings for each item is currently being tested. The DIPA interview and manual is freely available at http://medicine.tulane.edu/departments/psychiatry/research/dr-scheeringas-lab/manuals-measures-trainings.

The Preschool Age Psychiatric Assessment (PAPA; Egger & Angold, 2004) was developed to assess for parent-reported psychiatric disorders in children aged 2 to 5 years. The PAPA is based on the parent version of the Child and Adolescent Psychiatric Assessment and has been modified to include specific developmental modifications to aid the assessment of symptoms in 2- to 5-year-olds. In a community sample, the PAPA demonstrated fair to good test–retest reliability and intraclass correlations for most diagnostic modules (Bufferd, Dougherty, Carlson, & Klein, 2011; Egger et al., 2006; Wichstrøm et al., 2011), including PTSD (Egger et al., 2006). Information on the PAPA is available at http://devepi.duhs.duke.edu/papa.html.

Parent-Report Questionnaires

A variety of self-administered, parent-report questionnaires have been developed and are summarized in Table 8.2. These can be categorized as those that are narrowly focused and provide precise coverage of PTSD symptoms, such as the PTSD Symptoms in Preschool Children Scale (Levendosky et al., 2002), Preschool Posttraumatic Stress Symptoms Inventory (Graham-Bermann et al., 2008), and the Young Child PTSD Checklist (Scheeringa, 2010). Other questionnaires provide limited coverage of PTSD symptoms but include non-PTSD symptoms, such as the Trauma Symptom Checklist for Young Children (TSCYC; Briere, 2005; Briere et al., 2001; Pollio et al., 2008) and the Pediatric Emotional Distress Scale (PEDS; Saylor, Swenson, Stokes Reynolds, & Taylor, 1999; Spilsbury et al., 2005).

Screening is recommended as a simple, quick, and cost-effective method for identifying children who should continue to be monitored for risk or referred for more comprehensive targeted assessment or treatment following trauma exposure. Kramer, Hertli, and Landolt (2013) adapted the PEDS (PEDS Early Screener [PEDS-ES]) so that it could be used as an early screener for identifying the presence of PTSD symptoms within the first few weeks following a traumatic event and predicting which children were likely to develop persistent PTSD. Findings to date suggest that the PEDS-ES is a reliable and valid early screening tool (Kramer et al., 2013). In addition, Scheeringa developed a rapid, six-item screen, the Young Child PTSD Screen. A manuscript on the psychometrics of this screen is currently under review (Scheeringa, personal communication), but the screen is freely available at: http://medicine.tulane.edu/departments/psychiatry/research/dr-scheeringas-lab/manuals-measures-trainings.

Clinical Assessment

This section provides several recommendations on how to conduct best-practice assessment of trauma-related symptoms in young children. First, professionals need to be aware that young children can and do develop PTSD following trauma exposure. Given that developmental factors influence the manifestation of PTSD, utilization of the DSM-5 subtype for children 6 years and younger and appropriate assessment measures are needed.

Second, given the challenges of assessment with this age group, where possible, a comprehensive diagnostic interview should be used. This includes inquiring about possible exposure to all types of traumas, all 18 PTSD symptoms, plus additional symptoms that are common in young traumatized children (e.g., separation anxiety, aggression) and asking for examples, onsets, durations, and frequencies. Educational interviewing may be necessary to give respondents a frame of reference for the internalized and abstract items that comprise signs of PTSD (Scheeringa, 2011). The DIPA and PAPA are both promising clinician-administered diagnostic interviews that provide a developmentally sensitive measure of PTSD, as well as a range of other preschool emotional and behavioral disorders commonly seen following trauma. Interviews allow the most accurate assessments, providing either dichotomous diagnoses or continuous measures of the number of symptoms. A checklist with Likert-style responses can complement interviews by providing continuous measures with broader ranges that may be more sensitive to interventions and changes over time.

Ideally, assessments with infants, toddlers, and preschoolers should include a multimethod, multi-informant approach. However, this is particularly difficult to do. For example, as of yet, it is not feasible to administer interviews or questionnaires to children younger than 7 years of age because they have not mastered the multiple types of skills needed to do this (Scheeringa, 2011). When direct assessment with young children has been attempted the results have been discouraging. When 15 one- to three-year-old clinic children with PTSD symptoms were systematically examined during five types of observational sequences, only 12% of the symptoms known from parent report could be detected from observation or interaction with the children (Scheeringa, Zeanah, et al., 2011). Shahinfar and colleagues, using cartoon-based measures, used the Violence Exposure scale to measure exposure to family and community violence and the Levonn (Richters, Martinez, & Valla, 1990) to measure distress symptomatology in 3- to 4-year-old children (Shahinfar, Fox, & Leavitt, 2000). Data could be analyzed from less than half of the children (73 out of 155) who were judged to have understood the Violence Exposure scale. Further, there are few psychometrically sound questionnaires available (and none for children less than 3 years) to assess for PTSD symptoms in this age group. From the measures available, the TSCYC has a strength in that it provides a measure of trauma symptoms and comorbid conditions that can be compared to normative data. Additionally, there are no measures that have been validated when completed by another adult (e.g., teacher), making it difficult to conduct a multi-informant assessment.

Third, when children present with disruptive behavioral disorders (e.g., ODD, ADHD), it is important to screen for trauma exposure and the presence of PTSD symptoms. Additionally, because young children typically have trauma symptoms that extend beyond a diagnosis of PTSD, it is important to use assessments of comorbid conditions and other trauma-related symptoms (e.g., full DIPA interview). Fourth, research suggests that the impact of trauma must be considered within the context of the parent–child relationship. Therefore, assessments should also consider the quality of attachment and also directly inquire about any symptomatology that the child's caregivers may be experiencing.

Treatment

Cognitive behavioral therapy (CBT) is the only treatment modality with replications of randomized controlled trials (RCT) to treat posttraumatic problems in very young children. Three RCTs have demonstrated the effectiveness of CBT techniques in this age group. Cohen and Mannarino (1996) showed the superiority of a 12-session CBT protocol for 67 three- to six-year-old sexually abused children who were randomized to either CBT or nondirective supportive therapy. Scheeringa and colleagues (2011) showed the superiority of a 12-session CBT protocol to a wait-list condition for 64 three- to six-year-old children who had suffered a wide range of traumatic events. There was an 82.4% reduction in PTSD diagnosis for the treatment completers. The Scheeringa et al. (2010) group also assessed the feasibility of CBT techniques with young children and showed that the children understood and completed 83.5% of all tasks, with most of the problems in feasibility occurring with the younger (3 to 4-year-old) children on more abstract cognitive tasks.

Deblinger, Stauffer, and Steer (2001) compared supportive versus CBT group therapies for 2- to 8-year-old children who had experienced sexual abuse. Forty-four children and their nonoffending mothers were randomly allocated to receive 11 sessions of one of the therapies. Mothers who participated in the CBT group reported significantly greater reduction in their own problems compared to the supportive group. The children in the CBT group, however, did not demonstrate significantly greater reductions in PTSD symptoms, perhaps because children were not asked specifically to talk about their sexual abuse experiences due to the group format.

Child–parent psychotherapy (CPP) is a psychodynamic therapy for dyads that covers a broad range of topics over 50 weeks including parent–child interaction, normal development, and individual sessions for mothers in addition to creating a trauma narrative. Seventy-five 3- to 5-year-old children who had witnessed domestic violence were randomized to CPP or community treatment with case management. Children in the CPP group showed a greater reduction in PTSD symptoms immediately posttreatment (Lieberman, Van Horn, & Ippen, 2005).

Play therapy, which is a more feasible modality than CBT for 2-year-old children, appears to have achieved some symptom reduction in several case reports (Gaensbauer, 1997; Gaensbauer, Chatoor, Drell, Siegel, & Zeanah, 1995; Gaensbauer & Siegel, 1995). Several researchers have reported symptom reductions in case reports of individual 4- and 5-year-old children treated with eye movement desensitization and reprocessing (EMDR; Cocco & Sharpe, 1993; Greenwald, 1994; Tufnell, 2005), although the feasibility of cooperating with bilateral processing was not systematically documented. No RCT has been conducted with either play therapy or EMDR.

Despite the growing evidence base for the efficacy of CBT, very few young children who develop PTSD receive access to appropriate psychosocial services, and even when offered or directly referred to intervention programs, uptake and engagement are typically poor. Early identification and intervention programs for preventing the development of persistent PTSS after childhood trauma are therefore of considerable importance. Only one study has investigated any form of early intervention with children under 6 years of age (Kramer & Landolt, 2014). Unfortunately, the intervention was not found to be effective at reducing the presence of child PTSD, PTSS, or behavioral problems. Two parallel RCTs in Australia and Switzerland are currently investigating the effectiveness and feasibility of a two-session early intervention designed to prevent persistent PTSS in young preschool-aged children screened as at risk for PTSD following an unintentional injury (De Young, Haag, Kenardy, Kimble, & Landolt, 2016).

In regards to psychopharmacology, there are only two medications approved by the US Food and Drug Administration for PTSD, paroxetine and sertraline, and neither includes children in their accepted age ranges. Nevertheless, when psychopharmacology appears indicated in young children for intractable or severe cases, these types of medications, the selective serotonin reuptake inhibitors, would be obvious considerations because of their low side effect profile and ease of use. For youths with prominent arousal symptoms, the alpha-adrenergic agonist agents, such as clonidine and guanfacine, are often used in clinical practice. In fact, the only known psychopharmacological study in young children involved clonidine. In an uncontrolled study of clonidine in seven 3- to 6-year-old children in a day hospital setting, many of the children appeared to benefit. There has been an increasing amount of literature showing the effectiveness of prazosin, another type of alpha adrenergic agonist, for treatment of nightmares in adults with PTSD, and this could be another consideration for young children.

Clinical Case Example

The following case illustrates the importance of assessing a profile of comorbid syndromes, and difficult treatment decisions that can arise when there exist co-occurring syndromes. Robert, a 4-year-old male, was referred by his doctor to a specialty program that treated PTSD because he had witnessed repeated domestic violence since birth and was showing impairment with "out of control behavior at school." The assessment revealed six symptoms of PTSD (psychological distress from reminders, avoidance of reminders, intrusive recollections, nightmares, sleep difficulty, and irritability). He also manifested marked symptoms of attention-deficit/hyperactivity disorder (ADHD) with all nine of the hyperactivity/impulsivity symptoms and two inattention symptoms. It was decided to initially focus treatment on PTSD rather than ADHD because Robert showed significant mood and anxiety, suggesting that trauma responses may be the primary and underlying condition. He had multiple symptoms of depression, including sad mood, boredom, and expressed some notions of hopelessness and helplessness. He had significant separation anxiety and at times would appear excessively worried about minor things. Lastly, he also showed nearly all of the eight oppositional defiant disorder symptoms.

From the outset of counseling, Robert had difficulty remaining in one place and paying attention with the therapist. This made his therapist wonder if his ADHD ought to have been treated first so that he could make maximal use of the CBT techniques. Nevertheless, after beginning the CBT exposure sessions, he began to improve rather substantially on his symptoms of PTSD, depression, and anxiety; however, his ADHD symptoms never declined.

At the end of treatment with a 12-session CBT protocol, the severity and frequency of his symptoms improved by informal caregiver-report, and his sleep difficulty resolved, but the posttreatment PAPA interview indicated that he still had five PTSD symptoms. This illustrates how it would have been helpful to have a Likert-style checklist of PTSD severity to complement the interview and to capture the decrease in intensity of his symptoms. It was also evident that his ADHD symptoms were separate and persistent.

Following completion of his CBT treatment, stimulant medication was initiated for the ADHD symptoms, and, after a period for the stimulant dose to be adjusted, clonidine was added to target sleep disturbances. Because of some persisting PTSD symptoms, additional CBT sessions were added. With the improvement in his ADHD symptoms, it appeared that Robert was able to make even more effective use of his CBT skills, such as deep breathing and mental imagery relaxation. After this treatment for ADHD and additional CBT, his PTSD and depressive symptoms completely remitted. His ODD symptoms had improved but remained problematic.

Obtaining a careful timeline of the onsets of symptoms will usually reveal which symptoms pre-existed trauma and which were trauma-related, but in Robert's case his trauma experiences had been from birth, making it problematic to tell if his disruptive behaviors were of separate origin or trauma-related. In general, marked ADHD symptoms may be an indicator that they are not trauma-related. Robert's PTSD, depression, and ODD improved with CBT, but ADHD did not, which is consistent with the findings from a randomized trial of treating PTSD in preschool children (Scheeringa, Weems, et al., 2011). Furthermore, a profile that includes sleep difficulty may indicate that an adrenergic agent such as clonidine may be beneficial.

CONCLUSIONS

Trauma during early childhood is common and the inclusion of the DSM-5 subtype of "PTSD for children 6 years and younger" is an important advance in acceptance of developmental differences in psychiatric classification. As with older children, adolescents, and adults, young children are also at risk of developing a range of traumatic stress reactions. However, early childhood is associated with a unique set of vulnerabilities that may put young children at even greater risk of poor outcomes. Early and accurate assessment and treatment of posttrauma reactions is critical because of the detrimental short- and long-term effects that trauma can have on all aspects of functioning. However, due to developmental considerations, the unique salience of the parent–child relationship and limited psychometrically sound instruments and evidence-based treatments to choose from, the assessment and treatment of PTSD is particularly challenging in children under the age of 6 years. Fortunately, in recent years there has been an emergence of developmentally sensitive diagnostic criteria and assessment measures and this has greatly increased our understanding of the mental health needs of young traumatized children. However, although there are some promising measures and treatment options available, further research is urgently needed to investigate and develop evidence-based assessment measures and interventions for infants, toddlers, and preschoolers

REFERENCES

American Psychiatric Association. (2013). *Diagnostic and statistical manual of mental disorders* (5th ed.). Arlington, VA: American Psychiatric Publishing.

Amstadter, A. B., Nugent, N. R., & Koenen, K. C. (2009). Genetics of PTSD: Fear conditioning as a model for future research. *Psychiatric Annals, 39*(6), 358–367. doi:10.3928/00485713-20090526-01

Briere, J. (2005). *Trauma Symptom Checklist for Young Children (TSCYC): Professional manual.* Lutz, FL: Psychological Assessment Resources.

Briere, J., Johnson, K., Bissada, A., Damon, L., Crouch, J., Gil, E., . . . Ernst, V. (2001). The Trauma Symptom Checklist for Young Children (TSCYC): Reliability and association with abuse exposure in a multi-site study. *Child Abuse & Neglect, 25*(8), 1001–1014. doi:10.1016/s0145-2134(01)00253-8

Bufferd, S. J., Dougherty, L. R., Carlson, G. A., & Klein, D. N. (2011). Parent-reported mental health in preschoolers: Findings using a diagnostic interview. *Comprehensive Psychiatry*, *52*(4), 359–369. doi:10.1016/j.comppsych.2010.08.006

Choi, J., Jeong, B., Rohan, M. L., Polcari, A. M., & Teicher, M. H. (2009). Preliminary evidence for white matter tract abnormalities in young adults exposed to parental verbal abuse. *Biological Psychiatry*, *65*(3), 227–234. doi:10.1016/j.biopsych.2008.06.022

Cocco, N., & Sharpe, L. (1993). An auditory variant of eye movement desensitization in a case of childhood post-traumatic stress disorder. *Journal of Behavior Therapy and Experimental Psychiatry*, *24*(4), 373–377.

Cohen, E., & Gadassi, R. (2009). Posttraumatic stress disorder in young children exposed to terrorism: Validation of the alternative diagnostic criteria. *Journal of Child & Adolescent Trauma*, *2*(4), 229–241. doi:10.1080/19361520903317295

Cohen, J. A., & Mannarino, A. P. (1996). A treatment outcome study for sexually abused preschool children: Initial findings. *Journal of the American Academy of Child & Adolescent Psychiatry*, *35*(1), 42–50. doi:10.1097/00004583-199601000-00011

Cohen, J. A., & Scheeringa, M. S. (2009). Posttraumatic stress disorder diagnosis in children: Challenges and promises. *Dialogues in Clinical Neuroscience*, *11*(1), 91–99.

De Young, A. C., Haag, A.-C., Kenardy, J. A., Kimble, R. M., & Landolt, M. A. (2016). Coping with Accident Reactions (CARE) early intervention programme for preventing traumatic stress reactions in young injured children: Study protocol for two randomised controlled trials. *Trials*, *17*(1), 362. doi:10.1186/s13063-016-1490-2

De Young, A. C., Hendrikz, J., Kenardy, J. A., Cobham, V. E., & Kimble, R. M. (2014). Prospective evaluation of parent distress following pediatric burns and identification of risk factors for young child and parent posttraumatic stress disorder. *Journal of Child and Adolescent Psychopharmacology*, *24*(1), 9–17. doi:10.1089/cap.2013.0066

De Young, A. C., Kenardy, J. A., & Cobham, V. E. (2011). Diagnosis of posttraumatic stress disorder in preschool children. *Journal of Clinical Child & Adolescent Psychology*, *40*(3), 375–384. doi:10.1080/15374416.2011.563474

De Young, A. C., Kenardy, J. A., Cobham, V. E., & Kimble, R. (2012). Prevalence, comorbidity and course of trauma reactions in young burn-injured children. *Journal of Child Psychology & Psychiatry*, *53*(1), 56–63. doi:10.1111/j.1469-7610.2011.02431.x

Deblinger, E., Stauffer, L. B., & Steer, R. A. (2001). Comparative efficacies of supportive and cognitive behavioral group therapies for young children who have been sexually abused and their nonoffending mothers. *Child Maltreatment*, *6*(4), 332–343. doi:10.1177/1077559501006004006

DeVoe, E. R., Bannon, W. M. Jr., & Klein, T. P. (2006). Post-9/11 helpseeking by New York City parents on behalf of highly exposed young children. *American Journal of Orthopsychiatry*, *76*(2), 167–175.

Drury, S. S., Brett, Z. H., Henry, C., & Scheeringa, M. (2013). The association of a novel haplotype in the dopamine transporter with preschool age posttraumatic stress disorder. *Journal of Child and Adolescent Psychopharmacology*, *23*(4), 236–243. doi:10.1089/cap.2012.0072

Drury, S. S., Theall, K. P., Keats, B. J. B., & Scheeringa, M. (2009). The role of the dopamine transporter (DAT) in the development of PTSD in preschool children. *Journal of Traumatic Stress*, *22*(6), 534–539. doi:10.1002/jts.20475

Egger, H. L., & Angold, A. (2004). The Preschool Age Psychiatric Assessment (PAPA): A structured parent interview for diagnosing psychiatric disorders in preschool children. In R. DelCarmen-Wiggins & A. Carter (Eds.), *Handbook of infant, toddler, and preschool mental health assessment* (pp. 223–243). New York: Oxford University Press.

Egger, H. L., & Angold, A. (2006). Common emotional and behavioral disorders in preschool children: Presentation, nosology, and epidemiology. *Journal of Child Psychology & Psychiatry*, *47*(3–4), 313–337.

Egger, H. L., Erkanli, A., Keeler, G., Potts, E., Walter, B. K., & Angold, A. (2006). Test-retest reliability of the Preschool Age Psychiatric Assessment (PAPA). *Journal of the American Academy of Child & Adolescent Psychiatry*, *45*(5), 538–549.

Feldman, R., & Vengrober, A. (2011). Posttraumatic stress disorder in infants and young children exposed to war-related trauma. *Journal of the American Academy of Child & Adolescent Psychiatry*, *50*(7), 645–658. doi:10.1016/j.jaac.2011.03.001

Fivush, R. (1998). Children's recollections of traumatic and nontraumatic events. *Development and Psychopathology*, *10*(4), 699–716.

Gaensbauer, T. (1995). Trauma in the preverbal period. *Psychoanalytic Study of the Child*, *50*, 122–149.

Gaensbauer, T. J. (1997). DC: 0-3 Casebook. In A. F. Lieberman, S. Wieder, & E. Fenichel (Eds.), *DC: Zero to three* (pp. 31–46). Washington, DC: ZERO TO THREE: National Center for Infants, Toddlers, & Families.

Gaensbauer, T. J., Chatoor, I., Drell, M., Siegel, D., & Zeanah, C. H. (1995). Traumatic loss in a one-year-old girl. *Journal of the American Academy of Child & Adolescent Psychiatry, 34*(4), 520–528.

Gaensbauer, T. J., & Siegel, C. H. (1995). Therapeutic approaches to posttraumatic stress disorder in infants and toddlers. *Infant Mental Health Journal, 16*(4), 292–305.

Gigengack, M. R., van Meijel, E. P., Alisic, E., & Lindauer, R. J. (2015). Comparing three diagnostic algorithms of posttraumatic stress in young children exposed to accidental trauma: An exploratory study. *Child and Adolescent Psychiatry and Mental Health, 9*, 14. doi:10.1186/s13034-015-0046-7

Glass, S. P., Nejad, S. H., Fricchione, G. L., & Stoddard, F. J. (2018). Burn Patients. In T. A. Stern, O. Freudenreich, F. A. Smith, G. L. Fricchione, & J. F. Rosenbaum (Eds.), *Massachusetts General Hospital handbook of general hospital psychiatry* (7th ed., pp. 359–370). Philadelphia, PA: Mosby.

Graf, A., Schiestl, C., & Landolt, M. A. (2011). Posttraumatic stress and behavior problems in infants and toddlers with burns. *Journal of Pediatric Psychology, 36*(8), 923–931. doi:10.1093/jpepsy/jsr021

Graham-Bermann, S. A., Howell, K., Habarth, J., Krishnan, S., Loree, A., & Bermann, E. A. (2008). Toward assessing traumatic events and stress symptoms in preschool children from low-income families. *American Journal of Orthopsychiatry, 78*(2), 220–228.

Graham-Bermann, S. A., & Levendosky, A. A. (1997). The social functioning of preschool-age children whose mothers are emotionally and physically abused. *Journal of Emotional Abuse, 1*(1), 59–84.

Green, B. L., Korol, M., Grace, M. C., Vary, M. G., Leonard, A. C., Gleser, G. C., & Smitson-Cohen, S. (1991). Children and disaster: Age, gender, and parental effects on PTSD symptoms. *Journal of the American Academy of Child & Adolescent Psychiatry, 30*(6), 945–951.

Greenwald, R. (1994). Applying eye movement desensitization and reprocessing (EMDR) to the treatment of traumatized children: Five case studies. *Anxiety Disorders Practice Journal, 1*, 83–97.

Gunnar, M. R., & Fisher, P. A. (2006). Early Experience, Stress and Prevention Network. Bringing basic research on early experience and stress neurobiology to bear on preventive interventions for neglected and maltreated children. *Development and Psychopathology, 18*(3), 651–677. doi:10.1017/S0954579406060330

Hall, E., Saxe, G., Stoddard, F., Kaplow, J., Koenen, K., Chawla, N., . . . King, D. (2006). Posttraumatic stress symptoms in parents of children with acute burns. *Journal of Pediatric Psychology, 31*(4), 403–412.

Howe, M. L., Toth, S. L., & Cicchetti, D. (2006). Memory and developmental psychopathology. In D. Cicchetti & D. J. Cohen (Eds.), *Developmental psychopathology*, Vol. 2: *Developmental neuroscience* (2nd ed., pp. 629–655). Hoboken, NJ: John Wiley.

Hoyert, D. L., & Xu, J. (2012). Death: Preliminary data for 2011. *National Vital Statistics Reports 61(6)*, 40–42.

Ippen, C. G., Ford, J., Racusin, R., Acker, M., Bosquet, M., Rogers, K., . . . Edwards, J. (2002). *Traumatic Events Screening Inventory—Parent Report Revised*. Hanover, NH: U.S. Department of Veteran's Affairs, National Center for PTSD.

Kaufman-Shriqui, V., Werbeloff, N., Faroy, M., Meiri, G., Shahar, D. R., Fraser, D., . . . Harpaz-Rotem, I. (2013). Posttraumatic stress disorder among preschoolers exposed to ongoing missile attacks in the Gaza war. *Depression and Anxiety, 30*(5), 425–431. doi:10.1002/da.22121

Koenen, K. C., Uddin, M., Chang, S.-C., Aiello, A. E., Wildman, D. E., Goldmann, E., & Galea, S. (2011). SLC6A4 methylation modifies the effect of the number of traumatic events on risk for posttraumatic stress disorder. *Depression and Anxiety, 28*(8), 639–647. doi:10.1002/da.20825

Kramer, D. N., Hertli, M. B., & Landolt, M. A. (2013). Evaluation of an early risk screener for PTSD in preschool children after accidental injury. *Pediatrics, 132*(4), e945–e951. doi:10.1542/peds.2013-0713

Kramer, D. N., & Landolt, M. A. (2014). Early psychological intervention in accidentally injured children ages 2–16: A randomized controlled trial. *European Journal of Psychotraumatology, 5*. doi:10.3402/ejpt.v5.24402

Laor, N., Wolmer, L., Mayes, L. C., Golomb, A., Silverberg, D., Weizman, R., & Cohen, D. J. (1996). Israeli preschoolers under scud missile attacks: A developmental perspective on risk-modifying factors. *Archives of General Psychiatry, 53*(5), 416–423.

Lavigne, J. V., Gibbons, R. D., Christoffel, K. K., Arend, R., Rosenbaum, D., Binns, H., . . . Isaacs, C. (1996). Prevalence rates and correlates of psychiatric disorders among preschool children. *Journal of the American Academy of Child & Adolescent Psychiatry, 35*(2), 204–214. doi:10.1097/00004583-199602000-00014

Levendosky, A. A., Huth-Bocks, A. C., Semel, M. A., & Shapiro, D. L. (2002). Trauma symptoms in preschool-age children exposed to domestic violence. *Journal of Interpersonal Violence, 17*(2), 150–164.

Lieberman, A. F., Van Horn, P., & Ippen, C. G. (2005). Toward evidence-based treatment: Child-parent psychotherapy with preschoolers exposed to marital violence. *Journal of the American Academy of Child & Adolescent Psychiatry, 44*(12), 1241–1248. doi:10.1097/01.chi.0000181047.59702.58

Meiser-Stedman, R., Smith, P., Glucksman, E., Yule, W., & Dalgleish, T. (2008). The posttraumatic stress disorder diagnosis in preschool- and elementary school-age children exposed to motor vehicle accidents. *The American Journal of Psychiatry, 165*(10), 1326–1337.

Ohmi, H., Kojima, S., Awai, Y., Kamata, S., Sasaki, K., Tanaka, Y., . . . Hata, A. (2002). Post-traumatic stress disorder in pre-school aged children after a gas explosion. *European Journal of Pediatrics, 161*(12), 643–648.

Pollio, E. S., Glover-Orr, L. E., & Wherry, J. N. (2008). Assessing posttraumatic stress disorder using the Trauma Symptom Checklist for Young Children. *Journal of Child Sexual Abuse, 17*(1), 89–100. doi:10.1080/10538710701884557

Richters, J. E., Martinez, P., & Valla, J. (1990). *Levonn: A cartoon based interview for assessing children's distress symptoms.* Washington, DC: National Institute of Mental Health.

Salmon, K., & Bryant, R. A. (2002). Posttraumatic stress disorder in children: The influence of developmental factors. *Clinical Psychology Review, 22*(2), 163–188. doi:10.1016/s0272-7358(01)00086-1

Saylor, C. F., Swenson, C. C., Stokes Reynolds, S., & Taylor, M. (1999). The Pediatric Emotional Distress Scale: A brief screening measure for young children exposed to traumatic events. *Journal of Clinical Child Psychology, 28*(1), 70–81. doi:10.1207/s15374424jccp2801_6

Scheeringa, M. S. (2009). Posttraumatic stress disorder. In C. H. ZeanahJr. (Ed.), *Handbook of infant mental health* (3rd ed., pp. 345–361). New York: Guilford Press.

Scheeringa, M. S. (2010). Young Child PTSD Checklist (YCPC). New Orleans, LA: Tulane University.

Scheeringa, M. S. (2011). PTSD in children younger than the age of 13: Toward developmentally sensitive assessment and management. *Journal of Child & Adolescent Trauma, 4*(3), 181–197. doi:10.1080/19361521.2011.597079

Scheeringa, M. S., & Haslett, N. (2010). The reliability and criterion validity of the Diagnostic Infant and Preschool Assessment: A new diagnostic instrument for young children. *Child Psychiatry and Human Development, 41*(3), 299–312.

Scheeringa, M. S., Myers, L., Putnam, F. W., & Zeanah, C. H. (2012). Diagnosing PTSD in early childhood: An empirical assessment of four approaches. *Journal of Traumatic Stress, 25*(4), 359–367. doi:10.1002/jts.21723

Scheeringa, M. S., Myers, L., Putnam, F. W., & Zeanah, C. H. (2015). Maternal factors as moderators or mediators of PTSD symptoms in very young children: A two-year prospective study. *Journal of Family Violence, 30*(5), 633–642. doi:10.1007/s10896-015-9695-9

Scheeringa, M. S., Peebles, C. D., Cook, C. A., & Zeanah, C. H. (2001). Toward establishing procedural, criterion, and discriminant validity for PTSD in early childhood. *Journal of the American Academy of Child & Adolescent Psychiatry, 40*(1), 52–60.

Scheeringa, M. S., Weems, C. F., Cohen, J. A., Amaya-Jackson, L., & Guthrie, D. (2010). Trauma-focused cognitive-behavioral therapy for posttraumatic stress disorder in three through six year-old children: A randomized clinical trial. *Journal of Child Psychology and Psychiatry, 52*(8), 853–860. doi:10.1111/j.1469-7610.2010.02354.x

Scheeringa, M. S., Weems, C. F., Cohen, J. A., Amaya-Jackson, L., & Guthrie, D. (2011). Trauma-focused cognitive-behavioral therapy for posttraumatic stress disorder in three-through six year-old children: A randomized clinical trial. *Journal of Child Psychology and Psychiatry, 52*(8), 853–860. doi:10.1111/j.1469 7610.2010.02354.x

Scheeringa, M. S., Wright, M., Hunt, J. P., & Zeanah, C. H. (2006). Factors affecting the diagnosis and prediction of PTSD symptomatology in children and adolescents. *American Journal of Psychiatry, 163*(4), 644–651.

Scheeringa, M. S., & Zeanah, C. H. (1994). *Posttraumatic Stress Disorder Semi-structured Interview and Observational Record for Infants and Young Children.* New Orleans, LA: Department of Psychiatry and Neurology, Tulane University Health Sciences Center.

Scheeringa, M. S., & Zeanah, C. H. (1995). Symptom expression and trauma variables in children under 48 months of age. *Infant Mental Health Journal, 16*(4), 259–270.

Scheeringa, M. S., & Zeanah, C. H. (2008). Reconsideration of harm's way: Onsets and comorbidity patterns of disorders in preschool children and their caregivers following Hurricane Katrina. *Journal of Clinical Child & Adolescent Psychology, 37*(3), 508–518.

Scheeringa, M. S., Zeanah, C. H., & Cohen, J. A. (2011). PTSD in children and adolescents: Toward an empirically based algorithma. *Depression and Anxiety, 28*(9), 770–782. doi:10.1002/da.20736

Scheeringa, M. S., Zeanah, C. H., Drell, M. J., & Larrieu, J. A. (1995). Two approaches to the diagnosis of posttraumatic stress disorder in infancy and early childhood. *Journal of the American Academy of Child & Adolescent Psychiatry, 34*(2), 191–200.

Scheeringa, M. S., Zeanah, C. H., Myers, L., & Putnam, F. (2003). New findings on alternative criteria for PTSD in preschool children. *Journal of the American Academy of Child & Adolescent Psychiatry*, *42*(5), 561–570.

Scheeringa, M. S., Zeanah, C. H., Myers, L., & Putnam, F. (2004). Heart period and variability findings in preschool children with posttraumatic stress symptoms. *Biological Psychiatry*, *55*(7), 685–691.

Scheeringa, M. S., Zeanah, C. H., Myers, L., & Putnam, F. (2005). Predictive validity in a prospective follow-up of PTSD in preschool children. *Journal of the American Academy of Child & Adolescent Psychiatry*, *44*(9), 899–906.

Shahinfar, A., Fox, N. A., & Leavitt, L. A. (2000). Preschool children's exposure to violence: Relation of behavior problems to parent and child reports. *American Journal of Orthopsychiatry*, *70*(1), 115–125.

Spilsbury, J. C., Drotar, D., Burant, C., Flannery, D., Creeden, R., & Friedman, S. (2005). Psychometric properties of the Pediatric Emotional Distress Scale in a diverse sample of children exposed to interpersonal violence. *Journal of Clinical Child & Adolescent Psychology*, *34*(4), 758–764. doi:10.1207/s15374424jccp3404_17

Stoddard, F. J., Saxe, G., Ronfeldt, H., Drake, J. E., Burns, J., Edgren, C., & Sheridan, R. L. (2006). Acute stress symptoms in young children with burns. *Journal of the American Academy of Child & Adolescent Psychiatry*, *45*(1), 87–93.

Stoddard, F. J., Sorrentino, E., Drake, J. E., Murphy, J. M., Kim, A. J., Romo, S., . . . Sheridan, R. L. (2017). Posttraumatic stress disorder diagnosis in young children with burns. *Journal of Burn Care Research*, *38*(1), e343–e351. doi:10.1097/bcr.0000000000000386

Taylor, L., Zuckerman, B., Harik, V., & Groves, B. (1992). Exposure to violence among inner city parents and young children. *American Journal of Diseases of Children*, *14*(6), 487–494.

Tjaden, P., & Thoennes, N. (1998). *Prevalence, incidence, and consequences of violence against women: Findings from the National Violence Against Women Survey. Resaerch in brief.* Retrieved from https://www.ncjrs.gov/pdffiles/172837.pdf

Tufnell, G. (2005). Eye movement desensitization and reprocessing in the treatment of pre-adolescent children with post-traumatic symptoms. *Clinical Child Psychology and Psychiatry*, *10*(4), 587–600. doi:10.1177/1359104505056320

U.S. Department of Health and Services. (2009). *Child maltreatment 2007*. Retrieved from http://www.acf.hhs.gov/programs/cb/stats_research/index.htm

U.S. Department of Health and Services. (2012). Administration for Children and Families, Administration on Children, Youth and Families, Children's Bureau, Child Maltreatment Report 2011.

Wichstrøm, L., Berg-Nielsen, T. S., Angold, A., Egger, H. L., Solheim, E., & Sveen, T. H. (2011). Prevalence of psychiatric disorders in preschoolers. *Journal of Child Psychology & Psychiatry*, *53*(6), 695–705. doi:10.1111/j.1469-7610.2011.02514.x

9

Trauma in Late Life

KENNETH SAKAUYE AND JAMES E. NININGER

INTRODUCTION

Reaction to trauma in late life has characteristically been a two-edged sword. Frailty has characteristically been a functional definition of old age, but so has toughness and wisdom. Higher sensitivity to trauma, both physical and mental, and higher mortality have clearly been factors in the frail elderly. In primary care of the elderly, posttraumatic stress symptoms, depression, suicidal ideation, smoking, and at-risk drinking are common conditions as Rauch et al. (2006) found in a study of 2,718 adults over age 65. While posttraumatic stress disorder (PTSD) in the elderly has been studied, less is known about other common trauma- and stressor-related disorders (TSRDs) including adjustment disorder, acute stress disorder, and traumatic grief. Resilience, however, has been increasingly observed in studies of with lower rates of PTSD in elderly compared to younger cohorts after natural and manmade disasters (Sakauye et al., 2009; Siskind et al., 2016).

In the fifth edition of the *Diagnostic and Statistical Manual of Mental Disorders* (DSM-5; American Psychiatric Association, 2013), Criterion A for PTSD defines trauma as "exposure or actual or threatened death, serious injury, or sexual violence. "It must be directly experienced, witnessed, occur to a family member or friend, or be a repeated or extreme exposure to aversive details of a traumatic event. However, the strict definition of "trauma" from the Greek is "wound." Psychiatric wounds are manifest by behaviors and thoughts directly tied to the event. No event is always traumatic (i.e., always leads to injury), and, conversely, even a seemingly mild negative event can be traumatic to some individuals. Two presumed variables explaining the variance are (a) appraisal of the situation (i.e., whether one feels he or she remains in control) and (b) individual biological differences in responsiveness. A table of common traumatic stressors for elderly is given below in Table 9.1.

In the elderly, especially frail elderly or patients with dementia, less severe stresses can still be traumatic and cause significant problems. The manifestation of the traumatic injury is similar across all age groups, namely (a) intrusive thoughts (e.g., re-experiencing), (b) avoidance, (c) negative alterations in mood/cognition, and (d) alteration of arousal and reactivity, as well as subtypes of delayed depression or dissociation. Statistics suggest we are beginning a period of increased prevalence of TSRDs among older adults which may increase the prevalence of several age-related medical conditions including dementia (Palmer & Raskind, 2016).

Elder abuse and neglect is increasingly prevalent with elders, placing them at significant risk for TRSDs. This may relate to improving detection and reporting of elder abuse and neglect, with significant public health implications. Cooper et al. (2008) conducted a systematic review of 49 selected studies measuring elder abuse or neglect and found very high rates. Nearly a quarter of studies reported significant psychological abuse, and 5% of family caregivers reported physical abuse toward care recipients with dementia, but rates of reporting to adult protective services were low. General population studies found 6% of elders reporting abuse within the last month and 5.6% of couples reporting violence in their relationship in the last year. Cooper et al. conclude that only a small proportion of elder abuse is known to protective services. Acierno et al. (2010) assessed one-year prevalence of emotional, physical, sexual, and financial mistreatment and potential neglect of 5,777 adults 60 years or older in a randomly selected national sample. Their findings were that 17.1% of their sample were subject to one of these, with the highest being 4.6% emotional abuse, 5.1% potential neglect, and 5.2% financial abuse. They were alarmed at a high prevalence of potential neglect in community-residing, cognitively impaired older adults. They also pointed out that

TABLE 9.1. COMMON STRESSORS FOR ELDERLY

Losing one's home, possessions
Severe financial worries
Loss of friends (and social support network)
Fear of Falling
Loss of vision and hearing
Fear of pain and disability
Fear of helplessness
Fear of abandonment
Elder abuse
Loss of driver's license
Effects of racism (threats, mistreatment, seen as worthless)
Fear of pain

most investigations have not assessed financial exploitation and that it is the most likely form of exploitation. An unusual study (Laumann et al., 2008) of 3,005 community residing adults aged 57 to 85 years found prevalence of elder mistreatment to be "uncommon," with 9% verbal, 3.5% financial, and 0.2% physical mistreatment by a family member. Those without a romantic partner had higher rates, and African Americans had higher rates than whites or Latinos.

Catastrophic "traumas" experienced by the elderly include forced relocation from one's lifelong home to a nursing home (relocation trauma), elder abuse, financial loss (impoverishment), catastrophic illness, and untimely death of a child. For minority elderly, one might include the toll of lifelong racism and hate crimes such as assault (Sue et al., 2007). In general, perceived traumas, even if they do not appear severe, can still be sufficient to cause a variety of psychiatric disorders such as phobias, depression, "learned helplessness," anxiety disorders, and posttraumatic stress symptoms.

Case Example

Mrs. K was an elderly African American woman who was raised in the pre-civil rights South with only a fourth-grade education in a segregated school. She had been raised in a culture of violence and threats against blacks and lost her only son because a segregated white hospital refused care. She had panic attacks when admitted to a predominantly white hospital, worrying she might be killed. Upon further history, she had symptoms of hypervigilance, nightmares of her son's death, and anxiety problems since his death. Symptoms were revived by exposure to a potential threat.

An individual's reaction to a given trauma is determined by many variables including genetic predisposition, cultural background, medical health and experiences, and traumas from childhood through old age. The Harvard Study of Adult Development which began in 1938 following the emotional and physical health of 200 men beginning in their undergraduate days has now followed surviving members into their 90s. The variability of response, continued development of character and coping skills into old age, and often remarkable resilience in spite of significant difficulties in childhood and early adulthood is evident in these detailed longitudinal reports (Vaillant, 2012). Defense mechanisms utilized in stress also vary widely from individual to individual and may be adaptive or maladaptive. They can provide a period of repose and healing where normal mental mechanisms are put on hold in an uncontrollable situation. The different reactions of two octogenarians in New York City after 9/11 demonstrate reasons for a range of responses to trauma.

Case Example

Mrs. G was an 82-year-old German immigrant living in New York City when 9/11 occurred. She became quite depressed in part related to the fact that the event stirred up past memories of bombings and threats during World War II in Europe. The patient had felt that coming to the United States would ensure that she would never again have to be subject to attacks from outsiders and witness large-scale violence. The trauma revived disturbing memories which overwhelmed her. In contrast, Mrs. H, similar in age and living in New York City when 9/11 occurred, felt appropriately upset and sad after the attack on the World Trade Center but had not been subject to major traumas in the past. She did not relate to the trauma with as personal meaning and did not react in an abnormal manner.

Despite the huge body of literature on combat-related trauma and PTSD and disaster response, and much anecdotal information, there are relatively few research studies directly focused on psychological trauma in elderly. This chapter reviews information on the prevalence of trauma exposure and posttraumatic problems in the elderly, resilience, and suggested treatment approaches.

ASSESSMENT AND DIAGNOSIS

The core element in diagnosis is the psychiatric interview. An open-ended interview approach similar to the Cultural Formulation Interview (CFI) in the DSM-5 (American Psychiatric Association, 2013) is more clinically informative in the elderly than a structured interview approach like the Structured Clinical Interview (SCID) for DSM-5 (First, 2015).

The CFI mirrors the typical medical/psychiatric interview in starting with what is important to the patient (chief complaint) and allowing the patient to describe the problem, causal attribution, coping, what makes it better, what makes it worse, and what the support network is. At appropriate times in the interview, one should probe for details of specific symptoms, details about relationships, and values. The temporal relationship to a disturbing event usually becomes evident, as does degree of insight, coping mechanisms, and support systems. There are currently no confirmatory psychological tests or biological tests available to confirm a trauma-induced diagnosis.

Relevant Cultural Formulation Interview Questions

"Sometimes people have different ways of describing their problems to family, friends, or others in the community. How would you describe the problem to them?"

"Why do you think this is happening to you? What do you think are the causes? What do your family, friends or others in the community think is causing your problem?"

"Are there any kinds of stresses that make your problem worse?"

"How have you tried to cope?"

"Are there any kinds of support that make your problem better?"

"Sometimes people have particular ways of dealing with problems like this. What have you done on your own to cope?"

"Often people look for help from many different sources, including different kinds of doctors, helpers, or healers. In the past, what kinds of treatment, help, advice, or healing have you sought? Which were most helpful?"

(American Psychiatric Association, 2013)

After an acute traumatic event, patients must be screened for PTSD symptoms, pre-existing medical conditions, co-existing substance abuse or depression, psychosocial problems, sleep disturbance, anger, and irritability.

UNIQUE ASPECTS OF THE DISORDER IN THE ELDERLY

The cumulative risk of trauma exposure is extremely high in the elderly. In a German community study, using the PTSD module of the SCID for DSM-IV, trauma exposure was four-fold higher in elderly than in younger age groups. At least one major trauma was reported by 54.6% of individuals (Spitzer et al., 2008). The risk of trauma exposure should be expected to be even higher in US urban elderly, given higher crime rate statistics.

Despite the higher exposure to potentially traumatic events, the rate of PTSD seems lower in the elderly. A recent meta-analysis of studies of PTSD in older persons after human-induced disasters, like war zones or terrorist attacks, showed older adults were 2.85 times less likely to experience PTSD symptoms compared to younger adults. (Siskind et al., 2016) However, high-risk subpopulations like the frail elderly and elderly with dementia traditionally do not cope well and have the highest mortality rates after a disaster (Sakauye et al., 2009). It is not clear if PTSD occurs in the elderly with dementia, since memory encoding is abnormal.

Persistence of symptoms over the lifespan is often seen. The National Vietnam Veterans Longitudinal Study, which followed veterans 40 years after the Vietnam War, showed about 17% lifetime wartime PTSD, and 10.8% showed current plus subthreshold war-zone PTSD (waxed and waned). In addition, about one-third of these individuals showed a current major depressive disorder (Marmar et al., 2015). Another study using the Vet Registry of male twins who served during the Vietnam era showed the influence of age when serving and proximity to severe trauma (service in theater versus not). The younger veterans had a higher lifetime prevalence of PTSD than the older veterans, and the theater veterans had much higher rates of PTSD than non theater veterans. Unfortunately, this study could not estimate current prevalence of PTSD. (Goldberg, 2016). The context of stress is often important in how stress is perceived and reacted to. A recent study of 1,300 female military personnel, Red Cross workers, and others who served in Vietnam actually showed many felt positive experiences about this era, possibly because of group support or the fact that they did not feel helpless in their caregiving roles (Kaiser, 2017).

Trauma exposure during the lifespan increases the risk of suicidal ideation among older adults (Beristianos et al., 2016; Rauch, 2006). The difference between a good and a bad outcome seems to be related to a history of positive family relationships, a cohesive fighting unit at the time of trauma, desirable appraisals by the patient (positive attitude), fewer intervening stresses, and positive social support, based on the Veterans Administration (VA) Normative Aging Study (Kang et al., 2016).

One unusual trauma outcome in the elderly is delayed onset of PTSD. Patients may have had trauma years before symptoms appear. This is typically assumed to be due to successful psychological defenses of repression or denial until some reminder or change in life revives the old memories (Bonanno & Mancini, 2012).

Case Example

Mr. A is a Vietnam vet who did not seek treatment until age 62 when he retired. He stated he felt symptoms were triggered by his grandson's enlistment and entry into a war zone. Flashbacks, nightmares, and depression became intolerable. There were mild symptoms dating back to the initial trauma, a feeling that he was more emotionally labile and had no desire to maintain close relationships, but he said he "didn't know what to call it" and never sought treatment until symptoms were incapacitating.

NEUROBIOLOGICAL FACTORS

The recent renewed attention to positive psychiatry has emphasized the association of resilience with traits that are typically described as wisdom in normal elderly. These include a lower level of perceived stress in the face of adversity, placing value in the ability to adapt to circumstances, taking a positive attitude toward the future, and not requiring an absence of physical disability to be content (i.e., being able to feel well within an illness). Posttraumatic growth can be manifested by a greater appreciation of life, altered priorities, and closer interpersonal relationships (Jeste et al., 2015). Changes in neural circuitry are putatively associated with these behaviors in normal elderly, as summarized by Meeks and Jeste in a 2009 review. These neural pathway changes are associated with emotional homeostasis, conflict detection, processing self and socially relevant stimuli, effortful reasoning/executive functioning, processing ambiguity, pragmatic knowledge, tolerance of ambiguity, and reflection.

The original hypothesis of the central role of the hypothalamic-pituitary-adrenal (HPA) axis in stress responses from the 1950s has been confirmed. The response to fear or anger is thought to be the same as the response to a pleasant experience, namely HPA activation. However, extreme terror leads to a sustained physiologic response which has negative catabolic and immunosuppressive actions and if sustained can cause hippocampal neuronal loss (Vergne, 2014). Elevations in circulating glucocorticoids persist longer in older than in younger individuals, presumably due to a reduced effectiveness of the negative feedback loop. This would predict that elderly should have a greater risk of negative stress-induced changes, but this effect seems to be countered by compensatory protective changes, such as reduced amygdala activity, and related reduction in an intense fear response to stress (Vijg, 2015).

TREATMENT

The biopsychosocial model has always emphasized that treatment of any disorder should "treat the whole person." Related to trauma, one must remove the trauma, prevent retraumatization, provide treatments to restore health such as medication, and enhance the social network and coping skills. Treatment for elderly who are traumatized is similar to younger age groups with some special considerations described. The framework for treatment for all traumas has been mapped out by the Veterans Administration and Department of Defense in its *Clinical Practice Guideline for Management of Post-traumatic Stress* (VA/DoD Post-Traumatic Stress Management Working Group, 2010).

Medications

Cognitively Intact Elderly

As there are few studies of medication safety and efficacy for trauma-related disorders in the elderly, extrapolations from general adult populations must be made, guided by geriatric psychiatry prescribing guidelines. In most cases, efficacy is assumed to be similar, but adjustments are made for differences in pharmacokinetics due to body size, distribution, and unbound fraction of drug, altered metabolism, altered excretion, and drug-drug interactions.

The usual geriatric prescribing guideline is to

1. Apply sequential single medication trials (avoid polypharmacy).
2. Start at half the usual starting dose.

TABLE 9.2. GERIATRIC DOSING OF COMMON MEDICATIONS TO TREAT PTSD SYMPTOMS

Symptom Category	Most Common Medications (Generics)	Avoid	Geriatric Dosing (Common Usage)
Depressive symptoms	Common Order in Treatment Algorithms: SSRI first SNRI next Other category FDA-approved augmentation agents: Aripiprazole Rexulti Quetiapine	Not applicable	Start with 50% of usual starting dose and advance slowly
Panic attacks/ Generalized anxiety	Sertraline Venlafaxine	Benzodiazepines	Start with 50% of usual starting dose and advance slowly
PTSD symptoms of hyperarousal, irritability, and anger	Most Evidence: Sertraline Paroxetine Venlafaxine Less Evidence Fluoxetine Citalopram Fluvoxamine Amitriptyline/Nortriptyline May be Helpful Valproate Quetiapine Lamotrigine Propranolol	Benzodiazepines	Start with 50% of usual starting dose and advance slowly
Nightmares	Prazosin	Not applicable	Start with 1mg qhs

Note: PTSD = posttraumatic stress disorder; SSRI = selective serotonin reuptake inhibitors; SNRI = serotonin and norepinephrine reuptake inhibitors; FDA = Food and Drug Administration.
Adapted from VA/DoD Treatment Guidelines for PTSD.

3. Titrate to a minimum effective dose, or maximum recommended dose if there is no improvement. Wait at least five half-life intervals before the next dose adjustment to allow steady state to be achieved.
4. Be aware of published drug-drug interactions, and modify accordingly Avoid highly anticholinergic or highly sedating medications in the elderly, especially in patients with dementia (AGS American Geriatrics Society 2015 Beers Crieteria Update Expert Panel, 2015).

The medications used for treating PTSD and trauma act upon neurotransmitters related to the fear and anxiety circuitry of the brain, including serotonin, norepinephrine, GABA, and dopamine. Currently the strongest evidence for efficacy is for sertraline and venlafaxine which are considered first-line treatments at the VA. Use of other agents such as atypical antipsychotics, lamotrigine, propranolol, clonidine, or gabapentin has less evidence base. Medications not demonstrated to have benefit are risperidone, valproate, topiramate, guanfacine, and tiagbine (VA/DoD Post-Traumatic Stress Management Working Group, 2010). See Table 9.2.

In both younger and older patients with PTSD, the treatment guideline recommends that benzodiazepines be avoided. Benzodiazepines may interfere with the extinction of fear conditioning and actually potentiate the acquisition of fear responses (National Center for PTSD, 2015). In the elderly, benzodiazepines also have more pronounced negative effects on cognition and balance, and may lead to physical dependence (AGS American Geriatrics Society 2015 Beers Crieteria Update Expert Panel, 2015). Additionally there is a risk of unintentional overdose or withdrawal if administration of medicine is not monitored carefully.

In rapid eye movement (REM) sleep disorder, a person acts out dreams, such as fighting and kicking instead of remaining paralyzed as in normal REM. REM sleep disorder is seen more in the elderly, even in the absence of trauma exposure. Prazosin, an alpha blocker, can be used for such nightmares and seems to blunt the autonomic reactions associated with the nightmare. A similar effect has not been seen with other alpha blockers, such as those used for benign prostatic hypertrophy (BPH). Alpha blocker combination therapy has been approved for those with PTSD and BPH by the VA (VA Pharmacy Benefits Management Services, Medical Advisory Panel, VISN Pharmacist Executives, 2012). Starting doses of 1 mg at bedtime in the elderly can be gradually titrated to an effective dose. The patient must be warned about slow titration and low doses to avoid hypotension, especially in the presence of other alpha blockers or antihypertensive medications. Often the elderly will respond to doses as low as 1 to 2 mg at bedtime, whereas an average dose of 6 mg is more typical of younger patients who are not using use concomitant medications.

The newer neurobiological understanding of memory and associative learning has led to potential ways to make exposure therapies more effective. Fear extinction or erasure seems possible by pairing the recall of a traumatic event with administration of a noradrenergic blocker. A nonthreatening re-exposure to the traumatic memory after taking the medication being tested seems to disrupt the reconsolidation of the fear response to the event (Fitzgerald et al., 2015; Giustino et al., 2016). A number of medications are being tested for medication-assisted psychotherapy, ranging from propranolol and other adrenergic blockers to MDMA (3,4-ethylenedioxymethamphetamine, or Ecstasy), but efficacy and safety are not established.

Pharmacotherapy for Agitation in Patients with Dementia

The manifestation of catastrophic stress in patients with dementia is often an attempt to flee or a sign of fear. Often nonmedication approaches are sufficient and there are no Food and Drug Administration–approved medications for agitation in dementia. The American Psychiatric Association *Practice Guideline on the Use of Antipsychotics to Treat Agitation or Psychosis in Patients with Dementia* suggests restricting use of antipsychotics to individuals with dangerous agitation or psychosis (Reus et al., 2015; Reus et al., 2016). Since the 1987 Nursing Home Reform Act, the use of "chemical restraints" has been banned in nursing home care. The new extension to all care has been caused by the Black Box warning placed on antipsychotics due to the risk of QTc prolongation and Torsade de Pointe and a 1.8 times higher all-cause death rate compared to placebo in the studies of antipsychotics in Alzheimer's psychosis. Although the actual numbers of individuals affected is quite low, they do call for caution. The guideline recommends first assessing patients for the type, frequency, severity, pattern, and timing of symptoms. Severe aggression, risk of harm, or continuous symptoms often benefit from antipsychotics. Mild psychotic symptoms and benign hallucinations of seeing and talking to dead relatives, who may be comforting, often are better untreated. In addition, it is prudent to obtain a baseline EKG and repeat it annually to check QTc. Caution is usually exercised for QTc >450msec. The other caveat regarding medication choice is using the lowest effective dose and avoiding benzodiazepines and sedating antihistamines if possible (AGS American Geriatrics Society 2015 Beers Crieteria Update Expert Panel, 2015).

Psychotherapy

Although data on psychotherapy of stress disorders in the elderly is still sparse and anecdotal, clinical experience suggests treatment strategies that can benefit those with major neurocognitive disorders.

Cognitively Intact Elderly

After an acute trauma, patients must be reassured that what they are experiencing is common (normalize) and may need brief cognitive restructuring therapy to address themes in Box 9.1.

Persisting Symptoms

The *VA/DoD Clinical Practice Guideline for Management of Post-Traumatic Stress* (VA/DoD Post-Traumatic Stress Management Working Group, 2010) summarizes several evidence-based psychotherapeutic interventions, but these studies have not been compared head to head, lack a common treatment terminology, and have not

BOX 9.1. TYPES OF DISTORTIONS ADDRESSED IN COGNITIVE-RESTRUCTURING THERAPY

1. Catastrophizing and expecting the worst
2. Believing one is helpless and incapacitated
3. Rumination
4. Avoidance—I don't have time to think about this now
5. Self-Blame—I can't do anything right

Skills to Teach: Relaxation exercises (e.g. deep breathing or mindfulness)

been specifically studied in the aged. In general, the two categories of treatment are stress inoculation training or exposure and trauma-focused psychotherapies such as cognitive restructuring. Mindfulness-based approaches have often been viewed as preparatory to any therapy but may be a treatment in itself for this disorder. Mindfulness-based approaches may be more useful with the elderly, in part because the core beliefs underlying treatment (Box 9.2) fit what Meeks and Jeste (2009) have described as components of "wisdom."

There are many mindfulness-based treatments. Dialectical behavior therapy is one of the earlier models, with four skill modules—mindfulness skills, interpersonal effectiveness skills, emotion regulation skills, and distress tolerance skills. Mindfulness skills include not judging feelings as good or bad, not judging how one "should" feel, focusing on being able to describe an event, its effects and causes, and being flexible to accept things that are different from what one expected (Linehan, 2015).

Case Example

Mr. M is a 70-year-old Vietnam vet with chronic PTSD, depression, and war injuries. He was cognitively intact and others often commented on his youthful appearance. Like many vets with PTSD, he had never been in full remission. Before involvement in a mindfulness -based treatment, he spent most of his day bitter and angry about the thought that his sacrifice "ruined his life" and meant nothing to the people he fought for. He denied being depressed but felt just angry and bitter. He did not show significant neurovegetative features of depression. He enjoyed nothing and

BOX 9.2. CORE BELIEFS OF MINDFULNESS

1. A large part of psychological suffering is due to attempts to avoid internal negative experience (experiential avoidance).
2. Persons must accept themselves as they are, not how they wish things were or wish they could be.
3. Rather than teach people to try to better control their thoughts, feelings, sensations, and other private events, it is better to teach them to notice and accept them.
4. Acceptance is not resignation or passivity. It is just the first step to clarify values and increase psychological flexibility and take action in a constructive manner rather than avoid or react with rage.
5. Mindful awareness allows one to cope better rather than remain preoccupied with the past.

GOALS OF TREATMENT

1. Increase ability to focus attention
2. Improve ability to detach from thoughts, images, and sensations
3. Decrease reactivity to mental events
4. Avoid pushing away experiences or holding on to experiences
5. Be content with oneself and life, even in bad circumstances

Adapted from Linehan, 2015.

felt he could never be satisfied until he could be free from pain. He had been in exposure therapies in the past and felt they were countertherapeutic, making his symptoms worse. Mindfulness-based treatment, however, made more intuitive sense to him. Instead of trying to learn how to better control thoughts, feelings, sensations, and memories or avoid them, he learned to accept his current situation, to self-observe without needing to react, and to focus instead on improving interpersonal effectiveness and distress tolerance skills.

Cognitively Impaired Elderly

Encoding new memories is reduced. Reaction to trauma seems to be more "instinctive"—fight (aggression), flight (avoidance), or becoming immobilized. Memories of new traumatic events are very short-lived. If the individual is made to feel safe and protected, reactions are often minimal. Basic management approaches for agitation in dementia are listed in Box 9.3.

A systematic review of the effectiveness of nonpharmacological interventions for the management of neuropsychiatric symptoms indicated efficacy of interventions that address behavioral issues and unmet needs. Interventions included actions by caregivers and bright light therapy (Ayalon et al., 2006).

PREVENTION

There is significant risk of TRSDs, comorbid disorders, and complications to existing illness when caretakers fail to protect elders. Elders in community living, assisted living, and nursing homes are dependent on caretakers, institutions, the law, and Medicare and Medicaid regulations for protection and for help in responding to emergencies (Centers for Medicare and Medicaid Services, 2006). Fires in long-term care facilities are common although there are few deaths. Hurricane Katrina brought the problem of vulnerable elders to the fore in New Orleans, but it is far broader than this with increased elders in elder care facilities, and it is an international problem also. Studies have examined emergency preparedness of long-term care facilities (Code of Federal Regulations, 2001) and evacuation plans of nursing homes. Castle (2008) evaluated written emergency plans, staff training, written evacuation plans, and fire drills and concluded that evacuation routes was the least well addressed area, but few nursing homes received deficiency citations for this. A recent report identified the need for improvements in nursing home comprehensive emergency preparedness and response (Department of Health and Human Services, 2014). Lane et al. (2016) found progress in many tasks or overall planning and sheltering in place but deficiencies in evacuation standards, interfacing with emergency management officials, establishing back-up evacuation sites and routes, identifying resident care items, and obtaining copies of state and local emergency planning regulations. Others have noted inadequate backup supplies of medications (Eiring et al., 2012). Greater attention to these serious issues will protect elders in long-term care facilities and reduce the risk of TSRDs resulting from inadequate care in the event of emergencies affecting the facilities.

BOX 9.3. GENERAL TREATMENT APPROACH

Stimulus reduction / Remove the threat
Distraction (change the subject, engage in a positive activity)
Behavior modification (praise and reward good behaviors; do not punish bad behaviors)
Reassurance and support (should be from a trusted and familiar person)
Understand the meaning of nonverbal communication (what the patient wants to convey)

Adapted from Sakauye, 2008.

SUMMARY

More than 50% of elderly persons have experienced a potential trauma at some point in their lives. When trauma has occurred earlier in life, it has a greater potential to cause PTSD or other impairment and leads to a chronic disorder in about one-fourth of individuals. When the trauma occurs later in life, the person is often more resilient than younger persons. This does not apply to frail elderly or those with dementia who have always been considered the highest risk for injury resulting from trauma. In the absence of specific age-related data, there are general medication guidelines that apply to the elderly of avoiding medications that have the highest risk for elderly, starting at about one-half the usual starting dose, and titrating more slowly. The reason for caution is mainly from age-related pharmacokinetic effects and concomitant drug-drug interactions. For the elderly, mindfulness-based psychotherapy approaches may be the most useful, emphasizing wisdom, flexibility, and resilience. For frail elderly, establishing a predictable and safe environment with an immediate support network that the person feels safe in is paramount.

REFERENCES

Acierno R, Hernandez MA, Amstadter AB, et al. (2010). Prevalence and correlates of emotional, physical, sexual, and financial abuse and potential neglect in the United States: The National Elder Mistreatment Study. *American Journal of Public Health*, 100:292–297.

American Geriatrics Society 2015 Beers Criteria Update Expert Panel. (2015). American Geriatrics Society 2015 Updated Beers Criteria for Potentially Inappropriate Medication Use in the Elderly. *JAGS*, 63:2227–2246.

American Psychiatric Association. (2013). *Diagnostic and statistical manual of mental disorders* (5th ed). Washington, DC: American Psychiatric Publishing.

Ayalon L, Gum AM, Feliciano L, Arean PA. (2006). Effectiveness of nonpharmacological interventons for the management of neurpsychiatric symptoms in patients with dementia. *Archives of Internal Medicine*, 166:2182–2188.

Beristianos MM, Maguen S, Neylan TC, Byers AL. (2016). Trauma exposure and risk of suicidal ideation among older adults. *American Journal of Geriatric Psychiatry*, 24:639–643.

Bonanno GA, Mancini A. (2012). Beyond resilience and PTSD: Mapping the heterogeneity of responses to potential trauma. *Psychological Trauma: Theory, Research, Practice, and Policy*, 4:74–83.

Castle NG. (2008). Nursing home evacuation plans. *American Journal of Public Health*, Jul;98(7):1235–1240. doi:10.2105/AJPH.2006.107532.

Centers for Medicare and Medicaid Services. (2006). Survey & certification: Emergency preparedness checklist recommended tool for effective health care facility planning. Retrieved from https://www.cms.gov/medicare/provider-enrollment-and-certification/surveycertemergprep/downloads/sandc_epchecklist_provider.pdf.

Code of Federal Regulations. (2001). Title 42: Public Health 483.75(m) F518(1). Public Health Requirements for States and Long-Term Care Facilities: Administration. Retrieved from http://www.ecfr.gov/cgi-bin/text-idx?rgn=div5&node=42:5.0.1.1.2#se42.5.483_175

Cooper C, Selwood A, Livingston G. (2008). The prevalence of elder abuse and neglect: A systematic review. *Age & Ageing*, 37:151–160.

Department of Health and Human Services, Centers for Medicare and Medicaid Services. (2014). Memorandum to State Survey Agency Directors. February 28. Retrieved from http://www.cms.gov/Medicare/Provider-Enrollment-and-Certification/Survey CertificationGenInfo/Downloads/Survey-and-Cert-Letter-14-12.pdf

Eiring H, Blake SC, Howard DH. (2012). Nursing homes' preparedness plans and capabilities. *American Journal of Disaster Medicine*, 7(2):127–135.

First, M. W. (2015). *Structured Clinical Interview for DSM-5 Disorders—Clinician Version (SCID-5-CV)*. Arlington, VA: American Psychiatric Association Publishing.

Fitzgerald PJ, Giustino TF, Seemanna JR, Maren S. (2015). Noradrenergic blockade stabilizes prefonrtal activity and enables fear extinction under stress. *PNAS*, E3729–E3737. Advance online publication. http://www.pnas.org/content/112/28/E3729.full.pdf

Giustino TF, Fitzgerald PJ, Maren S. (2016). Revisiting propranolol and PTSD: Memory erasure or extinction enchancement? *Neurobiology of Learning and Memory*, 130:26–33.

Goldberg J, Magruder KM, Forsberg CW. (2016). Prevalence of post-traumatic stress disorder in aging Vietnam-Era veterans: Veterans Administration Cooperative Study 569: Course and consequences of post-traumatic stress disorder in Vietnam-era veteran twins. *American Journal of Geratric Psychiatry*, 24:181–191.

Jeste DV, Palmer BW, Rettew DC, Boardman S. (2015). Positive psychiatry: Its time has come. *Journal of Clinical Psychiatry*, 76:675–683.

Kaiser AP, Wang J, Davison EH, Park CL, Stellman JM. (2017). Stressful and positive experiences of women who served in Vietnam. *Journal of Women & Aging*, 29:26–38.

Kang S, Aldwin CM, Choun S, Spiro AA. (2016). A life-span perspective on combat exposure and PTSD symptoms in later life: Findings from the VA Normative Aging Study. *The Gerontogist*, 56:22–32.

Lane SJ, McGrady E. (2016). Nursing home self-assessment of implementation of emergency preparedness standards. *Prehospital and Disaster Medicine*, Aug;31(4):422–431. doi:10.1017/S1049023X16000492. PMID:27212562

Laumann EO, Leitsch SA, Waite LJ. (2008). Elder mistreatment in the United States: Prevalence estimates from a nationally representative study. *The Journals of Gerontology. Series B, Psychological Sciences and Social Sciences*, 63:S248–S254.

Linehan, M. (2015). *DBT skills training manual*, 2nd ed. New York: Guilford Press.

Marmar CR, Schlenger W, Henn-Haase C, et al. (2015). Course of posttraumatic stress disorder 40 years after the Vietnam War: Findings From the National Vietnam Veterans Longitudinal

Study. *Journal of the American Medical Association*, 72:875–881.

Meeks TW, Jeste DV. (2009). Neruobiology of wisdom: A literature review. *Archives of General Psychiatry*, 66:355–365.

National Center for PTSD. (2015). *National Center for PTSD white paper: Use of benzodiazepines for PTSD in VA*. Washington, DC: Department of Veterans Affairs/Department of Defense.

Palmer BW, Raskind MA. (2016). Posttraumatic stress disorder and aging. *American Journal of Geriatric Psychiatry*, 24:177–180.

Ramirez S, Liu X, Lin P-A, et al. (2013). Creating a false memory in the hippocampus. *Science*, 341:387–391.

Rauch SA, Morales KH, Zubritsky C, Knott K, Oslin D. (2006). Posttraumatic stress, depression, and health among older adults in primary care. *American Journal of Geriatric Psychiatry*, Apr;14(4):316–324.

Reus VI, Fochtmann LJ, Eyler AE, et al. (2015). *The American Psychiatric Association practice guideline on the use of antipsychotics to treat agitation or psychosis in patients with dementia*. Arlington, VA: American Psychiatric Association. Retrieved from psychiatryonline.org/doi/pdf/10.1175/appi.books.9780890426807

Reus VI, Fochtmann LJ, Eyler AE, et al. (2016). The American Psychiatric Association practice guideline on the use of antipsychotics to treat agiation or psychosis in patients with dementia. *American Journal of Psychiatry*, 173:543–546.

Sakauye K. (2008). *Geriatric psychiatry basics*. New York: W.W. Norton.

Sakauye KM, Streim JE, Kennedy GJ, et al. (2009). AAGP position statement: disaster preparedness for older Americans: Critical issues for the preservation of mental health. *American Journal of Geriatric Psychiatry*, 17:916–924.

Siskind DJ, Sawyer E, Lee I, et al. (2016). The mental health of older adults post human-induced disaster. *American Journal of Geriatric Psychiatry*, 24(5):379–388.

Spitzer C, Barnow S, Völzke H, John U, Freyberger HJ, Grabe HJ. (2008). Trauma and posttraumic stress disorder in the elderly: Findings from a German community study. *Journal of Clinical Psychiatry*, 69:693–700.

Sue DW, Capodilupo CM, Torino GC, et al. (2007). Racial microaggressions in everyday life: Implications for clinical practice. *American Psychologist*, 62:271–286.

VA Pharmacy Benefits Management Services, Medical Advisory Panel, VISN Pharmacist Executives. (2012, June). *Alpha-blocker combination therapy in PTSD and BPH: Recommendations for use*. Retrieved from www.pbm.va.gov.

VA/DoD Post-Traumatic Stress Management Working Group. (2010). *VA/DoD clinical practice guideline for management of post-traumatic stress*. Washington, DC: Department of Veterans Affairs and Department of Defense.

Vaillant G. (2012). *Triumphs of experience*. New York: Belknap Press.

Vergne D. (2014, September 24). How the brain responds to trauma. *Medscape*. Retrieved from www.medscape.com/viewarticle/831940_print

Vijg JC. (2015). *Molecular and cellular biology of aging*. Washington, DC: Gerontological Society of America.

10

Population Trauma

Disasters

FREDERICK J. STODDARD JR., ROBERT J. URSANO, AND STEPHEN J. COZZA

INTRODUCTION

Disaster is defined by the World Health Organization (1992) as "a severe disruption, ecological and psychosocial, which greatly exceeds the coping capacity of the affected community." Each disaster is unique, and some are preventable while others are not. For instance, while a shooting may be preventable, an earthquake or hurricane is not. Some are human-made such as a terrorist event, while others are due to natural events. Humanitarian emergencies are also a class of disasters. Since most but not all people and communities are resilient, the prevalence of trauma- and stressor-related disorders after disaster and what interventions are optimal is highly relevant to disaster recovery. Figure 10.1 illustrates an intervention pyramid from basic services and security, to specialized services, for mental health and psychosocial support in humanitarian emergencies.

Despite severe disasters such as the nuclear reactor disaster at Chernobyl in 1986, the Armenian earthquake of 1988 and the Southeast Asian tsunami of 2004, there has historically been limited focus on disaster research. Governments have primarily focused on continuity of operations. That changed in the United States with 9/11. The period since the attacks of September 11, 2001, has advanced the fields of disaster psychiatry, psychology (Watson et al., 2011) and mental health, and disaster medicine from a limited research literature to one which addresses issues of disaster global health and mental health (Katz et al., 2002; Pandya & Katz, 2004; Ursano, 2002; Stoddard & Katz, 2010; Stoddard, 2014; Cozza et al., 2014; Ursano, Fullerton, Weisaeth, & Raphael, 2017; Katz & Pandya, 2013; Ciottone & Biddinger, 2015). Disaster mental health is now the subject of extensive writing, with new research and many publications focused on natural disasters (Neria, Galea, & Norris, 2009); violence, especially the attacks of 9/11 (Neria et al., 2006); bioterrorism (Ursano et al., 2004; Hyams, 2002), nuclear terrorism (Institute of Medicine, 2009); cyberterrorism (Harries & Yellowlees, 2013; Albahar, 2017); treatment guidelines for posttraumatic stress disorder (PTSD; Foa et al., 2009); interventions (Ursano, Fullerton, & Norwood, 2003; Ritchie, Watson, & Friedman, 2006); resilience (Blumenfield & Ursano, 2008; Brenner, Bush, & Moses, 2010; Southwick & Charney, 2012); international disaster mental health and mental health research methods (Norris et al., 2006); and considerations of triage and surge capacity. Due to the scope of the topic, this chapter is only a brief introduction to the broad and evolving area of disaster mental health and psychosocial preparations and responses with particular focus on mental disorders and resilience (Ursano, Fullerton, Raphael, & Weisaeth 2017; Stoddard, Pandya, & Katz, 2011). Wars are themselves a type of human-made disaster. Wars frequently result in vast numbers of deaths or people who must flee their homes, such as the Syrian refugees, exceeding the numbers affected by natural or other human-made disasters. Climate change and its associated increase in natural disasters is also expected to add to the toll of disaster related behavioral health problems (Figure 10.2, Box 10.1) (Dodgen et al., 2016).

PTSD and depression are the most common outcomes after disaster, with a prevalence of 30% to 40% of disaster survivors with PTSD and similarly high rates of depression (Neria et al., 2008; Goldman & Galea, 2014; Flory & Yehuda, 2015). Governments have a central role in preparing and educating their populations, training those in public service, and establishing regulations,

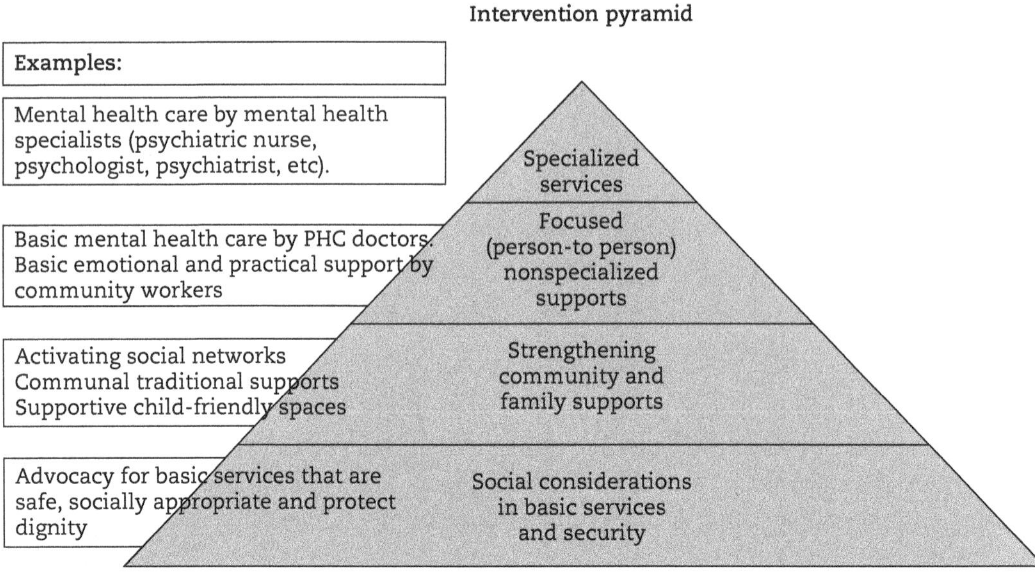

FIGURE 10.1. Intervention pyramid for mental health and psychosocial support in humanitarian emergencies. (IASC Reference Group for Mental Health and Psychosocial Support in Emergency Settings, What Should Humanitarian Health Actors Know? 2010, p. 3)

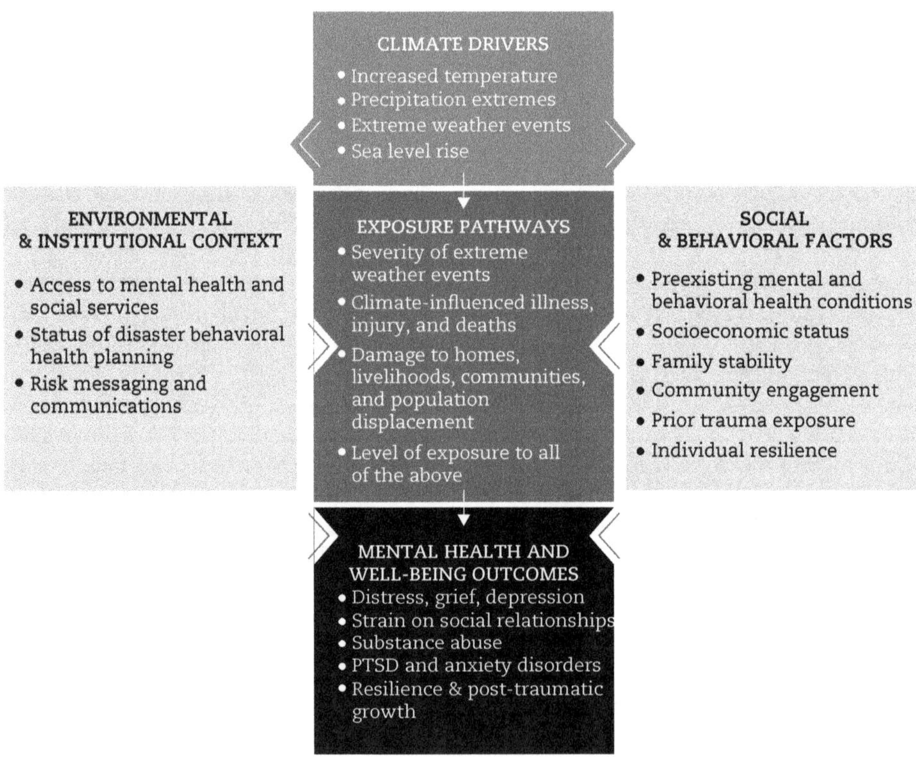

FIGURE 10.2. Diagram illustrating the key pathways by which humans are exposed to health threats from climate drivers and potential mental health and well-being outcomes. (US Global Change Research Program, 2016)

BOX 10.1. FOUR KEY FINDINGS FROM THE US GLOBAL CHANGE RESEARCH PROGRAM ON MENTAL HEALTH AND WELL-BEING (2016)

1. Exposure to disaster results in mental health consequences.
2. Specific groups of people are at high risk: children, the elderly, women (especially pregnant and postpartum women), people with pre-existing mental illness, the economically disadvantaged, the homeless, and first responders.
3. Climate change threats result in mental health consequences and social impacts.
4. Extreme heat increases risks for people with mental illness: higher risk for poor health with increased risk of disease and death for people with mental illness, including elderly and those taking prescription medications that impair the body's ability to regulate temperature.

policies, and procedures for possible disasters (Myers & Zunin, 2000). In addition, international policies and procedures are available through the World Health Organization (WHO). The WHO's (2013) "Emergency Response Framework" states:

> WHO's Member States face a broad range of emergencies resulting from various hazards and differing in scale, complexity and international consequences. These emergencies can have extensive political, economic, social and public health impacts, with potential long-term consequences sometimes persisting for years after the emergency. They may be caused by natural disasters, conflict, disease outbreaks, food contamination, or chemical or radio-nuclear spills, among other hazards. They can undermine decades of social development and hard-earned health gains, damage hospitals and other health infrastructure, weaken health systems and slow progress towards the Millennium Development Goals (MDGs). Preparing for and responding effectively to such emergencies are among the most pressing challenges facing the international community.

PREPAREDNESS

Preparedness for disaster varies greatly and is often based on how recent and frequent a nation experiences disasters. Coordination improves in response to lessons learned in real time and with disaster drills or tabletop exercises. The media can play an important preventive role for populations anticipating or responding to disasters, including epidemics such as Ebola or influenza (Centers for Disease Control and Prevention, 2015a,b), by providing constructive guidance informed by the principles of risk communication, which highlight "accurate timely helpful information, and minimizing information which may increase fear and anxiety"(Center for Mental Health Services, 2010; Stoddard, 2011; Centers for Disease Control and Prevention, 2017); alternatively, the media can increase fear and feelings of unsafety. In the past 20 years, long-term research studies have been conducted in the United States and internationally, providing lessons learned, improved guidance, and factors affecting the outcomes of survivors. While most individuals exposed to a disaster do not develop a trauma- or stressor-related disorder, some do, and in some disasters this includes a sizeable number of those directly exposed. Alternatively, exposed individuals may develop another disorder or behavioral risk behaviors—such as depression or increased substance use—or they may manifest resilience with posttraumatic growth (Charney, 2004).

HOW COMMUNITIES COPE

Important factors influencing how communities cope with disasters are whether there has been planning, preparation, and training for responders; whether there is community leadership (Reissman et al., 2005); and whether media responses aid members of the community in receiving accurate information and helpful guidance before, after, and long term. Underlying local community responses can be more beneficial than outside rescue operations, particularly over the longer term, as seen in the capacity for self-organization of local communities after the 2009 L'Aquila earthquake in central Italy (Imperiale & Vanclay, 2016). Resources related to disaster preparation, training, and responding are available at some websites (TRACIE, 2017) and include important information for leaders and emergency responders, as well as tools for planning and guidance, resources for self-care, and disaster behavioral health training opportunities. Mental health resources for leaders, employers, schools, parents, responders, and researchers for disasters are also available from the websites of the American Psychiatric Association, the American Academy of Child and Adolescent Psychiatry, the American Psychological Association, the National Association of Social Work, the American Red Cross, the Center for the Study of Traumatic Stress, the National Center for PTSD, and the Child Traumatic Stress Network.

HOW MASS TRAUMA AND STRESS AFFECT POPULATIONS

Recent disasters illustrate how severely traumatic and stressful events affect populations. In 1986, the Chernobyl nuclear disaster affected thousands, and its psychological and physical health effects on adults and children (Bromet, 2014) have persisted despite efforts to prevent them (Lucchini et al., 2017). In 1995, the Alfred P. Murrah Federal Building in Oklahoma City was truck-bombed by domestic terrorists who opposed the government, killing 168 people and injuring over 680 others. Subsequent research made clear that *proximity* to the site of the blast was associated with more PTSD and PTSD symptoms. The coordinated attacks by al-Qaeda on the World Trade Center (WTC) in 2001 with hijacked airplanes killed 2,996 people and injured over 6,000 others. This method and scale of attack was unexpected, and there was not preparation to prevent or fully respond to it. In 2010, the Haiti earthquake killed approximately 300,000 people with an equal number injured and over a million displaced, an event so traumatic that the country has still not fully recovered. As a result, Haiti and its people are more vulnerable to future disasters because of the earthquake's colossal cost of human life, the toll on the resilience of survivors, and destruction of infrastructure (Farmer, 2011). In 2011 in Japan, the Fukishima earthquake, tsunami, and the secondary Fukishima Daiichi nuclear disaster led the government to recommend that people evacuate from coastal areas. While a few people were seriously injured, no subsequent deaths occurred—indicating the moderate success of secondary prevention efforts after this huge disaster. However, rates of distress and PTSD were high and persistent; rates of PTSD decreased from 19% to 17.8% over three years for men and from 25.3% to 23.3% for women. Problem drinking remained steady for men at 20.4% over three years, as well as for women at 10.5%. These results indicate the need for *long-term interventions* post-disaster due to persistence of posttraumatic and other symptomatology (Oe et al., 2017).

Children

The impact of disasters on infants, children, and adolescents is likely to be stressful and may result in traumatic reactions in some, while for others, especially those with family and community support and resources, it can evoke resilience and lead to posttraumatic growth (La Greca et al., 2005). In high-income countries, mental health resources (including child and adolescent psychiatry) are more likely to become available soon after a disaster, compared with lower and middle-income countries where such resources are often scarce (Shibley & Stoddard, 2011). Evidence-based or promising practices, some applicable to all ages of children, are recommended by the National Child Traumatic Stress Network (www.nctsn.org). The first of these is *Psychological First Aid (PFA) for Children,* the goals of which includes contact and engagement, safety and comfort, stabilization, information gathering about current needs and concerns, practical assistance, connection with social supports, information on coping, and linkage with collaborative services (Brymer et al., 2006).

PFA for children differs from adult PFA in being more developmentally focused, and provides information for parents and providers to help them better understand and support children after a disaster. While initial efforts should focus on ensuring safety and securing food, water, shelter, and first aid to the survivors, developmentally targeted interventions are also essential (Gurwitch et al., 2002; Schreiber & Gurwitch, 2006; Allen et al., 2010), including reuniting children with their parents in a timely manner. Similar to adults, there are no data to support critical incident stress debriefing for children as the potential risks of exposing children to peers with extreme emotional responses and experiences outweigh potential benefits (Cohen et al., 2006).

It is very important that responders feel comfortable with children, listen to what they say, and attend to their nonverbal actions and behaviors since children usually express their feelings nonverbally. Key areas to observe are changes in sleep, appetite, play, mood, physical complaints, school achievement, and peer interactions. It is helpful to provide time and space for them to share feelings or stories through play, and they should never be forced to share thoughts or feelings. Parents and teachers should be educated regarding typical post-disaster behaviors and reactions of very young and older children and adolescents. These typically include regression and clinginess, oppositional behaviors, or disinhibition. Children should be told about the disaster and what is being done to keep them safe in language that is understandable and at a level that is developmentally appropriate. Young children have egocentric thoughts and need to be reassured that they are not to blame for the disaster or any resultant destruction or distress. Children look to adults on how to cope and behave, and first responders should encourage families to reestablish routines and model healthy coping. Decreasing distress and uncertainty and increasing constructive activities, hope, and resilient coping enhances recovery. Assuring connection or re-connection with their families and social supports is essential if at all possible. When they cannot rejoin their families, it is important to reassure them that responsible adults will care for them (Cohen et al., 2006). Supportive caregivers foster resilience reducing risk of developing PTSD symptoms. School is often a part of the nurturing recovery environment. Parental psychopathology and poor family functioning increase risk for psychological sequelae (Pine & Cohen, 2002). Parental protection and presence during and after the disaster and resilient parental reactions are critical protective factors (Masten et al., 1990; Laor & Wolmer, 2007). Many children, both girls and boys, are at increased risk of violence and abuse in disasters communities when displaced from their homes and families, especially when limited community resources are available to protect them (Sloand et al., 2017).

Skills for Psychological Recovery (SPR) is a selective/indicated prevention model utilizing skills-building components found helpful to adults and children later, after many posttrauma situations including disasters. SPR incorporates a range of assessments and interventions that may promote healthy recovery after PFA and in those that require greater support months after a disaster event.

Post-disaster school based responses are also important. Schools are trusted environments in the lives of children, therefore schools play an important role in children's post-disaster recovery (Klingman A 1993). Similarly, teachers are trusted adults in the lives of children who are uniquely engaged with children and can supplement the efforts of parents or other caring adults in supporting children's recovery. Traumatized and grieving parents may not be reliable reporters of children's mental health, often cannot or do not obtain evaluation for their children, and may not be able to give the support children require (Stoddard & Menninger, 2004). As a result, many children do not receive interventions from which they could benefit (Cohen et al., 2006). Mental health screening at schools can detect children who would not have been identified, and schools can be centers for post-disaster interventions. Health professionals should meet with teachers to ensure that they are adjusting well, recovering from their own traumatic exposures, and are prepared to reestablish classroom order and structure and meet the needs of children. The mental health team should aid teachers in addressing students' responses by providing psychoeducation about normal responses, modeling healthy coping, instilling self-efficacy and hope, expecting return to normalcy, and identifying children who need evaluation or treatment (Laor & Wolmer, 2007; Schreiber & Gurwitch, 2006). School interventions can be targeted to the entire class or to smaller groups of at-risk children (Klingman, 1993). One example includes a class activation program with a parent session that involves eight two-hour sessions on safety, psychoeducation, emotions after death and disaster, and future planning and which incorporates therapeutic techniques such as cognitive behavioral therapy (CBT), psychoeducation, and play. The result was reduced child dissociation and posttraumatic symptoms and improved adaptation three years later (Wolmer et al., 2003; Wolmer et al., 2005). Practitioners should remember that schools may be directly impacted by disasters, either disrupted or destroyed (e.g., after earthquakes in China and Haiti), making school-based post-disaster programming problematic or impossible.

Child and Adolescent Post-Disaster Treatment

Brief supportive therapy is one form of treatment. While most children and adolescents are resilient and respond well to the natural support systems in their families and communities, a minority require more specialized mental health treatment (Cohen et al., 2006). Children and adolescents with continued distress should be enrolled in a brief crisis-oriented supportive psychotherapy for, typically, one to six sessions. The intervention should be culturally informed and focus on psychoeducation, relaxation exercises, cognitive reframing, problem-solving, and coping mechanisms such as distraction, physical activities, and social activities (Goenjian et al., 1997).

A randomized study comparing meditation and relaxation to narrative exposure therapy in Sri Lanka after the tsunami revealed that both brief six session treatments were effective (Catani et al., 2009). This study is noteworthy as it targeted children already traumatized secondary to the civil war and other disasters.

Cognitive-behavioral therapies are also important. Children who demonstrate sustained PTSD symptoms despite early supportive interventions or brief treatment require formal psychotherapy. CBT has the largest evidence base and has been used in both individual and group formats, including school programs (Wethington et al., 2008). Treatment protocols typically last 10 to 16 weeks. Chemtob et al. (2002) described a decrease in child PTSD symptoms in a randomized controlled trial of CBT for individuals and groups compared to a control group. Goenjian et al. (1997) studied Armenian adolescents following a major earthquake, comparing trauma and grief-focused CBT with no intervention. The control group had worsening PTSD and depression and the treatment group improved in PTSD but had no change in depression. Several evidence-based CBT treatments have been developed and are relevant to the post-disaster treatment of children, including trauma-focused CBT (TF-CBT), Cognitive Behavioral Intervention for Trauma in Schools (CBITS), trauma systems therapy (TST), and parent–child interaction therapy (PCIT), and they are described here.

Trauma-focused cognitive-behavioral therapy (TF-CBT) is a specialized CBT treatment effective in trauma survivors (Cohen et al., 2006). It addresses the multiple domains of trauma impact including but not limited to PTSD, depression, anxiety, externalizing behavior problems, relationship and attachment problems, school problems, and cognitive problems. It includes skills for regulating affect, behavior, thoughts and relationships, trauma processing, and enhancing safety, trust, parenting skills, and family communication. It focuses on reconstructing the traumatic experience to desensitize the child and achieve mastery over the situation. It consists of psychoeducation, stress management and relaxation exercises, affect identification and modulation, cognitive restructuring, exposure therapies such as trauma narratives and drawings, identification of themes such as guilt and revenge, conjoint child and family sessions, and enhancing safety (Cohen, Mannarino, & Deblinger, 2006). TF-CBT training is available online (https://tfcbt.musc.edu/).

Trauma systems therapy (TST; Saxe et al., 2015) is a comprehensive model for treating traumatic stress in children and adolescents that adds to individually based approaches by specifically addressing the child's social environment and/or system of care. TST was designed to provide an integrated and highly coordinated system of services guided by the specific understanding of the nature of child traumatic stress. Specifically, this model conceptualizes the development of a "trauma system," which is comprised of two main elements: (a) a traumatized child who is not able to regulate emotional states and (b) a social environment and/or system of care that is not sufficiently able to help the child contain this dysregulation. A "trauma system" thus emerges when a failure of the natural systemic balance between the developing child and his or her social environment occurs. Healthy development requires a regulatory balance or "goodness of fit" between the child and his or her social environment such that the social environment is properly equipped to help the child. When the child enters service systems, this goodness of fit includes the system of care, such as school or social services departments. Given the presence of a trauma system, the essence of TST is to help children gain control over emotions and behavior via enhancing their capacity to regulate emotion and diminishing the ongoing stresses and threats in the social environment. TST was also designed to build the capacity of significant others in children's environment to help them control their emotional and behavioral responses. TST is a phase-based model; as such, a dual assessment is conducted of both the youth's emotional/behavioral regulation and the stability of the social environment. Utilizing the TST assessment grid, the youth is assessed as being in one of five phases (surviving, stabilizing, enduring, understanding, transcending). The TST phase determines the appropriate interventions to use at the time of assessment. Interventions address the stability of both the youth and the environment.

Cognitive Behavioral Intervention for Trauma in Schools (CBITS) is a skills-based, child group intervention that is aimed at relieving symptoms of PTSD, depression, and general anxiety among children exposed to multiple forms of trauma (Morsette et al., 2009; Jaycox et al., 2010). One unique aspect of CBITS is the focus on trauma from the child's perspective. For those children who have multiple traumas, CBITS recommends that the child be the one to choose, with help from the clinician, which trauma will be the focus of cognitive behavioral treatment. Frequently, although a clinician will perceive one trauma to be the most salient for a child, the child will associate greater impact from another trauma. In addition to the group sessions, participants receive one to three individual sessions (Box 10.2), usually held before the exposure exercises. CBITS also includes two parent education sessions and one teacher education session.

Parent–child interaction therapy (PCIT; Funderburk et al., 2011) is an evidence-based treatment for young children with emotional and behavioral disorders that places emphasis on improving the quality of the parent–child relationship and changing parent–child interaction patterns. Children and their caregivers are seen together in PCIT. Most of the session time is spent coaching caregivers in the application of specific therapy skills. Therapists typically coach from an observation room with a one-way mirror into the playroom, using a "bug-in-the-ear" system for communicating to the parents as they play with their child. Concluding each session, therapist and caregiver together decide which skill to focus on most during daily five-minute home practice sessions the following week. PCIT is an intervention that may be particularly helpful to disaster-exposed and distressed younger children who could benefit from greater understanding and closer engagement from a supportive parent (Hood & Eyberg, 2003).

Play therapy is a non-CBT intervention that is widely taught and practiced in the treatment of younger children. Play therapy does not have a formal research base in treating traumatized children. In fact, evidence suggests that nondirected play in traumatized children offers little to no therapeutic benefit, particularly if traumatic content is avoided. However, play therapy is likely an effective adjunctive medium by which less verbal or nonverbal children can safely explore traumatic experiences and responses as part of evidence-based treatments. Through play, children can share the trauma in displacement and, with the help of a psychotherapist, gain a sense of mastery that was lacking in their real-life experience. For example, a child in a burns hospital at the time of 9/11 drew a picture of bodies falling from buildings, alerting curious and attentive nurses that she had witnessed images of the disaster on TV and which prompted them to request a child psychiatric consultation. Through interactive play therapy, clinicians can help children learn words to name and express feelings of pain, fear, and terror and interpret the child's feelings and thoughts in order to process anxiety and helplessness, gain a greater self-awareness, and learn healthy coping techniques (Terr, 1990; Ablon, 1996).

Children and adolescent psychopharmacology is also a consideration (see also Chapter 23: Pharmacologic Treatment of Children). Psychopharmacological agents are not the primary intervention recommended for young children after a disaster. Similarly, most older children do not require psychotropic medications acutely after a disaster because they respond well to therapeutic interventions and family support. There is little evidence to support the use of psychopharmacological agents for children acutely after a disaster. However, medications used for pre-existing conditions should be continued. Occasionally, children have acute distress such as insomnia that significantly interferes with functioning. A child may benefit from diphenhydramine for difficulty falling asleep in the days after a disaster (Donnelly, 2003; Disaster Psychiatry Outreach, 2008), but the starting dose should be low and monitored closely. In the weeks after a disaster selective serotonin reuptake inhibitors may be indicated if a child displays symptoms of severe persistent depression or anxiety (Donnelly, 2003). Sertraline, fluoxetine, and imipramine are agents which may be effective in inpatient medical settings for acute stress disorder, PTSD, and depression in children (Stoddard et al., 2006). Adrenergic agents such as clonidine and guanfacine are occasionally used for hyperarousal and impulsivity but must be given under close observation due to potential adverse side effects (Donnelly, 2003). If a child displays intense aggression, severe mood dysregulation, psychotic symptoms, or self-injurious behavior or is a threat to self or others, he or she should be evaluated for psychiatric hospitalization and safety precautions be instituted. Psychiatrists can

BOX 10.2. CBITS SIX COGNITIVE BEHAVIORAL TECHNIQUES

- Education about reactions to trauma
- Relaxation training
- Cognitive therapy
- Real-life exposure
- Stress or trauma exposure
- Social problem-solving

http://www.nctsn.org/sites/default/files/assets/pdfs/cbits_general.pdf

evaluate for off-label use of atypical antipsychotics for severe agitation such as risperidone, olanzapine, or aripiprazole, or in younger children diphenhydramine or low-dose benzodiazapines (Stoddard et al., 2006). Clinicians must be aware that children often present with inattention, hyperactivity, and high levels of distraction after a disaster. This is most likely a reaction to the disaster, not a new diagnosis of attention deficit hyperactivity disorder.

Care for Youth after Disasters in Lower and Middle-Income Countries

Resources are very limited in lower and middle-income countries (LMICs), and alternatives to well-funded national disaster relief programs must be found. Several authors address this problem directly, from somewhat different perspectives but with similar conclusions. None are optimistic that the task is easy to provide mental health interventions to children and adolescents in LMICs, and all take a human ecological perspective. Saltzman et al. (2003) describe the need to build capacity of local service providers and to foster indigenous supports in order to develop a postwar trauma and grief intervention program for adolescents in Bosnia and Herzogovina. Their model was effective in reducing posttraumatic stress, depression, and grief symptoms among adolescents in their program. They felt their approach might be appropriate for terrorist and mass casualty events internationally and domestically. Raviola et al. (2012) and Farmer (2011) explain how children are more vulnerable in a resource-poor country like Haiti and that after the 2010 earthquake long-term mental health interventions required close collaborations with Haitians and international organizations, in order to gradually develop health and mental health resources. de Jong et al. (2015) propose four strategies to respond to the "plight of youth" in situations of violence and humanitarian emergencies. They highlight that although children and adolescents are 50% of the population in LMICs, they receive fewer mental health services than adults. They propose (a) a participatory public health approach to youth, (b) a systems approach to collaboratively engage public and private resources, (c) health care professionals to translate pre-trauma needs assessment into mental health and psychosocial support, (d) alignment of programs and prevention toward curative interventions in the public health system, and (e) research on the gap of effective treatment practices for youth in the LMIC, children at the bottom of the social pyramid.

Refugees

The scale of adversities and trauma to displaced persons and refugees from natural and manmade disasters and war is often overwhelming and can be difficult to grasp. Their status as shown in the following box was recognized after World War I and was expanded after World War II.

Nations' Definition of Refugee

"Grounded in Article 14 of the Universal Declaration of Human Rights 1948, which recognizes the right of persons to seek asylum from persecution in other countries, the United Nations Convention relating to the Status of Refugees, adopted in 1951, is the centrepiece of international refugee protection today . . . The 1967 Protocol . . . gave the Convention universal coverage. It has since been supplemented . . . via the progressive development of international human rights law."

It defines a refugee as one who: "owing to well founded fear of being persecuted for reasons of race, religion, nationality, membership of a particular social group or political opinion, is outside the country of his nationality and is unable or, owing to such fear, is unwilling to avail himself of the protection of that country; or who, not having a nationality and being outside the country of his former habitual residence as a result of such events, is unable or, owing to such fear, is unwilling to return to it."

Convention and protocol relating to the status of refugees. Geneva: Office of the United Nations High Commissioner for Refugees, UN Refugee Agency, 2010.

http://www.unhcr.org/en-us/protection/basic/3b66c2aa10/convention-protocol-relating-status-refugees.html

---

The tragic displacement of populations from their homes and countries goes back to ancient times. As the world population increases, more children, adults, and elderly people will be impacted. Huge natural disasters such as drought, hurricanes, earthquakes, tsunamis displace millions of people. Millions of children and adults were affected during the American Civil War, and worldwide during World War I, World War II, and since then in Korea, Vietnam, Cambodia, Laos, the Balkans, Africa, and the Middle East, Haiti,

Syria, and other regions and countries. Many who are displaced are especially vulnerable. In addition to severe poverty, they experience chronic combined effects of separation from their families and home, starvation, rape and other violent attack, untreated injuries, and diseases including mental disorders (Lindert et al., 2016). Many are also victims of human rights violations, rights which are protected by the Universal Declaration of Human Rights, adopted by the United Nations General Assembly in 1948 (Box 10.3).

Tragically, despite the Universal Declaration, refugees continue to experience extreme trauma and suffering. Many child and adult refugees from war and genocide have experienced atrocities such as torture or witnessing murders or abuse of others including of their own families. The history of human suffering experienced and the failure of nations to come to the aid of refugees has only been partially improved by efforts of the United Nations, wealthy nations, and private organizations.

FACTORS INFLUENCING SUSCEPTIBILITY AND RESILIENCE

The susceptibility and resilience of populations to trauma and stress varies widely. Major determinants include preparedness, socioeconomic status, and history of prior trauma (Nomura et al., 2016). In some circumstances, populations have been affected by disasters in close proximity to an earlier event, retraumatizing the community. As individuals, children, women, the disadvantaged, minorities, and the seriously mentally ill possess greater susceptibility.

Children as well as adults may be affected by highly stressful images of the human impact of disasters, and mental health professionals recommend limiting media exposure to potential traumatic imagery after disasters. There is some evidence from studies of children after the Oklahoma City bombing in 1995 (Pfefferbaum et al., 2001) and of adults after the Boston Marathon bombing in 2013 that post-disaster media exposure is associated with increased acute stress symptoms. The latter study found significantly higher stress symptomatology from six or more hours of bombing-related media exposure than direct exposure (Holman & Garfin, 2014). Since media exposure is excluded in *Diagnostic and Statistical Manual of Mental Disorders* (fifth edition; DSM-5) from Criterion A for PTSD (except work-related) and acute stress disorder as a potential traumatic stressor, further research on this is merited. Stress reactions with impairment secondary to media exposure are classified as adjustment disorders.

Normal responses are present for the majority of individuals following disaster, particularly varying reactions to loss, distress, acute stress reactions, acute grief, resilient and altruistic behavior, and other types of posttraumatic growth. Figure 10.3 illustrates the phases of emotional responses to disasters are described as a pre-disaster "warning" phase, a heroic "impact" phase, a honeymoon phase of "community cohesion," followed by phases of disillusionment, working through grief, and reconstruction.

Psychopathology can occur acutely after disasters. New onset disorders can also be delayed. Acute disorders that may occur include panic, acute stress, acute depression, impulsivity due to

BOX 10.3. PREAMBLE TO THE UNIVERSAL DECLARATION OF HUMAN RIGHTS

Whereas recognition of the inherent dignity and of the equal and inalienable rights of all members of the human family is the foundation of freedom, justice and peace in the world,

Whereas disregard and contempt for human rights have resulted in barbarous acts which have outraged the conscience of mankind, and the advent of a world in which human beings shall enjoy freedom of speech and belief and freedom from fear and want has been proclaimed as the highest aspiration of the common people,

Whereas it is essential, if man is not to be compelled to have recourse, as a last resort, to rebellion against tyranny and oppression, that human rights should be protected by the rule of law.

http://www.un.org/en/universal-declaration-human-rights/

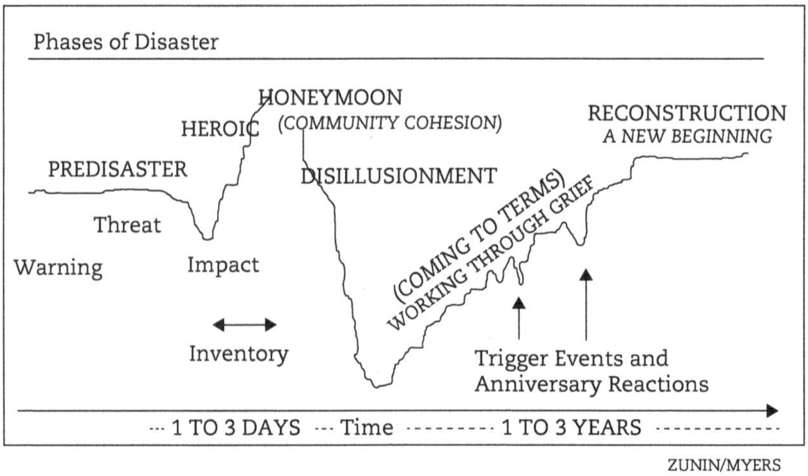

FIGURE 10.3. Phases of emotional response to disaster. (Myers and Zunin, 2000)

various disorders, substance use, suicidality, and an acute relapse of a preexisting mental illness including character disorders, such as borderline personality disorder or antisocial personality disorder. Postacute disorders and syndromes that have been carefully studied and found to occur weeks or months later include especially depression, PTSD, persistent complex bereavement disorder (traumatic grief), panic disorder, and substance-use disorders. Also present with major disasters are pain and suffering due to acute or long-term effects of injury. Of special interest are the factors conferring resilience to individuals and communities and which enhance the likelihood of posttraumatic emotional, interpersonal, and personal growth including the acquisition of new skills or competence. Such personal growth and development may occur for children, adolescents, adults, and the elderly and coexist with depression, PTSD, or other disorders and aid healing and recovery from them.

RESOURCES

Resources have a profound effect on response to disasters and the resilience of populations, their communities, and their nations, and each resource affects others. Resources include geographic location, human factors especially leadership and preparation, economic factors, systems infrastructure for response and recovery, and governmental factors including the political system. *Geographic location* may provide protection in the event of a disaster with proximity to emergency medical resources, or increased vulnerability such as the earthquake in 2010 in Haiti which lacked resources for early response and recovery from its long-term effects which were only partially made up by the huge international humanitarian response (Farmer, 2011). *Human factors* particularly entail planning, training, and readiness. Each of these involves varying groups from leaders to responders to citizens at large. Leadership, preparation, and training are key to limiting the degree of trauma exposure from disasters suffered by communities. Responsible leadership in government, business, and education anticipates risks, seeks to mitigate possible trauma from disasters, initiates constructive responses facilitates recovery, and informs and reassures the public. *Economic factors* affect all others. Preparations for early response and long-term recovery is usually greater in high-income countries. Disasters in LMIC are also often geographically remote from the limited assistance and vulnerable to disruptions in human, infrastructure, and political factors which might enhance resilience and recovery. *Systems infrastructure* for response and recovery affects how early and long-term responders function and how rapidly a population recovers. Communications are critical to a population at risk receiving early warning and accurate information during the disaster, and afterwards aiding recovery. When telephone, email, or Internet communications are inadequate or fail, responders are less able to coordinate their rescue and recovery efforts, and survivors and their families are less able to come together to support one another. If hospitals, schools, or offices are damaged, a return to normal may be impeded and there is risk of secondary traumatization due to lack of medical care, lost education, or economic losses. If modes of transportation are damaged, people cannot recover readily and return to normal activities such as work, school, or recreation. *Governmental factors* closely relate to human factors. National and local governmental structures such as a constitution, laws, executive, legislative and judicial branches, civil service, and funding for disaster relief help reestablish stability in the event of a disaster. As described in Chapter 19, the military often work together with emergency health and local public services as they are critical to maintaining and reestablishing public order and facilitating recovery.

Public Health and Mental Health

Luccini et al. (2017) assessed major international disasters including the industrial release of dioxin in Seveso, Italy, in 1976; the catastrophic nuclear accident in Chernobyl, Ukraine, in 1986; the terrorist attacks on the WTC, in Pennsylvania, and at the Pentagon on September 11, 2001; and the earthquake and tsunami leading to the Fukishima Daiichi nuclear disaster in 2011, to derive information for future preparedness and arrived at seven "lessons" (see Box 10.4). They simplified recommendations from prior work on preparedness such as that on psychological preparedness for terrorism by the Institute of Medicine (Butler et al., 2003).

The report by the Institute of Medicine (2003) committee "described interventions needed in the pre-event, event, and post-event phases. This report sought to limit the adverse psychological consequences of terrorism and to reduce the impact of any terrorist events by preparations which would facilitate growth and empowerment, minimize disruptions, and enhance community cohesion. This has special relevance because of the continuing terrorist threat and the possibility of intentional disaster caused by weapons of mass destruction requiring well planned psychiatric and overall public mental health preparation and responses (Stoddard, Gold et al., 2011). It, together with other writings, was a foundation for recommendations for exposure assessment, systematic emergency preparedness, and lifetime health care required after mass natural disasters or accidents as described by Lucchini et al. (2017).

> **BOX 10.4. LESSONS FOR FUTURE PREPAREDNESS FOR INTERNATIONAL DISASTERS**
>
> Lesson 1: Know who was there
> Lesson 2: Have public health input to the disaster response
> Lesson 3: Collect health and needs data rapidly
> Lesson 4: Take care of the affected
> Lesson 5: Emergency preparedness
> Lesson 6: Data driven, needs assessment, advocacy
>
> *Luccini et al. (2017)*

THE RANGE OF PSYCHOLOGICAL CONSEQUENCES OF DISASTERS

The range of psychological consequences of disasters shown in Figure 10.4 vary, with most individuals showing "normal" emotional or physiological reactions of distress (e.g., a sense of vulnerability or insomnia) but no abnormal reactions (such as increased substance use); these people are resilient in a disaster. Others manifest behavioral changes (e.g., increased smoking and alcohol use), while a minority develop psychiatric illness (e.g., major depression or PTSD). The three overlapping circles in the figure are intended to illustrate the breadth of behavioral changes after disaster and how these conditions may or may not overlap or coexist; that is, a person with insomnia and distress may go on to have PTSD later and also increase their use of alcohol and cigarettes, placing that individual in the center where the three circles overlap. There are other consequences of disasters of importance which may occur including acute stress disorder (Chapter 4), persistent complicated bereavement disorder or complicated grief (Chapter 6), as well as grief, pain and reactions to injury, panic disorder, bereavement, or personality disorder.

EARLY INTERVENTIONS

Early interventions involve initial mental health responses to a disaster, including via the media, through agency responses, and on-site interventions (Ritchie et al., 2006; Blumenfield & Ursano, 2008; O'Donnell et al., 2008). Evidence-informed PFA, a practical approach similar to physical first aid with similar goals, has largely replaced debriefing due to lack of evidence of the effectiveness of debriefing for adults (Center for Mental Health Services, 2002; Rose et al., 2009) or for children (Pfefferbaum et al., 2015).

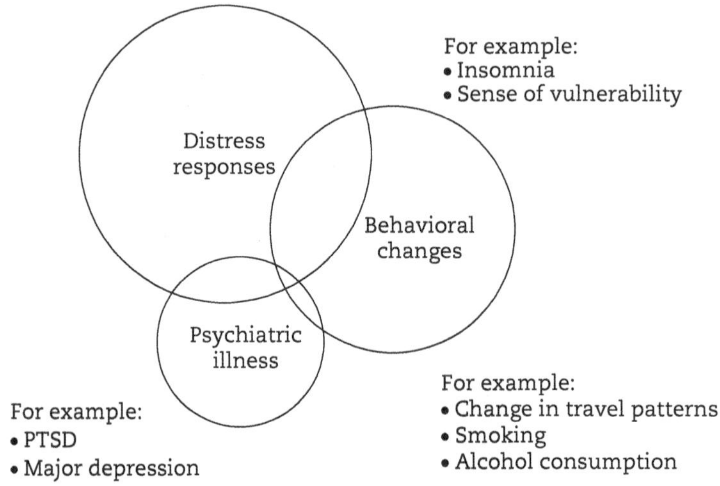

FIGURE 10.4. Psychological consequences of disaster and terrorism.

It is endorsed by key response agencies for early response to emotional needs of those affected by disaster and major traumatic events. The core elements of PFA are to establish contact and engagement, address basic needs for safety and comfort, provide stabilization, listen and gather information related to mental health needs and psychosocial issues, and provide reassurance and psychoeducation, practical information on coping and problem-solving, connection with social supports, and linkage to supports and formal services. (Kantor & Beckert, 2011; North & Pfefferbaum, 2013).

Mental Health Screening

Since disasters elicit a range of responses as evident in Figure 10.4, screening for mental health and illness responses should include a range of responses including those responding to distress, behavioral changes, and mental disorders. Emotional and behavioral responses to disasters and other stressors are not limited to PTSD. Screening in adults for *exposure* to stressful life events may be done with the Life Events Checklist for DSM-5 (Weathers et al., 2013), but this 17-item instrument does not specifically include acute grief or bereavement. Screening for *mental disorders* or *resilience* after disaster may be done with several instruments. Standard instruments for screening for mental disorders are the Kessler 6- or 10-item scales (Kessler et al., 2010; Stolk et al., 2014) and the General Health Questionnaire-28 item scale (GHQ-28; Goldberg & Hillier, 1979). For example, on the Kessler-6, the items for screening are nervous, hopeless, restless or fidgety, so depressed nothing could cheer one up, that everything is an effort, and either or both feeling worthless over one of two recall periods, the past month and the worst month. Chapter 19: Susceptibility, Resilience, and Trajectories includes instruments to screen for resilience. Screening for, evaluating, and seeking to strengthen resilience is of increasing importance in determining what is most helpful in both preventive and direct mental health services responses to reduce the impacts of traumatic stress (Charney, 2004).

Screening for PTSD and other trauma- and stressor-related disorders may include translations of the same instruments, the Kessler-6, or -10 which may have limitations (Stolk et al., 2014), and the GHQ-28, or others such as the Harvard Trauma Questionnaire developed to measure torture, trauma, and PTSD in Indochinese refugees (Mollica et al., 1992). An option for use in primary care is a multicomponent Health Information Technology screening tool for depression and PTSD, which are widely underdiagnosed, with four components: (a) web-based provider training, (b) multimedia electronic screening for depression and PTSD in the patient's language, (c) computer-generated risk assessment scores delivered to the provider, and (d) clinical decision support (Biegler et al., 2016).

Evidence-Based Interventions

Interventions for children and adolescents are briefly described earlier and in greater detail in Chapters 8, 21, and 23.

Acute, postacute, and long-term interventions for adults and the elderly are discussed in the chapters on psychotherapeutic and psychopharmacological treatment for adults and the elderly

(Chapters 8, 9, 19–25, and 28). Core established treatments for PTSD in adults include CBT, cognitive processing therapy, prolonged exposure therapy, eye movement desensitization and reprocessing, stress inoculation training, pharmacological treatment, complementary and alternative treatment, acceptance and commitment therapy, group treatment, couples treatment, PTSD coach, mindfulness, and telemental health interventions (U.S. Department of Veterans Affairs, 2017; Augusterfer et al., 2015). Many treatments in the other chapters are based on studies of stressors and trauma different from disasters and are largely the core evidence base applied for treatment after disasters when services are available, with the exception of interventions validated for disaster survivors. While this book addresses trauma- and stressor-related disorders, other disorders prevalent in disaster survivors, particularly affective and substance use disorders, also require treatment which often differs from that only for PTSD or related disorders. Those may be the primary disorders instead of PTSD, or they may be present also and require combined treatment. While the evidence base for treatments and other interventions after disasters has increased, the scale of the need for diagnosis and treatment interventions for millions of people worldwide complicates the emerging task of making possible and delivering optimal evidence-based care for diverse populations, with scarce resources, throughout the world.

Outcomes Research Evidence for Children, Adults, and Families

Injury is a huge burden in some disasters, particularly natural disasters such as earthquakes. For instance in 2010, the 7.0 magnitude earthquake in Haiti left a reported 222,750 dead, 300,000 injured, 1.5 million displaced, and more than 3 million "affected" (Doocy et al., 2013). Following that disaster, screening for PTSD, anxiety, and depression in children aged 7 to 18 years revealed a high prevalence of those disorders but lower than that of other children on the streets due to psychological or physical abuse at home (Derivois et al., 2017). Among police involved in the WTC rescue and recovery in 2001, rates of prior month full and partial WTC-related PTSD were 5.4% and 15.4%, respectively, with both groups needing mental health care (Pietrzak et al., 2012). Following the Florida hurricanes in 2004, state Department of Health workers were screened via electronic questionnaires and 4% were found to have probable PTSD and 3.8% probable depression, and these groups were at greater risk for high alcohol and tobacco use (Fullerton et al., 2013).

There are increasing numbers of long-term mental health interventions after disasters provided by various organizations, including extensive, long-term assessment and interventions. Related disasters are the attacks of 9/11 in New York, Pennsylvania, and Washington, D.C. (Neria et al., 2006) and the 2010 earthquake in Haiti (Raviola et al., 2012; Raviola et al., 2013). The mental health services responses to community disasters in the United States is reviewed by North and Pfefferbaum (2013).

Posttraumatic Stress in Responders

Responders are highly stressed and may manifest symptoms of PTSD. A study of 8,466 police who were involved in the WTC rescue and recovery effort found that those with full and subsyndromal (partial) PTSD more likely reported mental health care (Pietrzak et al., 2012). A subsequent study of 4,352 responders to the 9/11 WTC terrorist attacks examined PTSD subgroups ("latent PTSD symptom typologies") of those with probable DSM-IV PTSD, finding that those in the high symptom group (45%) had higher probability of all PTSD symptoms and were more likely to have depression, while those in the dysphoric group (31%) had higher emotional numbing and arousal (e.g., sleep disturbance) symptoms, and those (23%) in the "threat" group had more re-experiencing, avoidance, and anxious arousal. The authors suggest that this might inform assessment, risk stratification, and treatment approaches (Horn et al., 2016). Findings such as these inform the teaching of self-care and monitoring of levels of stress by supervisors in order to reduce the risk of PTSD symptoms and increase social supports for those responding to disasters.

CONCLUSIONS

The occurrence of a disaster is one of the major contributors for children, adults, and the elderly experiencing trauma- and stressor-related disorders. The numbers of people affected and the severity of symptoms relates in part to the circumstances since some reactions are rapid and relatively transient, while others are insidious and persisting. While many disaster survivors are resilient, a significant minority of people worldwide who survive a disaster manifest PTSD or comorbid depression, and many have comorbid substance use disorders. Interventions for disasters in the United States have been extensively studied, finding 11% to 38% of distressed individuals presenting for evaluation. However, there is inadequate evidence to recommend evidence-based psychosocial interventions such as psychological first aid, debriefing, crisis counseling, or psychoeducation (North & Pfefferbaum, 2013), although the evidence base for cognitive behavioral interventions is expanding. Further intervention research is necessary. International disasters in low to middle-income countries are especially vulnerable, and specific initiatives are currently recommended to address the needs in these countries to reduce the burden of mental illness and disability from the trauma of disaster.

Katz and Nathaniel (2002) wrote on disasters, psychiatry, and psychodynamics, observing that the mental health professional "who listens, who tolerates intense affects, who is attuned to the role of the unconscious, of fantasy and of impulse in peoples' response to disasters carries with them a psychological 'trauma tent'" like the tent at the disaster site which protects them. It resembles D. W. Winnicott's "holding environment" in early childhood and may be similarly psychologically protective for those the mental health professional works with at the disaster site. They reflect further that "It is the privilege of the psychiatrist and other mental health professional to simply be permitted access to the raw wound of survivor's grief and suffering. Of course, as with many areas of disaster psychiatry, much more remains to be learned about psychodynamic practice in the face of unfolding tragedy." This remains true.

REFERENCES

Ablon SL. The therapeutic action of play. *J Am Acad Child Adolesc Psychiatry*. 1996;35:545–549.

Albahar M. Cyber attacks and terrorism: A twenty-first century conundrum. *Sci Eng Ethics*. 2017 Jan 5. doi:10.1007/s11948-016-9864-0.

Allen B, Brymer MJ, Steinberg AM, Vernberg EM, Jacobs A, Speier A, Pynoos RS. Perceptions of use of psychological first aid among providers responding to Hurricanes Gustav and Ike. *J Trauma Stress*, 2010;23:509–513.

Augusterfer EF, Mollica RF, Lavelle J. A review of telemental health in international and post-disaster settings. *Int Rev Psychiatry*. 2015;27(6):540–546. doi:10.3109/09540261.2015.1082985

Biegler K, Mollica R, Sim SE, Nicholas E, Chandler M, Ngo-Metzger Q, Paigne K, Paigne S, Nguyen DV, Sorkin DH. Rationale and study protocol for a multi-component health information technology (HIT) screening tool for depression and post-traumatic stress disorder in the primary care setting. *Contemp Clin Trials*. 2016 Sep;50:66–76. doi:10.1016/j.cct.2016.07.001

Blumenfield M, Ursano RJ (Eds.). *Intervention and Resilience after Mass Trauma*. Cambridge UK: Cambridge University Press, 2008.

Brenner GH, Bush DH, Moses J (Eds.). *Creating Spiritual and Psychological Resilience: Integrating Care in Disaster Relief Work*. New York: Routledge, Taylor and Francis Group, 2010.

Bromet EJ. Emotional consequences of nuclear power plant disasters. *Health Phys*. 2014 Feb;106(2): 206–210. doi:10.1097/HP.0000000000000012. PMID: 24378494

Brymer M, Layne C, Jacobs A, et al. *Psychological First Aid Field Operations Guide* (2nd ed.). Los Angeles, CA: National Child Traumatic Stress Network and National Center for PTSD, 2006. Retrieved from http://www.nctsn.org/content/psychological-first-aid and http://www.ptsd.va.gov/professional/manuals/psych-first-aid.asp

Butler AS, Panzer AM, Goldfrank LR (Eds.). Committee on Responding to the Psychological Consequences of Terrorism Board on Neuroscience and Behavioral Health, Institute of Medicine. *Preparing for the Psychological Consequences of Terrorism: A Public Health Strategy*. Washington, DC. National Academy of Sciences Institute of Medicine, 2003.

Catani C, Kohiladevy M, Ruf M, et al. Treating children traumatized by war and tsunami: A comparison between exposure therapy and meditation-relaxation in North-East Sri Lanka. *BMC Psychiatry*. 2009;9:22.

CATS Consortium. Implementation of CBT for youth affected by the World Trade Center disaster: Matching need to treatment intensity and reducing trauma symptoms. *J Trauma Stress*. 2010 Dec;23(6):699–707. doi:10.1002/jts.20594

Centers for Disease Control and Prevention, Crisis and Emergency Risk Communication. CERC pandemic influenza training, 2015a. Retrieved from http://emergency.cdc.gov/cerc/CERConline/pandemic/index.html

Centers for Disease Control and Prevention. Recommendations about international travel for education purposes and the Ebola outbreak in West Africa, 2015b. Retrieved from http://wwwnc.cdc.gov/travel/page/advice-for-colleges-universities-and-students-about-ebola-in-west-africa

Centers for Disease Control and Prevention. Crisis and Emergency Risk Communication, 2017. Retrieved from https://emergency.cdc.gov/cerc/index.asp

Center for Mental Health Services. Communicating in a crisis: Risk communication guidelines for public officials. Rockville, MD: Substance Abuse and

Mental Health Administration, 2002. Retrieved from http://www.riskcommunication.samhsa.gov

Charney DS. Psychobiological mechanisms of resilience and vulnerability: Implications for successful adaptation to extreme stress. [Review] *Am J Psychiatry.* 2004;161(2):195–216.

Chemtob CM, Nakashima J, Hamada RS. Psychosocial intervention for postdisaster trauma symptoms in elementary school children: A controlled community field study. *Arch Ped Adolesc Med.* 2002;156:211–216.

Ciottone GR, Biddinger PD (Eds.). *Disaster Medicine*, 2nd ed. Philadelphia, PA: Elsevier, 2015.

Cohen JA, Mannarino AP, Deblinger E. *Treating Trauma and Traumatic Grief in Children and Adolescents.* New York: Guilford Press, 2006.

Cohen JA, Mannarino AP, Gibson LE, et al. Interventions for children and adolescents following disasters. In: Interventions Following Mass Violence and Disasters: Strategies for Mental Health Practice. Edited by EC Ritchie, PJ Watson, and MJ Friedman. New York: Guilford Press, 2006, pp. 227–256.

Cozza SJ, Cohen JA, Doherty JG (Eds.). *Disaster and Trauma, An Issue of Child and Adolescent Psychiatric Clinics of North America.* Amsterdam: W.B. Saunders 2014.

de Jong JT, Berckmoes LH, Kohrt BA, Song SJ, Tol WA, Reis R. A public health approach to address the mental health burden of youth in situations of political violence and humanitarian emergencies. *Curr Psychiatry Rep.* 2015 Jul;17(7):60. doi:10.1007/s11920-015-0590-0

Derivois D, Cenat JM, Joseph NE, Karray A, Chahraoui K. Prevalence and determinants of posttraumatic stress disorder, anxiety and depression symptoms in street children survivors of the 2010 earthquake in Haiti, four years after. *Child Abuse Negl.* 2017;67:174–181. doi:10.1016/j.chiabu.2017.02.034

Disaster Psychiatry Outreach. The essentials of disaster psychiatry: A training course for mental health professionals: Course syllabus, 2008. Retrieved from http://sites.google.com/a/disasterpsych.org/blog/File-Cabinet

Dodgen D, Donato D, Kelly N, et al. Mental health and well-being. In: *The Impacts of Climate Change on Human Health In the United States. A Scientific Assessment.* Washington, DC: U.S. Global Change Research Program, 2016, pp. 217–246.http://dx.doi.org/10.7930/J0TX3C9H

Donnelly CL. Pharmacologic treatment approaches for children and adolescents with posttraumatic stress disorder. *Child Adolesc Psychiatr Clin N Am.* 2003;12:251–269.

Doocy S, Jacquet G, Cherewick M, Kirsch TD. The injury burden of the 2010 Haiti earthquake: A stratified cluster survey. *Injury: Int. J Care Injured.* 2013;44:842–847.

Farmer P. *Haiti After the Earthquake.* New York: BBS Public Affairs, 2011.

Feder A, Mota N, Salim R, Rodriguez J, et al. Risk, coping and PTSD symptom trajectories in World Trade Center responders. *J Psychiatr Res.* 2016 Nov;82:68–79. doi:10.1016/j.jpsychires.2016.07.003

Flory JD, Yehuda R. Comorbidity between posttraumatic stress disorder and major depressive disorder: Alternative explanations and treatment considerations. *Dialogues Clin Neurosci.* 2015;17:141–150.

Foa EB, Keane TM, Friedman MJ, et al. (Eds.). *Effective Treatments for PTSD: Practice Guidelines from the International Society for Traumatic Stress Studies,* 2nd ed. New York: Guilford, 2009.

Fullerton CS, McKibben JBA, Reissman DB, Scharf T, Kowalki-Trakofler KM, Shulz JM, Ursano RJ. Posttraumatic stress disorder, depression, and alcohol and tobacco use in public health workers after the 2004 Florida hurricanes. *Disaster Med Public Health Preparedness* 2013;7:89–95.

Funderburk BW, Eyberg S. Parent-Child Interaction Therapy. In: *History of Psychotherapy: Continuity and Change*, 2nd ed. Edited by JC Norcross and DK Freedheim. Washington, DC: American Psychological Association, 2011, pp. 415–420

Goenjian AK, Karayan I, Pynoos RS, et. al: Outcome of psychotherapy among early adolescents after trauma. *Am J Psychiatry.* 1997;154:536–542.

Goldberg DP, Hillier VF. A scaled version of the General Health Questionnaire. *Psychol Med.* 1979;9:139–145.

Goldman E, Galea S. Mental health consequences of disasters. *Annual Rev Public Health.* 2014;35:169–183.

Gurwitch RH, Sitterle KA, Young BH, Pfefferbaum B. The aftermath of terrorism. In: *Helping Children Cope with Disasters and Terrorism.* Edited by AM La Greca. Washington, DC: American Psychological Association, 2002.

Harries D, Yellowlees PM. Cyberterrorism: Is the U.S. healthcare system safe? *Telemed J E Health.* 2013 Jan;19(1):61–66. doi:10.1089/tmj.2012.0022

Holman EA, Garfin DR, Silver RC. Media's role in broadcasting acute stress following the Boston Marathon bombings. *Proc Natl Acad Sci U S A.* 2014 Jan 7;111(1):93–98. doi:10.1073/pnas.1316265110

Hood KK, Eyberg SM. Outcomes of parent-child interaction therapy: Mothers' reports of maintenance three to six years after treatment. *J Clin Child Adolesc Psychol.* 2003;32:419–429.

Horn SR, Pietrzak RH, Schechter C, et al. Latent typologies of posttraumatic stress disorder in

World Trade Center responders. *J Psychiatr Res.* 2016 Dec;83:151–159. doi:10.1016/j.jpsychires.2016.08.018

Hyams KC, Murphy FM, Wessely S. Responding to chemical, biological or nuclear terrorism: The indirect and long-term health effects may present the greatest challenge. *J Health Polit Policy Law.* 2002;27(2):273–291.

Inter-Agency Standing Committee, Reference Group for Mental Health and Psychosocial Support in Emergency Settings. *Mental Health and Psychosocial Support in Humanitarian Emergencies: What Should Humanitarian Health Actors Know?* Geneva: Author, 2010.

Imperiale AJ, Vanclay F. Experiencing local community resilience in action: Learning from post-disaster communities. *J Rural Studies.* 2016;47:204–219.

Institute of Medicine. *Preparing for the Psychological Consequences of Terrorism. A Public Health Strategy.* Washington DC: Author, 2003.

Institute of Medicine. *Assessing Medical Preparedness to Respond to a Terrorist Nuclear Event: Workshop Report.* Washington, DC: National Academies Press, 2009.

Jaycox LH, Cohen JA, Mannarino AP, et al. Children's mental health care following Hurricane Katrina: A field trial of trauma-focused psychotherapies. *J Trauma Stress.* 2010;23(2):223–231.

Kantor EM, Beckert DR. Psychological first aid. In: *Disaster Psychiatry: Readiness, Evaluation and Treatment.* Edited by FJ Stoddard, A Pandya, and CL Katz. Washington, DC: American Psychiatric Publishing, 2011, pp. 203–212.

Katz CL, Nathaniel R. Disasters, psychiatry, and psychodynamics. *J Am Acad Psychoanalysis.* 2002;30(4):519–529.

Katz CL, Pandya A (Eds.). Disaster mental health: Around the world and across time. *Psychiatr Clin N Am.* 2013;36(3):iii–474.

Katz CL, Pellegrino L, Pandya A, Ng A, DeLisi LE. Research on psychiatric outcomes and interventions subsequent to disasters: A review of the literature. *Psychiatry Res.* 2002 Jul 31;110(3):201–217.

Kessler RC, Green JG, Gruber MJ, et al. Screening for serious mental illness in the general population with the K6 Screening Scale: Results from the WHO World Mental Health (WMH) survey initiative. *Int J Methods Psychiatr Res.* 2010 Jun;19(Suppl. 1):4–22. doi:10.1002/mpr.310

Klingman A. School based interventions following a disaster. In: *Children and Disasters.* Edited by CF Saylor. New York: Plenum Press, 1993, pp. 165–186.

La Greca AM, Silverman WK, Vernberg EM, Roberts MC. *Helping Children Cope with Disasters and Terrorism.* Washington, DC: National Child Traumatic Stress Network, 2005. www.nctsnet.org/

Laor N, Wolmer L. Children exposed to disaster: The role of the mental health professional. In *Lewis's Child and Adolescent Psychiatry.* Edited by A Martin and FR Volkmar. Philadelphia, PA: Lippincott Williams and Wilkins, 2007, pp. 727–739.

Lindert J, Carta MG, Schäfer I, Mollica RF. Refugees mental health—A public mental health challenge. *Eur J Public Health.* 2016 Jun;26(3):374–375. doi:10.1093/eurpub/ckw010. PMID: 27053728

Lucchini RG, Hashim D, Acquilla S, et al. A comparative assessment of major international disasters: The need for exposure assessment, systematic emergency preparedness, and lifetime health care. *BMC Public Health.* 2017 Jan 7;17(1):46. doi:10.1186/s12889-016-3939-3

Masten AS, Best KM, Garmezy N. Resilience and development: Contributions from the study of children who overcome adversity. *Dev Psychopathol.* 1990;2:425–444.

Mollica RF, Caspi-Yavin Y, Bollini P, Truong T, Tor S, Lavelle J. The Harvard Trauma Questionnaire: Validating a cross-cultural instrument for measuring torture, trauma, and posttraumatic stress disorder in Indochinese refugees. *J Nerv Ment Dis.* 1992;180:111–116.

Morsette A, Swaney G, Stolle D, Schuldberg D, van den Pol R, Young M. Cognitive Behavioral Intervention for Trauma in Schools (CBITS): School-based treatment on a rural American Indian reservation. *J Behav Ther Exp Psychiatry.* 2009;40(1), 169–178.

Myers D, Zunin L. Phases of disaster. In: *Training Manual for Mental Health and Human Service Workers in Major Disasters*, 2nd ed. Edited by D DeWolfe. (DHHS Publication No. ADM 90-538). Washington, DC: U.S. Government Printing Office, 2000.

Neria Y, Galea S, Norris FH (Eds.). *Mental Health and Disasters.* Cambridge, UK: Cambridge University Press, 2009.

Neria Y, Gross R, Marshall R, et al. (Eds.). *9/11: Mental Health in the Wake of Terrorist Attacks.* Cambridge, UK. Cambridge University Press, 2006.

Neria Y, Nandi A, Galea S. Posttraumatic stress disorder following disasters: A systematic review. *Psychol Med.* 2008;38(4):467–480.

Nomura S, Parsons AJQ, Hirabayashi M, Kinoshita R, Liao Y, Hodgson S. Social determinants of mid-to long-term disaster impacts on health: A systematic review. *Int J Disaster Risk Reduct.* 2016;16:53–67.

Norris FH, Galea S, Friedman MJ (Eds.). *Methods for Disaster Mental Health Research.* New York: Guilford Press, 2006.

North CS, Pfefferbaum B. Mental health response to community disasters: A systematic review. *JAMA*. 2013 Aug 7;310(5):507–518. doi:10.1001/jama.2013.107799

O'Donnell ML, Bryant RA, Creamer M, Carty J. Mental health following traumatic injury: Toward a health system model of early intervention. *Clin Psychol Rev*. 2008;28:387–406.

Oe M, Fujii S, Maeda M, Nagai M, et al. Three-year trend survey of psychological distress, post-traumatic stress, and problem drinking among residents in the evacuation zone after the Fukushima Daiichi Nuclear Power Plant accident. *Psychiatry Clin Neurosci*. 2016 Jun;70(6):245–252. doi:10.1111/pcn.12387

Oe M, Takahashi H, Maeda M, et al. Changes of posttraumatic stress responses in evacuated residents and their related factors. *Asia Pac J Public Health*. 2017 Mar;29(2 Suppl.):182S–192S. doi:10.1177/1010539516680733

Pandya A, Katz C. *Disaster Psychiatry: Intervening When Nightmares Come True*. Hillsdale, NJ: Analytic Press, 2004.

Pfefferbaum B, Nixon SJ, Tivis RD, Doughty DE, Pynoos RS, Gurwitch RH, Foy DW. Television exposure in children after a terrorist incident. *Psychiatry*. 2001 Fall;64(3):202–211.

Pietrzak RH, Schechter CB, Bromet EJ, et al. The burden of full and subsyndromal stress disorder among police involved in the World Trade Center rescue and recovery effort. *J Psychiatric Res*. 2012;46(7):835–842.

Pine DS, Cohen JA. Trauma in children and adolescents: Risk and treatment of psychiatric sequelae. *Biol Psychiatry*. 2002;51:519–531.

Raviola G, Eustache E, Oswald C, Belkin GS. Mental health response in Haiti in the aftermath of the 2010 earthquake: A case study for building long-term solutions. *Harv Rev Psychiatry*. 2012 Feb 15;20(1):68–77.

Raviola G, Severe J, Therosme T, Oswald C, Belkin G, Eustache E. The 2010 Haiti earthquake response. *Psychiatr Clin North Am*. 2013 Sep;36(3):431–450. doi:10.1016/j.psc.2013.05.006

Reissman DB, Spencer S, Tanielian TL, Stein BD. Integrating behavioral aspects into community preparedness and response systems. *J Aggress Maltreat Trauma*. 2005;10(3–4):707–720.

Ritchie EC, Watson PJ, Friedman MJ (Eds.). *Interventions Following Mass Violence and Disasters: Strategies for Mental Health Practice*. New York: Guildford Press, 2006.

Rose SC, Bisson J, Churchill R, Wessely S. Psychological debriefing for preventing posttraumatic stress disorder (PTSD): Review. *Cochrane Library*. 2009;1:1–46.

Saltzman WR, Layne CM, Steinberg AM, Arslanagic B, Pynoos RS. Developing a culturally and ecologically sound intervention program for youth exposed to war and terrorism. *Child Adolesc Psychiatr Clin N Am*. 2003;12:2:319–342.

Saxe GN, Ellis BH, Brown AD.4 *Trauma Systems Therapy for Children and Teens*, 2nd ed. New York: Guilford, 2015.

Schreiber M, Gurwitch R. *Listen, protect, and connect: Psychological first aid for children and parents*, 2006. Retrieved from www.ready.gov/kids/_downloads/PFA_SchoolCrisis.pdf, downloaded 3/15/08

Shibley HL, Stoddard FJ. Child and adolescent psychiatry interventions. In: *Disaster Psychiatry: Readiness, Evaluation and Treatment*. Edited by FJ Stoddard, A Pandya, and CL Katz. Washington, DC: American Psychiatric Publishing, 2011, pp. 287–312.

Sloand E, Killion C, Yarandi H, Sharps P, Lewis-O'Connor A, Hassan M, Gary F, Muller CN, Campbell D. Experiences of violence and abuse among internally displaced adolescent girls following a natural disaster. *J Adv Nurs*. 2017;73:3200–3208. doi:10.1111/jan.13316

Southwick SM, Charney DS. *Resilience: The Science of Mastering Life's Greatest Challenges*. Cambridge UK: Cambridge University Press, 2012.

Stoddard FJ. Communicating risk before, during and after a disaster. In: *Disaster Psychiatry: Readiness, Evaluation and Treatment*. Edited by FJ Stoddard, A Pandya, and CL Katz. Washington, DC: American Psychiatric Publishing, 2011, pp. 19–33.

Stoddard FJ. Outcomes of traumatic exposure. In: *Disaster and Trauma, An Issue of Child and Adolescent Psychiatric Clinics of North America*. Edited by SJ Cozza, JA Cohen, and JG Doherty. Amsterdam: W.B. Saunders, 2014, pp. 243–256.

Stoddard FJ, Gold J, Henderson SW, Merlino JP, Norwood A, Post JM, Shanfield S, Weine S, Katz CL. Psychiatry and terrorism. *J Nerv Ment Dis*. 2011;199(8):537–543.

Stoddard FJ, Katz CL, Merlino JP (Eds.). *Hidden Impact: What You Need to Know for the Next Disaster: A Practical Guide for Clinicians*. Sudbury/Boston: Jones and Bartlett, 2010.

Stoddard FJ, Menninger EW. Guidance for parents and other caretakers after disasters or terrorist attacks. In: *Disaster Psychiatry Handbook*. Edited by RCW Hall, AT Ng, and AE Norwood. Washington, DC: American Psychiatric Association, 2004, pp. 44–56.

Stoddard FJ, Pandya A, Katz CL (Eds.). *Disaster Psychiatry: Readiness, Evaluation and Treatment*. Washington, DC: American Psychiatric Publishing, 2011.

Stoddard F, Usher C, Abrams A. Psychopharmacology in pediatric critical care. *Child Adolesc Psychiatr Clin N Am.* 2006;15(3):611–655.

Stolk Y, Kaplan I, Szwarc J. Clinical use of the Kessler psychological distress scales with culturally diverse groups. *Int J Methods Psychiatr Res.* 2014 Jun;23(2):161–183. doi:10.1002/mpr.1426

Terr LC. *Too Scared to Cry—Psychic Trauma in Childhood.* New York: Basic Books, 1990.

TRACIE. Disaster behavioral health: Resources at your fingertips. 2017. Retrieved from https://asprtracie.hhs.gov/documents/aspr-tracie-dbh-resources-at-your-fingertips.pdf

Ursano RJ. Terrorism and mental health: Public health and primary care. In: *Report: Meeting the Mental Health Needs of the Country in the Wake of September 11, 2001.* Atlanta, GA: The Carter Center, 2002, pp. 64–68. http://www.cartercenter/org/documents/1441pdf

Ursano RJ, Fullerton CS, Norwood AE (Eds.). *Terrorism and Disaster: Individual and Community Mental Health Interventions.* Cambridge, UK: Cambridge University Press, 2003.

Ursano RJ, Fullerton CS, Vanced K, Kao TC. Posttraumatic stress disorder and identification in disaster workers. *Am J Psychiatry.* 1999; 156:353–359.

Ursano RJ, Fullerton CS, Weisaeth L, Raphael B (Eds.). *Textbook of Disaster Psychiatry,* 2nd ed. Cambridge, UK: Cambridge University Press, 2017. doi:10.1017/9781316481424

Ursano RJ, Norwood AE, Fullerton CS (Eds.). *Bioterrorism: Psychological and Public Health Interventions.* Cambridge, UK: Cambridge University Press, 2004.

U.S. Department of Veterans Affairs. PTSD and Telemental Health. National Center for PTSD, 2017. https://www.ptsd.va.gov/professional/treatment/overview/ptsd-telemental.asp

Watson PJ, Brymer M, Bonanno G. Post-disaster psychological intervention since 9/11. In: Special Issue: The 10th Anniversary of the September 11, 2001 Terrorist Attacks, 2011. *Am Psychologist.*

Weathers FW, Blake DD, Schnurr PP, Kaloupek DG, Marx BP, Keane TM. The Life Events Checklist for DSM-5 (LEC-5). National Center for PTSD, 2013. Retrieved from www.ptsd.va.gov

Wethington HR, Hahn RA, Fuqua-Whitley DS, et al. The effectiveness of interventions to reduce psychological harm from traumatic events among children and adolescents: A systematic review. *Am J Prev Med.* 2008;35:287–313.

Wolmer L, Laor N, Dedeoglu C, et al. Teacher mediated intervention after disaster: A controlled three year follow up of children's functioning. *J Child Psychol Psychiatry.* 2005;41:277–289.

Wolmer L, Laor N, Yazgan Y. School reactivation programs after disaster: Could teachers serve as clinical mediators? *Child Adolesc Psychiatr Clin N Am.* 2003;12:363–381.

World Health Organization. *Psychosocial Consequences of Disaster: Prevention and Management.* Geneva: World Health Organization, 1992. http://whqlibdoc.who.int/hq/1991/WHO_MNH_PSF_91.3_REV.1.pdf

World Health Organization. Emergency Response Framework. Geneva: World Health Organization, 2013. http://www.who.int/hac/about/erf_.pdf

Zhang Z, Ran MS, Li YH, Ou GJ, Gong RR, Li RH, Fan M, Jiang Z, Fang DZ. Prevalence of posttraumatic stress disorder among adolescents after the Wenchuan earthquake in China. *Psychol Med.* 2012 Aug;42(8):1687–1693. doi:10.1017/S0033291711002844 PMID:22152150

11

Culture and Trauma-Related Disorders

DEVON E. HINTON AND ROBERTO LEWIS-FERNÁNDEZ

INTRODUCTION

In the fifth edition of the *Diagnostic and Statistical Manual of Mental Disorders* (DSM-5; American Psychiatric Association, 2013), the trauma- and stressor-related disorders include a range of conditions: posttraumatic stress disorder (PTSD), acute stress disorder, adjustment disorders, reactive attachment disorder, and disinhibited social engagement disorder. This chapter examines the role of culture in trauma-related experiencing, focusing on PTSD because there is much cross-cultural data in this area. However, we propose a model and analytic approach that applies to the other trauma-related disorders as well.

In this chapter, we define "culture" in a broad sense, namely, as encompassing a group's particular interpretive systems, such as their understanding of how the mind and body function; healing traditions; religious systems; social structures; economic situation; security situation; and patterns of previous trauma (Perilla, Norris, & Lavizzo, 2002). At the same time, it must be understood that there is considerable variation within a group--not just one "culture"--and that these notions are in dynamic change (Mattingly & Garro, 2000). Our examples of cultural factors tend to prioritize intercultural variation over intracultural variation.

The rest of the chapter examines PTSD from a cross-cultural perspective. We first present a general model of culture and trauma-related disorder, which is applicable to all trauma-related disorders. Then, guided by that model, we review the cultural influence on the rates of PTSD and on the meaning and salience of particular PTSD symptoms, followed by a discussion of the content validity of the diagnostic category of PTSD in assessing trauma-related disorder across cultures. We conclude with reflections on the clinical utility of the PTSD construct when viewed in cultural context.

A MODEL OF THE EFFECT OF CULTURE ON TRAUMA-RELATED DISORDERS

According to current cognitive-behavioral models, if culture influences the interpretation and appraisal of trauma and trauma-related symptoms—for example, ideas about what disturbances of mind and body produce the symptoms—then culture would be expected to give rise to differences in the prominence of individual PTSD symptoms, in the comorbidity with PTSD of other symptoms or syndromes (e.g., panic attacks), and in the course of PTSD (Clark & Ehlers, 2004; Dunmore, Clark, & Ehlers, 2001; Ehlers, Mayou, & Bryant, 1998; Halligan, Michael, Clark, & Ehlers, 2003; Jobson & O'Kearney, 2009; Moser, Hajcak, Simons, & Foa, 2007). In Figure 11.1 we summarize our model of how trauma-related disorders are influenced by cultural context.

As depicted in the model, vulnerability to trauma will vary by such variables as current levels of stress and the local meanings of the trauma. The trauma may result in PTSD that causes such symptoms as anger, poor concentration, and nightmares. Trauma may also cause other DSM disorders like panic attacks and panic disorder that cause multiple symptoms, for example, somatic symptoms and surges of fear (Dell & O'Neil, 2009; Leskin & Sheikh, 2002; McQuaid, Pedrelli, McCahill, & Stein, 2001). In addition, trauma will result in arousal that will tend to produce somatic symptoms, for example, muscle tension, headache, and dizziness, and to produce other disorders like sleep paralysis.

These various trauma-caused symptoms will be locally interpreted in certain ways, attributed to disturbances in the mind, body, or spiritual state. For example, poor concentration may be considered evidence of a permanently disordered mind such as part of the syndrome of "thinking a lot," a syndrome found in many cultures (Hinton, Reis, &

de Jong, 2015; Kaiser et al., 2015); nightmares may be interpreted as being a visitation by a dead relative that is dangerous to the dreamer; startle may be attributed to a "weak heart" in Cambodian or Vietnamese contexts; and somatic symptoms like shaking may be attributed to a local cultural syndrome such as an *ataque de nervios* among Latino groups. As indicated in Figure 11.1, the attribution of symptoms to a certain "disorder" will increase symptoms by such mechanisms as catastrophic cognitions that produce arousal (e.g., causing symptoms by activation of the autonomic nervous system) and that produce hypervigilance (e.g., causing symptoms by the seeking out and focusing on certain symptoms), creating a looping effect.

The symptoms and the attribution of symptoms to a certain disorder—within the mental, physical, or spiritual domain—will contribute to a particular sociocultural course. That is, the symptoms and the disorder to which they are attributed will give rise potentially to the following (Hinton & Good, 2016):

- stigma (e.g., owing to self-labeling or other-labeling as being crazy as evidenced by certain symptoms, such as poor concentration or flashbacks);
- social network effects (e.g., owing to uncontrollable anger);
- economic effects (e.g., receiving disability, being unable to work because of poor concentration);
- help-seeking (e.g., from a curandero in Latin America or a Buddhist monk among Cambodian refugees);
- treatment in the health care system (e.g., of somatic symptoms by a primary care physician); and
- the use of an idiom of distress, namely, a locally sanctioned way of expressing distress, to signal being in a dire state—a final ethnobehavioral pathway (e.g., function of *ataque de nervios* or the complaint of *nervios* as an idiom of distress).

These sociocultural effects (what might be called sociocultural pragmatics) result in a certain sociocultural course of trauma-related disorders and may lead to a decrease or increase of distress and symptoms resulting from trauma-related disorder, as is shown in the looping depicted in the model.

PREVALENCE OF PTSD ACROSS CULTURES

As indicated by Figure 11.1, prevalence of PTSD would be expected to vary across groups owing to such contributing domains as type and degree of trauma exposure, the meaning of the traumatic event, level of stressors (e.g., poverty), and the cultural interpretation of the meaning of trauma-related symptoms. The following are examples of a range of rates: 1.7% of a community sample in post-conflict East Timor met DSM (fourth edition) PTSD criteria (Silove et al., 2008) as did 10% of inhabitants in a Senegalese refugee camp (Tang & Fox, 2001), 20% of tortured and imprisoned Tibetan refugees (Crescenzi et al., 2002), 59.7% of torture survivors in rural Nepal (Tol et al., 2007), and 62% of community-based Cambodian refugees in the United States (Marshall, Schell, Elliott, Berthold, & Chun, 2005). To clarify the role of culture in the onset and persistence of PTSD, some investigators have focused on cross-cultural conditional risk, that is, whether members of certain cultural groups display more or less vulnerability to meeting PTSD criteria after experiencing comparable traumatic stressors and after adjusting for certain predisposing or enabling characteristics like economic status.

The evidence of difference in conditional risk of PTSD is mixed, with some evidence for varying prevalence among certain groups (Alcantara, Casement, & Lewis-Fernandez, 2013; Alegria et al., 2013). Some studies have looked at possible protective mechanisms. Research among Tibetans has found low rates of PTSD despite substantial traumatic exposure, leading investigators to suggest that Tibetan religious traditions may be protective against PTSD (Holtz, 1998; Sachs, Rosenfeld, Lhewa, Rasmussen, & Keller, 2008). This hypothesis is supported by a mediation analysis in which coping activity, such as religious involvement, mediates the psychological effects of trauma exposure. However, another study did not find low rates in the Tibetan population (Sachs, et al., 2008).

A literature also tries to explain possible higher conditional risk in Latino populations (Alcantara, et al., 2013). For example, after the World Trade Center attack of 9/11 New Yorkers of Latino origin had significantly higher rates of PTSD than non-Latino whites 5 to 8 weeks after 9/11 and again two years after the disaster, including higher rates of new-onset PTSD in the intervening period (Adams & Boscarino, 2005). One possible explanation for the higher rate of post-9/11 PTSD among Latinos involves a higher prevalence of disaster-related panic attacks in this ethnic group--13.4% to 16.8%, depending on the Latino group, versus 5.5% among non-Latino whites (Adams & Boscarino, 2006; Galea et al., 2002; Galea et al., 2003)—since the presence of panic attacks during

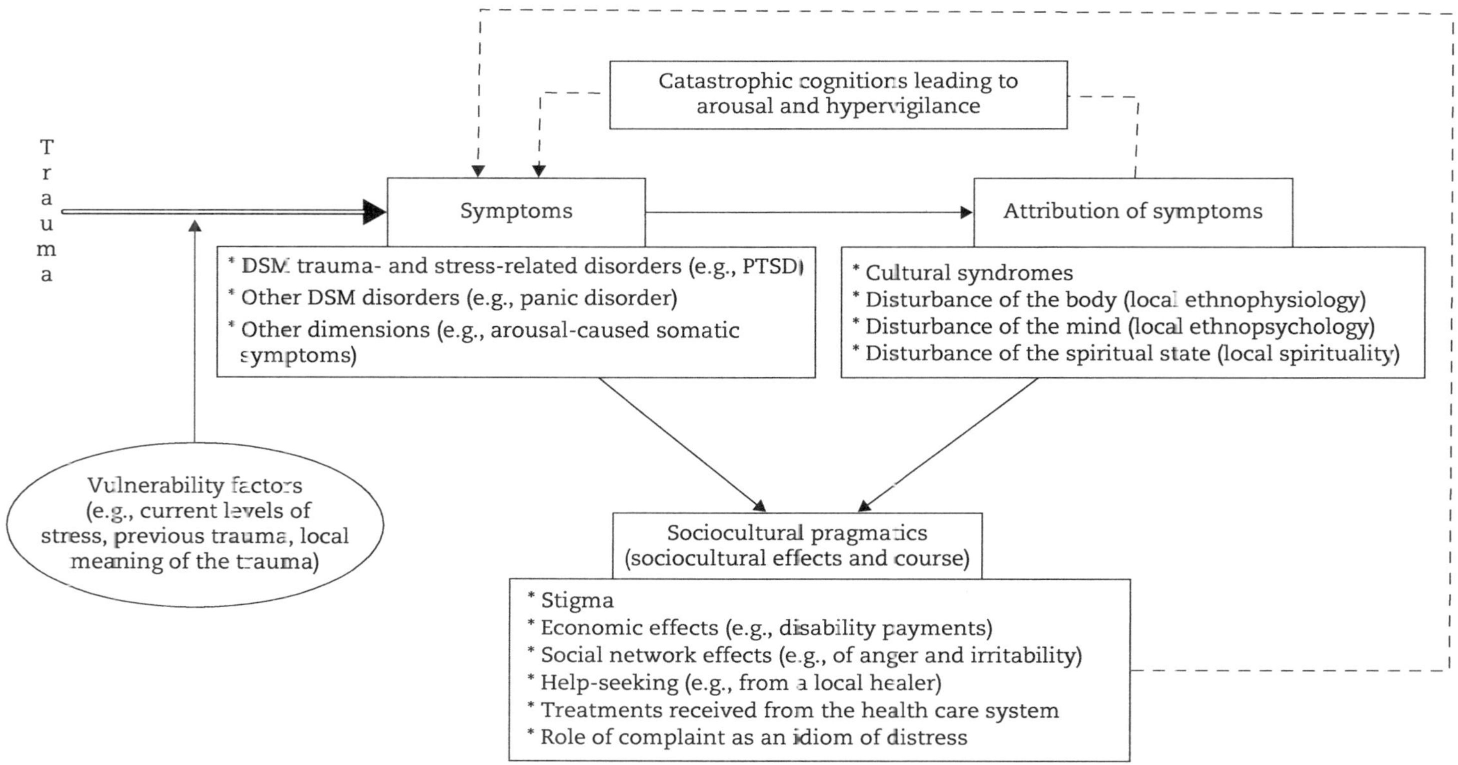

FIGURE 11.1. Cultural effects on trauma-related disorders: trauma in sociocultural context.

or after the disaster is an independent risk factor for post-9/11 PTSD. The higher rates of panic attacks and PTSD in Latino groups after 9/11 may result from the cultural syndrome of *ataque de nervios*. Endorsement of panic attack symptoms on research instruments like that in the 9/11 study may represent reports of *ataque de nervios* (attack of nerves), a cultural syndrome similar in phenomenology to panic attacks (Guarnaccia, Lewis-Fernández, & Marano, 2003; Lewis-Fernández et al., 2002). *Ataques* are associated in Latino cultures with overwhelming stress, especially a sudden, unexpected event such as a terrorist attack. *Ataques* may increase the experiencing of PTSD symptoms that overlap with *ataques* (e.g., arousal symptoms) because an *ataque* serves as an idiom of distress, thereby inflating rates of PTSD. Moreover, the cultural availability of *ataque* as a way of expressing peritraumatic distress may inadvertently facilitate the emergence of PTSD after a mass trauma by emphasizing a dissociative response (Hinton, Chong, Pollack, Barlow, & McNally, 2008; Lewis-Fernández et al., 2002), with peritraumatic dissociation possibly predisposing to PTSD (Candel & Merckelbach, 2004; Ozer, Best, Lipsey, & Weiss, 2003). Another possible explanation for the role of *ataque de nervios* is that it may increase catastrophic cognitions. According to this hypothesis, the concern that the trauma may predispose to *ataques*, in conjunction with the interpretation of fear and PTSD symptoms in terms of an *ataque*, may facilitate the emergence and continuation of PTSD by increasing arousal and the self-perception of vulnerability and disability (Hinton, Chong, et al., 2008; Hinton, Lewis-Fernández, & Pollack, 2009).

PTSD SYMPTOM MEANING AND SALIENCE IN CROSS-CULTURAL PERSPECTIVE

Due to the mechanism depicted in Figure 11.1, there will be cross-cultural differences in the local meaning of symptoms, leading to variation in salience of symptoms and therefore to variable endorsement of different DSM-5 PTSD criteria items (Hinton & Good, 2016). In each cultural setting, exposure to trauma may lead the person to scan for the presence of the feared symptoms and symptom sets that are thought to result from trauma in that culture and, when found, to the amplification of those particular symptoms through attentional and arousal mechanisms (Hinton et al., 2006; Hinton, Chhean, Fama, Pollack, & McNally, 2007; Hinton & Good, 2016). These concerns may vary across time and place; for example, concerns may focus on soul loss in various cultures or on the experience of shell shock during and after World War I in English-speaking populations. Even if there is not a specific folk illness thought to be caused by trauma in a culture, the symptoms caused by trauma will be interpreted according to the local conceptualization of the mind, body, and spiritual aspect of reality (Hinton & Good, 2016). Examples include the symptoms of startle and arousal that may be connected to a self-diagnosis of *susto* among Latino populations and arousal symptoms that may lead to the self-diagnosis of *khyâl* attack among Cambodian populations.

In respect to the DSM nightmare symptom, one study of American Indian combat veterans found higher rates compared to veterans of other racial/ethnic backgrounds, with the authors hypothesizing the cause to be the cultural meaning associated with distressing dreams in that group (Shore, Orton, & Manson, 2009). Higher rates of nightmares among Alaskan Natives were also found in a study comparing their PTSD symptoms with those of non-Hispanic whites following the Exxon Valdez disaster (Palinkas, Petterson, Russell, & Downs, 2004). Among Cambodian refugees, nightmares are often considered to indicate that the dreamer has a depleted and vulnerable bodily and spiritual status, that the dreamer has been attacked by a spirit, and that, in the case that the dreamer dreamed of a loved one, that the deceased loved one is in a purgatory-like state, with dreaming of the loved one also considered dangerous. Possibly as a result of these culturally specific interpretations, in one study of Cambodian refugees, having nightmares during the last month was extremely highly associated with the presence of PTSD, with an odds ratio of 126, 95% confidence level, 23.3–626.5 (Hinton et al., 2009).

Another DSM-5 PTSD criterion item is "Persistent, distorted cognitions about the cause or consequences of the traumatic event(s) that lead the individual to blame himself/herself or others." In many Buddhist and Hindu cultures there is the idea of karma, the notion that one encounters adverse events owing to bad karma resulting from one's past bad deeds in this and other lives. These cultural conceptualizations about karma may lead to increased self-blaming following a traumatic event (Hinton & Good, 2016).

The following DSM-5 PTSD criterion item would be expected to vary greatly across cultures: "Persistent and exaggerated negative beliefs or expectations about oneself, others, or the world" (e.g., "I am bad," "No one can be trusted," "The world is completely dangerous," "My whole nervous system is permanently ruined"). The sense of permanent damage may vary across cultures and be more salient owing to cultural interpretations. Many populations believe that psychological trauma may have a direct, markedly damaging effect on the body and mind, and this gives rise to the sense of foreshortened future. The Latin American folk illness of *susto* (fright) is thought to be provoked by various stressors, including those that are of traumatic proportion, and to have dangerous effects on health, which may be attributed to the loss of the person's soul (Rubel, O'Nell, & Collado-Ardón, 1984). The folk illness of *nervios* (nerves) is attributed to stress (including trauma) and is thought to bring about physical alterations of the nervous system (e.g., the anatomical nerves) that result in various physiological complications, for example, gastrointestinal, motor, and sensory pathology, as well as cognitive decline, for example, memory loss and poor concentration (Guarnaccia et al., 2003; Low, 1985). These views are echoed in other settings, such as Cambodia, Rwanda, and Vietnam where PTSD-related symptoms are thought to indicate the presence of dangerously disordered mental, physical, and spiritual states (Hagengimana & Hinton, 2009; Hinton & Good, 2016; Hinton, Hinton, Pham, Chau, & Tran, 2003; Hinton, Hinton, Um, Chea, & Sak, 2002).

Among traumatized refugees, in respect to the DSM-5 PTSD criterion item "persistent negative state," there may be a more depressive effect following trauma among refugees and certain groups for reason of bereavement (Hinton & Good, 2016). This may result from "cultural bereavement" (the loss of one's culture, such as the ability to participate in certain rituals or religious rites, the loss of language ability in the next generation), "social bereavement" (the loss of social connections due to distance and death), "person bereavement" (unresolved grief after a death, e.g., due to war or genocide), and "geographic bereavement" (nostalgia for the food, climate, and place of origin).

In respect to the DSM-5 arousal symptoms, we could expect to find elevated levels in cultural groups with high rates of comorbidity between PTSD and panic attacks, such as among Cambodian refugees (Hinton, Hofmann, Pitman, Pollack, & Barlow, 2008) and Rwandan genocide survivors (Hagengimana & Hinton, 2009; Hagengimana, Hinton, Bird, Pollack, & Pitman, 2003). Re-experiencing and other symptoms could also be more salient owing to increased arousal. For example, panic is highly comorbid with PTSD among Cambodian refugees, seemingly due in part to cultural syndromes; the following mechanism is likely: PTSD-caused arousal results in somatic symptoms that are often attributed to "*khyâl* attacks," activating "*khyâl* attack"-related catastrophic cognitions, which lead to panic. Among Cambodian populations, "*khyâl* attacks" are attributed to disturbed flow in the body of the wind-like *khyâl*, which can suddenly reverse flow and rise in the body to cause multiple symptoms and disasters, such as pushing on the heart and lungs to impede their functioning and entering the head to cause dizziness and tinnitus and possibly fatal syncope.

CONTENT VALIDITY OF PTSD IN ASSESSING TRAUMA-RELATED DISORDER ACROSS CULTURAL GROUPS

Culture may also affect the content validity of the PTSD criteria items, raising the question of whether the PTSD criteria capture the core experiences of trauma-related disorder in diverse cultural context, and specifically whether focusing exclusively on PTSD symptoms in trauma survivors neglects key complaints (Keane, Kaloupec, & Weathers, 1996). This has been called "category truncation," that is, the truncation of the true range of distress complaints relevant to a category, in this case, trauma-related experiencing (Hinton & Good, 2016). In particular, authors (Hinton & Lewis-Fernández, 2011) have argued that to attain full content validity in assessing trauma-related disorder across cultures, somatic symptoms and cultural syndromes must be assessed.

Somatic symptoms can be prominent for several reasons in particular cultural contexts (Hinton & Simons, 2015; Kirmayer & Bhugra, 2009; Kirmayer & Sartorius, 2007). The somatic symptoms may be prominent because they are part of cultural syndromes and are related to the local understanding of the functioning of mind, body, and spiritual state. They may also be prominent because the somatic symptoms serve as a locally sanctioned way of expressing distress. Some of the following are examples of somatic complaints that are a prominent part of the reaction to traumatic events in specific cultures (the list is by no means exhaustive): among Salvadorian and Senegalese refugees, a sense of bodily heat (Jenkins & Valiente, 1994; Tang & Fox, 2001); among tortured Bhutanese refugees, bodily pain (Van Ommeren, de Jong, et al., 2001); among Cambodian refugees, gastrointestinal distress, neck soreness, tinnitus, and orthostatic dizziness (Hinton, et al., 2007; Hinton, Chhean, Pich, Hofmann, & Barlow, 2006; Hinton, Chhean, Pich, Um, et al., 2006; Hinton, Hinton, Loeum, & Pollack, 2008; Hinton, Hofmann, et al., 2008; Hinton, Hofmann, Pollack, & Otto, 2009); and among Rwandan genocide survivors, sudden shortness of breath (Hagengimana & Hinton, 2009).

Just assessing for the diagnostic criteria for PTSD also neglects local cultural syndromes, leading to a reduction of content validity. As highlighted throughout the chapter, many trauma-related symptoms—startle, flashbacks, numbing, the somatic symptoms caused by arousal, and the emotions of fear or anger—may be locally interpreted as indicating the presence of a folk illness (often in the stereotypical form of a cultural "syndrome"), a specific dysregulation of mind, body, and spiritual state (Nichter, 1981). Examples of these local expressions that are common experiences associated with trauma in various cultural groups include the following (Hinton & Good, 2016; Hinton & Lewis-Fernández, 2011; Kohrt et al., 2014): among Latino populations, *susto* (fright), *nervios* (nerves), and *ataque de nervios* (attack of nerves) (Dickson-Goméz, 2002; Guarnaccia, Canino, Rubio-Stipec, & Bravo, 1993; Guarnaccia, et al., 2003; Lewis-Fernández, Garrido-Castillo, et al., 2002; Lewis-Fernández, Guarnaccia, et al., 2002; Lewis-Fernández et al. 2010; Norris, Perilla, & Murphy, 2001; Weller, Baer, Garcia de Alba Garcia, & Salcedo Rocha, 2008); among Cambodian refugees, "*khyâl* attacks" ("wind attacks" [*gaeut khyâl*]) and "weak heart" (*khsaoy beh doung*) (Hinton et al., 2002; Hinton, Pich, Marques, Nickerson, & Pollack, 2010); in Guinea Bissau and among Mozambique, Ugandan, and Bhutanese refugees, possession by a local supernatural being (de Jong & Reis, 2010; Duijl, Cardeña, & De Jong, 2005; Igreja, Kleijn, & Richters, 2006; Van Ommeren, Sharma, et al., 2001); among civil war victims in Sierra Leone, "hypertension" (*haypatɛnsi*) (Henry, 2006); among Rwandan genocide survivors, *ihahamuka*, literally, "lungs without breath," a syndrome characterized by the sudden onset of shortness of breath (Hagengimana & Hinton, 2009); among Quechua speakers of the Peruvian highlands, *llaki* ("sorrow/sadness") (Pedersen, Tremblay, Errazuriz, & Gamarra, 2008); among the Mandika, *masilango* ("extreme fear") (Fox, 2003); and among Gulf War veterans, the Gulf War Syndrome (Jones & Wessely, 2005).

CONCLUSION: REFLECTIONS ON CLINICAL UTILITY

In this chapter we proposed a model of how culture contributes to the specific patterning and interpretation of the symptoms of trauma-related disorder and then, guided by this model, we reviewed the evidence on cross-cultural prevalence of PTSD, focusing on conditional risk, the differences in symptom salience and meaning across cultures, and the content validity of the diagnostic category of PTSD in assessing trauma-related disorder across cultures. We showed the role that folk illnesses—and local ethnopsychologies, ethnophysiologies, and religious/spiritual ideas, more broadly—play in the patterning of PTSD symptoms. We showed the centrality of somatic symptoms and folk illnesses in the experiencing of trauma-related conditions, which if not evaluated leads to category truncation, a reduction in content validity.

The cross-cultural applicability of the PTSD category as currently specified has generated considerable debate, both in terms of its validity and its clinical utility (Cohn, Dyson, & Wessely, 2008; Jones et al., 2003; Summerfield, 1999). According to some leading investigators, while PTSD begins to describe a few key features of a universal trauma response, its clinical utility for negotiating more fine-grained aspects of healing practice lags behind that of more local forms of expressing trauma-related psychopathology, including folk illnesses (Kleinman & Kleinman, 1991; Young, 1995). Since these local expressions are more "experience-near," their clinical utility may be greater, in that they may be better able to promote empathy and communication, facilitate adherence, negotiate treatment, predict psychopathology, and indicate illness course (Miller et al., 2009).

In this chapter, we have tried to show that the PTSD category does have great utility, but that when doing research and clinical work with a cultural group, a broader model should be kept in mind, which is shown in Figure 11.1. To not consider trauma-related disorder and its symptoms in this way is to commit what we have called an "error of decontextualization" (Hinton & Good, 2016). This might also be called an "abstraction error," in which the evaluator just considers a symptom, a set of symptoms, or a diagnosis in the abstract, rather than as embedded in local meanings and in certain institutions and local practices.

The model of trauma-related disorder in cultural context (Figure 11.1) has important research and treatment implications. The model shows areas that need evaluation and that may be targeted in interventions. Trauma-related disorders and their symptoms should be considered to be part of a constellation of symptoms that constitute a dynamic network experienced in a particular sociocultural context (for recent reviews of the importance of network models in PTSD and psychopathology more generally, see Hofmann, Curtiss, & McNally, 2016; McNally, 2016). Local trauma-related symptoms and their meaning must be assessed at intake and covered in psychoeducation efforts; symptom reduction efforts should highlight these interpretations, such as when instructing the patient in applied muscle relaxation; catastrophic cognitions about trauma-related symptoms should be identified and modified; and the sociocultural course of PTSD needs to be profiled and addressed, such as the effects of trauma-related anger on the family, the role of the local presentations associated with trauma (e.g., *nervios* or *ataque de nervios*) as an idiom of distress emerging from a person's dire social context (e.g., poverty or spousal abuse), and the treatment of trauma symptoms in the health care system and through self-help (and the question of the efficacy of local healing traditions such as Buddhist meditation). In assessing trauma-related disorder, the diagnosis of PTSD has greater clinical utility in cross-cultural work when viewed from the perspective of the model presented in Figure 11.1. This model allows a contextualization of PTSD and trauma-related experiencing more generally.

REFERENCES

Adams, R. E., & Boscarino, J. A. (2005). Differences in mental health outcomes among Whites, African Americans, and Hispanics following a community disaster. *Psychiatry, 68*, 250–265.

Adams, R. E., & Boscarino, J. A. (2006). Predictors of PTSD and delayed PTSD after disaster: The impact of exposure and psychosocial resources. *Journal of Nervous and Mental Disease, 194*, 485–493.

Alcantara, C., Casement, M. D., & Lewis-Fernández, R. (2013). Conditional risk for PTSD among Latinos: A systematic review of racial/ethnic differences and sociocultural explanations. *Clinical Psychology Review, 33*(1), 107–119.

Alegria, M., Fortuna, L. R., Lin, J. Y., Norris, F. H., Gao, S., Takeuchi, D. T., et al. (2013). Prevalence, risk, and correlates of posttraumatic stress disorder across ethnic and racial minority groups in the United States. *Medical Care, 51*(12), 1114–1123.

American Psychiatric Association. (2013). *Diagnostic and statistical manual of mental disorders* (5th ed). Washington, DC: American Psychiatric Publishing.

Candel, I., & Merckelbach, H. (2004). Peritraumatic dissociation as a predictor of posttraumatic stress disorder: A critical review. *Comprehensive Psychiatry, 45*, 44–50.

Clark, D. M., & Ehlers, A. (2004). Posttraumatic stress disorder: From cognitive theory to therapy. In R. L. Leahy (Ed.), *Contemporary cognitive therapy* (pp. 141–160). New York: Guilford.

Cohn, S., Dyson, C., & Wessely, S. (2008). Early accounts of Gulf War illness and the construction of narratives in UK service personnel. *Social Science and Medicine, 67*, 1641–1649.

Crescenzi, A., Ketzer, E., Van Ommeren, M., Phuntsok, K., Komproe, I., & de Jong, J. (2002). Effect of political imprisonment and trauma history on recent Tibetan refugees in India. *Journal of Traumatic Stress, 15*, 369–375.

de Jong, J. T., & Reis, R. (2010). Kiyang-yang, a West-African postwar idiom of distress. *Culture, Medicine, and Psychiatry, 34*, 301–321.

Dell, P. F., & O'Neil, J. A. (Eds.). (2009). *Dissociation and the dissociative disorders: DSM-V and beyond.* New York: Routledge.

Dickson-Goméz, J. (2002). The sound of barking dogs: Violence and terror among Salvadoran families in the postwar. *Medical Anthropology Quarterly, 16*, 415–438.

Duijl, M. V., Cardeña, E., & De Jong, J. T. (2005). The validity of DSM-IV dissociative disorders categories in south-west Uganda. *Transcultural Psychiatry, 42*, 219–241.

Dunmore, E., Clark, D. M., & Ehlers, A. (2001). A prospective investigation of the role of cognitive factors in persistent posttraumatic stress disorder (PTSD) after physical and sexual assault. *Behaviour Research and Therapy, 39*, 1063–1084.

Ehlers, A., Mayou, R. A., & Bryant, B. (1998). Psychological predictors of chronic posttraumatic stress disorder after motor vehicle accidents. *Journal of Abnormal Psychology, 107*, 508–519.

Fox, S. H. (2003). The Mandinka nosological system in the context of post-trauma syndromes. *Transcultural Psychiatry, 40*, 488–506.

Galea, S., Ahern, J., Resnick, H. S., Kilpatrick, D. G., Bucuvalas, M. J., Gold, J., et al. (2002). Psychological sequelae of the September 11 terrorist attacks in New York City. *New England Journal of Medicine, 346*, 982–987.

Galea, S., Vlahov, D., Resnick, H., Ahern, J., Susser, E., Gold, J., et al. (2003). Trends of probable post-traumatic distress disorder in New York City after the September 11 terrorist attacks. *American Journal of Epidemiology, 158*, 514–524.

Guarnaccia, P. J., Canino, G., Rubio-Stipec, M., & Bravo, M. (1993). The prevalence of *ataques de nervios* in the Puerto Rico Disaster Study: The role of culture in psychiatric epidemiology. *Journal of Nervous and Mental Disease, 181*, 157–165.

Guarnaccia, P. J., Lewis-Fernández, R., & Marano, M. R. (2003). Toward a Puerto Rican popular nosology: *Nervios* and *ataque de nervios*. *Culture, Medicine, and Psychiatry, 27*, 339–366.

Hagengimana, A., & Hinton, D. E. (2009). Ihahamuka, a Rwandan syndrome of response to the genocide: Blocked flow, spirit assault, and shortness of breath. In D. E. Hinton & B. J. Good (Eds.), *Culture and panic disorder* (pp. 205–229). Stanford, CA: Stanford University Press.

Hagengimana, A., Hinton, D. E., Bird, B., Pollack, M. H., & Pitman, R. K. (2003). Somatic panic attack equivalents in a community sample of Rwandan widows who survived the genocide. *Psychiatry Research, 117*, 1–9.

Halligan, S. L., Michael, T., Clark, D. M., & Ehlers, A. (2003). Posttraumatic stress disorder following assault: The role of cognitive processing, trauma memory, and appraisal. *Journal of Consulting and Clinical Psychology, 71*, 410–431.

Henry, D. (2006). Violence and the body: Somatic expressions of trauma and vulnerability during war. *Medical Anthropology Quarterly, 20*, 379–415.

Hinton, D. E., Chhean, D., Fama, J. M., Pollack, M. H., & McNally, R. J. (2007). Gastrointestinal-focused panic attacks among Cambodian refugees: Associated psychopathology, flashbacks, and catastrophic cognitions. *Journal of Anxiety Disorders, 21*, 42–58.

Hinton, D. E., Chhean, D., Pich, V., Hofmann, S. G., & Barlow, D. (2006). Tinnitus among Cambodians: Relationship to PTSD severity. *Journal of Traumatic Stress, 19*, 541–546.

Hinton, D. E., Chhean, D., Pich, V., Um, K., Fama, J. M., & Pollack, M. H. (2006). Neck-focused panic attacks among Cambodian refugees; A logistic and linear regression analysis. *Journal of Anxiety Disorders, 20*, 119–138.

Hinton, D. E., Chong, R., Pollack, M. H., Barlow, D. H., & McNally, R. J. (2008). *Ataque de nervios*: Relationship to anxiety sensitivity and dissociation predisposition. *Depression and Anxiety, 25*, 489–495.

Hinton, D. E., & Good, B. J. (Eds.). (2016). *Culture and PTSD: Trauma in historical and global perspective*. Philadelphia: University of Pennsylvenia Press.

Hinton, D. E., Hinton, A., Chhean, D., Pich, V., Loeum, J. R., & Pollack, M. H. (2009). Nightmares among Cambodian refugees: The breaching of concentric ontological security. *Culture, Medicine, and Psychiatry, 33*, 219–265.

Hinton, D. E., Hinton, S. D., Loeum, J. R., & Pollack, M. H. (2008). The "multiplex model" of somatic symptoms: Application to tinnitus among traumatized Cambodian refugees. *Transcultural Psychiatry, 45*, 287–317.

Hinton, D. E., Hinton, S. D., Pham, T., Chau, H., & Tran, M. (2003). "Hit by the wind" and temperature-shift panic among Vietnamese refugees. *Transcultural Psychiatry, 40*, 342–376.

Hinton, D. E., Hinton, S. D., Um, K., Chea, A., & Sak, S. (2002). The Khmer "weak heart" syndrome: Fear of death from palpitations. *Transcultural Psychiatry, 39*, 323–344.

Hinton, D. E., Hofmann, S. G., Pitman, R. K., Pollack, M. H., & Barlow, D. H. (2008). The panic attack–PTSD model: Applicability to orthostatic panic among Cambodian refugees. *Cognitive Behaviour Therapy, 27*, 101–116.

Hinton, D. E., Hofmann, S. G., Pollack, M. H., & Otto, M. W. (2009). Mechanisms of efficacy of CBT for Cambodian refugees with PTSD: Improvement in emotion regulation and orthostatic blood pressure response. *CNS Neuroscience and Therapeutics, 15*(3), 255–263.

Hinton, D. E., & Lewis-Fernández, R. (2011). The cross-cultural validity of posttraumatic stress disorder: Implications for DSM-5. *Depression and Anxiety, 28*, 783–801.

Hinton, D. E., Lewis-Fernández, R., & Pollack, M. H. (2009). A model of the generation of *ataque de nervios*: The role of fear of negative affect and fear of arousal symptoms. *CNS Neuroscience and Therapeutics, 15*, 264–275.

Hinton, D. E., Pich, V., Marques, L., Nickerson, A., & Pollack, M. H. (2010). Khyâl attacks: A key idiom of distress among traumatized Cambodian refugees. *Culture, Medicine and Psychiatry, 34*, 244–278.

Hinton, D. E., Reis, R., & de Jong, J. T. (2015). The "thinking a lot" idiom of distress and PTSD: An examination of their relationship among traumatized Cambodian refugees using the "Thinking a Lot" Questionnaire. *Medical Anthropology Quarterly, 29*, 357–380.

Hinton, D. E., & Simons, N. (2015). Somatization, anxietydisorders (GAD, panic disorder, and PTSD), and the arousal complex in cultural context: The multiplex model and the cultural neuroscience of anxiety disorders. In L. J. Kirmayer, R. Lemelson, & C. Cummings (Eds.), *Revisioning psychiatry: Cultural phenomenology, critical neuroscience, and global mental health* (pp. 343–374). Cambridge, UK: Cambridge University Press.

Hofmann, S. G., Curtiss, J., & McNally, R. J. (2016). A complex network perspective on clinical science. *Perspectives Psychological Science, 11*(5), 597–605.

Holtz, T. H. (1998). Refugee trauma versus torture trauma: A retrospective controlled cohort study of Tibetan refugees. *Journal of Nervous and Mental Disease, 186*, 24–34.

Igreja, V., Kleijn, W., & Richters, A. (2006). When the war was over, little changed: Women's posttraumatic suffering after the war in Mozambique. *Journal of Nervous and Mental Disease, 194*, 502–509.

Jenkins, J. H., & Valiente, M. (1994). Bodily transactions of the passions: El calor (the heat) among Salvadoran women. In T. Csordas (Ed.), *The body as existential ground: Studies in culture, self, and experience* (pp. 163–182). Cambridge, UK: Cambridge University Press.

Jobson, L., & O'Kearney, R. T. (2009). Impact of cultural differences in self on cognitive appraisals in posttraumatic stress disorder. *Behavioural and Cognitive Psychotherapy, 37*, 249–266.

Jones, E., Vermaas, R. H., McCartney, H., Beech, C., Palmer, I., Hyams, K., et al. (2003). Flashbacks and post-traumatic stress disorder: The genesis of a 20th-century diagnosis. *British Journal of Psychiatry, 182*, 158–163.

Jones, E., & Wessely, S. (2005). *Shell shock to PTSD: Military psychiatry from 1900 to the Gulf War*. New York: Psychology Press.

Kaiser, B., Haroz, E., Kohrt, B., Bolton, P., Bass, J., & Hinton, D. E. (2015). Thinking too much: A systematic review of a common idiom of distress. *Social Science and Medicine, 147*, 170–183.

Keane, T. M., Kaloupec, D. G., & Weathers, F. W. (1996). Ethnocultural considerations on the assessment of PTSD. In A. J. Marsella, M. J. Friedman, E. T. Gerrity, & R. M. Scurfield (Eds.), *Ethnocultural aspects of posttraumatic stress disorder: Issues, research, and clinical applications* (pp. 183–208). Washington, DC: American Psychological Association.

Kirmayer, L. J., & Bhugra, D. (2009). Culture and mental illness: Social context and explanatory models. In I. M. Salloum & J. E. Mezzich (Eds.), *Psychiatric diagnosis: Patterns and prospects* (pp. 29–40). New York: Wiley.

Kirmayer, L. J., & Sartorius, N. (2007). Cultural models and somatic syndromes. *Psychosomatic Medicine, 69*, 832–840.

Kleinman, A., & Kleinman, J. (1991). Suffering and its professional transformation: Toward an ethnography of interpersonal experience. *Culture, Medicine, and Psychiatry, 15*, 275–301.

Kohrt, B. A., Rasmussen, A., Kaiser, B., Haroz, E. E., Maharjan, S. M., Mutamba, B. B., et al. (2014). Cultural concepts of distress and psychiatric disorders: Literature review and research recommendations for global mental health epidemiology. *International Journal of Epidemiology, 43*, 365–406.

Leskin, G. A., & Sheikh, J. I. (2002). Lifetime trauma history and panic disorder: Findings from the National Comorbidity Survey. *Journal of Anxiety Disorders, 16*, 599–603.

Lewis-Fernández, R., Garrido-Castillo, P., Bennasar, M. C., Parrilla, E. M., Laria, A. J., Ma, G., et al. (2002). Dissociation, childhood trauma, and *ataque de nervios* among Puerto Rican psychiatric outpatients. *American Journal of Psychiatry, 159*, 1603–1605.

Lewis-Fernández, R., Gorritz, M., Raggio, G. A., Peláez, C., Chen, H., & Guarnaccia, P. J. (2010). Association of trauma-related disorders and dissociation with four idioms of distress among Latino psychiatric outpatients. *Culture, Medicine, and Psychiatry, 34*, 219–243.

Lewis-Fernández, R., Guarnaccia, P. J., Martinez, I. E., Salmán, E., Schmidt, A., & Liebowitz, M. (2002). Comparative phenomenology of *ataques de nervios*, panic attacks, and panic disorder. *Culture, Medicine, and Psychiatry, 26*, 199–223.

Low, S. (1985). Culturally interpreted symptoms or culture-bound syndromes: A cross-cultural review of nerves. *Social Science and Medicine, 21*, 187–196.

Marshall, G. N., Schell, T. L., Elliott, M. N., Berthold, S. M., & Chun, C. A. (2005). Mental health of Cambodian refugees 2 decades after resettlement in the United States. *JAMA, 294*, 571–579.

Mattingly, C., & Garro, L. C. (Eds.). (2000). *Narrative and the cultural construction of illness*. Berkeley: University of California Press.

McNally, R. J. (2016). Can network analysis transform psychopathology? *Behavior Research Therapy, 86*, 95–104.

McQuaid, J. R., Pedrelli, P., McCahill, M. E., & Stein, M. B. (2001). Reported trauma, post-traumatic stress disorder and major depression among primary care patients. *Psychological Medicine, 31*, 1249–1257.

Miller, K. E., Omidian, P., Kulkarni, M., Yaqubi, A., Daudzai, H., & Rasmussen, A. (2009). The validity and clinical utility of post-traumatic stress disorder in Afghanistan. *Transcultural Psychiatry, 46*, 219–237.

Moser, J. S., Hajcak, G., Simons, R. F., & Foa, E. B. (2007). Posttraumatic stress disorder symptoms in trauma-exposed college students: The role of trauma-related cognitions, gender, and negative affect. *Journal of Anxiety Disorders, 21*, 1039–1049.

Nichter, M. (1981). Idioms of distress: Alternatives in the expression of psychosocial distress: A case from South India. *Culture, Medicine, and Psychiatry, 5*, 379–408.

Norris, F. H., Perilla, J. L., & Murphy, A. D. (2001). Postdisaster stress in the United States and Mexico: A cross-cultural test of the multicriterion conceptual model of posttraumatic stress disorder. *Journal of Abnormal Psychology, 110*, 553–563.

Ozer, E. J., Best, S. R., Lipsey, T. L., & Weiss, D. S. (2003). Predictors of posttraumatic stress disorder and symptoms in adults: A meta-analysis. *Psychological Bulletin, 129*, 52–73.

Palinkas, L. A., Petterson, J. S., Russell, J. C., & Downs, M. A. (2004). Ethnic differences in symptoms of posttraumatic stress after the Exxon Valdez oil spil. *Prehospital and Disaster Medicine, 19*, 102–112.

Pedersen, D., Tremblay, J., Errazuriz, C., & Gamarra, J. (2008). The sequelae of political violence: Assessing trauma, suffering and dislocation in the Peruvian highlands. *Social Science and Medicine, 67*, 205–217.

Perilla, J. L., Norris, F. H., & Lavizzo, E. A. (2002). Ethnicity, culture, and disaster response: Identifying and explaining ethnic differences in PTSD six months after Hurricane Andrew. *Journal of Social and Clinical Psychology, 21*, 20–45.

Rubel, A. J., O'Nell, C. W., & Collado-Ardón, R. (1984). *Susto: A folk illness*. Berkeley: University of California Press.

Sachs, E., Rosenfeld, B., Lhewa, D., Rasmussen, A., & Keller, A. (2008). Entering exile: Trauma, mental health, and coping among Tibetan refugees arriving in Dharamsala, India. *Journal of Traumatic Stress, 21*, 199–208.

Shore, J. H., Orton, H., & Manson, S. M. (2009). Trauma-related nightmares among American Indian veterans: Views from the dream catcher. *American Indian and Alaska Native Mental Health Research, 16*, 25–38.

Silove, D., Bateman, C. R., Brooks, R. T., Fonseca, C. A. Z., Steel, A., Rodger, J., et al. (2008). Estimating clinically relevant mental disorders in a rural and an urban setting in postconflict Timor Leste. *Archives of General Psychiatry, 65*, 1205–1212.

Summerfield, D. (1999). A critique of seven assumptions behind psychological trauma programs in war-affected areas. *Social Science and Medicine, 48*, 1449–1462.

Tang, S. S., & Fox, S. H. (2001). Traumatic experiences and the mental health of Senegalese refugees. *Journal of Nervous and Mental Disease, 189*, 507–512.

Tol, W. A., Komproe, I. H., Thapa, S. B., Jordans, M. J. D., Sharma, B., & Jong, J. T. V. M. D. (2007). Disability associated with psychiatric symptoms among torture survivors in rural Nepal. *Journal of Nervous and Mental Disease, 195*, 463–469.

Van Ommeren, M., de Jong, J. T., Sharma, B., Komproe, I., Thapa, S. B., & Cardeña, E. (2001). Psychiatric disorders among tortured Bhutanese refugees in Nepal. *Archives of General Psychiatry, 58*, 475–482.

Van Ommeren, M., Sharma, B., Komproe, Poudyal, B. N., Sharma, G. K., Cardeña, E., et al. (2001). Trauma and loss as determinants of medically unexplained epidemic illness in a Bhutanese refugee camp. *Psychological Medicine, 31*, 1259–1267.

Weller, S. C., Baer, R. D., Garcia de Alba Garcia, J., & Salcedo Rocha, A. L. (2008). *Susto* and *nervios*: Expressions for stress and depression. *Culture, Medicine, and Psychiatry, 32*, 406–420.

Young, A. (1995). *The harmony of illusions: Inventing post-traumatic stress disorder*. Princeton, NJ: Princeton University Press.

12

The Role of Stress in the Etiology of PTSD

EDWARD F. PACE-SCHOTT AND SAMUEL GAZECKI

INTRODUCTION

The fifth edition of the *Diagnostic and Statistical Manual of Mental Disorders* has clustered posttraumatic stress disorder (PTSD) symptomatology into four distinct categories, which include intrusive memories or nightmares of the traumatic event, avoidance of situations or stimuli associated with the event, persistent negativity of mood and cognition, and hyperarousal. Although these symptoms are quite common for anyone who has experienced a significantly traumatic event, symptom alleviation generally occurs within one month [1]. However, 10% to 30% of people who experience a traumatic event continue to have enduring symptoms [2]. In the past 15 years, advances in understanding the neurobiology of stress and anxiety have revealed underlying neural abnormities in patients with PTSD that might help explain why symptoms persist in some patients. This chapter focuses on research showing that abnormal hypothalamic-pituitary-adrenal (HPA) axis activity, abnormalities of the catecholamingergic/autonomic system, as well as atypical physiologic and neural circuit responses during fear extinction recall may be important biological factors for the etiology and maintenance of PTSD symptoms.

ETIOLOGIES OF PTSD: HOW ABNORMALITIES OF THE HPA AXIS PRECIPITATE PTSD SYMPTOMS

Due to its prominent role in facilitating a neuroendocrine response to stress, the study of the HPA axis following a particularly stressful (traumatic) event has been extensive. Definitions of stress might vary, but in the context of HPA activity as it relates to PTSD, stress is defined in this chapter "as an actual or anticipated disruption of homeostasis or an anticipated threat to well-being" [3]. Neurochemical factors that mediate the stress response in the HPA axis, such as corticotropin releasing factor (CRF) have consistently been found to function abnormally in PTSD patients [4].

The HPA axis works through the interplay of three endocrine components: the hypothalamus, the anterior pituitary gland, and the adrenal gland. Upon exposure to a stressor, parvocellular neurons of the hypothalamic paraventricular nucleus release CRF into the hypothalamo-pituitary portal circulation. This in turn stimulates the production of adrenocorticotropin releasing hormone (ACTH) from the anterior pituitary gland. ACTH then acts on the cortex of the adrenal gland to stimulate the release of glucocorticoids. Glucocorticoids might be thought of as the "terminating" hormone of this stress response, as they inhibit both the hypothalamus from producing CRF and the anterior pituitary from producing ACTH; that is to say, cortisol is the primary neurochemical signal that enables a negative feedback response to stress. So, having more cortisol released should lead to a less active hypothalamus and anterior pituitary gland, which will lead to less CRF and ACTH production and therefore a less active HPA axis as a whole.

Initial findings suggested that low basal cortisol levels might be a strong biomarker for PTSD. In a well-known study [5], mean cortisol level in urine was compared between Holocaust survivors that had developed PTSD and Holocaust survivors who had not developed PTSD; survivors who had developed PTSD had lower mean cortisol levels over a 24-hr time period. This finding was initially seen as counterintuitive, as it would be expected that activity of cortisol in people with PTSD would be similar to cortisol activity in those experiencing anxiety and depression [6], since anxiety and depression are often comorbid psychiatric diseases. However, repeated studies measuring mean cortisol output from peripheral systems (urine, saliva, blood, etc.) in patients with PTSD versus non-PTSD could not consistently replicate this finding [7–9]. Furthermore, a recent meta-analysis was done on cortisol levels between patients with PTSD and without PTSD, and there was no significant difference in cortisol levels found [10].

The next particularly fruitful line of studies in PTSD and stress research examined the effect that dexamethasone (DEX) has on the negative feedback mechanism of the HPA axis. DEX is a synthetic glucocorticoid that inhibits the production of ACTH at the level of the pituitary and therefore mimics the negative feedback produced by endogenous cortisol and acts as an inhibitor of feedback in the HPA axis as a whole. The dexamethasone suppression test uses DEX to observe how HPA axis activity is perturbed, and this test has been used to determine that people with PTSD have less cortisol production during this test. This signifies that the HPA axis in people with PTSD is more sensitive to the inhibitory effect that cortisol has on HPA axis activity [11]. This finding led to the hypothesis that glucocorticoid receptor (GR) sensitivity is enhanced in people with PTSD [12]. Since the inception of this hypothesis, the finding that GR sensitivity is increased in people with PTSD has been clearly supported [13], as has the finding that GR number is also increased in people with PTSD [14, 15]. This finding makes intuitive sense, given that cortisol is a primary neurochemical used to quell the activity of the sympathetic nervous system (SNS) during "fight-or-flight" situations. With a hypersensitivity of the GR leading to less overall cortisol output, there is less neurochemical available to stop SNS activity, and thus the stress response continues unabated.

Studies have examined catecholamine levels in people with PTSD, as levels of catecholamine are an index of SNS activity. It has been consistently found that people with PTSD demonstrate elevated catecholamine levels [7, 16–19]. This might suggest that trauma memories in people with PTSD might become overconsolidated and inappropriately expressed due to enhanced levels of distress [12, 20]; although people with PTSD have not been found to have elevated catecholamine levels directly after the time of trauma [21, 22]. Taken together, these findings might suggest that both GR sensitivity, quantity of GR, and elevated catecholamine levels are all acquired traits of PTSD, rather than risk factors for the development of PTSD.

Over the last decade, geneticists have uncovered some gene x environmental factors that might contribute to the development of PTSD. As it relates to stress and the HPA axis, it has been found that a glucocorticoid-regulating co-chaperone protein called FKBP5 significantly alters the probability of PTSD development following a traumatic experience [23–25]. Glucocorticoid receptors are located within the cytoplasm and are typically bound to the FKBP5 protein when not bound to cortisol. Upon the GR binding to a ligand, the FKBP5 protein detaches from the GR and the FKBP4 protein attaches to the GR. FBKP4 recruits dynein and enables the GR to translocate to the nucleus, wherein gene expression can be modified [26, 27]. The FKBP5 protein is thought to have a negative feedback relationship with GR sensitivity, such that higher expression levels of the FKBP5 protein will cause the GR to become less sensitive to the binding of a ligand. Moreover, studies have shown that overexpression of FKBP5 in vitro have led to a reduction in the affinity for cortisol to bind to GR [26–28]. This is consistent with the finding that persons with PTSD have been found to have a reduced expression of FKBP5 [29], which provides a genetic basis for why GRs are more sensitive in persons with PTSD.

More recently, research has begun to examine how the presence of a specific type of FKBP5 gene mutation might dictate structural and functional connectivity in persons with FKBP5. This research is especially amenable for looking at structures that heavily express GRs, as the presence of FKBP5 has been shown to significantly modulate the activity of GRs. Due to this, FKBP5 might be an agent in changing how structures communicate with one another, particularly by influencing dendritic remodeling and dendritic spine plasticity [30]. A recent study [31] examined whether the presence of an FKBP5 functional polymorphism with two "T" alleles would influence structural and functional connectivity between the hippocampus and anterior cingulate cortex (ACC), both of which are regions that may be functionally abnormal in PTSD. Indeed, one study [31] found that patients diagnosed with PTSD who express this functional polymorphism have a weaker structural connectivity between the hippocampus and prefrontal areas (a pathway known to be important for emotional regulation) as compared to persons exposed to trauma but who did not develop PTSD. Additionally, the functional connectivity was significantly impaired between the hippocampus and the ACC. Their finding is consistent with previous findings which showed that PTSD patients have a decreased structural and functional connectivity of the hippocampus-prefrontal pathway [32]. Thus, the authors conclude that they have successfully identified a gene that is a biomarker for a pre-risk factor. Identifying pre-risk factors have consistently been a challenge for PTSD research, but recent advances in genetics point to a promising road for answering this challenge.

THE INTERPLAY BETWEEN STRESS AND THE FEAR CIRCUITRY

Neuroimaging techniques have elucidated the neural mechanisms that underlie many of our emotional learning processes. Advances in functional magnetic resonance imaging, positron emission tomography, magnetoencephalography, and electroencephalography have allowed us to discover that associative fear learning may be impaired in PTSD. This finding has been researched using a fear-conditioning paradigm, with strong evidence indicating that the fear learning and expression processes function abnormally in people with PTSD. Moreover, stress is known to have a significant effect on fear learning and expression. First and foremost, it is a well-documented fact that chronic stress has been shown to substantially increase the probability of developing PTSD after experiencing a traumatic event [33]. How exactly these stress-induced effects on the brain make one more susceptible to developing PTSD is not entirely clear. However, studies have found that chronic stress modulates the volume of particular areas of the brain, primarily through chronic stress causing abnormal glucocorticoid activity, which lead to other abnormalities in downstream processes such as glutamatergic transmission, which is important for structural remodeling of dendrites and synapses [34]. The areas commonly affected include the prefrontal cortex, amygdala, and hippocampus [35, 36], all of which heavily express glucocorticoid receptors and are important structures for fear learning processes.

Neuroimaging studies looking at people with PTSD have discovered that there is a set of structures in the brain that communicate with each other when responding to a threatening situation or stimulus. This is known as the "fear circuit." Interestingly, studies have found that there are discrete sets of structures that do not activate nor communicate with each other normally in people with PTSD. The most replicated example of this abnormality is seen during fear extinction recall [37–39]. More recently, scientists have begun to examine how the stressed brain responds in persons without PTSD both during and after fear conditioning. Since PTSD can be thought of as a disorder of stress, it is thought that the stressed brain of someone without PTSD might serve as an adequate control for the PTSD brain. The stressed brain then will lend insight into how the brain of someone with PTSD might work during fear learning. Investigators have found that some processes in the stressed brain during fear learning parallel what is observed in patients with PTSD, which lends credence to the belief that PTSD is a disorder of stress.

In order to examine how the stressed brain processes fearful information, one study [40] used a single prolonged stress (SPS) test in rats before fear conditioning and then examined how acquisition and retention of both cued and contextual extinction was affected. SPS is a method used to stress an animal to such an extent that it exhibits symptoms similar to the PTSD phenotype (i.e., hyperarousal, changes in HPA function) [41]. In doing so, Knox et al. discovered that both cued and contextual fear extinction recall were impaired but not the extinction acquisition process. That is, the rats were able to extinguish the initial unconditioned stimulus (US)–conditioned stimulus (CS) association during the extinction training session but could not exhibit any memory of the extinction association when tested the following session. Additionally, it was found that fear renewal was also compromised. A possible explanation for this observation is that stress sensitizes the rat to fear learning, such that the rat more strongly encodes the initial CS-US contingency during the initial fear-learning phase. As a result, the initial CS-US contingency becomes more resistant to extinction relative to other types of CS-US associations [40].

This hypothesis has been substantiated using the stress enhanced fear-learning paradigm (SEFL), which is a method that entails spontaneously foot-shocking rats in order to induce stress prior to fear conditioning [42]. In one experiment [43], it was found that fear learning is greatly potentiated after SEFL; additionally, it was also found that the fear association was highly resistant to extinction. The extinction process was explored by presenting to the rat the extinguished context and extinguished cue individually. In either case, the rat continued to exhibit a conditioned response. Due to the fact that the rat continued to exhibit a conditioned response to the novel context in which extinction took place, it could be said that the US-CS contingency is resistant to extinction due to a *non*-associative sensitization of fear (because there was no prior association between fear response and context). This nonassociative sensitization is attributed to the stress response potentiating the initial US-CS contingency during the learning phase; similarly, it might be hypothesized that people develop PTSD because of an elevated stress response from the traumatic event, and this stress response potentiates the US-CS learning process.

Neuroimaging and psychophysiology studies of humans have reported results that are consistent with the findings in the animal literature. A canonical finding among psychophysiological studies is that persons diagnosed with PTSD do not exhibit a significantly different skin conductance response (SCR) to extinguished stimuli when compared to the SCR to unextinguished stimuli. Increased SCR is indicative of an increased SNS response and is commonly measured to evaluate associative learning to fearful stimuli. In comparison, people without a PTSD diagnosis demonstrate a significantly lower SCR to extinguished stimuli versus unextinguished stimuli [44], which suggests a learning difference between the two. This learning difference has been discovered to have a neural basis in the fear circuitry; persons with PTSD have a hypoactivation of the hippocampus and the bilateral vmPFC, as well as hyperactivation of the dorsal ACC during extinction recall (dACC) [38]. Moreover, the extent to which one retains the extinction memory has been found to positively co-vary with activation of the hippocampus and vmPFC and to negatively co-vary with activity of the dACC. Last, it has been found that persons with PTSD have a hyper¥activation of the dACC and hypoactivation of the vmPFC when exposed to the context in which the extinction training took place [45]. This differential responding to contextual information is taken to suggest that persons with PTSD might have an deficient ability to recognize safety cues, and this could be an explanation for why it seems that persons with PTSD generalize their fear response [46].

STRUCTURAL ABNORMALITIES OF FEAR EXTINCTION NETWORK

Structural abnormalities in patients with PTSD have also been consistently found by using structural magnetic resonance imaging. Studies have consistently found that chronic stress seems to be associated with a decreased hippocampus and vmPFC volume [47, 48]. This finding has also been found in PTSD populations, where reduced volume was found in the rostral vmPFC and additionally in the dACC [49–51]. Persons displaying PTSD were also found to have less total brain tissue and lower cerebral grey matter in the left ventral prefrontal regions. Within the context of fear learning, the hippocampus is thought to incorporate contextual cues from the environment to realize safety. Meanwhile, the vmPFC is thought to maintain the extinction of the conditioned emotional responses intact; the reduced ability to recognize contextual cues and maintain extinction memory trace intact is symptomatic of PTSD, and thus a diminution in the volume of these structures is consistent with the PTSD model [4].

Studies have been done to try to determine whether a change in the volume of these structures is an acquired trait or a pre-risk factor. A popular method for researching this question is to examine twins that have been exposed to the same type of trauma but are discordant for PTSD. One such study used this exact method and found that there was no significant difference in volume in the hippocampus. Additionally, the authors also compared the hippocampal volume of identical twins that did not have PTSD and only one of the twins had been exposed to trauma. When comparing the pair of twins with the PTSD to the non-PTSD pair of twins, they found that the twins who had an individual with PTSD had a smaller hippocampal volume [52]. This seems to suggest that volume size is a pre-risk factor when one pair of twins, which had an individual with PTSD, had a significantly smaller hippocampal volume. Additionally, there is evidence that hippocampal volume is subject to change and not predetermined. Research has demonstrated that hippocampal volume can change with treatment of 5-hydroxytryptamine (serotonin) [53]. Moreover, research has shown that aerobic exercise promotes structural growth, particularly in the hippocampus through brain derived neurotrophic factor (BDNF) [54]. There is evidence pointing in both directions as to whether decreased hippocampal volume is an acquired trait or a pre-risk factor for PTSD, and to this day the question still remains unanswered. Though, given the information presented in this chapter, it seems likely that stress—whether chronic or acute—is a factor in increasing the likelihood for developing PTSD after experiencing a traumatic event.

REFERENCES

1. Nemeroff, C. B., Bremner Jd Fau - Foa, E. B., Foa Eb Fau - Mayberg, H. S., Mayberg Hs Fau - North, C. S., North Cs Fau - Stein, M. B., and Stein, M. B. (2006). Posttraumatic stress disorder: a state-of-the-science review. Journal of Psychiatry Research. *Feb;40(1)*, 1–21.

2. Keane, T. M., Marshall, A. D., and Taft, C. T. (2006). Posttraumatic stress disorder: Etiology, epidemiology, and treatment outcome. *Annual Review of Clinical Psychology, 2*(1548-5943 (Print)), 161–197.
3. Daskalakis, N. P. (2016). New translational perspectives for blood-based biomarkers of PTSD: From glucocorticoid to immune mediators of stress susceptibility. *Experimental Neurology, 284(Pt B)*(2016 Oct), 133–140.
4. Pitman, R. K. (2012). Biological studies of post-traumatic stress disorder. *Nature Reviews Neuroscience, 13*, 769–787.
5. Yehuda, R., Kahana, B., Binder-Brynes, K., Southwick, S. M., Mason, J. W., and Giller, E. L. (1995). Low urinary cortisol excretion in Holocaust survivors with posttraumatic stress disorder. *American Journal of Psychiatry, 152*, 982–986.
6. Mason, J. W. J. (1986). Urinary free-cortisol levels in posttraumatic stress disorder patients. *Journal of Nervous and Mental Disease, 174*, 145–149.
7. Pitman, R. K., and Orr, S. P. (1990). Twenty-four hour urinary cortisol and catecholamine excretion in combat-related posttraumatic stress disorder. *Biological Psychiatry, 27(2)*(0006-3223 (Print)), 245–247.
8. Lemieux, A. M., and Coe, C. L. (1995). Abuse-related posttraumatic stress disorder: Evidence for chronic neuroendocrine activation in women. *Psychosomatic Medicine, 57(2)*(0033-3174 (Print)), 105–115.
9. Maes, M., Lin, A., van Hunsel, F., Van Gastel, A., Delmeire, L., et al. (1998). Increased 24-hour urinary cortisol excretion in patients with posttraumatic stress disorder and patients with major depression, but not in patients with fibromyalgia. *Acta Psychiatrica Scandinavica, 98(4)*(0001-690X (Print)), 328–335.
10. Meewisse, M. L., Reitsma, J. B., de Vries, G.-J., Gersons, B. P. R., and Olff, M. (2007). Cortisol and post-traumatic stress disorder in adults: Systematic review and meta-analysis. *British Journal of Psychiatry, 191*(0007-1250 (Print)), 387–392.
11. Yehuda, R., Southwick, S. M., Krystal, J. H., Bremner, D., Charney, D. S., and Mason, J. W. (1993). Enhanced suppression of cortisol following dexamethasone administration in posttraumatic stress disorder. *Journal of Psychiatry, 150(1)*(0002-953X (Print)), 83–86.
12. Yehuda, R. R. (2009). Status of glucocorticoid alterations in post-traumatic stress disorder. *Annals of the New York Academy of Sciences, 1179*, 56–69.
13. Yehuda, R., Golier, J. A. Yang, R.-K., and Tischler, L. (2004). Enhanced sensitivity to glucocorticoids in peripheral mononuclear leukocytes in posttraumatic stress disorder. *Biological Psychiatry, 55(11)*(0006-3223 (Print)), 1110–1116.
14. Yehuda, R., Boisoneau, D., Mason, J. W., and Giller, E. L. (1993). Glucocorticoid receptor number and cortisol excretion in mood, anxiety, and psychotic disorders. *Biological Psychiatry, 34(1-2)*(0006-3223 (Print)), 18–25.
15. Yehuda, R., Lowy, M. T., Southwick, S. M., Shaffer, D., and Giller, E. L. Jr. (1991). Lymphocyte glucocorticoid receptor number in posttraumatic stress disorder. *American Journal of Psychiatry, 148(4)* (0002-953X (Print)), 499–504.
16. Mason, J. W., Giller, E. L., Kosten, T. R., Ostroff, R. B., and Podd, L. (1986). Urinary free-cortisol levels in posttraumatic stress disorder patients. *The journal of nervous and mental disease, 174(3)* (0022-3018 (Print)), 145–149.
17. Simeon, D., Knutelska, M., Smith, L., Baker, B. R., and Hollander, E. (2007). A preliminary study of cortisol and norepinephrine reactivity to psychosocial stress in borderline personality disorder with high and low dissociation. *Psychiatric Research, 149(1-3)*(0165-1781 (Print)), 177–184.
18. Marshall, R. D., Blanco, C., Printz, D., Liebowitz, M. R., Klein, D. F., and Coplan, J. (2002). A pilot study of noradrenergic and HPA axis functioning in PTSD vs. panic disorder. *Psychiatric Research, 110(3)*(0165-1781 (Print)), 219–230.
19. Yehuda, R. (1998). Psychoneuroendocrinology of post-traumatic stress disorder. *Psychiatric Clinics of North America, 21(2)*(0193-953X (Print)), 359–379.
20. Cahill, L., Prins, B., Weber, M., and McGaugh, J. L. (1994). Beta-adrenergic activation and memory for emotional events. *Nature, 371(6499)* (0028-0836 (Print)), 702–704.
21. Shalev, A.Y. (2007). Stress hormones and post-traumatic stress disorder in civilian trauma victims: A longitudinal study. Part I: HPA axis responses. *International Journal of Neuropsychopharmacology, 11*, 365–372.
22. Videlock, E. J., Peleg, T., Segman, R., Yehuda, R., Pitman, R. K., and Shalev, A.Y. (2008). Stress hormones and post-traumatic stress disorder in civilian trauma victims: A longitudinal study. Part II: The adrenergic response. T*he International Journal of Neuropsychopharmacology, 11*(3), 365–372.
23. Binder, E. B., Bradley, R. G., Liu, W., Epstein, M. P., Deveau, T. C., Mercer, K. B., et al. (2008). Association of FKBP5 polymorphisms and childhood abuse with risk of posttraumatic stress disorder symptoms in adults. *The Journal of the*

American Medical Association, 299(11)(1538-3598 (Electronic)), 1291–1305.

24. Xie, P., Kranzler, H. R., Poling, J., Stein, M. B., Anton, R. F., Farrer, L. A., Farrer, L., and Gelernter, J. (2010). Interaction of FKBP5 with childhood adversity on risk for post-traumatic stress disor der.*Neuropsychopharmacology, 35(8)*(1740-634X (Electronic)), 1684–1692.
25. Mehta, D. D. (2011). Using polymorphisms in FKBP5 to define biologically distinct subtypes of posttraumatic stress disorder: Evidence from endocrine and gene expression studies. *Archives of General Psychiatry, 68*, 901–910.
26. Davies, T. H., Ning, Y. M., and Sanchez, E. R. (2002). A new first step in activation of steroid receptors: Hormone-induced switching of FKBP51 and FKBP52 immunophilins. *Journal of Biological Chemistry, 277(7)*(0021-9258 (Print)), 4597–4600.
27. Wochnik, G. M., Ruegg, J. Abel, G. A., Schmidt, U., Holsboer, F., and Rein, T. (2005). FK506-binding proteins 51 and 52 differentially regulate dynein interaction and nuclear translocation of the glucocorticoid receptor in mammalian cells. *Journal of Biological Chemistry, 280(6)*(0021-9258 (Print)), 4609–4616.
28. Matic, G., Milutinovic, D. V., Nestorov, J., Elakovic, I., Jovanovic, S. M., Perisic, T., et al. (2013). Lymphocyte glucocorticoid receptor expression level and hormone-binding properties differ between war trauma-exposed men with and without PTSD. *Progress in neuro-psychopharmacology & biological psychiatry, 43*(1878-4216 (Electronic)), 238–245.
29. Yehuda, R., Cai, G., Golier, J. A., Sarapas, C., Galea, S., Ising, M., et al. (2009). Gene expression patterns associated with posttraumatic stress disorder following exposure to the World Trade Center attacks. *Biological Psychiatry, 66(7)*(1873-2402 (Electronic)), 708–711.
30. Hall, B. S., Moda, R. N., and Liston, C. (2015). Glucocorticoid mechanisms of functional connectivity changes in stress-related neuropsychiatric disorders. *Neurobiology of Stress, 1*(2352-2895 (Print)), 174–183.
31. Fani, N., King, T. Z., Shin, J., Srivastava, A., Brewster, R. C., Jovanovic, T., Bradley, B., and Ressler, K. J. (2016). Structural and functional connectivity in posttraumatic stress disorder: Associations with FKBP5. *Depression and Anxiety, 33*, 300–307.
32. Fani, N., King, T. Z., Reiser, E., Binder, E. B., Jovanovic, T., Bradley, B., and Ressler, K. J. (2014). FKBP5 genotype and structural integrity of the posterior cingulum. *Neuropsychopharmacology, 39(5)*(1740-634X (Electronic)), 1206–1213.
33. Karstoft, K. I., Statnikov, A., Andersen, S. B., Madsen, T., and Galatzer-Levy, I. R. (2015). Early identification of posttraumatic stress following military deployment: Application of machine learning methods to a prospective study of Danish soldiers. *Journal of Affective Disorders, 184*(1573-2517 (Electronic)), 170–175.
34. Popoli, M., Yan, Z., McEwen, B. S., and Sanacora, G. (2011). The stressed synapse: The impact of stress and glucocorticoids on glutamate transmission. *Nature Reviews Neuroscience, 13(1)*(1471-0048 (Electronic)), 22–37.
35. McEwen, B. S., Nasca, C., and Gray, J. D. (2016). Stress effects on neuronal structure: Hippocampus, amygdala, and prefrontal cortex. *Neuropsychopharmacology, 41*, 3–23.
36. Rubin, T. G., Gray, J. D., and McEwen, B. S. (2014). Experience and the ever-changing brain: What the transcriptome can reveal. *BioEssays, 36*, 1072–1081.
37. Hofmann, S. G. (2007). Enhancing exposure-based therapy from a translational research perspective. *Behaviour Research and Therapy, 45(9)* (0005-7967 (Print)), 1987–2001.
38. Milad, M. R. (2009). Neurobiological basis of failure to recall extinction memory in posttraumatic stress disorder. *Biological Psychiatry, 66*, 1075–1082.
39. Bontempo, A., Panza, K. E., and Bloch, M. H. (2012). D-cycloserine augmentation of behavioral therapy for the treatment of anxiety disorders: A meta-analysis. *The Journal of Clinical Psychiatry, 73(4)*(1555-2101 (Electronic)), 533–537.
40. Knox, D., George, S. A., Fitzpatrick, C. J., Rabinak, C. A., Maren, S., and Liberzon, I. (2012). Single prolonged stress disrupts retention of extinguished fear in rats. Single prolonged stress disrupts retention of extinguished fear in rats. *Learning & Memory, 19(2)*(1549-5485 (Electronic)).
41. Kohda, K., Harada, K., Kato, K., Hoshino, A., Motohashi, J., Yamaji, T., Morinobu, S., Matsuoka, N., and Kato, N. (2007). Glucocorticoid receptor activation is involved in producing abnormal phenotypes of single-prolonged stress rats: A putative post-traumatic stress disorder model. *Neuroscience, 148*, 22–33.
42. Rau, V., DeCola, J. P., and Fanselow, M. S. (2005). Stress-induced enhancement of fear learning: An animal model of posttraumatic stress disorder. *Neuroscience & Biobehavioral Reviews, 29(8)* (0149-7634 (Print)), 1207–1223.
43. Long, V. A., and Fanselow, M. S. (2012). Stress-enhanced fear learning in rats is resistant to the effects of immediate massed extinction. *Stress, 15(6)*(1607-8888 (Electronic)), 627–636.

44. Milad, M. R., Orr, S. P., Lasko, N. B., Chang, Y., Rauch, S. L., and Pitman, R. K. (2008). Presence and acquired origin of reduced recall for fear extinction in PTSD: results of a twin study. *Journal of Psychiatric Research, 42*(7)(0022-3956 (Print)), 515–520.
45. Rougemont-Bucking, A., Linnman, C., Zeffiro, T. A., Zeidan, M. A., Lebron-Milad, K., Rodriguez-Romaguera, J., et al. (2011). Altered processing of contextual information during fear extinction in PTSD: An fMRI study. *CNS Neuroscience & Therapeutics, 17*(4)(1755-5949 (Electronic)), 227–236.
46. Milad, M. R., Rosenbaum, B. L., and Simon, N. M. (2014). Neuroscience of fear extinction: Implications for assessment and treatment of fear-based and anxiety related disorders. *Behaviour Research and Therapy, 62*, 17–23.
47. Kitayama, N., Vaccarino, V., Kutner, M., Weiss. P., and Bremner, J. D. (2005). Magnetic resonance imaging (MRI) measurement of hippocampal volume in posttraumatic stress disorder: a meta-analysis. *Journal of Affective Disorders, 88*(*1*) (0165-0327 (Print)), 79–86.
48. Bremner, J. D., Randall, P. Scott, T. M., Bronen, R. A., Seibyl, J. P., Southwick, S.M., et al. (1995). MRI-based measurement of hippocampal volume in patients with combat-related posttraumatic stress disorder. *American Journal of Psychiatry, 152*(*7*)(0002-953X (Print)), 973–981.
49. Carrion, V. G., Weems, C. F., Richert, K., Hoffman, B. C., and Reiss, A.L. (2010). Decreased prefrontal cortical volume associated with increased bedtime cortisol in traumatized youth.*Biological Psychiatry, 68*(*5*)(1873-2402 (Electronic)), 491–493.
50. Kitayama, N., Quinn, S., and Bremner, J. D. (2006). Smaller volume of anterior cingulate cortex in abuse-related posttraumatic stress disorder. *Journal of Affective Disorders, 90*(*2-3*) (0165-0327 (Print)), 171–174.
51. Kasai, K., Yamasue, H. Gilbertson, M. W., Shenton, M. E., Rauch, S. L., and Pitman, R. K. (2008). Evidence for acquired pregenual anterior cingulate gray matter loss from a twin study of combat-related posttraumatic stress disorder. *Biological Psychiatry, 63*(*6*)(1873-2402 (Electronic)), 550–556.
52. Gilbertson, M. W. M. W. (2002). Smaller hippocampal volume predicts pathologic vulnerability to psychological trauma. *Nature neuroscience, 5*(11), 1242–1247.
53. Vermetten, E., Vythilingam, M., Southwick, S. M., Charney, D. S., and Bremner, J. D. (2003). Long-term treatment with paroxetine increases verbal declarative memory and hippocampal volume in posttraumatic stress disorder. *Biological Psychiatry, 54*(*7*)(0006-3223 (Print)), 693–702.
54. Erickson, K. I., Voss, M. W., Prakash, R. S., Basak, C., Szabo, A., Chaddock, L., et al. (2011). Exercise training increases size of hippocampus and improves memory. *Annals of Neurosciences, 22*(*2*) (1091-6490 (Electronic)), 107.

13

Characterization, Conceptualization, and Treatment of Sleep Disturbances in PTSD

EDWARD F. PACE-SCHOTT AND RYAN BOTTARY

INTRODUCTION

Sleep disturbances have been recognized as a core feature of posttraumatic stress disorder (PTSD) since the disorder was first characterized in the third edition of the *Diagnostic and Statistical Manual of Mental Disorders* (DSM; American Psychiatric Association, 1980). Contemporary diagnostic criteria for PTSD in the fifth edition (DSM-5) designates sleep-related symptoms within two of the four diagnostic symptom clusters. Specifically, sleep-related diagnostic symptoms of PTSD include difficulties initiating and maintaining sleep (alterations in arousal and reactivity) and trauma-related recurrent, distressing dreams, or "nightmares" (intrusive symptoms) (American Psychiatric Association, 2013).

While not necessary for formal diagnosis based on DSM-5 criteria, sleep-related symptoms, especially insomnia and nightmares, are quite common in PTSD and have even been suggested to be the hallmark feature of the condition (Hartmann, 1998; Ross, Ball, Sullivan, & Caroff, 1989). Sleep avoidance, excessive movement during sleep, nocturnal panic attacks, and comorbid sleep disorders such as sleep-disordered breathing (SDB) have also been observed in PTSD (Germain, Buysse, & Nofzinger, 2008; Germain, Hall, Krakow, Shear, & Buysse, 2005; Krakow et al., 2001; Krakow, Hollifield, et al., 2000; Krakow, Ulibarri, Moore, & McIver, 2015). Further, sleep disturbances are a common residual symptom following first-line behavioral and pharmacological treatments for PTSD (Zayfert & DeViva, 2004).

Diagnostically relevant sleep disturbances and comorbid sleep disorders may contribute to both daytime and nighttime PTSD symptomatology (Pace-Schott, Germain, & Milad, 2015b). While sleep disturbances appear to play an important role in the development and maintenance of PTSD symptoms, first-line treatments do not address sleep specifically. This is to the disadvantage of patients seeking treatment as both behavioral and pharmacological interventions that treat sleep-related symptoms of PTSD have shown some benefit for both day and nighttime symptoms (Casement & Swanson, 2012; Ho, Chan, & Tang, 2016; Raskind et al., 2013). Additionally, treatment of certain comorbid sleep disorders, such as SDB, may potentially ameliorate PTSD symptoms in patients presenting with both conditions (Tamanna, Parker, Lyons, & Ullah, 2014).

In this chapter, we review the commonly observed sleep-related symptoms of PTSD, focusing on both subjective reports of sleep disturbance and objectively measured sleep abnormalities. Next, we summarize the contemporary theoretical pathways in which sleep disturbances and abnormalities may contribute to the development and maintenance of PTSD symptomatology. We conclude by touching upon clinically relevant sleep-related treatment considerations for patients with PTSD.

DEFINITION AND PHYSIOLOGICAL CHARACTERISTICS OF HEALTHY HUMAN SLEEP

Sleep is most generally defined as a transient, reversible state of relative behavioral quiescence, marked by progressively reduced responsiveness to the external environment and perceptual disengagement (Carskadon & Dement, 2017). Human sleep is divided into rapid eye movement (REM) and non-REM (NREM) sleep. NREM sleep is subdivided into stages N1, N2, and N3 (also referred to as slow wave sleep [SWS]), which correspond to progressive deepening of sleep (American Academy of Sleep Medicine, 2014).

The gold standard for measuring human sleep physiology is polysomnography (PSG), a montage of electrodes that record brain activity (electroencephalography [EEG]), eye movements (electrooculography [EOG]), and skeletal muscle tone (electromyography [EMG]). While standardized criteria have changed over time, sleep scoring largely relies on the qualitative assessment of dominant frequencies and amplitudes in EEG as well as characteristic EOG and EMG signals (American Academy of Sleep Medicine, 2014; Davis, Davis, Loomis, Harvey, & Hobart, 1937; Rechtschaffen & Kales, 1968; Woodward, Arsenault, Murray, & Bliwise, 2000).

Healthy young adults generally spend between 75% and 80% of total sleep time (TST) in NREM (N1, 2% to 5%; N2, 45% to 50%; N3, 13% to 23%) and the remaining 20% to 25% in REM sleep. Wakefulness during the sleep period, often referred to as wake after sleep onset (WASO), tends to be less than 5% of TST (Carskadon & Dement, 2017). Sleep stage distribution changes across the night, with the first half being composed largely of N2 and N3 sleep and the second half being rich in N2 and REM sleep with REM periods cycling roughly every 90 minutes and REM duration becoming progressively longer across the night (Brown, Basheer, McKenna, Strecker, & McCarley, 2012; Pace-Schott, 2008).

CHARACTERISTIC SLEEP DISTURBANCES IN PTSD

Sleep disturbance is a commonly reported symptom of PTSD (Pace-Schott et al., 2015b; Pigeon & Gallegos, 2015). Of diagnostic importance is the presence of insomnia and nightmares. However, SDB has also been shown to be a common sleep-related comorbidity in PTSD (Krakow et al., 2015). The following sections discuss these three common sleep-related phenomena and their relevance to the pathogenesis and maintenance of PTSD symptomatology. We then discuss evidence for objectively measured sleep abnormalities in PTSD.

Insomnia

Insomnia, or difficulty initiating and/or maintaining sleep, difficulty returning to sleep after waking, and non-restorative sleep, is a common sleep-related experience, with a 6% to 12% prevalence in the general population (Ohayon, 2002; Sinha, 2016). This figure is strikingly higher in trauma-exposed populations in which the prevalence has been observed to be as high as 60% to 90% (Pigeon & Gallegos, 2015). In fact, insomnia has been recognized as a normal and immediate reaction to stress and a common sleep-related disturbance following a traumatic experience (Lavie, 2001; Sinha, 2016; Wright et al., 2011). Further, higher degree of trauma exposure has been associated with greater amounts of sleep disturbance (Neylan et al., 1998). Conversely, PTSD severity has been shown to be an independent risk factor for insomnia (Hall Brown & Mellman, 2014). Insomnia symptom prevalence in PTSD has been reported to be up to 47% for civilian populations and 91% for combat veterans (Neylan et al., 1998; Ohayon & Shapiro, 2000; Pigeon & Gallegos, 2015). Insomnia is often a persistent symptom of PTSD. For example, in a sample of combat veterans with PTSD, 74% endorsed clinically relevant levels of insomnia that persisted for at least six months. Further, presence of insomnia conferred greater PTSD symptom severity at baseline and at six-month follow-up. Finally, a nearly eight-fold difference in persistence of PTSD was observed in individuals with insomnia compared to those without insomnia at six months (Pigeon, Campbell, Possemato, & Ouimette, 2013).

The high prevalence of insomnia in PTSD is not surprising given that it remains a diagnostic feature of the condition (American Psychiatric Association, 2013). However, early identification of insomnia may be of particular clinical importance as disturbed sleep prior to and following trauma exposure, as well as failure to normalize sleep disturbances posttrauma, has been shown to increase risk of developing PTSD. For example, in a prospective study of military personnel, Gehrman and colleagues (2013) showed that combat soldiers who endorsed predeployment insomnia symptoms were twice as likely to develop new-onset, postdeployment PTSD compared to those who did not. Additionally, individuals who reported both insomnia and short sleep duration (<6 hrs) before deployment were up to three times more likely to develop PTSD postdeployment. A study by Koren, Arnon, Lavie, and Klein (2002) that followed 102 motor vehicle accident survivors found that insomnia complaints were common at one week posttrauma. However, at one-month follow-up, those who met criteria for PTSD had greater insomnia severity than those who did not, and this difference was maintained for at least one year after trauma exposure. In another study of combat veterans, Wright and colleagues (2011) found that insomnia severity at four months postdeployment was a significant predictor of PTSD symptom severity at one-year postdeployment.

Trauma may produce an acute hyperarousal response mediated by central stress systems that results in difficulty initiating and maintaining sleep. Conversely, disrupted sleep may produce heightened daytime stress responses. This bidirectional relationship has been hypothesized to set up a positive feedback loop between trauma-induced hyperarousal and poor sleep and, if this pattern is maintained, may contribute to the development of further PTSD symptomatology (Pace-Schott et al., 2015b). Later, we will discuss the evidence linking treatment of insomnia in PTSD with improved clinical outcomes.

Nightmares

Nightmares are dysphoric dreams with lengthy, elaborate, and story-like sequences that seem real, incite anxiety and fear, and result in awakenings from sleep (American Psychiatric Association, 2013). Replicative nightmares, with content resembling an experienced trauma, are a common form of distressing dream mentation in PTSD and have been conceptualized as falling on the extreme end of a dream experience continuum (Phelps, Forbes, & Creamer, 2008; Schreuder, Kleijn, & Rooijmans, 2000). The occurrence of posttraumatic nightmares has been recognized since Freud and modern psychodynamic interpretations suggest that nightmares represent psychological attempts to integrate traumatic experiences into the psyche (Germain, 2013; Hartmann, 1998; Krakow, Hollifield, et al., 2000). Alternatively, posttraumatic nightmares have been conceptualized as episodic memories that have failed to become contextualized and integrated into existing memory stores (Nielsen & Carr, 2017).

Nightmares remain a core diagnostic feature of PTSD and, in addition to insomnia, have been regarded as one of the hallmark features of PTSD (Germain, 2013). Frequent nightmares have been observed in up to 19% of civilians and over 50% of veterans with PTSD, with the frequency of nightmares in the latter group being highly correlated with degree of combat exposure (Neylan et al., 1998; Ohayon & Shapiro, 2000). Nightmares in the early aftermath of a trauma have also been associated with subsequent problems initiating and maintaining sleep (Kobayashi, Sledjeski, Spoonster, Fallon, & Delahanty, 2008).

In a prospective military cohort study, van Liempt, van Zuiden, Westenberg, Super, and Vermetten (2013) found that self-reported pre-deployment nightmares predicted PTSD symptom development at six-months postdeployment. In another study, veterans who reported having nightmares had higher PTSD severity at both a postdeployment baseline assessment and six-month follow-up, at which time 41% of nightmare sufferers continued to meet criteria for PTSD, compared to less than 10% who did not experience nightmares (Pigeon et al., 2013).

Nightmares are regarded as largely a REM sleep phenomenon. However, nightmares may also arise in NREM sleep in individuals with PTSD (Germain, 2013). Nightmares disrupt sleep in two ways. First, recurrent nightmare experiences may produce heightened anticipatory anxiety surrounding sleep and result in difficulty initiating sleep or in varying degrees of sleep avoidance. Second, nightmares cause awakenings from sleep and heightened acute physiological arousal that may make returning to sleep difficult (Pigeon & Gallegos, 2015; Woodward, Arsenault, et al., 2000).

The pathophysiology of nightmares remains poorly understood (for a recent review see Nielsen & Carr 2017). This largely has to do with methodological limitations and the fact that nightmares are rarely observed under laboratory conditions (Germain, 2013). Despite this gap in knowledge, the observation that nightmares disrupt sleep makes them a target of clinical interest. Importantly, as we discuss later, treatment of nightmares has been shown to benefit both day and nighttime symptoms of PTSD.

Sleep-Disordered Breathing

SDB is a common sleep disorder with prevalence estimates of 9% to 24% in the general population (Krakow et al., 2015). The triad of symptoms associated with SDB, in order of decreasing severity of airflow restriction, includes (a) total cessation of breathing (apnea), (b) attenuated breathing (hypopnea), and (c) respiratory effort-related arousals. Further, distinct subtypes of SDB exist based on varying combinations of mechanical and central neurological abnormalities that contribute to suppression or cessation of breathing during sleep (Sunitha & Aravindkumar, 2009).

Reports of the prevalence of SDB in trauma-exposed individuals and those with established PTSD have been highly variable but suggest a higher prevalence than the general population (Krakow et al., 2015). Consideration of SDB is important in PTSD for three reasons: (a) respiratory events associated with SDB may awaken the patient, fragmenting sleep or producing a syndrome that resembles insomnia; (b) sleep breathing events trigger cortical arousal, possibly contributing to heightened nocturnal arousal and nightmares; and (c) REM sleep atonia confers greater susceptibility for upper airway collapse, a mechanical antecedent of breathing cessation, which may fragment REM sleep, a stage that appears to be of particular importance to pathogenesis of PTSD (Krakow et al., 2015; Pace-Schott et al., 2015b; Pigeon & Gallegos, 2015; Pillar, Malhotra, & Lavie, 2000).

The exact pathophysiological mechanism underlying the high comorbidity between PTSD and SDB is still unknown. However, several theories have been put forth to explain this relationship. The first is predicated on the notion that hypercapnia produced by deeper stages of sleep is homeostatically regulated via increase in ventilatory drive and stimulation of upper airway muscles, providing resistance to upper airway collapse, thus maintaining normal breathing during sleep. However, anxiety in PTSD may promote hyperventilation during sleep, inhibiting this process and resulting in apneic events (Pillar et al., 2000). Another model suggests that SDB serves as a chronic physical stressor, or "allostatic challenge." Activation of the hypothalamic-pituitary-adrenal axis combats increased demands placed on the body by SDB, subsequently increasing sympathetic tone and resulting in anxious symptoms (Gold, 2011). A contemporary model proposed by Krakow and colleagues (2015) hypothesizes that PTSD and SDB have a bidirectional relationship in that stress-induced sleep fragmentation may increase the risk of upper airway collapsibility, further fragmenting sleep and worsening PTSD symptoms.

While these theories still need to be substantiated, this evidence highlights the possible clinical importance of treating SDB in PTSD. Further, as we discuss later, some recent evidence suggests that treatment of SDB may be beneficial in reducing PTSD symptomatology in individuals with both conditions.

OBJECTIVE SLEEP ABNORMALITIES IN PTSD

Subjective sleep complaints, such as difficulty falling asleep, staying asleep, short sleep duration, and restless sleep, are commonly reported by individuals with PTSD (Kobayashi, Boarts, & Delahanty, 2007). However, such subjective complaints do not necessarily map onto objective physiological measures obtained during sleep in PTSD (Koren et al., 2002; Werner, Griffin, & Galovski, 2016). Further, evidence of objectively measured sleep-state differences have, to date, been somewhat equivocal (Kobayashi et al., 2007). Notwithstanding, several differences in objective measures of the sleep state have emerged. In a recent, large-scale meta-analysis of 20 PSG studies, Kobayashi, Boarts & Delahanty (2007) found that individuals with PTSD demonstrated more N1, less SWS, and greater REM density (REMD; the frequency of rapid eye movements during REM sleep), when compared to non PTSD controls. Additional moderator variables such as age, sex, and presence of substance use disorders (SUDs) were found to account for some of the sleep differences observed in PTSD. Specifically, younger individuals with PTSD showed greater reductions in TST compared to younger non-PTSD controls while older individuals with PTSD had less SWS and more REM compared to older non-PTSD controls. Additionally, males with PTSD were shown to have less TST and N2, longer sleep onset latency, and greater REMD compared to males without PTSD, with effect sizes much larger than in mixed-sex studies (Kobayashi et al., 2007). This last finding is of particular importance as lifetime prevalence of PTSD is twice as high in women compared to men (Kessler, Sonnega, Bromet, Hughes, & Nelson, 1995; Ohayon & Shapiro, 2000), and recent evidence suggests that less TST and REM percentage differentiate women, but not men, who develop PTSD following a traumatic accident from those who are resilient (Kobayashi & Mellman, 2012). Further, women who developed PTSD experience greater amounts of wakefulness during the night compared to men who developed PTSD (Kobayashi & Mellman, 2012).

In addition to age- and sex-dependent influences on PTSD-related sleep disturbances, Kobayashi and colleagues (2007) also found that individuals with PTSD and comorbid SUDs exhibited greater REM sleep abnormalities (i.e., increased REMD) compared to controls than those with PTSD alone. This is important due to the high rate of comorbid SUDs in PTSD with 35% to 52% of men, and 27% to 28% of women, with PTSD reporting drug and/or alcohol abuse or dependence (Kessler et al., 1995). Both acute exposure to, and withdrawal from, drugs and alcohol can significantly deteriorate sleep quality, and sleep complaints commonly persist beyond acute withdrawal (Brower, Krentzman, & Robinson, 2011; Vandrey, Babson, Herrmann, &

Bonn-Miller, 2014). Sleep disturbance has also been shown to increase the likelihood of developing SUDs and increase the risk of relapse in established SUDs (Brower, Aldrich, & Hall, 1998; Crum, Storr, Chan, & Ford, 2004). Individuals with comorbid PTSD and SUDs report greater sleep disturbances compared to those with PTSD alone (Saladin, Brady, Dansky, & Kilpatrick, 1995). Further, sleep disturbances, such as insomnia and nightmares, have been shown to persist in individuals with PTSD and SUDs despite targeted treatment of these comorbid conditions. Interestingly, improvements in sleep across treatment in those with comorbid PTSD and SUDs result in better PTSD outcomes (McHugh et al., 2014).

Converging evidence exists for REM sleep abnormalities being a prominent objectively measured feature of sleep in PTSD and possibly a hallmark feature of the disorder (Babson & Feldner, 2010; Germain, 2013; Kobayashi et al., 2007; Kobayashi, Lavela, Bell, & Mellman, 2016; Pace-Schott et al., 2015b; Ross et al., 1989). In a large-scale, community-based PSG study, individuals with diagnosed PTSD were observed to have more shifts from REM to light NREM (N1) sleep or to wakefulness compared to trauma-exposed individuals without PTSD (Breslau et al., 2004). Similarly, posttrauma REM abnormalities have been shown to predict greater likelihood of later developing PTSD symptoms. For example, Mellman, Bustamante, Fins, Pigeon, and Nolan (2002) and Mellman, Pigeon, Nowell, and Nolan (2007) found that among individuals who experienced a traumatic incident, greater REM sleep fragmentation in the early phase following the trauma differentiated those who went on to develop PTSD from those who did not.

Quantitative evaluation of sleep stage EEG micro-architecture also suggests the importance of REM sleep in PTSD. For example, REM sleep theta (4–8 Hz) power, which has been demonstrated to play a role in emotional memory processing (Cowdin, Kobayashi, & Mellman, 2014; Nishida, Pearsall, Buckner, & Walker, 2009; Walker & van der Helm, 2009), is diminished in trauma-exposed individuals with PTSD compared to those who are resilient (Cowdin et al., 2014). Additionally, beta-frequency (14–32 Hz) spectral power, a frequency band associated with cortical arousal, is increased during REM sleep in patients with PTSD compared to non-PTSD controls (Woodward, Murburg, & Bliwise, 2000). Conversely, REM beta power measured within one month of a traumatic event was negatively correlated with early symptoms of PTSD (Mellman et al., 2007). While this finding counters Woodward and colleagues' observation that REM sleep beta power is elevated in established PTSD, the authors concluded that increased REM beta power in the aftermath of a trauma may be an adaptive response that supports resiliency (Mellman et al., 2007). Stress-induced alterations of central neuromodulation may underlie the changes of REM sleep following trauma and in PTSD. For example, central norepinephrine (NE) both reaches its minimum level during REM sleep and, in the central nervous system, opposes REM sleep (Pace-Schott & Hobson, 2002). Elevated central levels of NE have been observed in patients with PTSD (Geracioti et al., 2001), and this may lead to REM suppression or fragmentation (Pace-Schott et al., 2015b). Elevated central levels of corticotropin releasing hormone (CRF) disrupt sleep in an animal model of unavoidable stress (Wellman, Yang, Ambrozewicz, Machida, & Sanford, 2013), and the elevated levels of central CRF seen in PTSD (Bremner et al., 1997) may cause similar effects on sleep in humans (reviewed in Pace-Schott et al., 2015b).

REM sleep abnormalities have also been measured in the peripheral (autonomic) nervous system. Greater sympathetic nervous system activation, as measured by heart rate variability, during REM sleep in the early phase following a trauma exposure has been shown to distinguish individuals who went on to subsequently develop PTSD from those who did not (Mellman, Knorr, Pigeon, Leiter, & Akay, 2004). In addition, in individuals with established PTSD, higher heart rate, a peripheral measure of increased sympathetic tone, during REM compared to NREM sleep, correlated with reduced REM percentage and increased latency to REM sleep (Woodward, Murburg, et al., 2000). Further, early evening REM and NREM heart rate has recently been shown to be elevated in individuals with PTSD compared to resilient controls (Kobayashi et al., 2016). Increased sympathetic tone, and subsequent sleep fragmentation, may be of particular importance in PTSD in light of basic research that has linked emotional memory regulation with sleep, the topic of the next section.

SLEEP AND EXTINCTION

One prominent theory regarding the pathogenesis and maintenance of PTSD involves conditioning and extinction of acquired fears (reviewed in Pace-Schott et al., 2015b). Fear conditioning involves creating fearful associations with neutral objects, places, or people that have been paired with an inherently aversive experience. Such associations may persist in the form of a fear memory. Extinction learning, on the other hand, involves creating new associations with the once feared object when it is repeatedly presented in the absence of the aversive outcome. The subsequent extinction memory trace competes with the fear memory, serving to regulate emotion.

Sleep appears to play an important role in the consolidation of emotional memories, their integration into long-term storage, and their adaptive regulation (Goldstein & Walker, 2014; Walker & van der Helm, 2009). Fear and extinction memories are specific types of emotional memory that may be similarly influenced by sleep (Kuriyama, Soshi, & Kim, 2010; Pace-Schott et al., 2009). REM sleep appears to be particularly important for processing and integrating emotional memories (Nishida et al., 2009), and this extends to fear and extinction memory (Pace-Schott, Germain, & Milad, 2015a; Spoormaker et al., 2012). Conversely, sleep deprivation appears to inhibit acquiring and consolidating both fear (Menz et al., 2013) and extinction memory (Straus, Acheson, Risbrough, & Drummond, 2017). In an interesting parallel to human studies, REM sleep is suppressed in rats both following fear conditioning as well as when they are later reintroduced to the conditioning context (Pawlyk, Jha, Brennan, Morrison, & Ross, 2005). In addition REM sleep deprivation impairs consolidation and recall of extinction memory (Fu et al., 2007). Therefore REM sleep disruption in PTSD might impair consolidation of the extinction of traumatic memories, thus allowing trauma-related conditioned fear memories to persist unopposed.

Retention of extinction memories is of great importance to patients with anxiety-related disorders, including PTSD, since both naturally occurring and therapeutic extinction are hypothesized to play an important role in opposing fearful associations (Craske et al., 2008; McNally, 2007). Sleep has been shown to play an important role in promoting the consolidation of therapeutic extinction memory that is acquired during exposure-based therapy (Kleim et al., 2014; Pace-Schott et al., 2015b; Pace-Schott, Verga, Bennett, & Spencer, 2012; Zalta et al., 2013). Retention of extinction memory has been shown to be impaired in PTSD (Milad et al., 2009), and some have hypothesized that this may be mediated by the sleep disturbances that are common in this condition (Germain, 2013; Pace-Schott et al., 2015b; Straus et al., 2017).

While the preliminary evidence detailed here suggests that sleep plays an important role in therapeutic success and may even enhance retention of extinction memories following exposure-based therapy, first-line treatments for PTSD do not currently target sleep problems. However, this is now changing. The next section discusses the evidence for the usefulness of sleep-targeted interventions for PTSD.

SLEEP-SPECIFIC TREATMENT APPROACHES FOR PTSD

Sleep disturbance has been shown to be a common residual symptom of traditional PTSD treatments (Davidson, Rothbaum, van der Kolk, Sikes, & Farfel, 2001; Germain et al., 2008; Zayfert & DeViva, 2004). Treatment of insomnia, nightmares, and sleep comorbidities in PTSD, such as SDB, have been shown to be useful for reducing both day and nighttime symptomatology (Casement & Swanson, 2012; Ho et al., 2016; Raskind et al., 2007; Tamanna et al., 2014). In this section, we give an overview of contemporary behavioral and biomedical interventions for the treatment of disordered sleep in PTSD.

Cognitive-Behavioral Therapy for Insomnia

Cognitive behavioral therapy for insomnia (CBT-I), as its name implies, is a targeted psychotherapeutic approach for the treatment of insomnia. The principal components of CBT-I include maintaining proper sleep hygiene, minimizing stimuli in the sleeping environment that interfere with sleep, restructuring negative sleep-related associations, and, paradoxically, initial periods of sleep restriction (Morin et al., 2006; Sloan et al., 1993). Several findings suggest that CBT-I is a highly effective and economical intervention that is generally well tolerated. Further, CBT-I has been shown to be superior to traditional pharmacological approaches in head-to-head comparisons (Ellenbogen & Pace-Schott, 2012; Ho et al., 2016; Jacobs, Pace-Schott, Stickgold, & Otto, 2004; Sivertsen et al., 2006; Smith et al., 2002).

Insomnia is a modifiable risk factor and a common residual symptom following cognitive behavioral treatments for PTSD (Germain, 2013; Zayfert & DeViva, 2004). Additionally, insomnia in PTSD can be complicated by factors like sleep avoidance caused by distress related to nightmares and rumination about the inability to initiate or maintain sleep. Further heightened physiological arousal that is common to both insomnia and PTSD may become more problematic around bedtime if the sleeping environment is the context in which the trauma took place (Pigeon & Gallegos, 2015; Zayfert & DeViva, 2004). Given the large overlap between insomnia and PTSD, recent work has attempted to understand the effectiveness of CBT-I for sleep complaints related to PTSD. In a recent report, individuals with PTSD who completed an eight-week CBT-I treatment, compared to wait-list controls, showed increased objectively measured TST, improvements in self-reported sleep quality (decreased sleep onset latency and WASO and increased sleep efficiency, TST, and daytime energy) with 41% of patients demonstrating remission in insomnia symptoms, reduction in disrupted nocturnal behaviors (including nightmares), and increased levels of psychosocial functioning up to six months posttreatment (Talbot et al., 2014). A recent meta-analysis revealed that CBT-I provides greater reduction in PTSD symptoms, shorter self-reported sleep latency and WASO, and greater sleep efficiency compared to both wait-list and psychoeducation control groups with moderate to large effect sizes (Ho et al., 2016).

Further research is necessary to establish when introduction of CBT-I may optimize PTSD treatment outcomes. Of additional importance is determining how CBT-I may be successfully integrated into existing behavioral treatments for PTSD or be an effective prelude to established therapies, such as exposure-based treatment, the latter having some preliminary support (Baddeley & Gros, 2013). Further, CBT-I has been shown to be highly beneficial for improving sleep quality in PTSD when combined with other sleep-targeted interventions, such as imagery rehearsal therapy, which is covered in the next section (Seda, Sanchez-Ortuno, Welsh, Halbower, & Edinger, 2015).

Imagery Rehearsal Therapy

Imagery rehearsal therapy (IRT) is a psychotherapeutic intervention for treating nightmares by targeting the problematic dream, altering the storyline by changing the most distressing elements, and rehearsing the new dream prior to sleep (Harb et al., 2013; Krakow, Hollifield, et al., 2000). The rationale is that new content will become incorporated into the dream, resulting in less dream-related distress. Based on several recent studies, IRT appears to beneficial for treating both sleep and daytime symptomatology in PTSD (Casement & Swanson, 2012; Krakow, Hollifield, et al., 2000; Thunker & Pietrowsky, 2012; van Schagen, Lancee, de Groot, Spoormaker, & van den Bout, 2015). In a recent meta-analysis, IRT was shown to improve sleep quality, reduce nightmare frequency, and decrease PTSD symptomatology for up to 12 months following treatment (Casement & Swanson, 2012). There is also evidence to suggest that it is superior to treatment as usual for nightmare frequency, nightmare distress, and psychopathology indices across many psychiatric conditions, including PTSD (van Schagen et al., 2015). Further, IRT appears to be just as effective for treating nightmares in PTSD as pharmacological approaches like prazosin, which is the focus of the next section (Seda et al., 2015).

Prazosin

Nightmares are a prominent and distressing symptom of PTSD and may predict poorer outcomes for the condition. Despite this, first-line pharmacological treatments for PTSD have shown little benefit for relieving this symptom (Brownlow, Harb, & Ross, 2015). However, prazosin, an antihypertensive medication that antagonizes postsynaptic alpha-1 adrenergic receptors, has shown much promise as a generally well-tolerated pharmacological therapy for nightmares in PTSD (Brownlow et al., 2015; Krystal, Stein, & Szabo, 2017). Prazosin has been shown to reduce nightmares, non-nightmare distressed awakenings, sleep quality, and overall PTSD symptoms in both military and civilian populations (Raskind et al., 2007; Raskind et al., 2013; Taylor et al., 2008; Thompson, Taylor, McFall, Barnes, & Raskind, 2008). Additionally, there is some evidence that prazosin may both increase and consolidate REM sleep, a sleep stage of particular importance to the pathogenesis of PTSD, and alleviate daytime distress associated with trauma-related cues (Taylor et al., 2008). Prazosin may exert its positive effects via correcting elevated noradrenergic tone, a possible pathophysiological mechanism contributing to hyperarousal in PTSD (Hendrickson & Raskind, 2016; Pace-Schott et al., 2015b).

Continuous Positive Airway Pressure Therapy

As mentioned earlier, SDB has been shown to be a fairly common sleep-related comorbidity in PTSD. Interestingly, use of continuous positive airway pressure (CPAP) therapy, the gold standard treatment for obstructive sleep apnea (OSA), has shown some promise for treating sleep-related complaints associated with PTSD in individuals who also experience SDB.

In an early retrospective study by Krakow, Lowry, et al. (2000), improvement in nightmares and PTSD symptoms was greater in PTSD patients treated with CPAP compared to those who were untreated. In a recent study by Tamanna and colleagues (2014), individuals with PTSD and OSA that were treated with CPAP demonstrated improvement in both daytime sleepiness and reduced nightmare frequency after six months of treatment. However, CPAP adherence and response has been reported to be lower in patients with PTSD (Collen, Lettieri, & Hoffman, 2012; El-Solh, Ayyar, Akinnusi, Relia, & Akinnusi, 2010; Lettieri, Williams, & Collen, 2016). This is particularly problematic, as both insomnia and nightmares, key sleep-related features in PTSD, have been shown to be collateral symptoms in OSA (Krakow et al., 2015). Further research is necessary to clarify the clinical usefulness of CPAP in the treatment of individuals with both PTSD and SDB and to better understand and overcome obstacles to CPAP adherence in PTSD populations.

CONCLUSIONS

Sleep disturbances are both diagnostically relevant and possibly an antecedent of PTSD. In this chapter, we reviewed the two diagnostic sleep complaints in PTSD, insomnia and nightmares, and discussed how these features may serve to both precipitate and maintain PTSD symptoms. We also briefly discussed how comorbid sleep disorders, such as SDB, may exacerbate diagnostic sleep disturbances and contribute to daytime symptoms in PTSD. An overview of objective sleep findings revealed converging evidence for REM sleep playing a crucial role in PTSD. Possible importance of fear conditioning and extinction in the pathogenesis of PTSD also provided a theoretical framework to understand how sleep disturbances may influence PTSD prognosis. We finished by reviewing contemporary behavioral and pharmacological sleep-targeted therapies for sleep-related symptoms in PTSD and concluded that that these treatments may be of great clinical importance to the treatment of PTSD.

REFERENCES

American Academy of Sleep Medicine. (2014). *International classification of sleep disorders* (3rd ed.). Darien, IL: American Academy of Sleep Medicine.

American Psychiatric Association. (1980). *Diagnostic and statistical manual of mental disorders* (3rd ed.). Washington, DC: American Psychiatric Association.

American Psychiatric Association. (2013). *Diagnostic and statistical manual for mental disorders* (5th ed.). Arlington, VA: American Psychiatric Association.

Babson, K. A., & Feldner, M. T. (2010). Temporal relations between sleep problems and both traumatic event exposure and PTSD: A critical review of the empirical literature. *J Anxiety Disord*, *24*(1), 1–15. doi:10.1016/j.janxdis.2009.08.002

Baddeley, J. L., & Gros, D. F. (2013). Cognitive behavioral therapy for insomnia as a preparatory treatment for exposure therapy for posttraumatic stress disorder. *Am J Psychother*, *67*(2), 203–214.

Bremner, J. D., Licinio, J., Darnell, A., Krystal, J. H., Owens, M. J., Southwick, S. M., . . . Charney, D. S. (1997). Elevated CSF corticotropin-releasing factor concentrations in posttraumatic stress disorder. *Am J Psychiatry*, *154*(5), 624–629. doi:10.1176/ajp.154.5.624

Breslau, N., Roth, T., Burduvali, E., Kapke, A., Schultz, L., & Roehrs, T. (2004). Sleep in lifetime posttraumatic stress disorder: A community-based polysomnographic study. (Comparative Study Research Support, U.S. Government, P.H.S.). *Arch Gen Psychiatry*, *61*(5), 508–516. doi:10.1001/archpsyc.61.5.508

Brower, K. J., Aldrich, M. S., & Hall, J. M. (1998). Polysomnographic and subjective sleep predictors of alcoholic relapse. *Alcohol Clin Exp Res*, *22*(8), 1864–1871.

Brower, K. J., Krentzman, A., & Robinson, E. A. (2011). Persistent insomnia, abstinence, and moderate drinking in alcohol-dependent individuals. *Am J Addict*, *20*(5), 435–440. doi:10.1111/j.1521-0391.2011.00152.x

Brown, R. E., Basheer, R., McKenna, J. T., Strecker, R. E., & McCarley, R. W. (2012). Control of sleep and wakefulness. *Physiol Rev*, *92*(3), 1087–1187. doi:10.1152/physrev.00032.2011

Brownlow, J. A., Harb, G. C., & Ross, R. J. (2015). Treatment of sleep disturbances in posttraumatic stress disorder: A review of the literature. *Curr Psychiatry Rep*, *17*(6), 41. doi:10.1007/s11920-015-0587-8

Carskadon, M., & Dement, W. (2017). Normal human sleep. An overview. In M. Kryger, T. Roth, & W. Dement (Eds.), *Principles and practice of sleep medicine* (6th ed., pp. 15–24). Philadelphia, PA: Elsevier.

Casement, M. D., & Swanson, L. M. (2012). A meta-analysis of imagery rehearsal for post-trauma nightmares: Effects on nightmare frequency, sleep quality, and posttraumatic stress. *Clin Psychol Rev*, *32*(6), 566–574. doi:10.1016/j.cpr.2012.06.002

Collen, J. F., Lettieri, C. J., & Hoffman, M. (2012). The impact of posttraumatic stress disorder on CPAP adherence in patients with obstructive sleep apnea. *J Clin Sleep Med*, *8*(6), 667–672. doi:10.5664/jcsm.2260

Cowdin, N., Kobayashi, I., & Mellman, T. A. (2014). Theta frequency activity during rapid eye movement (REM) sleep is greater in people with resilience versus PTSD. *Exp Brain Res, 232*(5), 1479–1485. doi:10.1007/s00221-014-3857-5

Craske, M. G., Kircanski, K., Zelikowsky, M., Mystkowski, J., Chowdhury, N., & Baker, A. (2008). Optimizing inhibitory learning during exposure therapy. *Behav Res Ther, 46*(1), 5–27. doi:10.1016/j.brat.2007.10.003

Crum, R. M., Storr, C. L., Chan, Y. F., & Ford, D. E. (2004). Sleep disturbance and risk for alcohol-related problems. *Am J Psychiatry, 161*(7), 1197–1203. doi:10.1176/appi.ajp.161.7.1197

Davidson, J. R., Rothbaum, B. O., van der Kolk, B. A., Sikes, C. R., & Farfel, G. M. (2001). Multicenter, double-blind comparison of sertraline and placebo in the treatment of posttraumatic stress disorder. *Arch Gen Psychiatry, 58*(5), 485–492.

Davis, H., Davis, P. A., Loomis, A. L., Harvey, E. N., & Hobart, G. (1937). Changes in human brain potentials during the onset of sleep. *Science, 86*(2237), 448–450. doi:10.1126/science.86.2237.448

El-Solh, A. A., Ayyar, L., Akinnusi, M., Relia, S., & Akinnusi, O. (2010). Positive airway pressure adherence in veterans with posttraumatic stress disorder. *Sleep, 33*(11), 1495–1500.

Ellenbogen, J. M., & Pace-Schott, E. F. (2012). Drug-induced sleep: Theoretical and practical considerations. *Pflugers Arch, 463*(1), 177–186. doi:10.1007/s00424-011-1033-3

Fu, J., Li, P., Ouyang, X., Gu, C., Song, Z., Gao, J., . . . Hu, B. (2007). Rapid eye movement sleep deprivation selectively impairs recall of fear extinction in hippocampus-independent tasks in rats. *Neuroscience, 144*(4), 1186–1192. doi:10.1016/j.neuroscience.2006.10.050

Gehrman, P., Seelig, A. D., Jacobson, I. G., Boyko, E. J., Hooper, T. I., Gackstetter, G. D., . . . Smith, T. C. (2013). Predeployment sleep duration and insomnia symptoms as risk factors for new-onset mental health disorders following military deployment. *Sleep, 36*(7), 1009–1018. doi:10.5665/sleep.2798

Geracioti, T. D.Jr., Baker, D. G., Ekhator, N. N., West, S. A., Hill, K. K., Bruce, A. B., . . . Kasckow, J. W. (2001). CSF norepinephrine concentrations in posttraumatic stress disorder. *Am J Psychiatry, 158*(8), 1227–1230. doi:10.1176/appi.ajp.158.8.1227

Germain, A. (2013). Sleep disturbances as the hallmark of PTSD: Where are we now? *Am J Psychiatry, 170*(4), 372–382. doi:10.1176/appi.ajp.2012.12040432

Germain, A., Buysse, D. J., & Nofzinger, E. (2008). Sleep-specific mechanisms underlying posttraumatic stress disorder: Integrative review and neurobiological hypotheses. *Sleep Med Rev, 12*(3), 185–195. doi:10.1016/j.smrv.2007.09.003

Germain, A., Hall, M., Krakow, B., Katherine Shear, M., & Buysse, D. J. (2005). A brief sleep scale for posttraumatic stress disorder: Pittsburgh Sleep Quality Index Addendum for PTSD. *J Anxiety Disord, 19*(2), 233–244. doi:10.1016/j.janxdis.2004.02.001

Gold, A. R. (2011). Functional somatic syndromes, anxiety disorders and the upper airway: A matter of paradigms. *Sleep Med Rev, 15*(6), 389–401. doi:10.1016/j.smrv.2010.11.004

Goldstein, A. N., & Walker, M. P. (2014). The role of sleep in emotional brain function. *Annu Rev Clin Psychol, 10*, 679–708. doi:10.1146/annurev-clinpsy-032813-153716

Hall Brown, T., & Mellman, T. A. (2014). The influence of PTSD, sleep fears, and neighborhood stress on insomnia and short sleep duration in urban, young adult, African Americans. *Behav Sleep Med, 12*(3), 198–206. doi:10.1080/15402002.2013.784704

Harb, G. C., Phelps, A. J., Forbes, D., Ross, R. J., Gehrman, P. R., & Cook, J. M. (2013). A critical review of the evidence base of imagery rehearsal for posttraumatic nightmares: Pointing the way for future research. *J Trauma Stress, 26*(5), 570–579. doi:10.1002/jts.21854

Hartmann, E. (1998). Nightmare after trauma as paradigm for all dreams: A new approach to the nature and functions of dreaming. *Psychiatry, 61*(3), 223–238.

Hendrickson, R. C., & Raskind, M. A. (2016). Noradrenergic dysregulation in the pathophysiology of PTSD. *Exp Neurol, 284*(Pt B), 181–195. doi:10.1016/j.expneurol.2016.05.014

Ho, F. Y., Chan, C. S., & Tang, K. N. (2016). Cognitive-behavioral therapy for sleep disturbances in treating posttraumatic stress disorder symptoms: A meta-analysis of randomized controlled trials. *Clin Psychol Rev, 43*, 90–102. doi:10.1016/j.cpr.2015.09.005

Jacobs, G. D., Pace-Schott, E. F., Stickgold, R., & Otto, M. W. (2004). Cognitive behavior therapy and pharmacotherapy for insomnia: A randomized controlled trial and direct comparison. *Arch Intern Med, 164*(17), 1888–1896. doi:10.1001/archinte.164.17.1888

Kessler, R. C., Sonnega, A., Bromet, E., Hughes, M., & Nelson, C. B. (1995). Posttraumatic stress disorder in the National Comorbidity Survey. *Arch Gen Psychiatry, 52*(12), 1048–1060.

Kleim, B., Wilhelm, F. H., Temp, L., Margraf, J., Wiederhold, B. K., & Rasch, B. (2014). Sleep enhances exposure therapy. *Psychol Med, 44*(7), 1511–1519. doi:10.1017/s0033291713001748

Kobayashi, I., Boarts, J. M., & Delahanty, D. L. (2007). Polysomnographically measured sleep abnormalities in PTSD: A meta-analytic review. *Psychophysiology, 44*(4), 660–669. doi:10.1111/j.1469-8986.2007.537.x

Kobayashi, I., Lavela, J., Bell, K., & Mellman, T. A. (2016). The impact of posttraumatic stress disorder versus resilience on nocturnal autonomic nervous system activity as functions of sleep stage and time of sleep. *Physiol Behav, 164*(Pt A), 11–18. doi:10.1016/j.physbeh.2016.05.005

Kobayashi, I., & Mellman, T. A. (2012). Gender differences in sleep during the aftermath of trauma and the development of posttraumatic stress disorder. [Research Support, National Institutes of Health, Extramural]. *Behav Sleep Med, 10*(3), 180–190. doi:10.1080/15402002.2011.654296

Kobayashi, I., Sledjeski, E. M., Spoonster, E., Fallon, W. F. Jr., & Delahanty, D. L. (2008). Effects of early nightmares on the development of sleep disturbances in motor vehicle accident victims. *J Trauma Stress, 21*(6), 548–555. doi:10.1002/jts.20368

Koren, D., Arnon, I., Lavie, P., & Klein, E. (2002). Sleep complaints as early predictors of posttraumatic stress disorder: A 1-year prospective study of injured survivors of motor vehicle accidents. *Am J Psychiatry, 159*(5), 855–857. doi:10.1176/appi.ajp.159.5.855

Krakow, B., Germain, A., Warner, T. D., Schrader, R., Koss, M., Hollifield, M., . . . Johnston, L. (2001). The relationship of sleep quality and posttraumatic stress to potential sleep disorders in sexual assault survivors with nightmares, insomnia, and PTSD. *J Trauma Stress, 14*(4), 647–665. doi:10.1023/a:1013029819358

Krakow, B., Hollifield, M., Schrader, R., Koss, M., Tandberg, D., Lauriello, J., . . . Kellner, R. (2000). A controlled study of imagery rehearsal for chronic nightmares in sexual assault survivors with PTSD: A preliminary report. *J Trauma Stress, 13*(4), 589–609. doi:10.1023/a:1007854015481

Krakow, B., Lowry, C., Germain, A., Gaddy, L., Hollifield, M., Koss, M., . . . Melendrez, D. (2000). A retrospective study on improvements in nightmares and post-traumatic stress disorder following treatment for co-morbid sleep-disordered breathing. *J Psychosom Res, 49*(5), 291–298.

Krakow, B. J., Ulibarri, V. A., Moore, B. A., & McIver, N. D. (2015). Posttraumatic stress disorder and sleep-disordered breathing: A review of comorbidity research. *Sleep Med Rev, 24*, 37–45. doi:10.1016/j.smrv.2014.11.001

Krystal, A., Stein, M., & Szabo, S. (2017). Psychiatric disorders. In M. Kryger, T. Roth, & W. Dement (Eds.), *Principles and practice of sleep medicine* (6th ed., pp. 1341–1351). Philadelphia, PA: Elsevier.

Kuriyama, K., Soshi, T., & Kim, Y. (2010). Sleep deprivation facilitates extinction of implicit fear generalization and physiological response to fear. *Biol Psychiatry, 68*(11), 991–998. doi:10.1016/j.biopsych.2010.08.015

Lavie, P. (2001). Sleep disturbances in the wake of traumatic events. *N Engl J Med, 345*(25), 1825–1832. doi:10.1056/NEJMra012893

Lettieri, C. J., Williams, S. G., & Collen, J. F. (2016). OSA syndrome and posttraumatic stress disorder: Clinical outcomes and impact of positive airway pressure therapy. *Chest, 149*(2), 483–490. doi:10.1378/chest.15-0693

McHugh, R. K., Hu, M. C., Campbell, A. N., Hilario, E. Y., Weiss, R. D., & Hien, D. A. (2014). Changes in sleep disruption in the treatment of co-occurring posttraumatic stress disorder and substance use disorders. *J Trauma Stress, 27*(1), 82–89. doi:10.1002/jts.21878

McNally, R. J. (2007). Mechanisms of exposure therapy: How neuroscience can improve psychological treatments for anxiety disorders. *Clin Psychol Rev, 27*(6), 750–759. doi:10.1016/j.cpr.2007.01.003

Mellman, T. A., Bustamante, V., Fins, A. I., Pigeon, W. R., & Nolan, B. (2002). REM sleep and the early development of posttraumatic stress disorder. *Am J Psychiatry, 159*(10), 1696–1701. doi:10.1176/appi.ajp.159.10.1696

Mellman, T. A., Knorr, B. R., Pigeon, W. R., Leiter, J. C., & Akay, M. (2004). Heart rate variability during sleep and the early development of posttraumatic stress disorder. *Biol Psychiatry, 55*(9), 953–956.

Mellman, T. A., Pigeon, W. R., Nowell, P. D., & Nolan, B. (2007). Relationships between REM sleep findings and PTSD symptoms during the early aftermath of trauma. *J Trauma Stress, 20*(5), 893–901. doi:10.1002/jts.20246

Menz, M. M., Rihm, J. S., Salari, N., Born, J., Kalisch, R., Pape, H. C., . . . Buchel, C. (2013). The role of sleep and sleep deprivation in consolidating fear memories. *Neuroimage, 75*, 87–96. doi:10.1016/j.neuroimage.2013.03.001

Milad, M. R., Pitman, R. K., Ellis, C. B., Gold, A. L., Shin, L. M., Lasko, N. B., . . . Rauch, S. L. (2009). Neurobiological basis of failure to recall extinction memory in posttraumatic stress disorder. *Biol Psychiatry, 66*(12), 1075–1082. doi:10.1016/j.biopsych.2009.06.026

Morin, C. M., Bootzin, R. R., Buysse, D. J., Edinger, J. D., Espie, C. A., & Lichstein, K. L. (2006). Psychological and behavioral treatment of insomnia: Update of the recent evidence (1998–2004). *Sleep, 29*(11), 1398–1414.

Neylan, T. C., Marmar, C. R., Metzler, T. J., Weiss, D. S., Zatzick, D. F., Delucchi, K. L., . . . Schoenfeld, F. B. (1998). Sleep disturbances in the Vietnam generation: Findings from a nationally representative sample of male Vietnam veterans. *Am J Psychiatry, 155*(7), 929–933. doi:10.1176/ajp.155.7.929

Nielsen, T., & Carr, M. (2017). Nightmares and nightmare function. In M. Kryger, T. Roth, & W. Dement (Eds.), *Principles and practice of sleep medicine* (6th ed.). Philadelphia: Elsevier.

Nishida, M., Pearsall, J., Buckner, R. L., & Walker, M. P. (2009). REM sleep, prefrontal theta, and the consolidation of human emotional memory. *Cereb Cortex, 19*(5), 1158–1166. doi:10.1093/cercor/bhn155

Ohayon, M. M. (2002). Epidemiology of insomnia: What we know and what we still need to learn. *Sleep Med Rev, 6*(2), 97–111.

Ohayon, M. M., & Shapiro, C. M. (2000). Sleep disturbances and psychiatric disorders associated with posttraumatic stress disorder in the general population. [Research Support, Non-U.S. Government]. *Comp Psychiatry, 41*(6), 469–478. doi:10.1053/comp.2000.16568

Pace-Schott, E. F. (2008). Sleep architecture. In L. Squire (Ed.), *Encyclopedia of neuroscience* (pp. 983–989). Oxford: Academic Press.

Pace-Schott, E. F., Germain, A., & Milad, M. R. (2015a). Effects of sleep on memory for conditioned fear and fear extinction. *Psychol Bull, 141*(4), 835–857. doi:10.1037/bul0000014

Pace-Schott, E. F., Germain, A., & Milad, M. R. (2015b). Sleep and REM sleep disturbance in the pathophysiology of PTSD: The role of extinction memory. *Biol Mood Anxiety Disord, 5*, 3. doi:10.1186/s13587-015-0018-9

Pace-Schott, E. F., & Hobson, J. A. (2002). The neurobiology of sleep: Genetics, cellular physiology and subcortical networks. *Nat Rev Neurosci, 3*(8), 591–605. doi:10.1038/nrn895

Pace-Schott, E. F., Milad, M. R., Orr, S. P., Rauch, S. L., Stickgold, R., & Pitman, R. K. (2009). Sleep promotes generalization of extinction of conditioned fear. *Sleep, 32*(1), 19–26.

Pace-Schott, E. F., Verga, P. W., Bennett, T. S., & Spencer, R. M. (2012). Sleep promotes consolidation and generalization of extinction learning in simulated exposure therapy for spider fear. *J Psychiatr Res, 46*(8), 1036–1044. doi:10.1016/j.jpsychires.2012.04.015

Pawlyk, A. C., Jha, S. K., Brennan, F. X., Morrison, A. R., & Ross, R. J. (2005). A rodent model of sleep disturbances in posttraumatic stress disorder: The role of context after fear conditioning. *Biol Psychiatry, 57*(3), 268–277. doi:10.1016/j.biopsych.2004.11.008

Phelps, A. J., Forbes, D., & Creamer, M. (2008). Understanding posttraumatic nightmares: an empirical and conceptual review. *Clin Psychol Rev, 28*(2), 338–355. doi:10.1016/j.cpr.2007.06.001

Pigeon, W. R., Campbell, C. E., Possemato, K., & Ouimette, P. (2013). Longitudinal relationships of insomnia, nightmares, and PTSD severity in recent combat veterans. *J Psychosom Res, 75*(6), 546–550. doi:10.1016/j.jpsychores.2013.09.004

Pigeon, W. R., & Gallegos, A. M. (2015). Posttraumatic Stress Disorder and Sleep. *Sleep Med Clin, 10*(1), 41–48. doi:10.1016/j.jsmc.2014.11.010

Pillar, G., Malhotra, A., & Lavie, P. (2000). Posttraumatic stress disorder and sleep-what a nightmare! *Sleep Med Rev, 4*(2), 183–200. doi:10.1053/smrv.1999.0095

Raskind, M. A., Peskind, E. R., Hoff, D. J., Hart, K. L., Holmes, H. A., Warren, D., . . . McFall, M. E. (2007). A parallel group placebo controlled study of prazosin for trauma nightmares and sleep disturbance in combat veterans with post-traumatic stress disorder. *Biol Psychiatry, 61*(8), 928–934. doi:10.1016/j.biopsych.2006.06.032

Raskind, M. A., Peterson, K., Williams, T., Hoff, D. J., Hart, K., Holmes, H., . . . Peskind, E. R. (2013). A trial of prazosin for combat trauma PTSD with nightmares in active-duty soldiers returned from Iraq and Afghanistan. *Am J Psychiatry, 170*(9), 1003–1010. doi:10.1176/appi.ajp.2013.12081133

Rechtschaffen, A., & Kales, A. (1968). *A manual of standardized terminology, techniques and scoring system for sleep stages of human subjects.* Los Angeles: University of California, Brain Information Service/Brain Research Institute.

Ross, R. J., Ball, W. A., Sullivan, K. A., & Caroff, S. N. (1989). Sleep disturbance as the hallmark of posttraumatic stress disorder. *Am J Psychiatry, 146*(6), 697–707. doi:10.1176/ajp.146.6.697

Saladin, M. E., Brady, K. T., Dansky, B. S., & Kilpatrick, D. G. (1995). Understanding comorbidity between PTSD and substance use disorders: Two preliminary investigations. *Addict Behav, 20*(5), 643–655.

Schreuder, B. J., Kleijn, W. C., & Rooijmans, H. G. (2000). Nocturnal re-experiencing more than forty years after war trauma. *J Trauma Stress, 13*(3), 453–463. doi:10.1023/a:1007733324351

Seda, G., Sanchez-Ortuno, M. M., Welsh, C. H., Halbower, A. C., & Edinger, J. D. (2015). Comparative meta-analysis of prazosin and imagery rehearsal therapy for nightmare frequency, sleep quality, and posttraumatic stress. *J Clin Sleep Med, 11*(1), 11–22. doi:10.5664/jcsm.4354

Sinha, S. S. (2016). Trauma-induced insomnia: A novel model for trauma and sleep research. *Sleep Med Rev*, *25*, 74–83. doi:10.1016/j.smrv.2015.01.008

Sivertsen, B., Omvik, S., Pallesen, S., Bjorvatn, B., Havik, O. E., Kvale, G., . . . Nordhus, I. H. (2006). Cognitive behavioral therapy vs zopiclone for treatment of chronic primary insomnia in older adults: A randomized controlled trial. *JAMA*, *295*(24), 2851–2858. doi:10.1001/jama.295.24.2851

Sloan, E. P., Hauri, P., Bootzin, R., Morin, C., Stevenson, M., & Shapiro, C. M. (1993). The nuts and bolts of behavioral therapy for insomnia. *J Psychosom Res*, *37*(Suppl. 1), 19–37.

Smith, M. T., Perlis, M. L., Park, A., Smith, M. S., Pennington, J., Giles, D. E., & Buysse, D. J. (2002). Comparative meta-analysis of pharmacotherapy and behavior therapy for persistent insomnia. *Am J Psychiatry*, *159*(1), 5–11. doi:10.1176/appi.ajp.159.1.5

Spoormaker, V. I., Schroter, M. S., Andrade, K. C., Dresler, M., Kiem, S. A., Goya-Maldonado, R., . . . Czisch, M. (2012). Effects of rapid eye movement sleep deprivation on fear extinction recall and prediction error signaling. *Hum Brain Mapp*, *33*(10), 2362–2376. doi:10.1002/hbm.21369

Straus, L. D., Acheson, D. T., Risbrough, V. B., & Drummond, S. P. A. (2017). Sleep deprivation disrupts recall of conditioned fear extinction. *Biol Psychiatry Cogn Neurosci Neuroim*, *2*(2), 123–129.

Sunitha, C., & Aravindkumar, S. (2009). Obstructive sleep apnea: Clinical and diagnostic features. *Indian J Dent Res*, *20*(4), 487–491. doi:10.4103/0970-9290.59457

Talbot, L. S., Maguen, S., Metzler, T. J., Schmitz, M., McCaslin, S. E., Richards, A., . . . Neylan, T. C. (2014). Cognitive behavioral therapy for insomnia in posttraumatic stress disorder: A randomized controlled trial. *Sleep*, *37*(2), 327–341. doi:10.5665/sleep.3408

Tamanna, S., Parker, J. D., Lyons, J., & Ullah, M. I. (2014). The effect of continuous positive air pressure (CPAP) on nightmares in patients with posttraumatic stress disorder (PTSD) and obstructive sleep apnea (OSA). *J Clin Sleep Med*, *10*(6), 631–636. doi:10.5664/jcsm.3786

Taylor, F. B., Martin, P., Thompson, C., Williams, J., Mellman, T. A., Gross, C., . . . Raskind, M. A. (2008). Prazosin effects on objective sleep measures and clinical symptoms in civilian trauma posttraumatic stress disorder: A placebo-controlled study. *Biol Psychiatry*, *63*(6), 629–632. doi:10.1016/j.biopsych.2007.07.001

Thompson, C. E., Taylor, F. B., McFall, M. E., Barnes, R. F., & Raskind, M. A. (2008). Nonnightmare distressed awakenings in veterans with posttraumatic stress disorder: Response to prazosin. *J Trauma Stress*, *21*(4), 417–420. doi:10.1002/jts.20351

Thunker, J., & Pietrowsky, R. (2012). Effectiveness of a manualized imagery rehearsal therapy for patients suffering from nightmare disorders with and without a comorbidity of depression or PTSD. *Behav Res Ther*, *50*(9), 558–564. doi:10.1016/j.brat.2012.05.006

van Liempt, S., van Zuiden, M., Westenberg, H., Super, A., & Vermetten, E. (2013). Impact of impaired sleep on the development of ptsd symptoms in combat veterans: A prospective longitudinal cohort study. *Depress Anxiety*. doi:10.1002/da.22054

van Schagen, A. M., Lancee, J., de Groot, I. W., Spoormaker, V. I., & van den Bout, J. (2015). Imagery rehearsal therapy in addition to treatment as usual for patients with diverse psychiatric diagnoses suffering from nightmares: A randomized controlled trial. *J Clin Psychiatry*, *76*(9), e1105–e1113. doi:10.4088/JCP.14m09216

Vandrey, R., Babson, K. A., Herrmann, E. S., & Bonn-Miller, M. O. (2014). Interactions between disordered sleep, post-traumatic stress disorder, and substance use disorders. *Int Rev Psychiatry*, *26*(2), 237–247. doi:10.3109/09540261.2014.901300

Walker, M. P., & van der Helm, E. (2009). Overnight therapy? The role of sleep in emotional brain processing. *Psychol Bull*, *135*(5), 731–748. doi:10.1037/a0016570

Wellman, L. L., Yang, L., Ambrozewicz, M. A., Machida, M., & Sanford, L. D. (2013). Basolateral amygdala and the regulation of fear-conditioned changes in sleep: Role of corticotropin-releasing factor. *Sleep*, *36*(4), 471–480. doi:10.5665/sleep.2526

Werner, K. B., Griffin, M. G., & Galovski, T. E. (2016). Objective and subjective measurement of sleep disturbance in female trauma survivors with posttraumatic stress disorder. *Psychiatry Res*, *240*, 234–240. doi:10.1016/j.psychres.2016.04.039

Woodward, S. H., Arsenault, N. J., Murray, C., & Bliwise, D. L. (2000). Laboratory sleep correlates of nightmare complaint in PTSD inpatients. *Biol Psychiatry*, *48*(11), 1081–1087.

Woodward, S. H., Murburg, M. M., & Bliwise, D. L. (2000). PTSD-related hyperarousal assessed during sleep. *Physiol Behav*, *70*(1-2), 197–203.

Wright, K. M., Britt, T. W., Bliese, P. D., Adler, A. B., Picchioni, D., & Moore, D. (2011). Insomnia as predictor versus outcome of PTSD and depression among Iraq combat veterans. *J Clin Psychol, 67*(12), 1240–1258. doi:10.1002/jclp.20845

Zalta, A. K., Dowd, S., Rosenfield, D., Smits, J. A., Otto, M. W., Simon, N. M., . . . Pollack, M. H. (2013). Sleep quality predicts treatment outcome in CBT for social anxiety disorder. *Depress Anxiety, 30*(11), 1114–1120. doi:10.1002/da.22170

Zayfert, C., & DeViva, J. C. (2004). Residual insomnia following cognitive behavioral therapy for PTSD. *J Trauma Stress, 17*(1), 69–73. doi:10.1023/B:JOTS.0000014679.31799.e7

14

The Neurochemistry and Epigenetics of PTSD

Implications for Therapeutics

ROBERT M. POST

INTRODUCTION

Traditional views of the neurochemistry of posttraumatic stress disorder (PTSD) focus on alterations in classical central nervous system neurotransmitters serotonin and norepinephrine and pathological reactivity in the hypothalamic-pituitary-adrenal (HPA) axis, and these are only briefly noted here. Instead, we wish to emphasize a series of new conceptualizations and neurochemical data that have recently been elucidated. One is the recognition of the symptoms and neurobiology of PTSD as a moving target, being very different in different stages of illness evolution. Differences are apparent in the neurochemistry involved in early life stressor-related vulnerabilities to PTSD, the acute stress reaction, compensation and resolution phases, or ongoing chronicity with sleep disturbance, nightmares, flashbacks, hyperarousal, and dulling and depression. The neurochemical abnormalities will vary as a function of this temporal unfolding and further as a function of the common acquisition and progression of comorbid syndromes of alcohol and substance abuse.

Critical to the understanding of these evolving neurochemical abnormalities is the consensus that epigenetic alterations underlie the long-term mechanisms of both normal and pathological memory. Events in the environment affect what chemical groups are placed on DNA, the histones around which DNA is wrapped, and the production of messenger RNA (mRNA), each of which alter how easily DNA is turned on or off (transcribed or silenced) or proteins encoded (translation). These epigenetic chemical alterations can last a lifetime and provide the mechanisms for the long-term changes in behavioral and biochemical reactivity. Dramatic new data now also suggest that epigenetic changes can be transmitted across generations based either on parental influences on the offspring, or in some instances even in the absence of behavioral contact with the parents.

A new phase of memory reconsolidation has recently been described which may also play a key role in PTSD symptom progression and treatment. After short-term (hippocampally based) memory is consolidated into long-term (cortically based) memory, long-term memory (after it is actively recalled) can enter a new modifiable state where it can be either further reconsolidated or modified, and even extinguished. This provides a mechanism for recall and re-experiencing either sensitizing stress reactivity further or helping to dissipate it therapeutically.

A final new theme explored here is the role of inflammation in the stress sensitizing process involved in PTSD. This provides multiple insights as to how alterations in cytokines from peripheral monocytes and white cells can access the brain and further produce inflammation that alters stress-related neurochemistry and behavior. These new views not only further the understanding of mechanisms involved in PTSD but also open a series of new possibilities for therapeutics.

CLASSICAL NEUROCHEMISTRY AND ENDOCRINOLOGY OF PTSD

Detailed and comprehensive reviews are available on this topic and provide key insights into understanding the pathophysiology of the range of symptoms involved in PTSD (1–5). The neuroendocrine system is reregulated in multiple ways. Corticotropin-releasing hormone (CRH) in cerebrospinal fluid is increased, while cortisol is decreased. An important element is increased reactivity in the noradrenergic (norepinephrine) system, seen as the mechanism for hyperstartle and hyperarousal. As described by Davis (6) and

LeDoux (7), hyperreactivity of the amygdala and its effects on efferent pathways appears to underlie multiple different aspects of conditioned fear and PTSD symptoms. Output from the basolateral nucleus to different brain areas is associated with different symptoms occurring in PTSD, that is, lateral hypothalamus (blood pressure elevation, tachycardia); dorsal nucleus of vagus (ulcers, bradycardia); parabrachial nucleus (respiratory distress); ventral tegmental area and locus coeruleus (activity, arousal, attention); nucleus reticularis pontis caudalis (hyperstartle); central gray (freezing); trigeminal, facial motor nucleus (facial expression of fear); paraventricular nucleus hypothalamus (CRH release) (6).

Brain-derived neurotrophic factor (BDNF) in the locus coeruleus is increased after stressors, potentially accounting for the long-lasting increases in noradrenergic responsiveness. The alpha 2 antagonist yohimbine, which increases norepinephrine (NE) releases, causes flashbacks and increased autonomic reactivity in patients with PTSD. The noradrenergic abnormalities are further validated by the success of the alpha 1 receptor antagonist prazosin which inhibits nightmares and many other aspects of the PTSD syndrome.

NE feeds back on the amygdala and amplifies the synaptic response to stimulation as revealed by recordings of synaptic effects in a model of learning and memory in an amygdala or hippocampal slice preparation—long-term potentiation (LTP). LTP is specific to the specific synapses stimulated (homosynapstic LTP), but clinically patients' reactivity to cues in the environment appear to broaden, generalize, and extend beyond those explicitly experienced in the trauma to many others in the environment. This can perhaps now be explained by the concept of heterosynaptic LTP where synapses beyond those originally stimulated are also potentiated. New data suggest that glial cells are involved in this process, such that gliotransmission can occur over multiple neurons and some distance (8).

A further mechanism of upregulation of amygdala responsivity is seen in the phenomenon of metaplasticity. In contrast to the hippocampus where low frequency stimulation produces long-term depression (LTD), 1 Hz stimulation of the amygdala for 15 minutes produces LTP and upregulation of the excitability of the specific synapses stimulated. However, if one gives a brief high burst of stimulation (about 100Hz such as might be associated with a traumatic event), the subsequent 1Hz stimulation of the amygdala slice no longer produces LTP but LTD instead (9). This switch from LTP to LTD is based on the influence of metabotropic type 2 glutamate receptors, which, if blocked, prevent the metaplastic switch from LTP to LTD. In this fashion a traumatic event associated with a high frequency signal in the amygdala could change its ability to respond to subsequent low-level stimulation in the usual mode.

There is yet another mechanism for altering amygdala reactivity with stressor recurrence. The peptide CRH shows increases in its levels in the amygdala with the repetition of stressors or trauma, while CRH in the hypothalamus (conveying endocrine reactivity via pituitary adrenocorticotropic hormone and then adrenal cortisol) is reduced. CRH in the amygdala is fear enhancing and anxiogenic (10). Repeated stressors in young animals lead to increases in the size of the amygdala in adulthood, while the hippocampus shows the opposite change and decreases in size (11).

Yehuda et al. (2, 12) describe the reregulation of the HPA axis in PTSD as involving increased negative feedback from the adrenal steroid cortisol on hippocampal glucocorticoid receptors (GR). As opposed to depression (where there is hypercortisolemia, down regulation of hippocampal GR receptors, and escape from dexamethasone suppression), in PTSD there is hypocortisolism, up regulation of hippocampal GR, and enhanced suppression of cortisol after dexamethasone (Figure 14.1). Increased levels of GR have been demonstrated in PTSD patients' white cells, as well as hippocampus in autopsy samples.

The epigenetic basis of this change has been demonstrated in animal and humans by the hypomethylation of the GR DNA promoter and consequent increased levels of GR (13, 14) in those with trauma histories. Epigenetic changes (alterations in DNA methylation and acetylation of histones around which DNA is wrapped) are more abundant in patients with histories of adversity and stressors in childhood than in those without abuse (15).

EPIGENETIC BASIS FOR LONG-LASTING BEHAVIORAL AND BIOCHEMICAL RESPONSIVITY TO STRESSORS

Epigenetic (meaning above genetic) refers to chemical changes induced by environmental in DNA, histones, and mRNA that do not affect inherited gene sequences but rather alter the transcriptional activity of DNA, that is, how

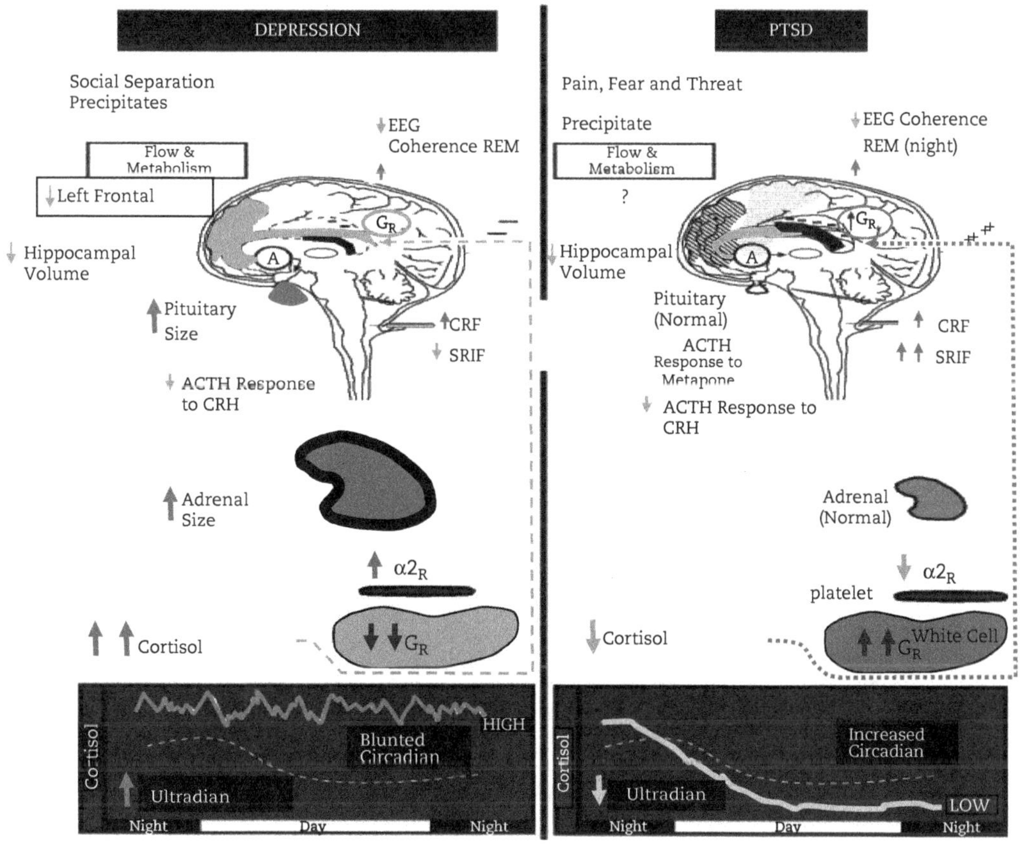

FIGURE 14.1. Overlapping and differential neurobiology of depression and PTSD. (See front matter.)
After Yehuda et al., 2010.

easily genes are turned on or off (Figure 14.2). Methylation of DNA and histones tends to inhibit gene transcription, while acetylation of histones loosens DNA winding and enhances transcription (16, 17). Epigenetic alterations are critical to normal functions of learning and memory as well as pathological aspects of learned fear (18).

The long-lasting epigenetic effects of early experience, ranging from subtle to traumatic influences on behavior, are readily illustrated in animal models (14, 19, 20). If newborn rat pups are mishandled by their mother, they develop lifelong deficits in levels of BDNF in their frontal cortex and associated behavioral changes (20). These changes are associated with methylation of the DNA promoter for BDNF, and if methylation is blocked by an inhibitor zebularine, the BDNF deficits are prevented. These persistent neurochemical changes induced by neonatal adversity provide a mechanistic insight to the well-documented observations that the experience of childhood adversity is one of the major risk factors for the later occurrence of PTSD after adult trauma (21). The early stress appears to sensitize the organism to the effects of later stressors (Table 14.1, Figure 14.3). Early life stressors also interact with one's genetic variation in increasing the incidence of depression or PTSD in response to adult social or traumatic stressor, respectively. This increase in vulnerability to depression has been shown in those who inherit the short form of the serotonin transporter (22), a variant of the GR chaperone FKBP5 (23), and a polymorphism of the CRH receptor 1 (24). Many similar genetic-environmental interactions would be expected in PTSD in light of the small percentage of people who experience trauma who then go on to develop PTSD; people may have genetic backgrounds that make them more or less vulnerable to this type of stressor sensitization.

Stressors later in life (such as the experience of 10 days of repeated defeat stress by a small mouse threatened by a large aggressive mouse which induces an anxious and depressive-like state) lead to decreases in BDNF in hippocampus but increases in BDNF in the ventral striatum

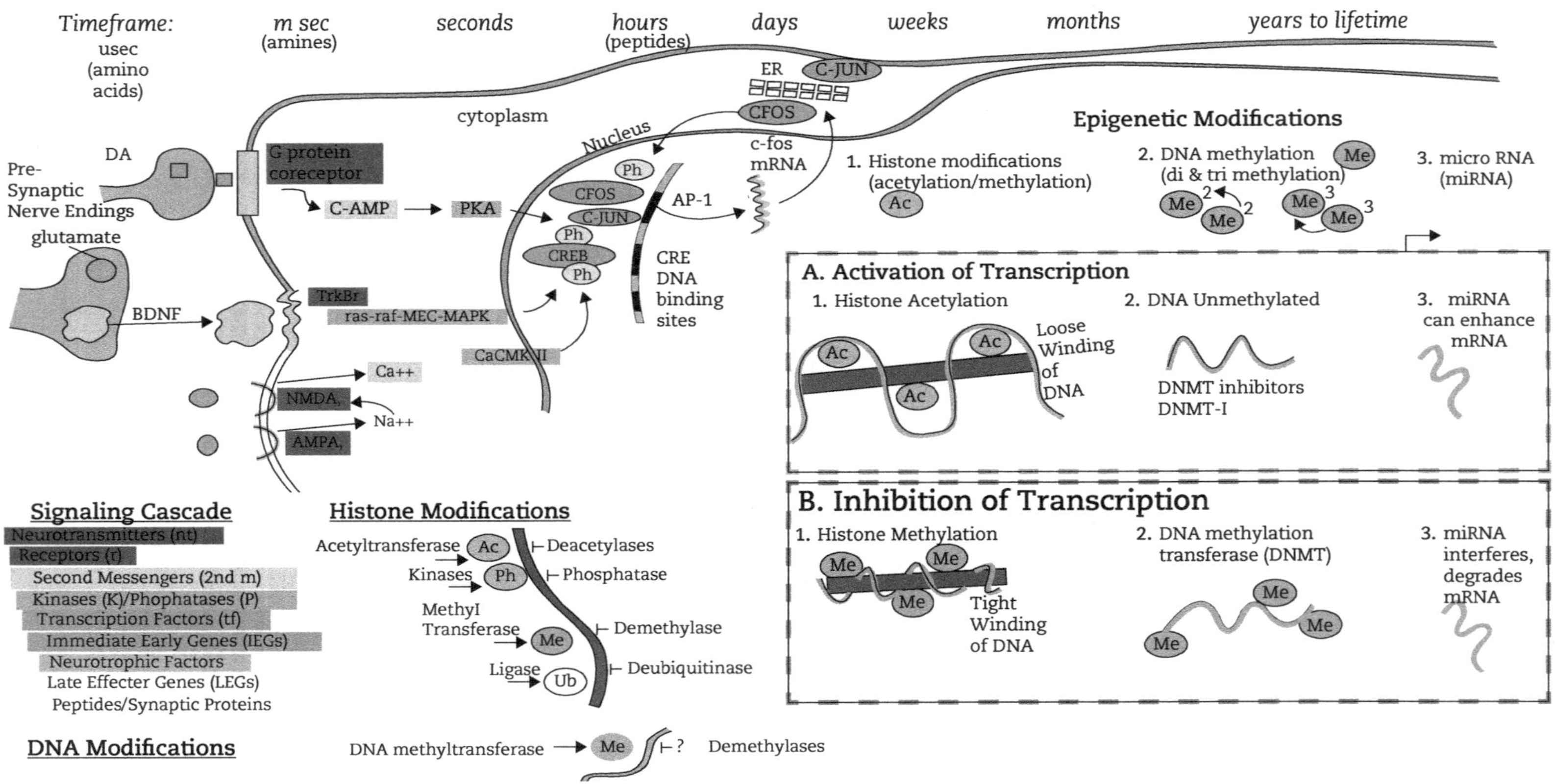

FIGURE 14.2. Epigenetic mechanisms of synaptic plasticity and long term effects. (See front matter.)

or nucleus accumbens (NAc). If either of these BDNF changes are prevented, the defeat stress behaviors do not emerge (25, 26). These same opposing BDNF alterations in hippocampus and NAc are seen in human depression (27).

The BDNF decreases in the hippocampus in the mouse model of defeat stress involve a suppressive triple methylation of histone H3 at lysine 27 (H3K27me3). This methyl mark persists even when antidepressants are given to increase hippocampal BDNF and reverse the defeat stress behavior. This may be an example of why continuous antidepressants are required to prevent depressive recurrences in humans, as they normalize the BDNF decrements in the hippocampus by other chemical pathways but leave the more permanent vulnerability marks (such as H3K27me3) unchanged. This raises the prospect that some lasting epigenetic changes in depression and PTSD may ultimately be amenable to more complete amelioration once treatment is targeted at the appropriate stress-induced epigenetic changes.

Patients with mood disorders and PTSD are particularly prone to develop problems with alcohol and drug abuse, in part as an attempt to treat some of their residual symptoms. However, this can add another level of neurochemical and behavioral abnormalities (17). For example, if one repeatedly uses cocaine, reactivity to it can increase or sensitize, and people can develop increased anxiety, dysphoric activation, panic attacks, paranoia, and outright psychosis (28). Animals given the same dose of cocaine show increased motor hyperactivity and stereotypy, what is known as behavioral sensitization (Table 14.1). This sensitization to cocaine has an epigenetic basis, as it too is associated with increases in BDNF in the NAc, and if the DNA methylation inhibitor zebularine is given, the sensitization is blocked (29). Cocaine-sensitized animals show cross sensitization to stressors, and vice versa, suggesting that each type of sensitization can exacerbate the other (28, 30, 31). The literature is strong in documenting that early stress predisposes to cocaine and other drug self-administration in animals and man (32–35).

Alcohol abuse is also highly comorbid with PTSD, and it can cause illness progression based on the number of alcohol withdrawal episodes. More episodes of alcohol withdrawal can kindle panic attacks or seizures (36) just the way that repeated electrical or chemical stimulation of the amygdala can lead to the development of full-blown seizures to a previously subthreshold stimulus (37). Following enough of these triggered amygdala-kindled seizures, seizures can begin to emerge spontaneously. The neurochemistry and neuroanatomy of the amygdala-kindled memory trace evolves in association with seizure development, generalization, and progression. cFos as a measure of neuronal activation and neuropeptides, such as thyrotropin-releasing hormone and CRH, are initially induced unilaterally, then bilaterally in limbic regions, and then spread to the cortex bilaterally (38–40). However, when spontaneous seizures occur, the original amygdala focus and spread to hippocampus is no longer apparent, suggesting a further migration of the amygdala-kindled memory trace with the progression to spontaneity.

This progression from seizures regularly triggered by amygdala stimulation to those that occur spontaneously may have some parallels to the evolution of flashbacks in PTSD from those that are regularly triggered by trauma cues to those that can start to occur more spontaneously in the absence of obvious triggers (42) (Figure 14.3). Multiple types of sensitization and kindling-like processes are evident in the longitudinal course of the development PTSD in Israeli prisoners of war (POWs) held during the Yom Kippur of 1973 and followed prospectively for the next 35 years (43). The occurrence and persistence of PTSD symptoms was related to the presence of trauma in the POWs' childhood, number and severity of both war and POW camp traumas, number of deployments, and for late-onset PTSD occurring in about 16% of the former POWs (without a previous PTSD diagnosis), exposure to the number of bombings occurring in Israel during the Palestinian intifadas, suggesting these repeated delayed traumatic experiences could also kindle delayed-onset PTSD.

In any event, it is important to note that the neurochemistry and epigenetic marks associated with PTSD will vary not only as a function of the number, severity, and intermittency of the inducing trauma itself but will be further complicated in a progressive fashion by the comorbid abuse of alcohol, cocaine, heroin, marijuana, and related drugs. Many of these drugs of abuse are associated with an increased level of the excitatory glutamate signaling in the NAc when drug-associated cues occur (28, 43, 44). If this glutamate signal in the NAc is dampened, these habits have less strength and automaticity, allowing more cortical control and the ability to refrain from drug use.

The drug N-acetylcysteine (NAC), which is available without prescription from health food stores, dampens the stimulus-induced glutamate

TABLE 14.1 SENSITIZATION AND KINDLING: INCREASED BEHAVIORAL REACTIVITY TO REPETITION OF THE SAME STIMULUS

I. STRESS SENSITIZATION: Greater stressor response upon repetition		RESULT
A. Psychosocial Stressors and Losses	——————>	Trigger Depression
B. Trauma and Threats to Life of Limb	——————>	Trigger PTSD
II. AFFECTIVE EPISODE AND FLASHBACK SENSITIZATION		
1. Repeated episodes and flashbacks	——————>	Faster recurrences
2. More repetitions (kindling-like)	——————>	Spontaneous recurrences
III. COAINE SENSITIZATION upon repeated doses		
A. Hyperactivity in animals	——————>	Greater hyperactivity and Stereotypy
B. Hypomanic-like Behavior in humans	——————>	Full-blown Mania
C. Euphoria	——————>	Dysphoria
D. Mania	——————>	Paranoid Psychosis
IV. CROSS SENSITIZATION		
A. Stress Sensitization crosses to	——————>	Episode and Cocaine Sensitization
B. Episode Sensitization crosses to	——————>	Stressor and cocaine sensitization
C. Cocaine Sensitization crosses to	——————>	Stressor and Episode Sensitization
V. KINDLING: Repeated Brain Stimulation		
A. Electrical Stimulation	——————>	Development of full-blown seizures & seizures become spontaneous
B. Pharmacological Stimulation (local anesthetics cocaine & lidocaine)	——————>	

signal in the NAc by increasing the growth of glutamate transporters on glial cells which remove glutamate from the synapse. Remarkably, NAC is able to lessen the craving for multiple drugs, including cocaine, alcohol, nicotine, and marijuana; decrease depression and anxiety in bipolar disorder (45); decrease obsessive-compulsive disorder symptoms as an adjunct to selective serotonin reuptake inhibitors; lessen trichotillomania and other habits, and improve multiple components of the PTSD syndrome (28, 35, 46). Given its properties as an anti-oxidant and glutathione precursor and safety and tolerability in all of the placebo-controlled studies noted, it would appear appropriate for NAC to have an increasing role in the treatment of PTSD and its multiple comorbidities.

TRANSGENERATIONAL TRANSMISSION OF STRESS VULNERABILITY VIA TWO EPIGENETIC ROUTES

Intergenerational transmission of the vulnerability to stress can occur through two expected routes—genetic and the epigenetic impact of parental behaviors on the offspring (19, 47)—and a third entirely unexpected mechanism. The epigenetic effects of some parental experiences can be transmitted to the next generation in the absence of any contact with the offspring (12, 48–52). For example, a male rat conditioned to an odor and a shock will have offspring more responsive to that specific odor and will even have increased numbers of receptors sensitive to that smell (53). A male rat with given THC will have offspring which prefer heroin (51). It is thought that some epigenetic marks escape erasure at conception or that double-stranded RNA in blood can get access to sperm. Some of these transgenerational effects can increase responsivity (12, 53) in the next generation or decrease it (52), and in some instances effects can extend across multiple generations and be sex dependent. Thus, it would appear that vulnerability to PTSD could be transmitted across generations via genetic and two different types of epigenetic mechanisms (17).

IMMUNE MECHANISMS OF STRESS SENSITIZATION

So far in this review we have focused on mechanisms in the brain conveying the potential

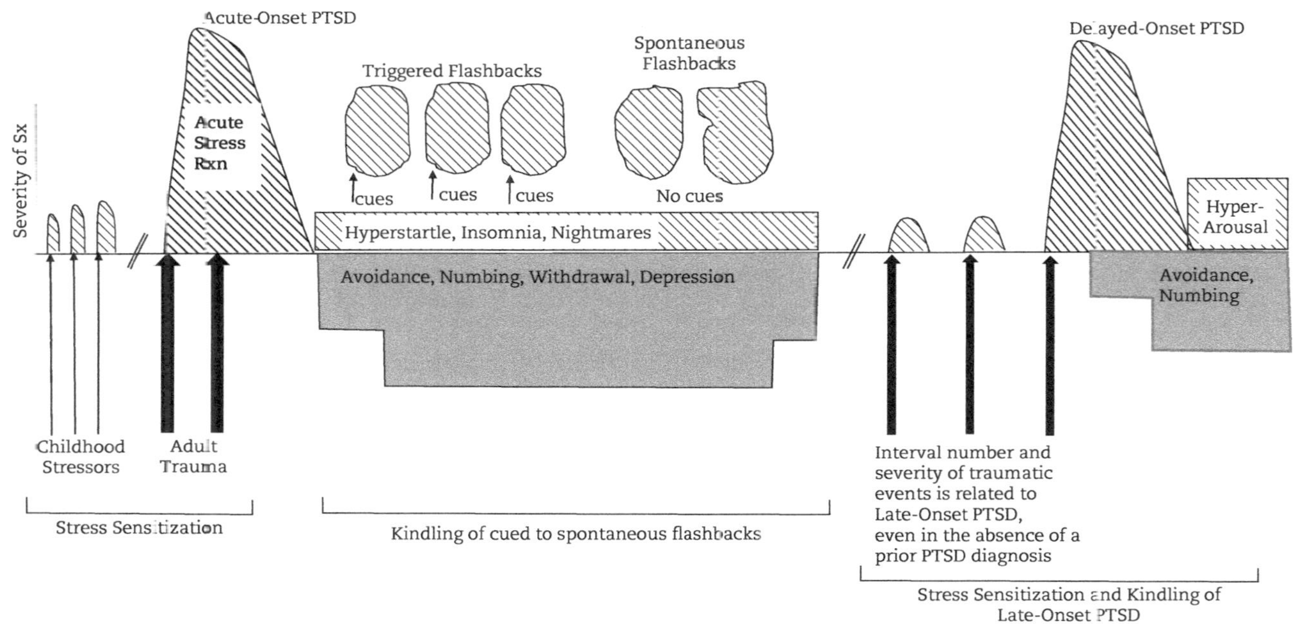

FIGURE 14.3. Stress sensitization and kindling-like effects in the evolution of acute and delayed onset PTSD.

for increased reactivity to stressors (sensitization) rather than what might be considered more adaptive down-regulation of responsivity or tolerance. Recently, new mechanisms in the periphery have been found to play a role in up-regulating biochemical and behavioral reactivity to repeated stressors. Inflammation has been recognized as occurring is a significant proportion of patients with PTSD. This is evident in the increased levels of the inflammatory cytokines Il-1, Il-6, and tumor necrosis factor (TNF) alpha, and the acute phase reactant C-reactive protein. These increases in inflammatory cytokines can be associated with depression, anxiety, loss of energy, and other sickness-related behaviors (54–57).

The model of defeat stress in a mouse has many parallels to symptoms and behaviors that occur not only in depression but also in PTSD (56). A small mouse repeatedly exposed to a larger, more aggressive animal (but protected from being killed by a plastic barrier) for ten days renders the animal anxious (tested on an elevated plus maze), withdrawn and asocial (not exploring novel objects), and showing generalization of trauma cues (not exploring another friendly animal) and other PTSD-like symptoms. Thus the model has some face and ecological validity as a repeated life-threatening stressor that could mimic what an animal might naturally face in the wild.

As we noted, this model gave us insights into some of the biochemistry and epigenetic changes associated with the defeat stress depressive and PTSD-like behaviors. In this section, we show that this model reveals several potential pathways by which immune cells (lymphocytes and monocytes) in the periphery traffic to the brain, exacerbate inflammatory processes, and produce biochemical alterations and anxiety-related behaviors (Figure 14.4). In the defeat stress paradigm, white cells secrete Il-6, and if this is prevented or inhibited with Il-6 antibodies, the defeat stress behaviors do not occur (58).

Similarly, monocytes from bone marrow are released into circulation (stimulated by norepinephrine secretion from sympathetic nerves), traverse to the brain, gain access to it via endothelial cells surrounding blood vessels, stimulate macrophages, and activate microglia to secrete further cytokines, including Il-1B, which induce a range of defeat stress behaviors (56). Again, if the monocyte trafficking to the brain is prevented, the behaviors do not occur. The details of this brain to periphery and back to the brain pathway have been elegantly elucidated by Weber et al. (56) and by Menard et al. (59). They include activation of "danger signals" in the brain via glutamate and the gliotransmitter adenosine triphosphate (ATP) from astrocytes. ATP activates P2X7R and macrophages and microglia release Il-1B which leads to the induction of TNF alpha via the NLRP 3 inflammasome. Mature Il-1B in the hippocampus is associated with increased anhedonia and decreased neurogenesis.

This inflammatory pathway and monocyte activation provides another mode of amplification of biochemical and behavioral reactivity with repeated stressors. It requires 3 days of defeat stress to induce a subclinical syndrome (and some monocyte activation) and 10 days of defeat stress for full activation and the behavioral syndrome (56). The body is registering the events and reacting with up-regulation of the responses. If an animal also had a prior 10-day defeat stress experience and superficially had recovered, a new set of defeat stress experiences leads to additional changes. The first defeat stress experience produced primed monocytes from the bone marrow, some of which are stored in the spleen. Upon the second round of stressors, these monocytes are released from spleen, traffic to the brain, and increase the inflammatory cascade further. Again, if the monocytes from the spleen are intercepted, the defeat stress behaviors do not occur.

Thus we have seen evidence that white cells from lymph nodes and monocytes from bone marrow and then the spleen are the conveyors of some of the PTSD-like defeat stress behaviors. It appears that appreciation of danger signals in the brain have multiple routes to influence behavioral reactivity, including the amygdala and multiple other brain regions, peptides such as CRH, neurotransmitters such as glutamate and NE, and NE release from sympathetic nerves to mobilize monocytes in bone marrow and spleen. These cells then traffic back to the brain to influence a range of cells including endothelial cells, astroglia, macrophages, microglia, and neurons again.

It appears that this multiplicity of organs and cell types are crucial players in this extraordinary interplay of brain and body. Certainly, these diverse systems in their proper functioning must serve some evolutionary beneficial and protective role, and the points where positive adaptions to the environment begin to go awry and become pathological are ones that deserve intense study for their heuristic value and the potential for therapeutic intervention (60). The clarification of some of the inflammatory pathways involved in stressor responsivity raises important questions of what role each type of anti-inflammatory agents

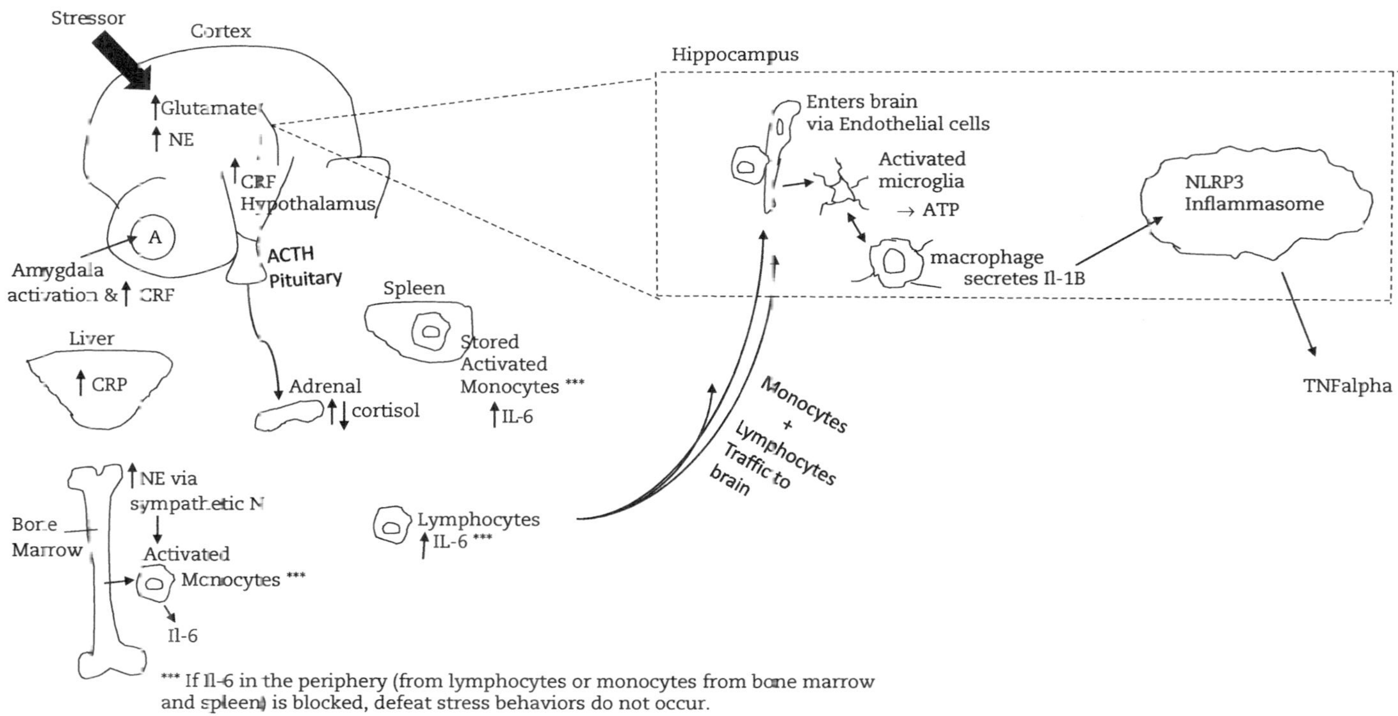

FIGURE 14.4. Role of inflammation in periphery and brain in defeat stress-induced biochemistry and behavior.

*** If Il-6 in the periphery (from lymphocytes or monocytes from bone marrow and spleen) is blocked, defeat stress behaviors do not occur.

might play in the treatment of some aspects of the PTSD syndrome. Again, a critical issue is the question of when in the pathophysiological sequence of the unfolding of the PTSD syndrome anti-inflammatory agents might be helpful. Among other anti-inflammatory drugs, the antibiotic minocycline with its potential antidepressant, anticonvulsant/antikindling (60), neuroprotective effects, and ability to inhibit microglial activation would be of interest for further study.

INSULIN RESISTANCE AS ANOTHER CONSEQUENCE OF STRESS SENSITIZATION: ROLE OF GLUTAMATE

Insulin resistance is a key component of the metabolic syndrome which is common in patients with depression and PTSD. It often develops in adulthood after sensitizing stressors earlier in life (62, 63). The double hit of early and later stressors increases glutamate release in the hippocampus via a down-regulation of the inhibitory metabotropic type 2 glutamate (mGlu2) receptor (64). Agents such as acetyl-l-carnitine that regulate metabolic factors, enhance mitochondrial function, and reduce glutamate overflow up-regulate the inhibitory mGlu2 receptors. Acetyl-L-carnitine increases levels of acetylated H3K27 bound to the DNA promoter for mGlu2 and also increases acetylation of NF-κB-p65 subunit, thereby enhancing the transcription of the gene encoding for the mGlu2 receptor, which is increased in hippocampus and prefrontal cortex.

Acetyl-L-carnitine also increases brain and serum levels of BDNF, and its behavioral effects in models of depression are evident in three days, while it took two weeks for the effects of the traditional tricyclic antidepressant chlorimpramine to become manifest. Therefore, acetyl-L-carnitine might rapidly ameliorate depression and could also be considered for treatment of insulin resistance in depressed subjects (65, 66). It is of interest that defeat stress, as noted, increases the suppressive tri-methyation mark of H3K27 in a long-lasting fashion (27), while in contrast, acetyl-L-carnitine acetylates and activates H3K27. It would be interesting to see whether acetyl-L-carnitine could more permanently reduce the vulnerability to repeated defeat stress experiences in animals and humans and preclude the necessity for long-term antidepressant treatment.

Lau et al. (67) also examined the effects of chronic stress on the medial amygdala and found, in contrast to other areas of the amygdala, the neurons and dendrites appeared to shrink. Treatment with acetyl-L-carnitine reversed these anatomical changes and the associated behavioral abnormalities, including social avoidance. Acetyl-L-carnitine also safely ameliorated arterial hypertension, insulin resistance, impaired glucose tolerance, and hypoadiponectinemia in subjects at increased cardiovascular risk (68).

Thus several types of glutamatergic mechanisms would appear to be promising targets of PTSD therapeutics. Given the preliminary evidence of acetyl-L-carnitine's effectiveness in depression (69), and its ability to rapidly up-regulate metabotropic glutamate receptors which are needed to inhibit glutamate release, acetyl-L-carnitine deserves further study in both depression and PTSD and as a potential protection against PTSD and aspects of the metabolic syndrome. As noted, NAC also decreases synaptic glutamate but does this via increasing glutamate transporters and glutamate transport into glial cells (44). The glutamate N-methyl-D-aspartic-acid (NMDA) receptor antagonist ketamine exerts rapid onset antidepressant effects, reverses some of the synaptic deficits of chronic stress (70), and may also have positive clinical effects in PTSD (71). The role of glutamate in PTSD is further supported by the findings that, in the hippocampus, a marker of neuronal integrity N-acetyl aspartate is reduced and glutamate levels are increased compared to trauma exposed non-PTSD controls (72).

THE NEUROCHEMISTRY OF RECONSOLIDATION: IMPLICATIONS FOR PATHOPHYSIOLOGY AND THERAPEUTICS

The mysteries of the mechanisms of memory formation are just beginning to be revealed. Until the past two decades, it was thought that short-term memory was consolidated in a process that required new protein synthesis into the long-term memory engram which was transferred from the hippocampus to the cerebral cortex. However, a further new phase of memory reconsolidation has been revealed which also requires new protein synthesis (73, 74). If a long-term memory is actively recalled and brought into consciousness along with its original emotional content, the memory becomes fragile and subject in a phase of reconsolidation, which either results in further reinforcement of the original version of the memory or, if there is new contradictory input, to modification or even extinction of the original memory (Figure 14.5). The reconsolidation window opens about five minutes to several hours after active recall, and, in contrast to successful extinction training within the reconsolidation window, attempts at memory revision either outside of the window or without the active recall are without lasting effect.

Agren et al. (75) showed a dramatic effect of extinction in the reconsolidation window on the encoding of a fear memory trace in the amygdala. Volunteers were conditioned to the pairing of a specific picture and the induction of a mild shock. As imaged on fMRI, amygdala activity remained high and changes in skin conductance persisted when extinction training was performed at six hours after recall of the picture-shock association; that is, extinction training outside of the reconsolidation window was ineffective in modifying the conditioned fear association. However, when the same extinction training occurred immediately following the recall (i.e., within the reconsolidation window), the amygdala and its efferent pathways no longer showed increased activity on the fMRI upon presentation of the picture alone, and skin conductance changes were no longer observed, as if the amygdala-based memory trace was abolished or erased.

Extinction work in the reconsolidation window has been used to treat anxiety disorders and PTSD with some initial success, but with the caution that it must be done in such a way as not to rekindle and enhance the original trauma memory upon recall (74). The technique of eye movement desensitization and reprocessing (EMDR) utilizes many of the principles of work in the reconsolidation window, first engendering active recall, and then working through and modifying traumatic memories in the safety of the therapeutic interaction (76–78).

Some of the same processes and principles have been used to more permanently extinguish the positive memories of the drug "high" and therefore prevent a relapse of craving that can occur spontaneously or with stress or cues of the drug experience. Such preliminary work using extinction training in the reconsolidation window in the study of Xue et al. (79) in both animals and humans has been successful in preventing reinstatement and relapse to cocaine and heroin use over long periods of time.

It is clear that epigenetic processes are involved in the normal processes of learning and memory and appear to involve both changes in DNA methylation and histone chemical marks (18, 80). How these changes relate to the different components of memory reconsolidation and extinction remain to be more clearly delineated. However, it already is apparent that epigenetic manipulations such as the use of histone deacetylase inhibitors can

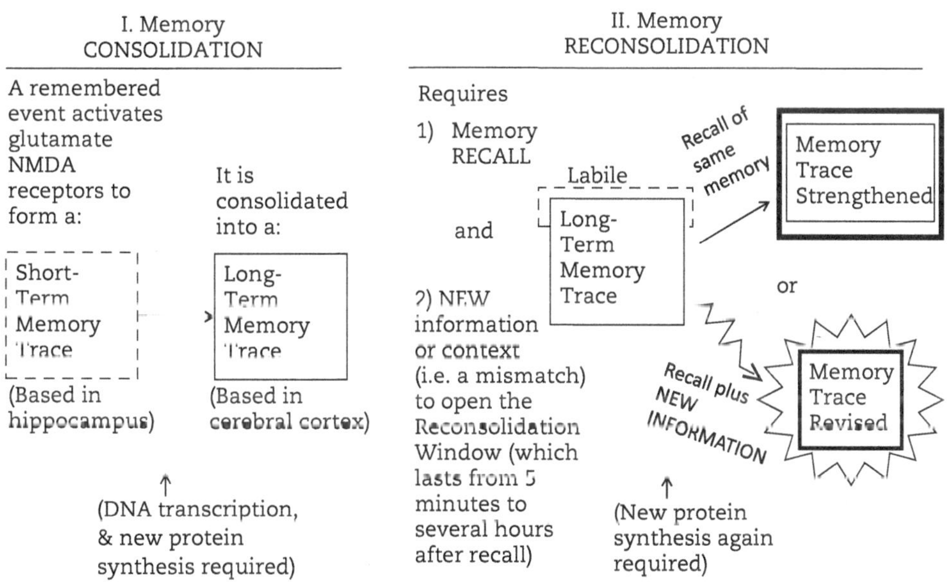

FIGURE 14.5. Opening the reconsolidation window renders a long-term memory trace labile and subject to permanent revision.

enhance extinction learning. Valproate is a nonspecific histone deacetylase inhibitor (HDAC-I) and has been shown in animals to increase BDNF isoforms that are specific for enhancing extinction learning (81, 82). More specific HDAC-Is are being studied in animals and appear promising. Vagal nerve stimulation in animals has also been shown to enhance the new learning involved in extinction, and work in humans will soon follow. The neurochemical mechanisms of this effect will be of great interest.

Potentially complicating these efforts is the view that epigenetic marks of stress-related memories not only vary as a function of the phase of syndrome evolution but, as in kindling of seizures, the epigenetic marks of conditioned fear migrate anatomically over time as well. Morris and Monteggia (83) found that different epigenetic marks were evident in different brain areas as a function of the duration of time after a fear learning event. It has been estimated that 100 million cells are involved in a simple avoidance learning task in the cat. Given the likely many-fold greater impact of a life-and-death stressor involved in the precipitation of PTSD, one could envision the firing, synaptic plasticity, and epigenetic marking of billions of neurons in brain and these further changing and migrating as a function of consolidation, reconsolidation, and other temporally based events, creating an immense and ongoing revision of brain functioning. Preventing or reversing the transition from adaptive hyper-alertness, avoidance, and trauma replay to the enduring dysfunction, disabilities, and comorbidities of chronic PTSD is a daunting task, but one that now has great possibilities given the initial understanding of some of the varied neurochemical mechanisms involved.

SUMMARY AND CONCLUSIONS

The neurochemistry of PTSD in the 21st century is revealing new biological mechanisms and accordingly, new targets for therapeutics. Sensitization to stressors involves not only changes in classical neurotransmitters in brain but memory-like mechanisms that involve epigenetic alterations that propel increased responsivity to recurrent stressors rather than tolerance and down regulation. Amplification of stress responsivity is seen at multiple levels of the central nervous system and periphery. Amygdala responses increase with stressor recurrence, as do CRH and immune mechanisms. Immunological sensitization involves an exquisite interplay of potentiating inflammatory mechanisms in both the brain (involving neurons, astrocytes, endothelial cells, macrophages, and microglia) and the periphery (involving lymphocytes and monocytes from bone marrow and spleen) which traffic to the brain and further engender biochemical and behavioral changes. If lymphocyte Il-6 actions or monocyte trafficking to brain is blocked, animals undergoing the repeated defeat stress paradigm do not show the expected behavioral alterations mimicking symptoms of anxiety, depression, and PTSD.

Promising treatments have evolved from the understanding of the neurochemistry of PTSD. The alpha 1 receptor antagonist has changed the treatment of PTSD via targeting the noradrenergic system. N-acetylcysteine dampens glutamate hyperreactivity in the NAc and appears valuable in multiple aspects of PTSD symptoms and its alcohol and substance abuse comorbidities. Acetyl-L-carnitine holds promise in addressing depression and some aspects of metabolic syndrome (such high blood pressure and insulin resistance) so prominent in PTSD. Targeting inflammation presents a rich new set of possibilities for therapeutics, but major conundrums persist as to when in the unfolding sequence of immunological and behavioral changes they should be applied. Long-term memory processes involved in the replay of nightmares, flashbacks, hyperstartle, and avoidance have an epigenetic basis, and more specifically and discretely manipulating epigenetic mechanisms holds the promise of memory modulation and reversal. While these are awaited in the future, neuropsychological manipulations of the extinction process in the reconsolidation window are already being used to treat conditioned fear and modulate the traumatic memories of PTSD.

One critical focus of therapeutics of PTSD has not progressed as rapidly as hoped. The study of prevention of PTSD by altering the acute neurochemistry that develops in the time immediately following a trauma, or what would be considered secondary prevention of PTSD, is just beginning to be explored. It is hoped that the understanding of the unfolding of acute PTSD symptoms and neurochemistry will lead to novel ways of intercepting these processes and alter the long-lasting sequelae of traumatic events.

Another major goal for the future is finding ways of psychologically and/or pharmacologically immunizing individuals against the effects of future trauma. This would be of great importance for rescue workers and soldiers who will knowingly very likely be exposed to major catastrophes and the traumas of wars, and such pre-exposure treatment would fall under the rubric of primary prevention. Again, it might be useful to remind one of the lessons of sensitization and kindling where different early, mid, and late phases of these progressively evolving syndromes have very different neuroanatomical and neurochemical substrates, and a drug or manipulation effective in one phase is not necessarily effective in another. The timing of a given intervention in relationship to phase of PTSD evolution may be central to its effectiveness.

REFERENCES

1. Heim C, Nemeroff CB. Neurobiology of posttraumatic stress disorder. *CNS Spectrums.* 2009; 14:13–24.
2. Yehuda R, Flory JD, Pratchett LC, Buxbaum J, Ising M, Holsboer F. Putative biological mechanisms for the association between early life adversity and the subsequent development of PTSD. *Psychopharmacology.* 2010; 212:405–417.
3. Pitman RK, Rasmusson AM, Koenen KC, Shin LM, Orr SP, Gilbertson MW, et al. Biological studies of post-traumatic stress disorder. *Nature Reviews Neuroscience.* 2012; 13:769–787.
4. Friedman MJ, Keane TM, Resick PA. *Handbook of PTSD.* 2nd ed. New York: Guilford Publications; 2015.
5. Yehuda R, Hoge CW, McFarlane AC, Vermetten E, Lanius RA, Nievergelt CM, et al. Post-traumatic stress disorder. *Natures Reviews: Disease Primers.* 2015; 1:15057.
6. Davis M. Neurobiology of fear responses: The role of the amygdala. *The Journal of Neuropsychiatry and Clinical Neurosciences.* 1997; 9:382–402.
7. LeDoux J. The emotional brain, fear, and the amygdala. *Cellular and Molecular Neurobiology.* 2003; 23:727–738.
8. Kronschlager MT, Drdla-Schutting R, Gassner M, Honsek SD, Teuchmann HL, Sandkuhler J. Gliogenic LTP spreads widely in nociceptive pathways. *Science.* 2016; 354:1144–1148.
9. Li H, Weiss SR, Chuang DM, Post RM, Rogawski MA. Bidirectional synaptic plasticity in the rat basolateral amygdala: characterization of an activity-dependent switch sensitive to the presynaptic metabotropic glutamate receptor antagonist 2S-alpha-ethylglutamic acid. *The Journal of Neuroscience.* 1998; 18:1662–1670.
10. Kalin NH, Shelton SE, Davidson RJ. The role of the central nucleus of the amygdala in mediating fear and anxiety in the primate. *The Journal of Neuroscience.* 2004; 24:5506–5515.
11. Lupien SJ, McEwen BS, Gunnar MR, Heim C. Effects of stress throughout the lifespan on the brain, behaviour and cognition. *Nature Reviews Neuroscience.* 2009; 10:434–445.
12. Yehuda R, Daskalakis NP, Lehrner A, Desarnaud F, Bader HN, Makotkine I, et al. Influences of maternal and paternal PTSD on epigenetic regulation of the glucocorticoid receptor gene in Holocaust survivor offspring. *The American Journal of Psychiatry.* 2014; 171:872–880.
13. McGowan PO, Sasaki A, D'Alessio AC, Dymov S, Labonte B, Szyf M, et al. Epigenetic regulation of the glucocorticoid receptor in human brain associates with childhood abuse. *Nature Neuroscience.* 2009; 12:342–348.
14. Suderman M, McGowan PO, Sasaki A, Huang TC, Hallett MT, Meaney MJ, et al. Conserved epigenetic sensitivity to early life experience in the rat and human hippocampus. *Proceedings of the National Academy of Sciences of the United States of America.* 2012; 109(Suppl 2):17266–17272.
15. Mehta D, Klengel T, Conneely KN, Smith AK, Altmann A, Pace TW, et al. Childhood maltreatment is associated with distinct genomic and epigenetic profiles in posttraumatic stress disorder. *Proceedings of the National Academy of Sciences of the United States of America.* 2013; 110:8302–8307.
16. Nestler EJ. Epigenetic mechanisms of depression. *JAMA Psychiatry.* 2014; 71:454–456.
17. Post RM. Epigenetic basis of sensitization to stress, affective episodes, and stimulants: Implications for illness progression and prevention. *Bipolar Disorders.* 2016; 18:315–324.
18. Zovkic IB, Sweatt JD. Epigenetic mechanisms in learned fear: implications for PTSD. *Neuropsychopharmacology.* 2013; 38:77–93.
19. Weaver IC, Cervoni N, Champagne FA, D'Alessio AC, Sharma S, Seckl JR, et al. Epigenetic programming by maternal behavior. *Nature Neuroscience.* 2004; 7:847–854.
20. Roth TL, Lubin FD, Funk AJ, Sweatt JD. Lasting epigenetic influence of early-life adversity on the BDNF gene. *Biological Psychiatry.* 2009; 65:760–769.
21. Binder EB, Bradley RG, Liu W, Epstein MP, Deveau TC, Mercer KB, et al. Association of FKBP5 polymorphisms and childhood abuse with risk of posttraumatic stress disorder symptoms in adults. *JAMA.* 2008; 299:1291–1305.
22. Caspi A, Sugden K, Moffitt TE, Taylor A, Craig IW, Harrington H, et al. Influence of life stress on depression: Moderation by a polymorphism in the 5-HTT gene. *Science.* 2003; 301:386–389.
23. Klengel T, Mehta D, Anacker C, Rex-Haffner M, Pruessner JC, Pariante CM, et al. Allele-specific

FKBP5 DNA demethylation mediates gene-childhood trauma interactions. *Nature Neuroscience.* 2013; 16:33–41.
24. Bradley RG, Binder EB, Epstein MP, Tang Y, Nair HP, Liu W, et al. Influence of child abuse on adult depression: Moderation by the corticotropin-releasing hormone receptor gene. *Archives of General Psychiatry.* 2008; 65:190–200.
25. Berton O, McClung CA, Dileone RJ, Krishnan V, Renthal W, Russo SJ, et al. Essential role of BDNF in the mesolimbic dopamine pathway in social defeat stress. *Science.* 2006; 311:864–868.
26. Tsankova NM, Berton O, Renthal W, Kumar A, Neve RL, Nestler EJ. Sustained hippocampal chromatin regulation in a mouse model of depression and antidepressant action. *Nature Neuroscience.* 2006; 9:519–525.
27. Krishnan V, Han MH, Graham DL, Berton O, Renthal W, Russo SJ, et al. Molecular adaptations underlying susceptibility and resistance to social defeat in brain reward regions. *Cell.* 2007; 131:391–404.
28. Post RM, Kalivas P. Bipolar disorder and substance misuse: Pathological and therapeutic implications of their comorbidity and cross-sensitisation. *The British Journal of Psychiatry.* 2013; 202:172–176.
29. Anier K, Malinovskaja K, Aonurm-Helm A, Zharkovsky A, Kalda A. DNA methylation regulates cocaine-induced behavioral sensitization in mice. *Neuropsychopharmacolog.* 2010; 35:2450–2461.
30. Sakae DY, Marti F, Lecca S, Vorspan F, Martin-Garcia E, Morel LJ, et al. The absence of VGLUT3 predisposes to cocaine abuse by increasing dopamine and glutamate signaling in the nucleus accumbens. *Molecular Psychiatry.* 2015; 20:1448–1459.
31. Miczek KA, Takahashi A, Gobrogge KL, Hwa LS, de Almeida RM. Escalated aggression in animal models: Shedding new light on mesocorticolimbic circuits. *Current Opinion in Behavioral Science.* 2015; 3:90–95.
32. Roberts JS, Barber M, Brown TM, Cupples LA, Farrer LA, LaRusse SA, et al. Who seeks genetic susceptibility testing for Alzheimer's disease? Findings from a multisite, randomized clinical trial. *Genetics in Medicine.* 2004; 6:197–203.
33. Covington HE 3rd, Maze I, Sun H, Bomze HM, DeMaio KD, Wu EY, et al. A role for repressive histone methylation in cocaine-induced vulnerability to stress. *Neuron.* 2011; 71:656–670.
34. Esparza MA, Bollati F, Garcia-Keller C, Virgolini MB, Lopez LM, Brusco A, et al. Stress-induced sensitization to cocaine: Actin cytoskeleton remodeling within mesocorticolimbic nuclei. *The European Journal of Neuroscience.* 2012; 36:3103–117.
35. Post RM. Mechanisms of sensitization to stress, affective episodes, and abused substances: Implications for treatment and prevention. In: *Neurobiology of addictions.* New York: Oxford University Press, 2016: 315–346.
36. Ballenger JC, Post RM. Kindling as a model for alcohol withdrawal syndromes. *The British Journal of Psychiatry.* 1978; 133:1–14.
37. Goddard GV, McIntyre DC, Leech CK. A permanent change in brain function resulting from daily electrical stimulation. *Experimental Neurology.* 1969; 25:295–330.
38. Clark M, Post RM, Weiss SR, Cain CJ, Nakajima T. Regional expression of c-fos mRNA in rat brain during the evolution of amygdala kindled seizures. *Molecular Brain Research.* 1991; 11:55–64.
39. Rosen JB, Cain CJ, Weiss SR, Post RM. Alterations in mRNA of enkephalin, dynorphin and thyrotropin releasing hormone during amygdala kindling: An in situ hybridization study. *Molecular Brain Research.* 1992; 15:247–255.
40. Rosen JB, Abramowitz J, Post RM. Colocalization of TRH mRNA and fos-like immunoreactivity in limbic structures following amygdala kindling. *Molecular and Cellular Neurosciences.* 1993; 4:335–342.
41. Post R, Weiss S, Smith M. Sensitization and kindling: Implications for the evolving neural substrate of PTSD. In: Friedman MJ, Charney DS, Deutch AY, eds. *Neurobiology and clinical consequences of stress: From normal adaptation to PTSD.* New York: Lippincott-Raven, 1995: 203–224.
42. Solomon Z1, Horesh D, Ein-Dor T, Ohry A. Predictors of PTSD trajectories following captivity: A 35-year longitudinal study. *Psychiatry Research.* 2012 Oct 30;199(3):188–194. doi:10.1016/j.psychres.2012.03.035
43. Kalivas PW. Addiction as a pathology in prefrontal cortical regulation of corticostriatal habit circuitry. *Neurotoxicity Research.* 2008; 14:185–189.
44. Kalivas BC, Kalivas PW. Corticostriatal circuitry in regulating diseases characterized by intrusive thinking. *Dialogues in Clinical Neuroscience.* 2016; 18:65–76.
45. Berk M, Copolov DL, Dean O, Lu K, Jeavons S, Schapkaitz I, et al. N-acetyl cysteine for depressive symptoms in bipolar disorder—a double-blind randomized placebo-controlled trial. *Biological Psychiatry.* 2008; 64:468–475.
46. Back SE, McCauley JL, Korte KJ, Gros DF, Leavitt V, Gray KM, et al. A double-blind, randomized, controlled pilot trial of N-acetylcysteine in veterans with posttraumatic stress disorder and substance use disorders. *The Journal of Clinical Psychiatry.* 2016; 77:e1439–e46.

47. Meaney MJ, Aitken DH, Bodnoff SR, Iny LJ, Tatarewicz JE, Sapolsky RM. Early postnatal handling alters glucocorticoid receptor concentrations in selected brain regions. *Behavioral Neuroscience.* 2013; 127:637–641.
48. Bale TL. Lifetime stress experience: Transgenerational epigenetics and germ cell programming. *Dialogues in Clinical Neuroscience.* 2014; 16:297–305.
49. Rodgers AB, Bale TL. Germ cell origins of posttraumatic stress disorder risk: The transgenerational impact of parental stress experience. *Biological Psychiatry.* 2015; 78:307–314.
50. Dietz DM, Nestler EJ. From father to offspring: Paternal transmission of depressive-like behaviors. *Neuropsychopharmacology.* 2012; 37:311–312.
51. Szutorisz H, DiNieri JA, Sweet E, Egervari G, Michaelides M, Carter JM, et al. Parental THC exposure leads to compulsive heroin-seeking and altered striatal synaptic plasticity in the subsequent generation. *Neuropsychopharmacology.* 2014; 39:1315–1323.
52. Vassoler FM, White SL, Schmidt HD, Sadri-Vakili G, Pierce RC. Epigenetic inheritance of a cocaine-resistance phenotype. *Nature Neuroscience.* 2013; 16:42–47.
53. Dias BG, Ressler KJ. Parental olfactory experience influences behavior and neural structure in subsequent generations. *Nature Neuroscience.* 2014; 17:89–96.
54. Fleshner M, Frank M, Maier SF. Danger signals and inflammasomes: Stress-evoked sterile inflammation in mood disorders. *Neuropsychopharmacology.* 2017; 42:36–45.
55. Miller AH, Haroon E, Felger JC. Therapeutic implications of brain-immune interactions: Treatment in translation. *Neuropsychopharmacology.* 2017; 42:334–359.
56. Weber MD, Godbout JP, Sheridan JF. Repeated social defeat, neuroinflammation, and behavior: Monocytes carry the signal. *Neuropsychopharmacology.* 2017; 42:46–61.
57. Michopoulos V, Powers A, Gillespie CF, Ressler KJ, Jovanovic T. Inflammation in fear- and anxiety-based disorders: PTSD, GAD, and beyond. *Neuropsychopharmacology.* 2017; 42:254–270.
58. Hodes GE, Kana V, Menard C, Merad M, Russo SJ. Neuroimmune mechanisms of depression. *Nature Neuroscience.* 2015; 18:1386–1393.
59. Menard C, Pfau ML, Hodes GE, Russo SJ. Immune and neuroendocrine mechanisms of stress vulnerability and resilience. *Neuropsychopharmacology.* 2017; 42:62–80.
60. Raison CL, Miller AH. Pathogen-host defense in the evolution of depression: Insights into epidemiology, genetics, bioregional differences and female preponderance. *Neuropsychopharmacology.* 2017; 42:5–27.
61. Beheshti Nasr SM, Moghimi A, Mohammad-Zadeh M, Shamsizadeh A, Noorbakhsh SM. The effect of minocycline on seizures induced by amygdala kindling in rats. *Seizure.* 2013; 22:670–674.
62. Shonkoff JP, Garner AS, Committee on Psychosocial Aspects of Child and Family Health, Committee on Early Childhood, Adoption, and Dependent Care, and Section on Developmental and Behavioral Pediatrics, Siegal, B. S., et al. The lifelong effects of early childhood adversity and toxic stress. *Pediatrics.* 2012; 129:e232–e246.
63. Danese A, S JL. Psychoneuroimmunology of early-life stress: the hidden wounds of childhood trauma? *Neuropsychopharmacology.* 2017; 42:99–114.
64. Nasca C, Zelli D, Bigio B, Piccinin S, Scaccianoce S, Nistico R, et al. Stress dynamically regulates behavior and glutamatergic gene expression in hippocampus by opening a window of epigenetic plasticity. *Proceedings of the National Academy of Sciences of the United States of America.* 2015; 112:14960–14965.
65. Nasca C, Xenos D, Barone Y, Caruso A, Scaccianoce S, Matrisciano F, et al. L-acetylcarnitine causes rapid antidepressant effects through the epigenetic induction of mGlu2 receptors. *Proceedings of the National Academy of Sciences of the United States of America.* 2013; 110:4804–4809.
66. Bigio B, Mathe AA, Sousa VC, Zelli D, Svenningsson P, McEwen BS, et al. Epigenetics and energetics in ventral hippocampus mediate rapid antidepressant action: Implications for treatment resistance. *Proceedings of the National Academy of Sciences of the United States of America.* 2016; 113:7906–7911.
67. Lau T, Bigio B, Zelli D, McEwen BS, Nasca C. Stress-induced structural plasticity of medial amygdala stellate neurons and rapid prevention by a candidate antidepressant. *Molecular Psychiatry.* 2017; 22:227–234.
68. Ruggenenti P, Cattaneo D, Loriga G, Ledda F, Motterlini N, Gherardi G, et al. Ameliorating hypertension and insulin resistance in subjects at increased cardiovascular risk: Effects of acetyl-L-carnitine therapy. *Hypertension.* 2009; 54:567–574.
69. Wang SM, Han C, Lee SJ, Patkar AA, Masand PS, Pae CU. A review of current evidence for acetyl-l-carnitine in the treatment of depression. *Journal of Psychiatric Research.* 2014; 53:30–37.
70. Li N, Liu RJ, Dwyer JM, Banasr M, Lee B, Son H, et al. Glutamate N-methyl-D-aspartate receptor antagonists rapidly reverse behavioral and synaptic deficits caused by chronic stress exposure. *Biological Psychiatry.* 2011; 69:754–761.

71. Feder A, Parides MK, Murrough JW, Perez AM, Morgan JE, Saxena S, et al. Efficacy of intravenous ketamine for treatment of chronic posttraumatic stress disorder: A randomized clinical trial. *JAMA Psychiatry*. 2014; 71:681–688.
72. Rosso IM, Crowley DJ, Silveri MM, Rauch SL, Jensen JE. Hippocampus glutamate and N-acetyl aspartate markers of excitotoxic neuronal compromise in posttraumatic stress disorder. *Neuropsychopharmacology*. 2017; 42(8):1698–1705.
73. Nader K, Schafe GE, Le Doux JE. Fear memories require protein synthesis in the amygdala for reconsolidation after retrieval. *Nature*. 2000; 406:722–726.
74. Nader K, Hardt O, Lanius R. Memory as a new therapeutic target. *Dialogues in Clinical Neuroscience*. 2013; 15:475–486.
75. Agren T, Engman J, Frick A, Bjorkstrand J, Larsson EM, Furmark T, et al. Disruption of reconsolidation erases a fear memory trace in the human amygdala. *Science*. 2012; 337:1550–1552.
76. Hogberg G, Pagani M, Sundin O, Soares J, Aberg-Wistedt A, Tarnell B, et al. Treatment of post-traumatic stress disorder with eye movement desensitization and reprocessing: Outcome is stable in 35-month follow-up. *Psychiatry Research*. 2008; 159:101–108.
77. Hogberg G, Nardo D, Hallstrom T, Pagani M. Affective psychotherapy in post-traumatic reactions guided by affective neuroscience: Memory reconsolidation and play. *Psychology Research and Behavior Management*. 2011; 4:87–96.
78. Post RM, Kegan R. Prevention of recurrent affective episodes using extinction training in the reconsolidation window: A testable psychotherapeutic strategy. *Psychiatry Research*. 2017; 249:327–336.
79. Xue YX, Luo YX, Wu P, Shi HS, Xue LF, Chen C, et al. A memory retrieval-extinction procedure to prevent drug craving and relapse. *Science*. 2012; 336:241–245.
80. Day JJ, Sweatt JD. Epigenetic mechanisms in cognition. *Neuron*. 2011; 70:813–829.
81. Bredy TW, Barad M. The histone deacetylase inhibitor valproic acid enhances acquisition, extinction, and reconsolidation of conditioned fear. *Learning and Memory*. 2008; 15:39–45.
82. Bredy TW, Wu H, Crego C, Zellhoefer J, Sun YE, Barad M. Histone modifications around individual BDNF gene promoters in prefrontal cortex are associated with extinction of conditioned fear. *Learning and Memory*. 2007; 14:268–276.
83. Morris MJ, Monteggia LM. Role of DNA methylation and the DNA methyltransferases in learning and memory. *Dialogues in Clinical Neuroscience*. 2014; 16:359–371.

15

Neurobiology and Neuroimaging of PTSD

MOHAMMED R. MILAD AND KYLIE N. MOORE

INTRODUCTION

Trauma- and stress-related disorders, such as posttraumatic stress disorder (PTSD), are some of the most common and most incapacitating neuropsychiatric disorders. Research efforts within the past two decades sought to shed light upon the psychological and neurobiological mechanisms underlying the pathology and symptomatology of PTSD. A robust body of evidence indicates that PTSD is a brain-based disorder. Emerging tools in neuroscience, including the advent of advanced neuroimaging techniques, have made it possible to translate preliminary findings from rodent studies into humans models of (pathological) stress, both in healthy and clinical populations.

One current model in this field of research suggests that impaired extinction of conditioned fear in the events following a traumatic incident may contribute to the etiology and symptomology of PTSD (Pace-Schott et al., 2015; Mineka and Oehlberg, 2008; Graham and Milad, 2011). Emerging evidence is now suggesting that PTSD symptom severity might be associated with greater fear conditioning and impaired fear extinction. Extinction learning occurs when the conditioned responses to a conditioned stimulus decrease when the reinforcing stimulus is eliminated. Extinction is thought to create a new association that "competes" with the previously learned fear association that eventually reduces conditioned fear expression. Individuals with PTSD may, however, experience impaired fear extinction and consequently continue to exhibit enhanced fear expression. Translational models of Pavlovian fear conditioning and extinction are used extensively in laboratory studies and are thought to mirror the process of fear acquisition occurring in cases of PTSD (Shin and Liberzon, 2010). Laboratory fear conditioning paradigms involve the repeated pairing of a previously neutral conditioned stimulus (CS) with an aversive unconditioned stimulus (UCS) to elicit a conditioned fear response to the presentation of the CS alone. Accordingly, in laboratory settings, individuals with impaired fear extinction (e.g., PTSD patients) maintain a conditioned fear response, despite repeated exposure to a CS in the absence of the UCS.

The regulation of the expression of fear is postulated to occur as a result of cortical influence over the amygdala. In this chapter, we provide a broad overview of the fear circuitry implicated in the development and maintenance of PTSD. We first review evidence from animal models of fear conditioning and extinction that unveiled the neural structures incorporated in the fear circuitry. We then explore the translation of these findings to healthy human models of fear conditioning and finally examine the neural dysfunctions highlighted by neuroimaging studies of PTSD in order to conceptualize mechanisms of fear extinction and the role of impaired fear extinction in contributing to the pathology of PTSD. We end with the potential therapeutic interventions for the treatment of PTSD in the scope of this model but with a note of caution regarding some of its limitations.

RODENT STUDIES

The neural regions responsible for mediating fear extinction and expression are well characterized in a multitude of studies examining the effects of lesions, activation/inactivation techniques, and electrophysiological and optogenetic tools to study the fear circuitry in animals. Though these experiments have generated a wealth of knowledge, animal models of fear conditioning primarily implicate the amygdala, medial prefrontal cortex, and hippocampus in neural mechanisms of fear.

The amygdala is widely accepted as a "hub of fear" (Milad and Quirk, 2012). Early studies in rodents demonstrated that lesions of the amygdala prevented the acquisition and expression of conditioned fear responses (Hitchcock and Davis, 1986; reviewed in Milad and Quirk, 2012). The role of the amygdala as a crucial component of conditioned fear responses has been solidified in numerous studies conducted within the last two decades (see Zuj et al., 2016; VanElzakker et al., 2014; Milad and Quirk, 2012; Graham and Milad, 2011; Pape and Pare, 2010; Shin and Liberzon, 2010; LeDoux, 2000). Recently, research efforts have utilized various neuroimaging and optogenetic tools in addition to molecular approaches in order to better understand the amygdala's complex circuitry and its role in conditioned fear. The amygdala is known to contain multiple neuroanatomical subregions (including the basolateral nucleus, the lateral nucleus, and the central nucleus) as well as multiple anatomically and functionally distinct subnuclei and neuron populations within these regions (Herry et al., 2010; Haubensak et al., 2010; Ciocchi et al., 2010). Though a detailed explanation of the intricacies of the amygdala circuitry may not be relevant in the scope of this chapter, a cursory understanding is necessary to fully grasp the complexities of the amygdala's role in fear conditioning. There is compelling evidence that discrete populations of intercalated neurons are a key component of fear conditioning and extinction. It is important to note that these distinct subpopulations of neurons may be differentially recruited in the encoding and subsequent maintenance of a CS-US association (Herry et al., 2010), thereby assuming distinct but cooperative roles in the mechanisms of fear conditioning and extinction. These neuron populations are known to project to neural regions such as the medial prefrontal cortex (mPFC) and hippocampus in addition to exhibiting reciprocal connections between amygdala subdivisions including the basolateral complex of the amygdala and the central amygdala (Herry et al., 2010; Haubensak et al., 2010; Ciocchi et al., 2010).

The basolateral complex of the amygdala was specifically implicated as the primary neural structure involved in the convergence of relevant information about conditioned and unconditioned stimuli (Graham and Milad, 2011). In rodent models, acquisition and expression of fear responses are disrupted by interfering with the functioning of the basolateral amygdala (LeDoux, 2007), demonstrating the key role of the basolateral amygdala in fear conditioning. In addition to communicating with other amygdala substructures, the basolateral amygdala is known to maintain connections with various regions of the rodent mPFC that may be associated with disparate aspects of fear conditioning, namely fear extinction and fear expression (VanElzakker, 2016; Holmes and Singewald, 2013; Milad and Quirk, 2002).

Current theories of fear extinction posit that extinction processes are potentiated by connections between the infralimbic (IL) region of the rodent mPFC and the central amygdala (Herry et al., 2010). Rodents with IL lesions demonstrated the capacity to acquire fear extinction but had difficulty retrieving the extinction memory the following day (Kim et al., 2015; Quirk et al., 2000; reviewed in Quirk and Mueller, 2008). Accordingly, future studies sought to distinguish between various components of extinction processes (acquisition, consolidation, and retrieval of the fear extinction memory). Single-cell recordings demonstrated that IL cells fired to a conditioned tone during phases of extinction retrieval, but not during conditioning phases (Milad and Quirk, 2002). Stimulation of IL cells was also associated with reduced conditioned fear responses in rodents (Milad and Quirk, 2002) by inhibiting the central amygdala (Herry et al., 2010), indicating that activation of the IL cortex may enhance recall of fear extinction memories.

Recent evidence suggests that a separate area of the rodent mPFC, the prelimbic system (PL), is associated with the expression of learned fear and may play an opposite role to the IL in fear conditioning (Zuj et al., 2016; Holmes and Singewald, 2013; Graham and Milad, 2011). In a study by Corcoran and Quirk (2007), rodent PLs were pharmacologically inactivated during instances of fear learning and fear expression. The inactivation of rodent PL was associated with reductions in the display of fearful behavior (freezing) but not with the formation of fearful memories, indicating that the PL is involved in the expression but not acquisition, of fear. Similarly, Burgos-Robles et al. (2009) demonstrated that fear responses (freezing behavior) to a conditioned tone were correlated with increased neuronal activity in the PL and that these responses persisted even after extinction training, indicating a failure to express extinction memory. Together, evidence from rodent studies suggest that a bidirectional feedback loop between the PL and the amygdala transform a transient "fear signal" to a sustained signal, maintaining the expression of fear (reviewed in Milad and Quirk, 2012). Microstimulation of rodent PL increased fear responses to conditioned stimuli but hindered extinction (Vidal-Gonzalez et al., 2006), providing evidence that the PL not only drives the expression of fear but opposes extinction as well.

The dual role of the rodent prefrontal cortex in modulating fear conditioning is evidenced by studies demonstrating the IL's role in fear extinction and the PL's role in fear expression. Whereas the IL's inhibitory projections target the central nucleus of the amygdala, PL's excitatory projections target the basal nucleus of the amygdala (Milad and Quirk, 2012; Greco and Liberzon, 2016). Through these distinct projections to the amygdala, correlated activity between the PL and IL is able to influence the expression or extinction of fear memories, possibly mediated by a circuit comprised of the limbic network and hippocampus. Peters and colleagues (2010) demonstrated that a single infusion of BDNF, a key mediator of synaptic plasticity, into the rodent hippocampus was able to pharmacologically induce extinction rather than simply facilitating extinction, as no extinction training was required. Results from this study highlighted the importance of hippocampal-limbic projections in potentiating extinction memories and paved the way for future research examining the hippocampus' role in mechanisms of fear. Recent work suggests that the hippocampus may act as a contextual modulator of fear responses (VanElzakker et al., 2014). Rodents demonstrated context-specific freezing behavior when hippocampal activity was unaltered; however, disrupting normal hippocampal activity resulted in a reduction of fearful behavior in response to a conditioned tone in both extinguished and unextinguished contexts (Corcoran and Maren, 2001). These results suggest that the hippocampus plays a pivotal role in identification of safe versus unsafe contexts and that disruption of normal hippocampal activity can influence fear extinction and expression processes in rodents.

Overall, there is a robust body of evidence suggesting that interactions between the amygdala, medial prefrontal cortex, and hippocampus form the basis of neural circuits contributing to rodent models of fear. Advances in this field, accordingly, will help us arrive at a more complete understanding of the general mechanisms underlying fear conditioning and extinction. Familiarity with animal models of fear conditioning may facilitate the improvement of clinical aspects of the treatment of PTSD, such as the development of novel pharmacological innovations that are able to target specific neuron populations within the fear circuitry.

HUMAN STUDIES

During the last two decades, rodent studies have delineated critical neural networks involved in fear learning and extinction, enabling translational efforts from work in rodents to human models of fear conditioning and extinction. Human models of fear learning have used classical fear conditioning and extinction paradigm with some variations from one lab to another (see Figure 15.1). Some of the studies examining fear extinction have focused on examining the neural correlates of fear extinction using neuroimaging techniques. Functional magnetic resonance imaging (fMRI) enables investigators to use blood-oxygen-level dependent (BOLD) signal to identify neural networks involved in the execution of various tasks, including fear conditioning and extinction. In human studies, neuroimaging findings are often tied to measures of physiological arousal, such as skin conductance response (SCR), electromyographic response, and heart rate response. Collectively, neuroimaging tools have been enormously useful in translating rodent work in fear to humans and have provided evidence that in humans there exists a neural network responsible for mediating fear extinction mechanisms. Neuroimaging findings in fear conditioning and extinction studies replicate elementary findings from rodent studies, demonstrating that human limbic and prefrontal brain structures work together during extinction processes. Key structures involved include the amygdala, the hippocampus, and the prefrontal cortical regions including the ventromedial prefrontal cortex (vmPFC) and the dorsal anterior cingulate cortex (dACC).

The amygdala's role in fear conditioning is well documented in humans. Located deep within in the temporal lobe of human brains, it is an integral part of the limbic system and is known to play a role in fear expression and learning as well as emotional regulation (Zuj et al., 2016; VanElzakker et al., 2014; Ehrlich et al., 2009). Specific to the content of this review, the amygdala also has a robust role in fear conditioning. Activation of the amygdala is known to be enhanced during fear conditioning in both the acquisition and early extinction of fear (see Zuj et al., 2016; Milad, Wright, et al., 2007; Phelps et al., 2004) and is known to co-occur with increases in SCR (VanElzakker et al., 2014). During fear conditioning, information about conditioned and unconditioned stimuli converges at the basolateral complex of the amygdala. Projections from the basolateral complex of the amygdala then "carry" this information to structures responsible for arousal of the sympathetic nervous system (Zuj et al., 2016; Graham and Milad, 2011; LeDoux, 2000).

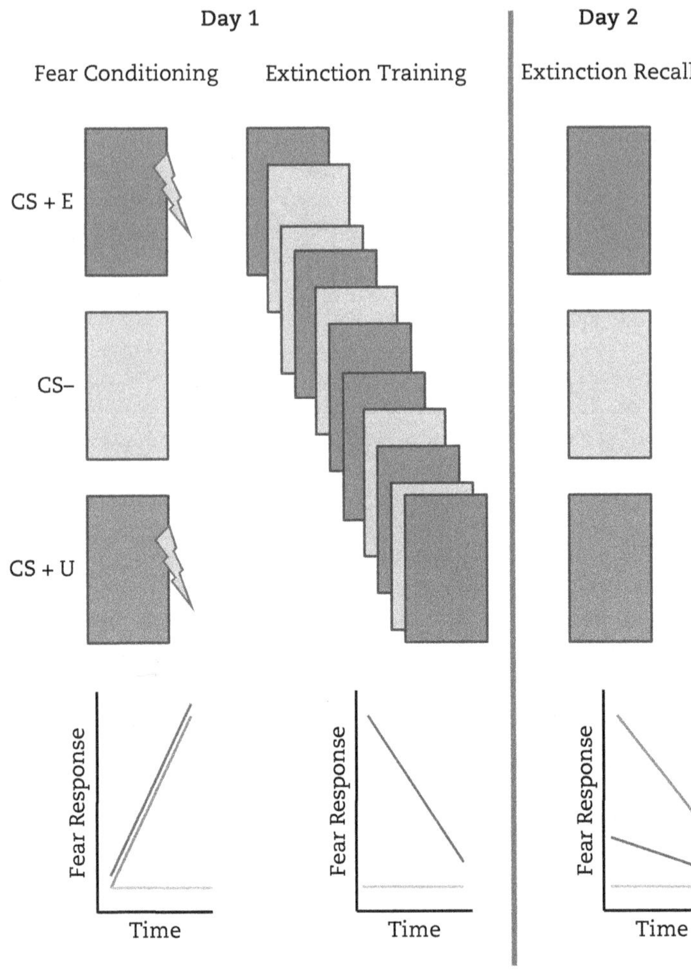

FIGURE 15.1. Schematic illustration of a typical fear conditioning and extinction paradigm conducted in humans. CS: conditioned stimulus, Plus sign notates the pairing of the CS with an electric shock (bolt sign in figure). CS+E: extinguished CS+, CS+U: unextinguished CS+, CS–: stimulus not paired with the shock. Lower panel illustrates typical conditioned responses across the different phases of the experiment for the different types of CSs. (See front matter.)

Neuroimaging studies in healthy humans have demonstrated that the dACC is the functional homolog to the PL cortex in rodents. Numerous studies reported increased activation of dACC during fear conditioning (see Zuj et al., 2016), suggesting that the dACC may be involved in the expression of fear. The dACC in humans extends excitatory projections to the basolateral amygdala that may be involved in the expression of conditioned fear (VanElzakker et al., 2014). Milad, Quirk, and colleagues (2007) demonstrated that the cortical thickness and activation of the dACC was positively correlated with SCR to conditioned stimuli during fear acquisition, indicating a role for the human dACC in the expression of fear responses.

The functional homolog to the rodent IL in humans was identified in an fMRI study done by Phelps and colleagues (2004). This group examined fear extinction mechanisms in healthy humans by using fMRI. Activation of the vmPFC was correlated with the recall of extinction learning (Phelps et al., 2004), suggesting that the human vmPFC was the functional homolog to the rodent IL. Using a paradigm that enabled the comparison of extinction recall and conditioning recall to extend theories of the rodent IL and fear expression into the human brain, Milad, Wright, and colleagues (2007) investigated the role of the vmPFC in recall of fear extinction in healthy humans. The vmPFC displayed significant activation during extinction learning, and the magnitude of vmPFC activation to the extinguished stimulus during recall was positively correlated with the magnitude of extinction retention (Milad, Wright, et al., 2007), indicating that stronger activation of the vmPFC was associated with a greater capacity to inhibit conditioned responses during extinction recall. Overall, vmPFC thickness and activation correlated with recall of extinction learning (Milad, Wright, et al., 2007). Recently, Motzkin et al. (2015) demonstrated that vmPFC lesions in humans disabled the inhibition of amygdala activity, providing further evidence for the role for the vmPFC in enhancing extinction recall.

This extinction recall is also associated with increased hippocampal activation, suggesting an important role for the human hippocampus in differentiating between acquisition and extinction contexts (Milad, Wright, et al., 2007). Hippocampal inactivation selectively impairs conditioned fear responses to context but not to innate fear responses to unconditioned stimuli (reviewed in Smith and Bulkin, 2014). Indeed, recent studies have provided further evidence that the human hippocampus is responsible for integrating contextual information in fear conditioning and extinction recall (Maren et al., 2013; Myers and Davis, 2007; Kalisch et al., 2006). Lang et al. (2009) used fMRI to investigate the role of various prefrontal and limbic structures in a contextual conditioning and extinction paradigm, demonstrating that interactions between the amygdala, prefrontal cortex, and hippocampus play a critical role in contextual learning of fear conditioning and fear extinction. Hermann and colleagues (2016) corroborate these findings, demonstrating that hippocampal activation distinguished conditioned responding in a novel context from extinction context responses. Enhanced activation of the hippocampus was also associated with stronger extinction recall as evidenced by reduced conditioned SCRs (Hermann et al., 2016) as well as the renewal of an extinguished fear response in a different retrieval context (Lissek et al., 2016). In context-only presentations, persons who do or do not show renewal of a fear response exhibited no significant difference in hippocampal involvement (suggesting the processing of novel information). On the other hand, presentations of a context *and* a cue elicited greater hippocampal activation in persons who later exhibited renewal compared to those who did not exhibit renewal (Lissek et al., 2016). Together, these results suggest a role for the hippocampus in the contextual processing of fear memories and moderating the recall and renewal of fear extinction.

CLINICAL STUDIES AND APPLICATIONS

As evidenced, animal models of fear conditioning and extinction prompted investigations into the human neural circuitry involved in fear. Because findings from animal studies and human neuroimaging endeavors are relevant to the etiology, maintenance, and treatment of PTSD, many investigators seek to further clarify the role of the neural circuitry of fear conditioning and extinction in a clinical PTSD population. Research efforts explore whether de novo conditioning is present in PTSD and if deficiencies in the neural circuitry involved in fear conditioning and extinction are related to the etiology and/or symptoms of PTSD.

Early psychophysiological findings in PTSD patients suggest that this population is hyperconditionable (Pitman, 1989). There is now a wealth of evidence suggesting that impairments in the acquisition and expression of extinguished fear are present in PTSD (Maren and Holmes, 2016; Blechert et al., 2007; Milad et al., 2006, Rauch et al., 2006; Orr et al., 2000). In instances of extinction training post-fear conditioning, patients with PTSD exhibit enhanced de novo conditional responding on various psychophysiological measures, such as heart rate, skin conductance, and acoustic startle paradigms (see Maren and Holmes, 2016, for references). It is proposed that this enhanced conditional responding in extinction phases is the result of a loss of differential responding, or an ability to differentiate appropriate responses to the CS+ or CS–, indicating that impairments in extinction may reflect an overgeneralization of fear (Grillon and Morgan, 1999). Additionally, subjects with PTSD demonstrate deficiencies in the appropriate maintenance of extinguished responding over an interval of retention (see Figure 15.2) (Milad et al., 2008, 2009). This finding provides evidence to support the claim that PTSD patients may experience deficits in the ability to appropriately retrieve memories of fear extinction (Maren and Holmes, 2016).

Neuroimaging studies in populations with PTSD explore these intriguing results and seek to further identify potential deficiencies within neural networks of fear that may contribute to the etiology and symptomatology of PTSD. Specifically, functional neuroimaging studies have demonstrated that individuals with PTSD may experience altered activity in the amygdala, vmPFC, dACC, and hippocampus (see Figure 15.3) (Pitman et al., 2012), such that neural regions responsible for generating fear responses

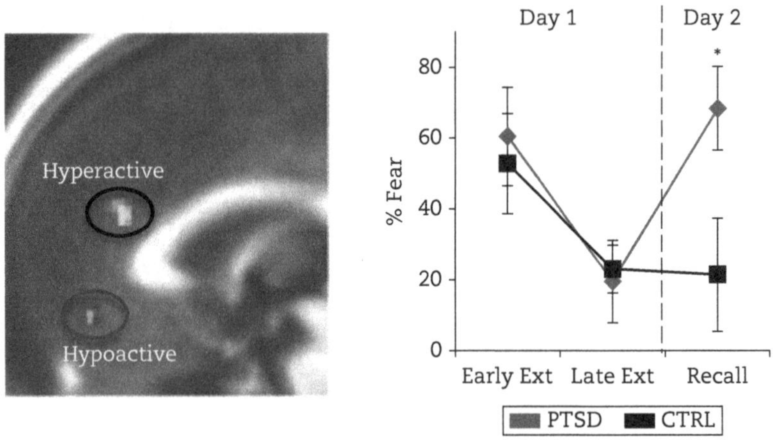

FIGURE 15.2. Fear extinction is impaired in PTSD patients. Left: activations of the ventromedial prefrontal cortex (vmPFC; lower circle) and dorsal anterior cingulate cortex (dACC; upper circle) in PTSD vs. controls (CTRL). Right: % of conditioned fear responses across the different phases of the experiment for the two groups. Ext: Extinction. Asterisk denotes a significance level of $p < 0.05$. (Adapted from Milad et al., 2009.) (See front matter.)

may be overactive, while the activity of structures involved in the inhibition conditioned fear may be suppressed.

The amygdala is consistently implicated in the pathophysiology of PTSD and is known to be hyperresponsive in cases of PTSD. Numerous studies rely upon the presentation of fearful faces to patients with PTSD, with variations in the duration of exposure, and have demonstrated increased amygdala responsiveness in PTSD (Garfinkel and Liberzon, 2009). Additionally, functional neuroimaging studies reveal that subjects with PTSD, compared to control populations, exhibit enhanced amygdala activation in response to both trauma-related and generic stimuli as well as in instances of acquiring conditioned fear (see Pitman et al., 2012).

Recently, enhanced neuroimaging techniques have been used to examine the strength of the connectivity between regions such as the

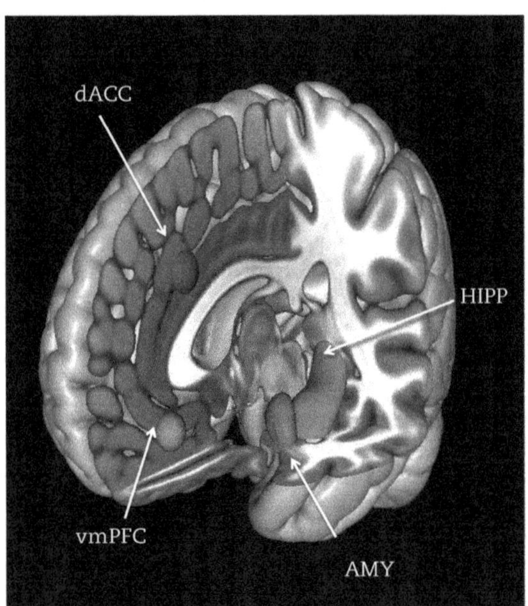

FIGURE 15.3. Illustration of key nodes of the fear extinction network in the human brain. vmPFC: ventromedial prefrontal cortex, dACC: dorsal anterior cingulate cortex, HIPP: hippocampus, AMY: amygdala. (See front matter.)

amygdala and the vmPFC. One such study sought to correlate the strength of this connection with self-reported measures of anxiety. Diffusion tensor imaging methods identified a structural white matter pathway between the amygdala and the PFC, and researchers demonstrated that the strength of this connection was inversely correlated with trait levels of anxiety, such that a stronger pathway connection predicted lower levels of anxiety (Kim and Whalen, 2009).

Ventromedial prefrontal cortex areas show decreased activation in subjects with PTSD during tasks that require attention to both trauma-related and trauma-unrelated stimuli (see Pitman et al., 2012). Ventromedial prefrontal cortex activity was positively coupled with resting-state amygdala activity in persons with low levels of reported trait anxiety and negatively coupled to amygdala activity at rest in those with high levels of anxiety (Kim et al., 2011). Accordingly, vmPFC activation during instances of recollection of traumatic events was negatively correlated with the severity of PTSD symptoms (Pitman et al., 2012). Furthermore, Milad et al. (2009) demonstrated that decreased BOLD responses in the vmPFC were associated with impaired extinction retrieval in patients with PTSD, providing further evidence that vmPFC activity may be reduced in PTSD cases.

Increased activation in the dACC of PTSD patients, relative to control participants with and without exposure to trauma, has been demonstrated in instances of fear conditioning, reduced recall of extinction learning, and a variety of auditory oddball tasks (Pitman et al., 2012). Specifically, individuals with PTSD exhibited hyperactivity in the dACC during fear acquisition, extinction learning, and extinction recall (Rougemont-Bucking et al., 2011; Milad et al., 2009). The multitude of studies in PTSD populations, demonstrating dACC hyperactivity in response to fearful stimuli, implicates the dACC as a neural correlate of extinction impairment.

Findings from neuroimaging studies of the hippocampus in patients with PTSD are varied. Some studies report less and others report more activation in the hippocampus of PTSD patients in comparison to control populations (Pitman et al., 2012). These disparities may be attributed to differences in experimental paradigms or analyses employed in laboratory settings. Regardless, it has been shown in a PTSD population that failure to recall extinction learning is correlated with inhibited activation in the hippocampus (Milad et al., 2009). Recent studies support an enhanced role for the hippocampus in PTSD, suggesting that the loss of context-appropriate engagement of inhibitory regulation via the prefrontal-amygdala circuits is instrumental in the manifestation of impaired extinction in PTSD (Garfinkel et al., 2014; Rougemont-Bucking et al., 2011). Patients with PTSD exhibited impairments in fear renewal outside the context of extinction in addition to expected deficits in extinction retrieval (Garfinkel et al., 2014), supporting previous claims of hippocampal dysfunction in PTSD. Similarly, in addition to enhanced amygdala activity and decreased vmPFC activity, PTSD patients exhibited reduced hippocampal activation to the extinguished stimulus (CS−) during renewal in comparison to combat-exposed controls (Garfinkel et al., 2014). These results suggest that the hippocampus plays an important role in extinction deficits in patients with PTSD, such that the ability to use contextual information in the determination of appropriate fear expression may be impaired (Maren and Holmes, 2016).

Overall, neurocircuitry models of PTSD emphasize the role of the amygdala and its interactions with the vmPFC, dACC, and hippocampus. The vmPFC fails to inhibit the hyperresponsive amygdala and the dACC promotes fear expression, resulting in an increased attentional bias toward threat, increased fear responses, impaired extinction, and an inability to appropriately regulate emotion (Rauch et al., 2006; Pitman et al., 2012). Abnormalities in hippocampal functioning may underlie deficits in the ability to identify safe versus threatening contexts and contribute to memory impairments for neural material (Rauch et al., 2006; Pitman et al., 2012). Deficiencies in the neurocircuitry involved in mediating fear-learning processes are supported by evidence for the generalization of extinction and impairment of extinction recall in PTSD populations. Accordingly, the fear extinction model conceptualizes a physiological pathway for the pathology of PTSD as a process of fear conditioning and (impaired) extinction.

However, there are some limitations to the fear extinction model as an appropriate model for the pathology of PTSD, including inconsistent findings of amygdala activity during trauma-related stimuli presentation in PTSD patients as well as vmPFC hyperactivity in instances of symptom provocation in PTSD patients compared to trauma exposed and trauma non-exposed controls (Bremner et al., 1999; Lanius et al., 2001; Lanius et al., 2002; Zubieta et al., 1999). Though the reason for these inconsistencies is unclear,

Graham and Milad (2011) note differences between symptom provocation tasks and fear extinction tasks, suggesting that the former employs functions of fear processing while the latter relies upon processes of fear inhibition. Additionally, the fear extinction model does not account for all possible presentations of PTSD symptoms. This model, by nature, is intimately associated with alterations in arousal and reactivity in response to a fearful stimulus and does not necessarily account for the presence of intrusion or avoidance symptoms or alterations in cognitions and mood that are known to be present in PTSD. Nevertheless, data from rodent studies of fear conditioning and neuroimaging findings in both healthy humans and PTSD populations indicate that impaired fear extinction has a critical role in the etiology of PTSD and that this model is a valuable tool in understanding the psychopathology of PTSD.

A recent review (LeDoux and Pine, 2016) proposes a "two-systems" framework that seeks to distinguish neural mechanisms underlying the conscious feeling of fear from the nonconscious behavioral and physical responses to threat. Authors note that the conflation of these distinct circuits has hindered the extension of fear circuitry research into clinical applications and the development of novel treatments for trauma and anxiety disorders. Although the fear extinction model may not account for the full symptomatology of PTSD, fear conditioning and extinction are key concepts in the most effective treatment for PTSD. Exposure therapy, widely accepted as the gold standard for PTSD treatment, is predicated upon extinguishing a learned fear association (Zuj et al., 2016). Recent PTSD treatment effect studies on functional brain changes may reaffirm the role of the neural circuitry involved in fear extinction as a key modulator of PTSD symptoms. After psychotherapy treatment, PTSD patients exhibited increased neural activation in areas such as the medial PFC (King et al., 2013), hippocampus, and dACC as well as decreased activation in the amygdala (as compared to pretreatment activity) during symptom provocation, and these changes in neural activity were associated with a decrease in PTSD symptoms (reviewed in Thomaes et al., 2014). Other neuroimaging studies report posttreatment normalization of activity in the amygdala and prefrontal cortex after virtual reality exposure therapy and prolonged exposure therapy in military members deployed to Iraq or Afghanistan (Roy et al., 2010). Collectively, these findings suggest that psychosocial interventions have the potential to alter the functioning of the neural circuitry involved in fear conditioning, providing concrete biological evidence for the efficacy of these treatments for PTSD. Results from these studies also provide a framework for the formulation of effective pharmacological treatment options. The NMDA receptor partial agonist, d-cycloserine, has been shown to promote extinction in rodents and to aid clinical improvement in response to cognitive behavioral therapy in many anxiety disorders (Ganasen et al., 2010). Additionally, recent research has demonstrated that 3,4-methylenedioxymethamphetamine (MDMA) is able to effectively stimulate fear extinction learning in rodents (Young et al., 2015). Mithoefer and colleagues (2011) demonstrated that MDMA worked as an adjunct in the facilitation of psychotherapy in individuals with treatment-resistant PTSD. MDMA-assisted therapy proved to be more effective than placebo-assisted therapy, with those who had been administered MDMA exhibiting a significant decrease in PTSD symptoms.

SUMMARY

As can be noted from the literature reviewed, there has been extensive focus on understanding the function of the fear and threat-detection networks in the human brain and the implications of the interactions of these brain regions to psychopathology in general and PTSD in particular. There is continuing evidence to point to PTSD as biologically based disorder. Together, findings suggest that pharmacological interventions can prove to be useful adjuncts to psychological therapy for PTSD and that these treatment methods may work to rectify consequences resulting from impaired fear extinction. Regardless of the mechanism of action, it is evident that psychological and pharmacological interventions are crucial for treating PTSD and related anxiety disorders characterized by dysfunctions in fear learning. Despite tremendous progress in the field, more research is necessary to continually advance our understanding of these disorders and develop the best possible treatment strategies for those afflicted by PTSD and other related conditions

REFERENCES

Blechert, J., Michael, T., Vriends, N., Margraf, J., & Wilhelm, F. H. (2007). Fear conditioning in posttraumatic stress disorder: Evidence for delayed extinction of autonomic, experiential, and behavioural responses. *Behaviour Research and Therapy*, *45*(9), 2019–2033.

Bremner, J. D., Narayan, M., Staib, L. H., Southwick, S. M., McGlashan, T., & Charney, D. S. (1999). Neural correlates of memories of childhood sexual abuse in women with and without posttraumatic stress disorder. *American Journal of Psychiatry, 156*(11), 1787–1795.

Burgos-Robles, A., Vidal-Gonzalez, I., & Quirk, G. J. (2009). Sustained conditioned responses in prelimbic prefrontal neurons are correlated with fear expression and extinction failure. *The Journal of Neuroscience, 29*(26), 8474–8482.

Ciocchi, S., Herry, C., Grenier, F., Wolff, S. B., Letzkus, J. J., Vlachos, I., . . . Müller, C. (2010). Encoding of conditioned fear in central amygdala inhibitory circuits. *Nature, 468*(7321), 277–282.

Corcoran, K. A., & Maren, S. (2001). Hippocampal inactivation disrupts contextual retrieval of fear memory after extinction. *The Journal of Neuroscience, 21*(5), 1720–1726.

Corcoran, K. A., & Quirk, G. J. (2007). Activity in prelimbic cortex is necessary for the expression of learned, but not innate, fears. *The Journal of Neuroscience, 27*(4), 840–844.

Ehrlich, I., Humeau, Y., Grenier, F., Ciocchi, S., Herry, C., & Lüthi, A. (2009). Amygdala inhibitory circuits and the control of fear memory. *Neuron, 62*(6), 757–771.

Ganasen, K. A., Ipser, J. C., & Stein, D. J. (2010). Augmentation of cognitive behavioral therapy with pharmacotherapy. *Psychiatric Clinics of North America, 33*(3), 687–699.

Garfinkel, S. N., Abelson, J. L., King, A. P., Sripada, R. K., Wang, X., Gaines, L. M., & Liberzon, I. (2014). Impaired contextual modulation of memories in PTSD: An fMRI and psychophysiological study of extinction retention and fear renewal. *The Journal of Neuroscience, 34*(40), 13435–13443.

Garfinkel, S. N., & Liberzon, I. (2009). Neurobiology of PTSD: A review of neuroimaging findings. *Psychiatric Annals, 39*(6), 370–381.

Graham, B. M., & Milad, M. R. (2011). The study of fear extinction: Implications for anxiety disorders. *American Journal of Psychiatry, 168*(12), 1255–1265.

Greco, J. A., & Liberzon, I. (2016). Neuroimaging of fear-associated learning. *Neuropsychopharmacology, 41*(1), 320–334.

Grillon, C., & Morgan, C. A. III. (1999). Fear-potentiated startle conditioning to explicit and contextual cues in Gulf War veterans with posttraumatic stress disorder. *Journal of Abnormal Psychology, 108*(1), 134–142.

Haubensak, W., Kunwar, P. S., Cai, H., Ciocchi, S., Wall, N. R., Ponnusamy, R., . . . Fanselow, M. S. (2010). Genetic dissection of an amygdala microcircuit that gates conditioned fear. *Nature, 468*(7321), 270–276.

Hermann, A., Stark, R., Milad, M. R., & Merz, C. J. (2016). Renewal of conditioned fear in a novel context is associated with hippocampal activation and connectivity. *Social Cognitive and Affective Neuroscience, 11*, 1411–1421.

Herry, C., Ferraguti, F., Singewald, N., Letzkus, J. J., Ehrlich, I., & Lüthi, A. (2010). Neuronal circuits of fear extinction. *European Journal of Neuroscience, 31*(4), 599–612.

Hitchcock, J., & Davis, M. (1986). Lesions of the amygdala, but not of the cerebellum or red nucleus, block conditioned fear as measured with the potentiated startle paradigm. *Behavioral Neuroscience, 100*(1), 11–22.

Holmes, A., & Singewald, N. (2013). Individual differences in recovery from traumatic fear. *Trends in Neurosciences, 36*(1), 23–31.

Kalisch, R., Korenfeld, E., Stephan, K. E., Weiskopf, N., Seymour, B., & Dolan, R. J. (2006). Context-dependent human extinction memory is mediated by a ventromedial prefrontal and hippocampal network. *The Journal of Neuroscience, 26*(37), 9503–9511.

Kim, H. S., Cho, H. Y., Augustine, G. J., & Han, J. H. (2015). Selective control of fear expression by optogenetic manipulation of infralimbic cortex after extinction. *Neuropsychopharmacology, 41*(5), 1261–1273.

Kim, M. J., Loucks, R. A., Palmer, A. L., Brown, A. C., Solomon, K. M., Marchante, A. N., & Whalen, P. J. (2011). The structural and functional connectivity of the amygdala: From normal emotion to pathological anxiety. *Behavioural Brain Research, 223*(2), 403–410.

Kim, M. J., & Whalen, P. J. (2009). The structural integrity of an amygdala-prefrontal pathway predicts trait anxiety. *The Journal of Neuroscience, 29*(37), 11614–11618.

King, A. P., Erickson, T. M., Giardino, N. D., Favorite, T., Rauch, S. A., Robinson, E., . . . Liberzon, I. (2013). A pilot study of group mindfulness-based cognitive therapy (MBCT) for combat veterans with posttraumatic stress disorder (PTSD). *Depression and Anxiety, 30*(7), 638–645.

Lang, S., Kroll, A., Lipinski, S. J., Wessa, M., Ridder, S., Christmann, C., . . . Flor, H. (2009). Context conditioning and extinction in humans: Differential contribution of the hippocampus, amygdala and prefrontal cortex. *European Journal of Neuroscience, 29*(4), 823–832.

Lanius, R. A., Williamson, P. C., Boksman, K., Densmore, M., Gupta, M., Neufeld, R. W., . . . Menon, R. S. (2002). Brain activation during script-driven imagery induced dissociative responses in PTSD: A functional magnetic resonance imaging investigation. *Biological Psychiatry, 52*(4), 305–311.

Lanius, R. A., Williamson, P. C., Densmore, M., Boksman, K., Gupta, M. A., Neufeld, R. W., . . . Menon, R. S. (2001). Neural correlates of traumatic memories in posttraumatic stress disorder: A functional MRI investigation. *American Journal of Psychiatry, 158*(11), 1920–1922.

LeDoux, J. (2000). Emotion circuits in the brain. *Annual Review of Neuroscience, 23*, 155–184.

LeDoux, J. (2007). The amygdala. *Current Biology, 17*(20), R868–R874.

LeDoux, J. E., & Pine, D. S. (2016). Using neuroscience to help understand fear and anxiety: A two-system framework. *American Journal of Psychiatry, 173*(11), 1083–1093.

Lissek, S., Glaubitz, B., Schmidt-Wilcke, T., & Tegenthoff, M. (2016). Hippocampal context processing during acquisition of a predictive learning task is associated with renewal in extinction recall. *Journal of Cognitive Neuroscience, 28*(5), 747–762.

Maren, S., & Holmes, A. (2016). Stress and fear extinction. *Neuropsychopharmacology, 41*(1), 58–79.

Maren, S., Phan, K. L., & Liberzon, I. (2013). The contextual brain: Implications for fear conditioning, extinction and psychopathology. *Nature Reviews Neuroscience, 14*(6), 417–428.

Milad, M. R., Orr, S. P., Lasko, N. B., Chang, Y., Rauch, S. L., & Pitman, R. K. (2008). Presence and acquired origin of reduced recall for fear extinction in PTSD: Results of a twin study. *Journal of Psychiatric Research, 42*(7), 515–520.

Milad, M. R., Pitman, R. K., Ellis, C. B., Gold, A. L., Shin, L. M., Lasko, N. B., . . . Rauch, S. L. (2009). Neurobiological basis of failure to recall extinction memory in posttraumatic stress disorder. *Biological Psychiatry, 66*(12), 1075–1082.

Milad, M. R., & Quirk, G. J. (2002). Neurons in medial prefrontal cortex signal memory for fear extinction. *Nature, 420*(6911), 70–74.

Milad, M. R., & Quirk, G. J. (2012). Fear extinction as a model for translational neuroscience: Ten years of progress. *Annual Review of Psychology, 63*, 129–151.

Milad, M. R., Quirk, G. J., Pitman, R. K., Orr, S. P., Fischl, B., & Rauch, S. L. (2007). A role for the human dorsal anterior cingulate cortex in fear expression. *Biological Psychiatry, 62*(10), 1191–1194.

Milad, M. R., Rauch, S. L., Pitman, R. K., & Quirk, G. J. (2006). Fear extinction in rats: implications for human brain imaging and anxiety disorders. *Biological Psychology, 73*(1), 61–71.

Milad, M. R., Wright, C. I., Orr, S. P., Pitman, R. K., Quirk, G. J., & Rauch, S. L. (2007). Recall of fear extinction in humans activates the ventromedial prefrontal cortex and hippocampus in concert. *Biological Psychiatry, 62*(5), 446–454.

Mineka, S., & Oehlberg, K. (2008). The relevance of recent developments in classical conditioning to understanding the etiology and maintenance of anxiety disorders. *Acta Psychologica, 127*(3), 567–580.

Mithoefer, M. C., Wagner, M. T., Mithoefer, A. T., Jerome, L., & Doblin, R. (2011). The safety and efficacy of ±3, 4-methylenedioxymethamphetamine-assisted psychotherapy in subjects with chronic, treatment-resistant posttraumatic stress disorder: The first randomized controlled pilot study. *Journal of Psychopharmacology, 25*(4), 439–452.

Motzkin, J. C., Philippi, C. L., Wolf, R. C., Baskaya, M. K., & Koenigs, M. (2015). Ventromedial prefrontal cortex is critical for the regulation of amygdala activity in humans. *Biological Psychiatry, 77*(3), 276–284.

Myers, K. M., & Davis, M. (2007). Mechanisms of fear extinction. *Molecular Psychiatry, 12*(2), 120–150.

Orr, S. P., Metzger, L. J., Lasko, N. B., Macklin, M. L., Peri, T., & Pitman, R. K. (2000). De novo conditioning in trauma-exposed individuals with and without posttraumatic stress disorder. *Journal of Abnormal Psychology, 109*(2), 290–298.

Pace-Schott, E. F., Germain, A., & Milad, M. R. (2015). Sleep and REM sleep disturbance in the pathophysiology of PTSD: The role of extinction memory. *Biology of Mood & Anxiety Disorders, 5*(1), 1–19.

Pape, H. C., & Pare, D. (2010). Plastic synaptic networks of the amygdala for the acquisition, expression, and extinction of conditioned fear. *Physiological Reviews, 90*(2), 419–463.

Peters, J., Dieppa-Perea, L. M., Melendez, L. M., & Quirk, G. J. (2010). Induction of fear extinction with hippocampal-infralimbic BDNF. *Science, 328*(5983), 1288–1290.

Phelps, E. A., Delgado, M. R., Nearing, K. I., & LeDoux, J. E. (2004). Extinction learning in humans: Role of the amygdala and vmPFC. *Neuron, 43*(6), 897–905.

Pitman, R. K. (1989). Post-traumatic stress disorder, hormones, and memory. *Biological Psychiatry, 26*(3), 221–223.

Pitman, R. K., Rasmusson, A. M., Koenen, K. C., Shin, L. M., Orr, S. P., Gilbertson, M. W., . . . Liberzon, I. (2012). Biological studies of post-traumatic stress disorder. *Nature Reviews Neuroscience, 13*(11), 769–787.

Quirk, G. J., & Mueller, D. (2008). Neural mechanisms of extinction learning and retrieval. *Neuropsychopharmacology, 33*(1), 56–72.

Quirk, G. J., Russo, G. K., Barron, J. L., & Lebron, K. (2000). The role of ventromedial prefrontal cortex in the recovery of extinguished fear. *The Journal of Neuroscience, 20*(16), 6225–6231.

Rauch, S. L., Shin, L. M., & Phelps, E. A. (2006). Neurocircuitry models of posttraumatic stress disorder and extinction: Human neuroimaging research—past, present, and future. *Biological Psychiatry, 60*(4), 376–382.

Rougemont-Bücking, A., Linnman, C., Zeffiro, T. A., Zeidan, M. A., Lebron-Milad, K., Rodriguez-Romaguera, J., . . . Milad, M. R. (2011). Altered processing of contextual information during fear extinction in PTSD: An fMRI study. *CNS Neuroscience & Therapeutics, 17*(4), 227–236.

Roy, M. J., Francis, J., Friedlander, J., Banks-Williams, L., Lande, R. G., Taylor, P., . . . Patt, I. (2010). Improvement in cerebral function with treatment of posttraumatic stress disorder. *Annals of the New York Academy of Sciences, 1208*(1), 142–149.

Shin, L. M., & Liberzon, I. (2010). The neurocircuitry of fear, stress, and anxiety disorders. *Neuropsychopharmacology, 35*(1), 169–191.

Smith, D. M., & Bulkin, D. A. (2014). The form and function of hippocampal context representations. *Neuroscience & Biobehavioral Reviews, 40*, 52–61.

Thomaes, K., Dorrepaal, E., Draijer, N., Jansma, E. P., Veltman, D. J., & van Balkom, A. J. (2014). Can pharmacological and psychological treatment change brain structure and function in PTSD? A systematic review. *Journal of Psychiatric Research, 50*, 1–15.

VanElzakker, M. B. (2016). Posttraumatic stress disorder. In W. D. Pfaff & D. N. Volkow (Eds.), *Neuroscience in the 21st century* (pp. 1–31). New York: Springer.

VanElzakker, M. B., Dahlgren, M. K., Davis, F. C., Dubois, S., & Shin, L. M. (2014). From Pavlov to PTSD: The extinction of conditioned fear in rodents, humans, and anxiety disorders. *Neurobiology of Learning and Memory, 113*, 3–18.

Vidal-Gonzalez, I., Vidal-Gonzalez, B., Rauch, S. L., & Quirk, G. J. (2006). Microstimulation reveals opposing influences of prelimbic and infralimbic cortex on the expression of conditioned fear. *Learning & Memory, 13*(6), 728–733.

Young, M. B., Andero, R., Ressler, K. J., & Howell, L. L. (2015). 3, 4-methylenedioxymethamphetamine facilitates fear extinction learning. *Translational Psychiatry, 5*(9), e634.

Zubieta, J. K., Chinitz, J. A., Lombardi, U., Fig, L. M., Cameron, O. G., & Liberzon, I. (1999). Medial frontal cortex involvement in PTSD symptoms: A SPECT study. *Journal of Psychiatric Research, 33*(3), 259–264.

Zuj, D. V., Palmer, M. A., Lommen, M. J., & Felmingham, K. L. (2016). The centrality of fear extinction in linking risk factors to PTSD: A narrative review. *Neuroscience & Biobehavioral Reviews, 69*, 15–35.

16

PTSD in Women

Sex Differences and Gonadal Hormones

LISA Y. MAENG AND MOHAMMED R. MILAD

INTRODUCTION

Prevalence Rates of PTSD in Women

Posttraumatic stress disorder (PTSD), as defined by the *Diagnostic and Statistical Manual of Mental Disorders* (fifth edition [DSM-V]; American Psychiatric Association, 2013), is a debilitating psychiatric condition that can develop from exposure, either direct or indirect, to psychological or physical trauma, or sexual abuse. Some symptoms include recurring thoughts about the trauma, reckless or destructive behavior, persistent negative mood, and hyperarousal, which can persist from months to years. Numerous epidemiological studies have been conducted to examine the prevalence of trauma exposure and PTSD across different populations, using a variety of surveys and definitions. Some studies have indicated that roughly 69% of a sample of 1,000 adults have been exposed to at least one traumatic event within their lifetime (Norris, 1992). Similarly, in another study examining a sample of US women, lifetime exposure to any type of traumatic event was also 69% (Resnick, Kilpatrick, Dansky, Saunders, & Best, 1993). Although, as these findings demonstrate, over half of the population (~55%–70%) will experience a traumatic event in their lifetime, only a small percentage of these trauma-exposed individuals will go on to have PTSD (American Psychiatric Association, 2000). One study reported that PTSD has a lifetime prevalence of 8.3% among a national sample of 2,953 adults in the United States (Kilpatrick et al., 2013).

Although the risk factors for PTSD include young age, early life trauma, and pre-existing mental illnesses (Atwoli, Stein, Koenen, & McLaughlin, 2015), this chapter focuses primarily on the influence of sex, specifically the female sex. Prevalence rates suggest women are especially vulnerable to developing PTSD (McLean, Asnaani, Litz, & Hofmann, 2011). One study found that when men and women experience a trauma event, women demonstrate an 11.0% lifetime prevalence rate compared to 5.4% in men; this disproportionate rate is seen in response to having experienced multiple types of trauma as well, with 12.8% of women experiencing PTSD symptoms after a combination of traumatic events compared to 5.7% of men (Kilpatrick et al., 2013). Interestingly, although more men experienced trauma than women (61% versus 51%), a nationwide sample of US adults found that twice as many women have PTSD (and with more persistent symptoms) compared to men (Breslau, 2009; Breslau et al., 1998; Kessler, Sonnega, Bromet, Hughes, & Nelson, 1995; Tolin & Foa, 2006). Despite changes to the diagnostic criteria and examinations across different populations of people, the prevalence of PTSD remains consistently twice as high in women compared to men, strengthening the claim that there is a true, reliable difference in how PTSD affects men and women.

Sex Differences in PTSD

In addition to the clear sex difference in the incidence of PTSD, men and women also experience the disorder differently in terms of clinical presentation (Tolin & Foa, 2006). Women are more likely to seek treatment for PTSD (Roberts, Gilman, Breslau, Breslau, & Koenen, 2011), which might influence the reported prevalence rates, but this does not impact the way men and women are differentially affected by the disorder. In fact, compared to men, women experience PTSD symptoms that are more severe, persist longer, and provide a worse quality of life (Christiansen & Hansen, 2015; Norris, 1992; Seedat, Stein, & Carey, 2005). In addition to the differing degrees to which individuals suffer from PTSD symptoms, the predominant symptom types differ as well; women report more depression and somatic symptoms, whereas men describe more aggression and anger (Blain, Galovski, & Robinson, 2010). One of the inevitable hurdles in PTSD research is that the types of trauma that can lead to the onset of these PTSD symptoms are multitudinous. This makes it difficult to conclude whether findings related to one type of stressor hold true for all. Additionally, even while controlling for trauma type, the sex differences in PTSD remain (Tolin & Foa, 2006). These differences extend beyond severity and symptoms to include disparities in response to treatment, but very few studies have been conducted to elucidate the deterrents at this stage of the PTSD trajectory (Blain et al., 2010; Galovski, Blain, Chappuis, & Fletcher, 2013).

There has been a growing interest in PTSD in women with support for identifying potential biomarkers to address the disparity in prevalence and highlight the need for sex-specific treatments. In this chapter, we review and discuss the neural and hormonal underpinnings of the female response to stress and fear as they relate to PTSD. We hope to shed light on why women are more at risk for developing PTSD before ending with some discussion on the implications of these findings for treatment.

PTSD Neurobiology in Women

Individuals with PTSD exhibit abnormalities in brain regions that are critical for learning, memory, and emotion regulation. These brain areas include the prefrontal cortex, amygdala, and hippocampus (Nutt & Malizia, 2004), and the alterations in these regions are structural and functional in nature. Specifically, PTSD patients exhibit decreased volume within the hippocampus as well as in certain cortico-limbic areas (Bremner, 1999; Karl et al., 2006; Liberzon & Sripada, 2008; Woon, Sood, & Hedges, 2010). Corticolimbic connectivity appears to be disrupted in individuals with PTSD, with hypoactivation within the prefrontal cortex and hyperactivation within the amygdala, suggesting the loss of top-down prefrontal control of the amygdala for emotion regulation (Shin, Rauch, & Pitman, 2006). In one study that investigated brain differences between civilian trauma-exposed women with and without PTSD, amygdala activation in response to fearful stimuli was found to be greater in women with PTSD. Additionally, this amygdala activation was positively correlated with PTSD hyperarousal symptom severity (Stevens et al., 2013). Consistent with previous reports, functional connectivity between the amygdala and prefrontal cortex was also reduced in the PTSD group. Brown et al. (2016) found that brain activation differences within the amygdala and hippocampus were associated with negative affect in PTSD women compared to healthy controls; however, since the results of this study compared PTSD patients and healthy women who had not experienced trauma, these findings may differ from those comparing PTSD with trauma-exposed individuals.

As mentioned previously, more studies investigating the neurocircuitry involved in recovery from PTSD are necessary to determine how treatment can rescue dysfunctional connections in the brain and how renewed function is associated with symptom reduction. Dickie et al. (2011) provides some insight into this, reporting that amygdala and ventromedial prefrontal cortex activity were related to symptom severity, whereas recovery seemed to be signified by changes in hippocampus and subgenual anterior cingulate cortex functional activity. However, sex was not used as a variable in this study, so whether men and women have different brain responses to recovery from PTSD was not addressed.

The answers to the following questions remain unclear: (a) Were the previous results in brain activations, when sex was not accounted for, driven by women? (b) If the PTSD-related changes are within the same brain regions in men and women, why do more women have PTSD? Studies conducted in healthy adults have begun to answer these questions, finding sex differences in fronto-limbic connectivity during negative emotion processing (Lungu, Potvin, Tikàsz, & Mendrek, 2015; Stevens & Hamann, 2012). These data suggest that the brain regions affected by PTSD have inherent sex differences in connectivity that are demonstrated even in the absence of disease. One approach to delineating these differences in PTSD has been to investigate the neural mechanisms underlying the symptoms and behaviors that women appear predisposed to.

Rumination, PTSD, and Women

One such behavior is rumination, a coping style that women tend to use more frequently than men when dealing with stress (Nolen-Hoeksema, 2012; Nolen-Hoeksema & Aldao, 2011). Although it is predominantly linked with depression, rumination, as uncontrollable, negatively valenced repetitive thinking, has also been connected to PTSD, with more rumination occurring in people with PTSD than those without (Michael, Halligan, Clark, & Ehlers, 2007). Increased ruminative behavior involves the same brain regions that are affected in PTSD (Buchholz et al., 2016), and in a cohort of women with PTSD, those with higher levels of rumination exhibited a positive correlation with orbital frontal activation. This suggests that difficulty inhibiting responses to fearful stimuli correlates with greater recruitment of the brain areas involved in cognitive control (Buchholz et al., 2016). These brain networks, which include the hippocampus, medial prefrontal cortex, and amygdala, were found to have altered functional connectivity in a study that examined women with PTSD and repeated exposure to a traumatic memory (Cisler et al., 2014). Together, these findings indicate that not only are there neural correlates of PTSD symptoms but that some of these neural correlates are specifically associated with PTSD in women. One explanation for this specific association may be the responsivity these regions have to the natural fluctuations in gonadal hormones that occur across the menstrual cycle.

GONADAL HORMONES

Ovarian Hormones: PTSD Symptomology in Women

It is increasingly recognized that changes in gonadal hormone levels can influence the same neurobiology affected in PTSD—in particular, the amygdala, prefrontal cortex, and hippocampus (Sundström Poromaa & Gingnell, 2014; Toffoletto, Lanzenberger, Gingnell, Sundström-Poromaa, & Comasco, 2014). Toffoletto et al. compiled over 30 functional magnetic resonance imaging (fMRI) studies reporting differences in brain activation across the phases of the menstrual cycle in healthy women, finding interactions between ovarian hormone level and emotion and cognitive processing within the medial prefrontal areas and the amygdala. This indicates a role for gonadal hormones in examining the behaviors modulated by these regions and in the development or treatment of PTSD psychopathology.

The two main phases of the menstrual cycle are the follicular and luteal phases, during which ovarian hormones fluctuate from low (early follicular/late luteal phase for estrogen and entire follicular phase for progesterone) to high levels (late follicular and mid-luteal phases for estrogen and mid- to late luteal phase for progesterone). Interestingly, as these gonadal hormones fluctuate across a woman's normal menstrual cycle, they appear to modulate psychiatric symptoms, exacerbating them during periods of low ovarian hormone levels (Bryant et al., 2011; Ferree, Kamat, & Cahill, 2011; Hendrick, Altshuler, & Burt, 1996). Few studies have directly examined PTSD symptoms across the menstrual cycle; however, one study did investigate the relationship between menstrual cycle phase and recurring traumatic memories, which is a feature of PTSD (Bryant et al., 2011). Bryant and colleagues demonstrated that in a cohort of women who had experienced trauma one to two weeks prior to the assessment, the women who experienced the trauma during the late luteal phase (when estrogen is low), as well as those women who were assessed during this phase, were more likely to have flashbacks compared to the women in other phases. Another recent study examined the effects of the menstrual cycle on not just one symptom, but a broader range of PTSD symptoms at 2 different phases of the menstrual cycle in trauma-exposed non-PTSD and PTSD women (Nillni et al., 2015). Regardless of diagnosis, women reported more depressive symptoms during the low-estrogen early follicular phase of their menstrual cycles compared to those assessed during the mid-luteal higher estrogen phase. Phobic anxiety was more severe in women with PTSD during the early follicular phase than the mid-luteal phase; however, menstrual phase did not have an effect on this fear and avoidance-related measure in women without PTSD (Nillni et al., 2015).

Together, these data suggest that decreasing or low levels of naturally fluctuating ovarian hormones (i.e., estrogen and progesterone) can modulate fear-related symptoms in women. This and other emerging evidence suggest that the higher prevalence of PTSD in women may be due to greater vulnerability to the adverse effects of stress and general inability to regulate fear responses. In this way, gonadal hormone levels can significantly influence the development and maintenance of PTSD. The neurocircuitry altered in PTSD is similarly influenced by stress and is critically engaged during fear regulation. In the following sections, we review how women respond behaviorally and neurobiologically to stress and fear with modulation by gonadal hormones such as estrogen and progesterone.

Ovarian Hormones: The Stressed Female Brain

PTSD is now defined as a stress disorder (DSM-V; American Psychiatric Association, 2013), and understanding the maladaptive response to stressful life events that can precipitate into PTSD psychopathology is integral to understanding its etiology. The brain systems involved in stress responses (i.e., hippocampus, medial prefrontal cortex, amygdala, cingulate cortex) include regions that are critical for learning and memory and overlap with the altered neurocircuitry in PTSD (Vermetten & Bremner, 2002). Numerous studies have consistently suggested that individuals with PTSD have a dysregulated hypothalamic-pituitary-adrenal (HPA) axis, a neurobiological system that modulates stress hormones and reactions to trauma (Cohen et al., 2006; Marshall & Garakani, 2002; Vermetten & Bremner, 2002; Yehuda, Teicher, Trestman, Levengood, & Siever, 1996). Some studies report elevated levels of cortisol in individuals with PTSD, whereas others have reported a blunted HPA axis response, having lower levels of baseline stress hormones (Marshall & Garakani, 2002).

The heightened vulnerability to PTSD seen in women may be related to differences in these responses to stress. In fact, studies in both animals and humans have revealed sex differences in HPA axis responsivity to stress (Kudielka & Kirschbaum, 2005). In animals, females exhibit greater HPA axis reactivity to stress exposure compared to males (Handa, Burgess, Kerr, & O'Keefe, 1994). Sex differences are also observed at the receptor level, where corticotropin-releasing factor receptor signaling has been found to be differentially responsive to stress exposure in females compared to males (Bangasser et al., 2010). Some animal models also demonstrate that females are more negatively affected by stress exposure than males, exhibiting an impairment in associative learning after acute stress and engaging different neurocircuits to mediate their responses to stress (Maeng, Waddell, & Shors, 2010). In healthy men and women, men appear to have higher basal levels of cortisol and higher cortisol response to psychosocial stress (Paris et al., 2010; Stephens, Mahon, McCaul, & Wand, 2016).

The HPA axis and activity within the critical brain regions involved in the response to stress also appear to be modulated by naturally circulating levels of gonadal hormones (Albert, Pruessner, & Newhouse, 2015; Duchesne & Pruessner, 2013; Kajantie & Phillips, 2006; Kirschbaum, Kudielka, Gaab, Schommer, & Hellhammer, 1999; Ossewaarde et al., 2010). For instance, women who underwent a psychosocial stress task during the high estrogen phase of their menstrual cycles exhibited less subjective stress, as well as less deactivation of the hippocampus, compared to women in the low estrogen phase (Albert et al., 2015). In an fMRI study, women stressed in the low estrogen phase had higher negative affect scores and exhibited greater activation of the amygdala and medial prefrontal cortex (Ossewaarde et al., 2010). Together, these findings emphasize how stress vulnerability in women can depend on the hormonal milieu during phases of the menstrual cycle and how the regions that are affected by stressful experience and gonadal hormonal status are also affected in individuals with PTSD.

Rodent studies have indicated similar interactions, with a stress-induced impairment in associative learning observed when female rats are exposed to a stressor during the diestrus phase of the rodent estrous cycle, when estrogen levels are low and rising (Shors, Lewczyk, Pacynski, Mathew, & Pickett, 1998; Wood & Shors, 1998). This is consistent with the increased stress sensitivity that is observed during the low estrogen menstrual phase in women, supporting the idea that these interactions (stress, menstrual phase, neurobiology) may contribute to the greater risk of PTSD in women and that women may be most vulnerable to developing PTSD when trauma is experienced during the phases of the menstrual cycle when estrogen levels are low.

Ovarian Hormones: Fear Regulation and PTSD

Fear conditioning and extinction protocols model signature features of fear regulation in PTSD. In fear conditioning, the subject learns that a neutral conditioned stimulus (CS), such as a light or tone, predicts an aversive unconditioned stimulus (US), such as a mild footshock, and expresses conditioned responses (CR) to CS presentations that follow. This process mimics the fear learning that takes place following a traumatic event in PTSD, and the measures of fear that are frequently used are conditioned freezing in rodents and skin conductance response or fear-potentiated startle in humans. During fear extinction, the subject learns that the CS no longer predicts the aversive US and exhibits a reduction in CR to the CS. The neurobiology of fear extinction has been studied extensively and implicated in the etiology of anxiety and stress-related disorders such as PTSD (Dias, Banerjee, Goodman, & Ressler, 2013; Hofmann, 2008). Increasing evidence suggests that individuals with PTSD exhibit impaired fear extinction, the ability to learn to no longer fear a stimulus (Milad et al., 2009; Pitman et al., 2012).

Interestingly, sex differences are also observed in fear conditioning and extinction in individuals with PTSD (Felmingham et al., 2010; Glover et al., 2012; Hwang et al., 2015; Inslicht et al., 2013; Shvil et al., 2014). One study reported that women with PTSD exhibited enhanced fear conditioning compared to men with PTSD (Inslicht et al., 2013). In contrast, neural activations and psychophysiological responses that were associated with poor extinction memory recall were exhibited in men but not in women with PTSD (Shvil et al., 2014). These mixed findings regarding sex differences in fear conditioning and extinction may be partly explained by the influence of gonadal hormones, as women in their high estrogen phase showed more differences in brain activations compared to men, with greater activations in general within the fear network (Hwang et al., 2015). Consistent with findings regarding changes in stress sensitivity across the menstrual cycle as well as those of Milad et al. (2010), Pineles and colleagues (2016) demonstrated that healthy non-PTSD, but trauma-exposed women exhibited better fear extinction memory during the high estrogen phase compared to the low estrogen phase. In women with PTSD, extinction retention was impaired during the mid-luteal phase and was associated with high levels of progesterone (Pineles et al., 2016). These findings suggest that although estrogen is often the focus of studies involving the menstrual cycle, progesterone may also play an important role in PTSD symptomology.

Rodent studies are increasingly highlighting a role for gonadal hormones, particularly estrogen, in fear conditioning and extinction processes. The estrous cycle consists of four to five days with four distinct phases: proestrus, estrus, metestrus, and diestrus. During the proestrus phase, estrogen and progesterone levels peak as ovulation occurs. Ovarian hormone levels decrease during the subsequent estrus and metestrus phases before rising again as the cycle progresses to late diestrus and proestrus. The fluctuations or varying hormonal statuses appear to differentially affect fear processes and related neurocircuitry. Similar to the enhanced fear conditioning observed in women with PTSD (Inslicht et al., 2013), estrogen has been found to enhance fear learning in ovariectomized rodents. Ovariectomized female mice given estrogen exhibited enhanced fear conditioning (Jasnow, Schulkin, & Pfaff, 2006; Morgan & Pfaff, 2001), which was associated with increased corticotropin-releasing hormone mRNA expression in the central amygdala (Jasnow et al., 2006). Similarly, estrogen administration also increased fear-potentiated startle in ovariectomized female rats (Hiroi & Neumaier, 2006). In contrast, estrogen replacement in ovariectomized female rats reduced contextual fear conditioning (Gupta, Sen, Diepenhorst, Rudick, & Maren, 2001). Mixed findings here may be attributed to the use of ovariectomized females that may have altered estrogen receptor density and function, producing varying dose-dependent effects of estrogen replacement and making interpretation of the results difficult. The inverted U-shaped dose-effect relationship of estrogen administration may influence results; some doses produce protective effects, while other doses may induce impairments (Barha, Dalton, & Galea, 2010; Inagaki, Gautreaux, & Luine, 2010).

In our studies, we report that naturally cycling high and low estrogen females do not exhibit significant differences in fear conditioning; however, we do find differences in extinction memory recall in both naturally cycling female rats and women (Milad, Igoe, Lebron-Milad, & Novales, 2009; Zeidan et al., 2011). Fear extinction, or learning to no longer fear a previously feared conditioned stimulus, is an integral process to the treatment of PTSD in which there is a failure to naturally extinguish or recover from the trauma (Foa, 2000). Prolonged exposure therapy, currently an effective treatment for PTSD, is based upon these fear extinction processes, and it appears to be most effective for women with PTSD (Foa, 1997; Foa & Street, 2001; Foa, Gillihan, & Bryant, 2013; Rachamim, Nacasch, Shafran, Tzur, & Gilboa-Schechtman, 2009). However, many rodent fear extinction studies do not control for estrous phase, which may be an oversight that could lead to faulty interpretation of findings. Without knowing the potential effects of naturally fluctuating ovarian hormone levels on extinction learning and memory, important sex differences may not be apparent even if they do exist, obscuring our understanding of important aspects of stress- and fear-related behaviors. For instance, Milad et al. (2009) did not observe sex differences in auditory-cued fear conditioning, extinction, and recall in male and female rats until the females were grouped by estrous phase during extinction training, and sex differences in fear expression were observed during extinction recall. Female rats that underwent extinction learning in the low estrogen metestrus phase exhibited poor extinction memory relative to male rats and to females extinguished during the high estrogen proestrus phase (Milad, Igoe, Lebron-Milad, & Novales, 2009; Rey, Lipps, & Shansky, 2014). Moreover, replacing estrogen and progesterone in low estrogen females, before and within 4 hours after extinction training, rescued fear extinction memory and altered neuronal activity within the fear network, suggesting that estrous phase and gonadal hormones do significantly influence extinction memory consolidation (Milad et al., 2009; Zeidan et al., 2011; Maeng et al., 2017). These findings further support the role of ovarian hormones in fear learning and memory consolidation processes (also reviewed in Maeng & Milad, 2015).

Although current treatment regimens such as prolonged exposure therapy, cognitive behavior therapy, and pharmacotherapy have been fairly successful in treating PTSD, women are still unequivocally more negatively impacted by the disorder relative to men. Why this condition persists continues to be up for debate. Further scrutiny of the symptomatology and behavioral profiles unique to, or more commonly manifested by, women with PTSD may reveal differentiating characteristics that we may not have recognized but are critical to improving our understanding of the disorder. We have discussed exploring rumination in women with PTSD as one step in this direction. There is also evidence that, upon closer examination, female rodents express fear differently from males, demonstrating a form of darting rather than the freezing behavior which has been the standard measure across most fear conditioning and extinction paradigms (Gruene, Flick, Stefano, Shea, & Shansky, 2015). Although no differences were observed across the estrous phases in this study, it is still possible that gonadal hormones influence these behaviors and the fear neurocircuitry involved in this female-specific expression of fear. This finding has important implications for future studies and further corroborates the need to examine clinical and behavioral profiles that are specific to females with PTSD or other female-dominant psychiatric disorders. The accumulating evidence in both rodents and humans, as presented in this chapter, indicates that the oscillatory nature of ovarian hormone levels (mostly "lower" vs. "higher") across the phases of the menstrual cycle and across the female lifespan are contributing factors in (a) the risk for developing PTSD after exposure to trauma, (b) the progression or maintenance of PTSD symptoms, and (c) how the individual responds to treatment.

CONCLUSION

Gonadal hormone fluctuations during the menstrual cycle can modulate a woman's sensitivity to stress and her ability to regulate fear, therefore playing a prominent role in the pathophysiology of PTSD. Still, the heightened vulnerability to PTSD seen in women calls for further investigation. Some questions that have yet to be tested are (a) whether gonadal hormones such as estrogen and progesterone can be used to augment and improve PTSD treatments, such as prolonged exposure therapy, that rely on fear extinction processes; (b) whether treatment during specific hormonal phases of the menstrual cycle would be beneficial for response to the treatment; (c) how gonadal hormones may influence coping behaviors and the underlying neurobiology that are specific to women with PTSD; and (d) how other gonadal hormone changes across a woman's lifespan outside of the menstrual cycle (such as pregnancy and menopause) influence the neurobiology of fear extinction and PTSD.

Although it is difficult to control or predict a traumatic event during distinct menstrual phases of increased vulnerability, we can use this line of research to answer the aforementioned questions and design sex-specific PTSD interventions that target specific phases and perhaps administer pharmacological or exposure-based cognitive behavioral therapies accordingly. Converging evidence suggests that taking the influence of gonadal hormones and menstrual cycle into consideration in the treatment of PTSD may help to address the greater risk and prevalence of PTSD in women with a more nuanced approach.

REFERENCES

Albert, K., Pruessner, J., & Newhouse, P. (2015). Estradiol levels modulate brain activity and negative responses to psychosocial stress across the menstrual cycle. *Psychoneuroendocrinology*, *59*, 14–24. http://doi.org/10.1016/j.psyneuen.2015.04.022

American Psychiatric Association. (2000). *The diagnostic and statistical manual of mental disorders* (4th ed., text revision). Washington, DC: American Psychiatric Publishing.

American Psychiatric Association. (2013). *Diagnostic and statistical manual of mental disorders* (5th ed.). Washington, DC: Author.

Atwoli, L., Stein, D. J., Koenen, K. C., & McLaughlin, K. A. (2015). Epidemiology of posttraumatic stress disorder: Prevalence, correlates and consequences. *Current Opinion in Psychiatry*, *28*(4), 307–311. http://doi.org/10.1097/YCO.0000000000000167

Bangasser, D. A., Curtis, A., Reyes, B. A. S., Bethea, T. T., Parastatidis, I., Ischiropoulos, H., . . . Valentino, R. J. (2010). Sex differences in corticotropin-releasing factor receptor signaling and trafficking: Potential role in female vulnerability to stress-related psychopathology. *Molecular Psychiatry*, *15*(9), 877, 896–904. http://doi.org/10.1038/mp.2010.66

Barha, C. K., Dalton, G. L., & Galea, L. A. (2010). Low doses of 17alpha-estradiol and 17beta-estradiol facilitate, whereas higher doses of estrone and 17alpha- and 17beta-estradiol impair, contextual fear conditioning in adult female rats. *Neuropsychopharmacology*, *35*(2), 547–559. http://doi.org/10.1038/npp.2009.161

Blain, L. M., Galovski, T. E., & Robinson, T. (2010). Gender differences in recovery from posttraumatic stress disorder: A critical review. *Aggression and Violent Behavior*, *15*(6), 463–474. http://doi.org/10.1016/j.avb.2010.09.001

Bremner, J. D. (1999). Alterations in brain structure and function associated with post-traumatic stress disorder. *Seminars in Clinical Neuropsychiatry*, *4*(4), 249–255.

Breslau, N. (2009). The epidemiology of trauma, PTSD, and other posttrauma disorders. *Trauma, Violence & Abuse*, *10*(3), 198–210. http://doi.org/10.1177/1524838009334448

Breslau, N., Kessler, R. C., Chilcoat, H. D., Schultz, L. R., Davis, G. C., & Andreski, P. (1998). Trauma and posttraumatic stress disorder in the community: The 1996 Detroit Area Survey of Trauma. *Archives of General Psychiatry*, *55*(7), 626–632.

Brown, W. J., Wojtalik, J. A., Dewey, D., Bruce, S. E., Yang, Z., & Sheline, Y. I. (2016). Affect and neural activity in women with PTSD during a task of emotional interference. *Journal of Affective Disorders*, *204*, 9–15. http://doi.org/10.1016/j.jad.2016.05.065

Bryant, R. A., Felmingham, K. L., Silove, D., Creamer, M., O'Donnell, M., & McFarlane, A. C. (2011). The association between menstrual cycle and traumatic memories. *Journal of Affective Disorders*, *131*(1–3), 398–401. http://doi.org/10.1016/j.jad.2010.10.049

Buchholz, K. R., Bruce, S. E., Koucky, E. M., Artime, T. M., Wojtalik, J. A., Brown, W. J., & Sheline, Y. I. (2016). Neural correlates of trait rumination during an emotion interference task in women with PTSD. *Journal of Traumatic Stress*, *29*(4), 317–324. http://doi.org/10.1002/jts.22112

Christiansen, D. M., & Hansen, M. (2015). Accounting for sex differences in PTSD: A multivariable mediation model. *European Journal of Psychotraumatology*, *6*, 1–10. http://doi.org/10.3402/ejpt.v6.26068

Cisler, J. M., Steele, J. S., Lenow, J. K., Smitherman, S., Everett, B., Messias, E., & Kilts, C. D. (2014). Functional reorganization of neural networks during repeated exposure to the traumatic memory in posttraumatic stress disorder: An exploratory fMRI study. *Journal of Psychiatric Research*, *48*(1), 47–55. http://doi.org/10.1016/j.jpsychires.2013.09.013

Cohen, H., Zohar, J., Gidron, Y., Matar, M. A., Belkind, D., Loewenthal, U., . . . Kaplan, Z. (2006). Blunted HPA axis response to stress influences susceptibility to posttraumatic stress response in rats. *Biological Psychiatry*, *59*(12), 1208–1218. http://doi.org/10.1016/j.biopsych.2005.12.003

Dias, B. G., Banerjee, S. B., Goodman, J. V., & Ressler, K. J. (2013). Towards new approaches to disorders of fear and anxiety. *Current Opinion in Neurobiology*, *23*(3), 346–352. http://doi.org/10.1016/j.conb.2013.01.013

Dickie, E. W., Brunet, A., Akerib, V., & Armony, J. L. (2011). Neural correlates of recovery from post-traumatic stress disorder: A longitudinal fMRI investigation of memory encoding. *Neuropsychologia*, *49*(7), 1771–1778. http://doi.org/10.1016/j.neuropsychologia.2011.02.055

Duchesne, A., & Pruessner, J. C. (2013). Association between subjective and cortisol stress response depends on the menstrual cycle phase. *Psychoneuroendocrinology*, *38*(12), 3155–3159. http://doi.org/10.1016/j.psyneuen.2013.08.009

Felmingham, K., Williams, L. M., Kemp, A. H., Liddell, B., Falconer, E., Peduto, A., & Bryant, R. (2010). Neural responses to masked fear faces: Sex differences and trauma exposure in posttraumatic stress disorder. *Journal of Abnormal Psychology*, *119*(1), 241–247. http://doi.org/10.1037/a0017551

Ferree, N. K., Kamat, R., & Cahill, L. (2011). Influences of menstrual cycle position and sex hormone levels on spontaneous intrusive recollections following emotional stimuli. *Consciousness and Cognition*, *20*(4), 1154–1162. http://doi.org/10.1016/j.concog.2011.02.003

Foa, E. B. (1997). Trauma and women: Course, predictors, and treatment. *The Journal of Clinical Psychiatry*, *58*(Suppl. 9), 25–28.

Foa, E. B. (2000). Psychosocial treatment of posttraumatic stress disorder. *The Journal of Clinical Psychiatry*, *61*(Suppl. 5), 43–48.

Foa, E. B., Gillihan, S. J., & Bryant, R. A. (2013). Challenges and successes in dissemination of evidence-based treatments for posttraumatic stress: Lessons learned from prolonged exposure therapy for PTSD. *Psychological Science in the Public Interest*, *14*(2), 65–111. http://doi.org/10.1177/1529100612468841

Foa, E. B., & Street, G. P. (2001). Women and traumatic events. *The Journal of Clinical Psychiatry*, *62*(Suppl. 17), 29–34.

Galovski, T. E., Blain, L. M., Chappuis, C., & Fletcher, T. (2013). Sex differences in recovery from PTSD in male and female interpersonal assault survivors. *Behaviour Research and Therapy*, *51*(6), 247–255. http://doi.org/10.1016/j.brat.2013.02.002

Glover, E. M., Jovanovic, T., Mercer, K. B., Kerley, K., Bradley, B., Ressler, K. J., & Norrholm, S. D. (2012). Estrogen levels are associated with extinction deficits in women with posttraumatic stress disorder. *Biological Psychiatry*, *72*(1), 19–24. http://doi.org/10.1016/j.biopsych.2012.02.031

Gruene, T. M., Flick, K., Stefano, A., Shea, S. D., & Shansky, R. M. (2015). Sexually divergent expression of active and passive conditioned fear responses in rats. *eLife*, *4*. http://doi.org/10.7554/eLife.11352

Gupta, R. R., Sen, S., Diepenhorst, L. L., Rudick, C. N., & Maren, S. (2001). Estrogen modulates sexually dimorphic contextual fear conditioning and hippocampal long-term potentiation (LTP) in rats. *Brain Research*, *888*(2), 356–365.

Handa, R. J., Burgess, L. H., Kerr, J. E., & O'Keefe, J. A. (1994). Gonadal steroid hormone receptors and sex differences in the hypothalamo-pituitary-adrenal axis. *Hormones and Behavior*, *28*(4), 464–476. http://doi.org/10.1006/hbeh.1994.1044

Hendrick, V., Altshuler, L. L., & Burt, V. K. (1996). Course of psychiatric disorders across the menstrual cycle. *Harvard Review of Psychiatry*, *4*(4), 200–207.

Hiroi, R., & Neumaier, J. F. (2006). Differential effects of ovarian steroids on anxiety versus fear as measured by open field test and fear-potentiated startle. *Behavioural Brain Research*, *166*(1), 93–100. http://doi.org/10.1016/j.bbr.2005.07.021

Hofmann, S. G. (2008). Cognitive processes during fear acquisition and extinction in animals and humans: Implications for exposure therapy of anxiety disorders. *Clinical Psychology Review*, *28*(2), 199–210. http://doi.org/10.1016/j.cpr.2007.04.009

Hwang, M. J., Zsido, R. G., Song, H., Pace-Schott, E. F., Miller, K. K., Lebron-Milad, K., . . . Milad, M. R. (2015). Contribution of estradiol levels and hormonal contraceptives to sex differences within the fear network during fear conditioning and extinction. *BMC Psychiatry*, *15*, 295. http://doi.org/10.1186/s12888-015-0673-9

Inagaki, T., Gautreaux, C., & Luine, V. (2010). Acute estrogen treatment facilitates recognition memory consolidation and alters monoamine levels in memory-related brain areas. *Hormones and Behavior*, *58*(3), 415–426. http://doi.org/10.1016/j.yhbeh.2010.05.013

Inslicht, S. S., Metzler, T. J., Garcia, N. M., Pineles, S. L., Milad, M. R., Orr, S. P., . . . Neylan, T. C. (2013). Sex differences in fear conditioning in posttraumatic stress disorder. *Journal of Psychiatric Research*, *47*(1), 64–71. http://doi.org/10.1016/j.jpsychires.2012.08.027

Jasnow, A. M., Schulkin, J., & Pfaff, D. W. (2006). Estrogen facilitates fear conditioning and increases corticotropin-releasing hormone mRNA expression in the central amygdala in female mice. *Hormones and Behavior*, *49*(2), 197–205. http://doi.org/10.1016/j.yhbeh.2005.06.005

Kajantie, E., & Phillips, D. I. W. (2006). The effects of sex and hormonal status on the physiological response to acute psychosocial stress. *Psychoneuroendocrinology*, *31*(2), 151–178. http://doi.org/10.1016/j.psyneuen.2005.07.002

Karl, A., Schaefer, M., Malta, L. S., Dörfel, D., Rohleder, N., & Werner, A. (2006). A meta-analysis of structural brain abnormalities in PTSD. *Neuroscience & Biobehavioral Reviews*, *30*(7), 1004–1031. http://doi.org/10.1016/j.neubiorev.2006.03.004

Kessler, R. C., Sonnega, A., Bromet, E., Hughes, M., & Nelson, C. B. (1995). Posttraumatic stress disorder in the National Comorbidity Survey. *Archives of General Psychiatry*, *52*(12), 1048–1060.

Kilpatrick, D. G., Resnick, H. S., Milanak, M. E., Miller, M. W., Keyes, K. M., & Friedman, M. J. (2013). National estimates of exposure to traumatic events and PTSD prevalence using DSM-IV and DSM-5 criteria. *Journal of Traumatic Stress*, *26*(5), 537–547. http://doi.org/10.1002/jts.21848

Kirschbaum, C., Kudielka, B. M., Gaab, J., Schommer, N. C., & Hellhammer, D. H. (1999). Impact of gender, menstrual cycle phase, and oral contraceptives on the activity of the hypothalamus-pituitary-adrenal axis. *Psychosomatic Medicine*, *61*(2), 154–162.

Kudielka, B. M., & Kirschbaum, C. (2005). Sex differences in HPA axis responses to stress: A review. *Biological Psychology*, *69*(1), 113–132. http://doi.org/10.1016/j.biopsycho.2004.11.009

Liberzon, I., & Sripada, C. S. (2008). The functional neuroanatomy of PTSD: A critical review. *Progress in Brain Research*, *167*, 151–169. http://doi.org/10.1016/S0079-6123(07)67011-3

Lungu, O., Potvin, S., Tikàsz, A., & Mendrek, A. (2015). Sex differences in effective fronto-limbic connectivity during negative emotion processing. *Psychoneuroendocrinology*, *62*, 180–188. http://doi.org/10.1016/j.psyneuen.2015.08.012

Maeng, L.Y., Cover, K. K., Taha, M. B., Landau, A. J., Milad, M. R., & Lebron-Milad, K. (2017). Estradiol shifts interactions between the infralimbic cortex and central amygdala to enhance fear extinction memory. *Journal of Neuroscience Research*, *95*(1–2), 163–175.

Maeng, L. Y., & Milad, M. R. (2015). Sex differences in anxiety disorders: Interactions between fear, stress, and gonadal hormones. *Hormones and Behavior*, *76*, 106–117. http://doi.org/10.1016/j.yhbeh.2015.04.002

Maeng, L. Y., Waddell, J., & Shors, T. J. (2010). The prefrontal cortex communicates with the amygdala to impair learning after acute stress in females but not in males. *The Journal of Neuroscience*, *30*(48), 16188–16196. http://doi.org/10.1523/JNEUROSCI.2265-10.2010

Marshall, R. D., & Garakani, A. (2002). Psychobiology of the acute stress response and its relationship to the psychobiology of post-traumatic stress disorder. *Psychiatric Clinics of North America, 25*(2), 385–395.

McLean, C. P., Asnaani, A., Litz, B. T., & Hofmann, S. G. (2011). Gender differences in anxiety disorders: Prevalence, course of illness, comorbidity and burden of illness. *Journal of Psychiatric Research, 45*(8), 1027–1035. http://doi.org/10.1016/j.jpsychires.2011.03.006

Michael, T., Halligan, S. L., Clark, D. M., & Ehlers, A. (2007). Rumination in posttraumatic stress disorder. *Depression and Anxiety, 24*(5), 307–317. http://doi.org/10.1002/da.20228

Milad, M. R., Igoe, S. A., Lebron-Milad, K., & Novales, J. E. (2009). Estrous cycle phase and gonadal hormones influence conditioned fear extinction. *Neuroscience, 164*(3), 887–895. http://doi.org/10.1016/j.neuroscience.2009.09.011

Milad, M. R., Pitman, R. K., Ellis, C. B., Gold, A. L., Shin, L. M., Lasko, N. B., . . . Rauch, S. L. (2009). Neurobiological basis of failure to recall extinction memory in posttraumatic stress disorder. *Biological Psychiatry, 66*(12), 1075–1082. http://doi.org/10.1016/j.biopsych.2009.06.026

Milad, M. R., Zeidan, M. A., Contero, A., Pitman, R. K., Klibanski, A., Rauch, S. L., & Goldstein, J. M. (2010). The influence of gonadal hormones on conditioned fear extinction in healthy humans. *Neuroscience, 168*(3), 652–658. http://doi.org/10.1016/j.neuroscience.2010.04.030

Morgan, M. A., & Pfaff, D. W. (2001). Effects of estrogen on activity and fear-related behaviors in mice. *Hormones and Behavior, 40*(4), 472–482. http://doi.org/10.1006/hbeh.2001.1716

Nillni, Y. I., Pineles, S. L., Patton, S. C., Rouse, M. H., Sawyer, A. T., & Rasmusson, A. M. (2015). Menstrual cycle effects on psychological symptoms in women with PTSD. *Journal of Traumatic Stress, 28*(1), 1–7. http://doi.org/10.1002/jts.21984

Nolen-Hoeksema, S. (2012). Emotion regulation and psychopathology: The role of gender. *Annual Review of Clinical Psychology, 8*, 161–187. http://doi.org/10.1146/annurev-clinpsy-032511-143109

Nolen-Hoeksema, S., & Aldao, A. (2011). Gender and age differences in emotion regulation strategies and their relationship to depressive symptoms, *51*, 704–708.

Norris, F. H. (1992). Epidemiology of trauma: Frequency and impact of different potentially traumatic events on different demographic groups. *Journal of Consulting and Clinical Psychology, 60*(3), 409–418. http://doi.org/10.1037/0022-006X.60.3.409

Nutt, D. J., & Malizia, A. L. (2004). Structural and functional brain changes in posttraumatic stress disorder. *The Journal of Clinical Psychiatry, 65*(Suppl. 1), 11–17.

Ossewaarde, L., Hermans, E. J., van Wingen, G. A., Kooijman, S. C., Johansson, I.-M., Bäckström, T., & Fernández, G. (2010). Neural mechanisms underlying changes in stress-sensitivity across the menstrual cycle. *Psychoneuroendocrinology, 35*(1), 47–55. http://doi.org/10.1016/j.psyneuen.2009.08.011

Paris, J. J., Franco, C., Sodano, R., Freidenberg, B., Gordis, E., Anderson, D. A., . . . Frye, C. A. (2010). Sex differences in salivary cortisol in response to acute stressors among healthy participants, in recreational or pathological gamblers, and in those with posttraumatic stress disorder. *Hormones and Behavior, 57*(1), 35–45. http://doi.org/10.1016/j.yhbeh.2009.06.003

Pineles, S. L., Nillni, Y. I., King, M. W., Patton, S. C., Bauer, M. R., Mostoufi, S. M., . . . Orr, S. P. (2016). Extinction retention and the menstrual cycle: Different associations for women with posttraumatic stress disorder. *Journal of Abnormal Psychology, 125*(3), 349–355. http://doi.org/10.1037/abn0000138

Pitman, R. K., Rasmusson, A. M., Koenen, K. C., Shin, L. M., Orr, S. P., Gilbertson, M. W., . . . Liberzon, I. (2012). Biological studies of post-traumatic stress disorder. *Nature Reviews Neuroscience, 13*(11), 769–787. http://doi.org/10.1038/nrn3339

Rachamim, L., Nacasch, N., Shafran, N., Tzur, D., & Gilboa-Schechtman, E. (2009). Exposure-based therapy for post-traumatic stress disorder in children and adults. *Israel Journal of Psychiatry and Related Sciences, 46*(4), 274–281.

Resnick, H. S., Kilpatrick, D. G., Dansky, B. S., Saunders, B. E., & Best, C. L. (1993). Prevalence of civilian trauma and posttraumatic stress disorder in a representative national sample of women. *Journal of Consulting and Clinical Psychology, 61*(6), 984–991. http://doi.org/http://dx.doi.org/10.1037//0022-006X.61.6.984

Rey, C. D., Lipps, J., & Shansky, R. M. (2014). Dopamine D1 receptor activation rescues extinction impairments in low-estrogen female rats and induces cortical layer-specific activation changes in prefrontal-amygdala circuits. *Neuropsychopharmacology, 39*(5), 1282–1289. http://doi.org/10.1038/npp.2013.338

Roberts, A. L., Gilman, S. E., Breslau, J., Breslau, N., & Koenen, K. C. (2011). Race/ethnic differences in exposure to traumatic events, development of post-traumatic stress disorder, and treatment-seeking for post-traumatic stress disorder in the

United States. *Psychological Medicine*, *41*(1), 71–83. http://doi.org/10.1017/S0033291710000401

Seedat, S., Stein, D. J., & Carey, P. D. (2005). Post-traumatic stress disorder in women: Epidemiological and treatment issues. *CNS Drugs*, *19*(5), 411–427.

Shin, L. M., Rauch, S. L., & Pitman, R. K. (2006). Amygdala, medial prefrontal cortex, and hippocampal function in PTSD. *Annals of the New York Academy of Sciences*, *1071*, 67–79. http://doi.org/10.1196/annals.1364.007

Shors, T. J., Lewczyk, C., Pacynski, M., Mathew, P. R., & Pickett, J. (1998). Stages of estrous mediate the stress-induced impairment of associative learning in the female rat. *Neuroreport*, *9*(3), 419–423.

Shvil, E., Sullivan, G. M., Schafer, S., Markowitz, J. C., Campeas, M., Wager, T. D., . . . Neria, Y. (2014). Sex differences in extinction recall in posttraumatic stress disorder: A pilot fMRI study. *Neurobiology of Learning and Memory*, *113*, 101–108. http://doi.org/10.1016/j.nlm.2014.02.003

Stephens, M. A. C., Mahon, P. B., McCaul, M. E., & Wand, G. S. (2016). Hypothalamic-pituitary-adrenal axis response to acute psychosocial stress: Effects of biological sex and circulating sex hormones. *Psychoneuroendocrinology*, *66*, 47–55. http://doi.org/10.1016/j.psyneuen.2015.12.021

Stevens, J. S., & Hamann, S. (2012). Sex differences in brain activation to emotional stimuli: A meta-analysis of neuroimaging studies. *Neuropsychologia*, *50*(7), 1578–1593. http://doi.org/10.1016/j.neuropsychologia.2012.03.011

Stevens, J. S., Jovanovic, T., Fani, N., Ely, T. D., Glover, E. M., Bradley, B., & Ressler, K. J. (2013). Disrupted amygdala-prefrontal functional connectivity in civilian women with posttraumatic stress disorder. *Journal of Psychiatric Research*, *47*(10), 1469–1478. http://doi.org/10.1016/j.jpsychires.2013.05.031

Sundström Poromaa, I., & Gingnell, M. (2014). Menstrual cycle influence on cognitive function and emotion processing—from a reproductive perspective. *Frontiers in Neuroscience*, *8*, 380. http://doi.org/10.3389/fnins.2014.00380

Toffoletto, S., Lanzenberger, R., Gingnell, M., Sundström-Poromaa, I., & Comasco, E. (2014). Emotional and cognitive functional imaging of estrogen and progesterone effects in the female human brain: A systematic review. *Psychoneuroendocrinology*, *50*, 28–52. http://doi.org/10.1016/j.psyneuen.2014.07.025

Tolin, D. F., & Foa, E. B. (2006). Sex differences in trauma and posttraumatic stress disorder: A quantitative review of 25 years of research. *Psychological Bulletin*, *132*(6), 959–992. http://doi.org/10.1037/0033-2909.132.6.959

Vermetten, E., & Bremner, J. D. (2002). Circuits and systems in stress. II. Applications to neurobiology and treatment in posttraumatic stress disorder. *Depression and Anxiety*, *16*(1), 14–38. http://doi.org/10.1002/da.10017

Wood, G. E., & Shors, T. J. (1998). Stress facilitates classical conditioning in males, but impairs classical conditioning in females through activational effects of ovarian hormones. *Proceedings of the National Academy of Sciences of the United States of America*, *95*(7), 4066–4071.

Woon, F. L., Sood, S., & Hedges, D. W. (2010). Hippocampal volume deficits associated with exposure to psychological trauma and posttraumatic stress disorder in adults: A meta-analysis. *Progress in Neuro-Psychopharmacology and Biological Psychiatry*, *34*(7), 1181–1188. http://doi.org/10.1016/j.pnpbp.2010.06.016

Yehuda, R., Teicher, M. H., Trestman, R. L., Levengood, R. A., & Siever, L. J. (1996). Cortisol regulation in posttraumatic stress disorder and major depression: A chronobiological analysis. *Biological Psychiatry*, *40*(2), 79–88. http://doi.org/10.1016/0006-3223(95)00451-3

Zeidan, M. A., Igoe, S. A., Linnman, C., Vitalo, A., Levine, J. B., Klibanski, A., . . . Milad, M. R. (2011). Estradiol modulates medial prefrontal cortex and amygdala activity during fear extinction in women and female rats. *Biological Psychiatry*, *70*(10), 920–927. http://doi.org/10.1016/j.biopsych.2011.05.016

17

Genetics and Gene–Environment Interaction

TORSTEN KLENGEL, LAUREN A. M. LEBOIS, SHEILA GAYNOR, AND GUIA GUFFANTI

ROLE OF GENE–ENVIRONMENT INTERACTIONS IN TRAUMA AND STRESSOR-RELATED DISORDERS

Studies of gene–environment interactions (GxE) aim to describe how genetic and environmental factors jointly influence the risk of developing a disease.[1] The identification of genetic variants that contribute differently to phenotypic expression depending on the specific environmental variation may improve our understanding of the biology of complex diseases, as well as potential interventions and preventive strategies for those diseases. In addition, knowledge of GxE is crucial for replicating findings of association studies across different populations, unraveling unexplained genetic heritability and advancing individualized medicine.

Environmental factors are key determinants influencing risk for disease across all disciplines of medicine.[2] It has been suggested that disorders such as schizophrenia, bipolar, and autism spectrum disorders share a stronger genetic load while major depression and anxiety disorders may result from a stronger contribution of the environment.

Trauma and stress-related disorders make an excellent case for GxE interactions since exposure to trauma and stress are well-established risk factors toward the disorder, but are not sufficient to explain etiopathogenesis.[3] Exposure to traumatic events is a prerequisite of posttraumatic stress disorder (PTSD) diagnosis, but the majority of individuals who are exposed to even a severe traumatic event do not develop PTSD. Why some individuals are vulnerable and others are resilient remains an open question. While genetic factors may play a significant role, it is conceivable that the complex interplay between genetic and environmental factors contribute to the observed inter-individual variability.

DEFINITION OF GXE INTERACTION

In biology, interaction effects can come in a wide variety. This is especially true when considering GxE interactions. Even the term "interaction" assumes different meaning depending on the definition used by biologists, epidemiologists, statisticians, and human geneticists. In the context of medical genetics and epidemiology, a GxE interaction is defined as a "joint effect of one or more genes with one or more environmental factors that cannot be readily explained by their separate marginal effects."[4] The assumptions of the different interpretations of the concept of interaction have great implications for the analytical approaches used to identify them.

In the literature, discussion about interactions has been confused by the use of the same terminology applied to different concepts underlying the definition of biological and statistical interaction.

Biological interaction is defined as the joint effect of two factors that act together in a direct physical or chemical reaction to cause disease.[5] This concept generally applies to the cellular or molecular level but can also have implications for statistical interactions at the population level. A biological interaction implies that the effect of one risk factor depends upon the presence or absence of another. PTSD by definition corresponds to this definition as its development depends on the exposure to trauma upon the presence of specific genetic risk factors.

Statistical interaction is defined as the "departure" from independence of the effects of different risk factors in the way that they combine to cause disease without necessarily implying any particular biological mode of action. Effects can be additive or multiplicative for disease risk, and exponential or logarithmic for continuous traits, for example, symptoms count. Based on the statistical interaction definition, risk factors are said to interact if the effect of one risk factor depends on the level of the other risk factor.[6]

Statistical interactions are often divided into quantitative and qualitative types. Quantitative interactions imply that the effect of one factor goes in the same direction at different levels of the other but differ in magnitude.[1] For example, compared to noncarriers of the susceptible genotype of a specific genetic risk factor, risk carriers have additive or multiplicative increased risk of disease development. Qualitative interactions imply that the effect of risk factors goes in opposite directions. For example, exposure is deleterious in carriers of the susceptible genotype of a specific genetic risk factor, but exposure is not detrimental in noncarriers.

Two of the most studied genetic risk factors in the literature of GxE interactions in PTSD represent examples of qualitative and quantitative interactions, respectively. We fully review their biological context and implications in the following sections.

First, the risk allele of gene *FKBP5* (FK506 binding protein 5), is implicated in a possible statistical quantitative GxE interaction effect in PTSD. Genetic association analyses found that the combination of FKBP5 susceptible genotype and exposure to trauma increases the risk of PTSD severity with every additional copy of risk variant.[7] This is an example of a quantitative interaction. However, recent evidence shows that FKBP5 "risk" genotypes may have protective effects in distinct environments pointing towards a mixture of quantitative and qualitative interaction.

Second, the short (S) allele of gene *SLC6A4* (solute carrier family 6), also known as neurotransmitter serotonin transporter, *5-HTTLPR*, is implicated in a possible statistical qualitative GxE interaction effect in PTSD. The serotonin transporter regulates synaptic 5-HT reuptake and thereby influences emotional behavior. The S allele, also referred to as the risk allele, was found to be associated with decreased PTSD risk in environments with low crime and unemployment rates but with increased PTSD risk in opposite environments.[8] This is an example of qualitative interaction.

The study of GxE interactions requires information on both components of the relationship in addition to the different phenotypic outcomes. In the following section, we review the fundamentals of clinical diagnosis of PTSD and its intermediate phenotypes as well as the "E" environmental and "G" genetic components commonly used in GxE studies of PTSD.

CLINICAL OUTCOMES AND ENDOPHENOTYPES

When conducting a GxE analysis, it is important to be aware of the variety of possible psychopathological phenotypes commonly associated with trauma, for example trauma-spectrum disorders and dissociative disorders. Substance use disorders, mood disorders, anxiety disorders, eating disorders, and somatoform disorders are also commonly co-occurring with trauma-spectrum and dissociative disorders. Here, we focus on PTSD, its subtypes, and dissociative identity disorder (DID).

Posttraumatic Stress Disorder

Classic PTSD or the re-experiencing subtype of PTSD has been most widely studied. Its four major symptom categories include (1) intrusive re-experiencing symptoms, that is, re-living the traumatic memories (e.g., nightmares, flashbacks); (2) avoidance symptoms or staying away from situations, feelings, or people that are reminders of the trauma; (3) negative alterations in mood/cognition symptoms, that is, beliefs and thoughts about the world and people are changed in a negative way (e.g., distorted negative thoughts about one's self, gaps in memory); and (4) hyperarousal and reactivity symptoms, that is, heightened alertness toward one's environment manifested in, for example, an exaggerated startle response/sleep difficulties.[9]

Dissociative Subtype of PTSD

The dissociative subtype of PTSD includes the four aforementioned symptom categories, but individuals also experience moderate to severe disruptions in perceptual and cognitive experience, that is, dissociation.[9] The two major categories of dissociation associated with this PTSD subtype are depersonalization, feelings of detachment from one's sense of self, body, or emotions, and derealization, feelings of detachment from the environment or people and objects in the environment.[9] Derealization may also involve changes in one's visual perception of the environment (e.g., objects changing in size or shape, feeling like surroundings appear movie or video game-like).[9]

Dissociative Identity Disorder

DID is a childhood-onset disorder in which the typical identity-related developmental trajectory is disrupted.[10] In DSM-5, DID is categorized in the class, Dissociative Disorder, next to but not part of Trauma- and Stressor-Related Disorders

(American Psychological Association, 2013, p. 291). DID is characterized by the aforementioned PTSD dissociative subtype symptoms (i.e., intrusions, avoidance, negative alterations in mood/cognition, hyperarousal, depersonalization, derealization), in addition to symptoms of identity alteration and amnesia. Identity confusion is uncertainty about one's sense of self or who one is, and identity alteration is the presence of at least two distinct self or personality states with their own pattern of perceiving, relating to, and thinking about the environment and self (American Psychiatric Association, 2013). Amnesia can be the loss of memory for personal information, everyday events, or aspects of the traumatic experiences (American Psychiatric Association, 2013).

NEURAL ENDOPHENOTYPES

There are a number of key brain regions that consistently demonstrate either structural or functional differences or both in PTSD and DID, including the ventromedial prefrontal cortex (vmPFC), amygdala, insula, hippocampus (HP), and the anterior cingulate cortex (ACC). These regions are broadly involved in memory function, visceral state experience, and emotion regulation and production. These processes are often affected in trauma spectrum and stress-related disorders. More specifically, the vmPFC is involved in cognitive control and appraising the self-relevance of a stimulus.[11] It performs an inhibitory role on the amygdala.[12] The amygdala is involved in the detection of salient information, fear conditioning, and emotional processing.[12,13] The insula is involved in the perception of pain and self-referential processing, including visceral state awareness.[14] The HP is involved in memory for consciously recalled events and the context of experience.[15,16] The ACC is involved in emotion production and regulation.[17] Its function is often divided on the dorsal/ventral plane. The dorsal ACC (dACC) is commonly activated when processing pain, during fear learning, response selection and error detection.[17,18] The ventral ACC (vACC) is often involved in visceral state awareness and conflict monitoring.[17,18]

In classic re-experiencing PTSD, the observed functional pattern is one of decreased vmPFC activity, while the amygdala, insula, and dACC have increased activity.[18–20] The HP demonstrates mixed hyper and hypoactivity.[18] In the dissociative subtype of PTSD, the opposite pattern is observed. That is, the vmPFC is hyperactive, while the amygdala and insula are hypoactive.[19,20] In DID, both of these brain activity patterns are detected depending on the current identity state.[21,22]

THE "E": OVERVIEW OF ENVIRONMENTAL EXPOSURE ASSESSMENT

A relevant aspect of GxE interaction analysis is how to define and measure the "E"—environmental component. Most environmental factors relevant to GxE studies of trauma- and stress-related disorders have degrees of exposure intensity that are modified by qualitative factors, such as type of trauma or stress, as well as temporal factors, such as age at exposure or duration of exposure.

Trauma Exposures and Sex Differences

In the US National Comorbidity Study, rape was the trauma exposure most likely to be associated with PTSD for both males and females.[23] This was compared to all other categories assessed, including molestation, physical attack, combat experience, threat with a weapon, life-threatening accident, natural disaster (including fire, flood), witnessing someone be badly injured or killed, childhood parental neglect, and childhood physical abuse. Although rape had the greatest likelihood of being associated with PTSD for both sexes, a number of sex differences emerged in the probability of developing PTSD given the exposure type. For males, combat exposure, childhood neglect, and childhood physical abuse were next most associated with subsequent PTSD diagnoses. For females, rape was followed by molestation, physical attack, threat with a weapon, and childhood physical abuse as most likely to result in PTSD. Males and females were also more likely to experience different types of trauma. Compared to females, males were more likely to be exposed to potential traumatic events overall, and in particular, to experience a physical attack, a life-threatening accident, or a natural disaster; witness someone being badly injured or killed; and be threatened with a weapon. Females were more likely to experience rape, molestation, neglect by a parent, and childhood physical abuse.

Childhood Maltreatment

Childhood maltreatment is an important factor to assess in GxE studies of trauma and stressor-related disorders. Exposure to trauma or maltreatment in childhood, in particular, results in a wide range of negative mental health outcomes including the risk for suicide, depression, anxiety disorder, personality disorders, and psychosis.[24] It is important to consider that childhood abuse also results in a higher risk for somatic diseases including cardiovascular and metabolic diseases. Childhood maltreatment is commonly categorized into five types: emotional, physical, and sexual abuse, emotional neglect, and physical neglect. It is important to note, however, that these categories have considerable overlap, for example, sexual abuse also includes an element of emotional abuse. That aside, emotional abuse by itself may cause more severe pathological symptoms compared to other categories of maltreatment, even familial sexual abuse.[25,26] The dominant pattern emerging is that, the more *types* of childhood maltreatment an individual experiences, the more severe their pathological symptoms.[26–30]

Sensitive Periods

When investigating the influence of environmental factors on disease risk, it is vitally important to consider developmental processes. Different environmental factors modulate disease risk in distinct phases of the life cycle. The prenatal period and childhood may be among the most vulnerable times for the influence of mental health risk factors and within those periods there may be specific sensitive periods tied to particular outcomes.[31] Recent evidence even suggests an influence of the environment in the ancestral generations on disease risk of the unborn offspring.[32]

The type of environmental exposure as well as its timing in development may be especially key components when considering their effect on neural endophenotypes associated with mental disorders,[33] given different brain regions experience different developmental trajectories and periods of plasticity.[34] Preliminary evidence in a sample of women with repeated childhood sexual abuse demonstrated hippocampal volume was maximally reduced when sexual abuse occurred between ages 3 and 5 and ages 11 and 13.[35] The corpus callosum volume was most reduced when sexual abuse occurred between ages 9 and 10, and frontal cortex volume was most reduced when sexual abuse occurred between ages 14 and 16.[35] There was no discernable sensitive period for the amygdala associated with altered volume in this sample. In a follow-up study from the same group, Khan et al.[36] showed that nonverbal emotional abuse in males and peer emotional abuse in females at 14 years of age were the most significant predictors of lifetime depression, more important across age-specific models than by number or type of maltreatment. In addition, suicidal ideation was predicted by nonverbal emotional abuse in males and peer emotional abuse at age 14, but most importantly by parental verbal abuse at age 5 in males and sexual abuse at age 18 in females.[36]

Resilience

The number of possible factors influencing mental health outcomes is overwhelming. Although the current literature focuses particularly on environmental risk factors, it is important to keep in mind that positive or protective environmental factors also influence disease risk and may counterbalance some risk factors.[37]

THE "G": OVERVIEW OF INFORMATION ON GENETIC PREDISPOSITION

While most humans are exposed to stressful or even traumatic life events across their lifetime, only a minority of the affected individuals develops any disease.[38] It has been estimated that genetic factors explain up to 30% of the risk of developing PTSD. This estimate was observed in a male sample of Vietnam era veterans. The proportion of the risk attributable to genetic factors (i.e., heritability) has been estimated up to 72% in a community-based sample of young adult twins.[39] Genetic predisposition is inferred from direct analysis of the DNA sequence. The search for genetic risk factors starts with the identification of DNA variants derived from a mutational process leading to the substitution of a nucleotide for another (single nucleotide polymorphisms [SNPs]) and present to some appreciable degree in the general population. The two alternative nucleotides found at the same genomic location of a single DNA variant are also called "alleles." By definition a "risk" allele is considered the DNA variant less frequent in the general population. However, in the context of GxE this connotation needs careful revision, as a risk allele for a certain disorder in strongly context dependent and might be a protective allele in a different environmental condition. Multiple alleles on the same chromosomes with the tendency to be transmitted together from one generation to another form a haplotype. Depending on the frequency of the variant in the general population, we can distinguish between common (> 1%–5%) and rare (< 1%–5%) single nucleotide variants (SNVs). The presence of none, one or two copies (i.e., alleles) of the "mutated" or "polymorphic" variant at a specific location in the genome defines the genetic profile of an individual (i.e., the genotype). As of 8 June 2015, dbSNP, the database of variants from the National

Center for Biotechnology Information, listed 149,735,377 SNVs in humans' DNA. Current microarray platforms allow investigating up to 5 million genetic variants per subjects in one experiment. Most common variants do not alter gene function. Deleterious variants are more likely to be rare variants, which are not the main target of microarray approaches. This type of variant is detected using sequencing techniques that reveal the sequence of all nucleotides in the individual DNA. Recently, reduction techniques such as the polygenic risk scoring (PRS) have been used in GxE analyses to define the genetic component. PRS aims to summarize the genetic effect among an ensemble of variants selected based on biological (e.g., biological pathways) or statistical (e.g., significance threshold) criteria.

EXAMPLES OF GXE STUDIES AND POTENTIAL MOLECULAR MECHANISMS

A growing body of literature addresses the interaction of childhood and adult trauma exposure with genes previously implicated in underlying molecular mechanisms on risk for stress-related disorders. To date, 21 studies examined GxE interactions reporting a significant GxE interaction.[40] Sample sizes of these studies ranged between few hundreds to few thousands. A significant GxE interaction was found in PTSD studies that examined *SLC6A4*,[41–49] *FKBP5*,[7,36,50] *GABRA2*,[51] *RGS2*,[52] *COMT*,[53] RORA,[36] APOE,[54,55] OXTR,[56] COBL,[57] and ADCYAP1R1.[58]

We focus on selected examples to illustrate methodical challenges and provide an outlook on potential mechanisms underlying GxE interactions. Given the broad literature on exposure to maltreatment or abuse in childhood, we focus on this type and exposure age in the following paragraphs.

Although first theoretical and experimental principles of GxE emerged early in the last century, groundbreaking studies by Caspi and Moffitt first combined the influence of the environment in childhood and the influence of genetic variations towards stress-related disorders in a statistical framework of GxE.[59,60] They described the interactive effects of single nucleotide polymorphisms at the monoamine oxidase A (*MAO-A*) locus and the serotonin transporter locus (*SLC6A4*) with childhood adversities toward the risk to developing antisocial behavior and depression. These studies suggested that the influence of the environment represented by childhood maltreatment is not uniform toward the development of psychiatric disorders but moderated by the genetic disposition with so-called risk alleles leading to a higher risk of disease compared to so-called protective alleles associated with no or a reduced risk in response to maltreatment exposure. Subsequent studies showed that environmental factors differentially influence GxE depending on social context, timing, or severity of the trauma. Further studies investigated other candidate loci from the monoamine transmitter system, neurotropic factors and the hypothalamus-pituitary adrenal axis that were associated with stress-related phenotypes.[61]

Serotonin Transporter-Linked Polymorphic Region

The 5-HTTLPR is a polymorphic repeat region in the promoter of the serotonin transporter gene (*SCL6A4*). Although a number of variants of the GC-rich repeat region have been described, most studies differentiate between the short and long allele. Discovered in the early 1990s, the 5-HTTLPR was implicated in the risk for developing depression by affecting the gene expression of *SLC6A4*.[62] In 2003, the first evidence emerged that the 5-HTTLPR differentially influences the response to childhood maltreatment on the risk for developing depression in adulthood.[59] These findings did not remain without controversy and multiple studies and meta-analyses were published on GxE of the 5-HTTLPR.[63,64] The initial finding showed that individuals homozygous for the short allele also showed an increased risk for depression in adulthood compared to carriers of the long allele. However, a vivid debate resulted from following replication and nonreplication studies, and it became clearer that the definition of the environmental stressor is a pivotal determinant for the replication of this interaction. It became apparent that, in particular, childhood sexual and physical abuse was a strong predictor for replication of the initial finding while more global constructs of environmental risk such as "life stress" yielded a weaker replication or nonreplication overall. Studies on Hurricane Katrina represent another example of GxE study complexity. Here, the interaction of the 5-HTTLPR with the natural disaster on the risk to develop PTSD was apparent only in individuals living in areas with a low socioeconomic status compared to exposed individuals living in a more advantageous context with higher socioeconomic status.[65] Thus, not only the specific trauma or stressor is important but also the broader socioeconomic context that might put individuals at risk for specific negative events. The 5-HTTLPR GxE also illustrate that a certain genotype is not necessarily a "risk" or "protective" but a function of a specific environmental exposure. Studies on PTSD have recently shown that either the short allele of the 5-HTTLPR can have protective effects when studying emotional abuse or the long allele can confer risk for PTSD in a sample of European ancestry.[44,66] In summary, findings from the well-studied 5-HTTLPR GxE are not uniform, highlighting the need to study GxE in larger populations with distinct environmental exposures, with varying exposure timing and in different ethnicities to gain more insight into the relationship of genetic variation and environmental factors.

Besides the conceptual and statistical considerations, knowledge about the molecular underpinnings of the statistical findings might also provide a better understanding of GxE and of the pathophysiology of mental disorders.

FK506 Binding Protein 5

Another well-established example of a GxE study is the interaction of the *FKBP5* gene with childhood abuse on the risk for PTSD, depression, suicidal behavior, and aggression.[67] FKBP5 acts as a regulator of the glucocorticoid receptor (GR) and the hypothalamus-pituitary-adrenal (HPA) axis. It performs this regulation by modulating the central stress hormone axis with negative feedback loops, which are critical for cortisol secretion. The dysregulation of the HPA axis and its feedback loops are a key finding in multiple studies on the pathophysiology of stress-related psychiatric disorders. First shown by Binder et al.,[7] childhood abuse exposure leads to higher PTSD symptom levels in adulthood in individuals carrying a risk haplotype of *FKBP5* including the SNPs rs3800373, rs9296158, rs9470080, and rs1360780 compared to individuals carrying the protective haplotype.[7] Of note, although this interaction appeared robust related to childhood abuse exposure, no interaction of any SNP in *FKBP5* with adult trauma on adult psychopathology was observed. This GxE was later replicated by Xie et al.,[50] and further studies suggested that *FKBP5* SNPs interact with childhood abuse not only on PTSD but also on general health, intermediate phenotypes such as amygdala reactivity, and the risk to develop major depressive disorder, aggressive behavior, and suicidal ideation.

The genetic variants implicated in the GxE of *FKBP5* and childhood abuse are in high linkage disequilibrium and distributed across the entire gene locus. Most of them are located in noncoding regions and therefore possess no obvious relevant effects on protein structure and function. Hence it is difficult to determine the functional variant that mediates the biological effects. Extending previous findings from 2008, Klengel et al.[68] hypothesized that the functional genetic variant may be located in or close to known regulatory glucocorticoid response elements (GREs) mediating the effect of GR-activation on the transcriptional activation of FKBP5. In fact, a SNP in intron 2 of *FKBP5* named rs1360780 influences the enhancer properties of the adjacent GRE as shown by luciferase reporter assays. Further studies using chromatin conformation capture (3C) revealed that the downstream enhancer regions in intron 2 and intron 7 form a three-dimensional structure with the promoter region leading to a contact of the intron 2 GRE enhancer region with the promoter region in risk allele carriers but not in individuals harboring the protective genotype. This loop formation and interaction of the enhancer with the promoter site leads to a stronger transcriptional activation of *FKBP5* in risk allele carriers compared to protective genotype carriers.

However, besides the genetic predisposition in *FKBP5*, childhood abuse also induces long-lasting epigenetic changes that influence the risk for developing PTSD. When stratifying individuals according to childhood trauma exposure and *FKBP5* rs1360780 genotype an allele specific DNA methylation change became evident. Trauma-exposed risk allele carriers showed a reduced methylation in and around the GRE in intron 7 of *FKBP5* compared to trauma-exposed carriers of the protective genotype that retained a stable methylation pattern and were similar to nontrauma-exposed individuals irrespective of their genotype. This result is the first example of a genotype-dependent epigenetic modification in response to childhood trauma. It highlights that the long-lasting epigenetic effects of childhood abuse are genotype dependent paralleling previous statistical GxE. The functional consequence of demethylation in and around intron 7 GREs is an enhanced transcriptional activation and subsequently a reduced GR sensitivity to cortisol with higher cortisol level over time, which is in turn a risk factor for stress-related psychiatric disorders. A major limitation of most psychiatric epigenetic studies is the investigation of DNA methylation in peripheral blood, a heterogeneous tissue that may not be informative for pathophysiologic mechanisms in the brain. However, for *FKBP5* stress-induced demethylation, similar mechanisms may be in place in multiple tissues including neuronal tissue as shown by experiments in human hippocampal progenitor cells.

Genome-wide allele-specific epigenetic changes in response to environmental exposure are supported by the study of Teh et al.[69] The authors investigated the genome and epigenome of neonates and found over 1,400 regions that were highly variable across individuals. A quarter of these were best explained by genetic variation only, while three-quarters were explained by an interaction between genotype and in utero environment, suggesting that allele-specific environmental effects occur throughout the genome and will accumulate with age.

APPROACHES FOR GXE ASSOCIATION ANALYSIS

The goal of genetic association studies is to identify whether specific alleles correlate with a particular phenotypic effect in the individuals of the examined population. In the context of a GxE association analysis, the goal is to test whether this relationship is influenced by environmental risk factors. Traditionally GxE interactions were investigated using candidate-SNP/gene studies. This is an hypothesis-driven approach assuming that the causative genetic risk factor lays within a gene whose biological function is known and fits the assumptions about the pathophysiology of the trait under study.

Statistical Model

Whether the focus of the study is a candidate SNP or the whole genome, the statistical model to study GxE interactions usually relies on linear or logistic regression. Regression models are typically fit for a single variant, environment and their interaction. Consider that we have an environmental factorE, which in the simplest settings is a binary variable indicating whether an individual was exposed or unexposed.[70] Additionally, we have some genetic variant G, which could be binary, indicating whether the individual is a carrier or otherwise. The GxE interaction is statistically defined as the product of the E and G variables. We can consider fitting a generalized linear model as follows:

$$g \cdot p = \beta 0 + \beta 1 G + \beta 2 E + \beta 3 GE$$

where we have the disease probability p. The regression link function, g, corresponds to the scale of the outcome, that is, whether one considers the risk or log odds of disease. Scaling is particularly important when assessing interactions as changing the scale can either conceal or spuriously create a GxE interaction. Determining the appropriate scale must be done with respect to a particular problem. The effects of the model are dependent on the region of the environmental distribution that is sampled.

The interaction between the gene and environment is represented through the coefficient of the interaction term, β_3. Thus in order to test for the GxE interaction, the statistical hypothesis of $H_0 : \beta_3 = 0$ is tested. If one is simply modeling the risk of disease in a linear regression this tests for an additive interaction, meaning that when both gene and environment act simultaneously the excess risk is equal to the sum of their excess risks. Alternatively, if one models the log odds of disease in a logistic regression this tests for a multiplicative interaction. Here, the relative risk for both gene and environment acting simultaneously is equal to the product of the relative risk of each.

GWAS Methods

Despite the current interest in this area and the introduction of a variety of methodological approaches, no commonly accepted or "standard" set of methods has been established to study GxE on a genome-wide scale. Since the main problem pertaining to interaction testing in the context of genome-wide association studies (GWAS) is multiple hypotheses testing, most methods focus on strategies to reduce the "search space" for likely interactions that could involve as many as millions of genetic variants. Current approaches can be roughly divided into two categories: (a) the model-free methods such as the multifactor dimensionality reduction method, based on permutation testing to assess the statistical significance of their findings,[71] and (b) the model-based method, either fully parametric or semi-parametric.[72–75] Both approaches exploit multistage strategies to prioritize a set of SNPs for further analysis, either to decrease the computational burden that comes with the permutation-framework or to decrease the number of model-based hypotheses to test for interactions. Despite the appeal of multistage approaches to increase statistical power by decreasing the multiple testing burden, the criterion to prioritize SNPs in the first stage for determining which variants are tested in the second stage, without using arbitrary levels of significance, remains a critical issue. This is likely related to the fact that most traditional statistical methods applied to GWAS were not developed to detect purely interactive effects; as a consequence, interaction effects are usually identified by following up SNPs that had already exhibited a main effect. Excluding unlikely interactions on an a priori basis in this manner might increase power by decreasing the type I error rate, but at the cost of increasing the Type II error rate, essentially missing genetic variants that show only a marginal effect on the trait of interest. This is particularly true for studies of modest sample sizes, for which the need of new statistical and computational methods to detect interactions is a strong priority.

Statistical Power

In GWAS, the statistical power to detect GxE interactions is a critical issue, along with sample size requirements.[76,77] The standard statistical approach for testing interactions would proceed by testing the hypothesis $H_0 : \beta_3 = 0$, in the notation of the previous statistical methods section. This test can have low power if the genetic effect is limited to those who are exposed (or unexposed). Information of the genetic effect of those who are unexposed is effectively ignored. The test can further have low power if the environmental effect among the unexposed and among the exposed with the variant is associated with higher trait levels and lower trait levels, respectively.

Approaches to increase the power for detecting a GxE interaction have been proposed.[78] Whereas a case-control analysis oftentimes has low power to detect interaction, a case-only approach typically has the maximum power if one assumes that the genetic variant and environmental exposure are independently distributed.[79] However, this assumption results in the case-only analysis having large type 1 error if violated. There have been multiple proposals of hybrid approaches that combine both case-only and case-control analyses. Further, if one is interested in identifying markers related to a phenotype, one may increase the power by using a "joint" test to simultaneously test for the genetic effect under the null hypothesis $H_0 : \beta_1 = \beta_3 = 0$, which allows one to leverage the effect in both exposure subgroups. The sample sizes required to detect the GxE interaction reliably and with appropriate power can be prohibitively large. One must consider the type of GxE interaction, the type 1 rate, and the study design when determining the mostly highly powered and appropriate test.

Replication

The gold standard rule to reliably identify disease-causing genetic variants is to conduct large studies and to replicate the unequivocal statistically significant finding in an independent sample. In GxE studies, this is further complicated by the difficulty in finding studies measuring the "environmental" component in the exact same way.

CHALLENGES OF GXE STUDIES

Although the importance of the interaction of environment and genetic predispositions underlying PTSD and other psychiatric disorders is widely acknowledged, methodological limitations circumvent widespread application of GxE interaction analysis. Specifically, the four most pervasive limitations relate to the (a) lack of replication, which has raised questions about possible inconsistent results; (b) small sample size, which lead to a lack of statistical power, known to be responsible for false positive results; (c) lack of inclusion of confounding factors such as gender, ethnicity, and age in GxE statistical models[80,81] in most earlier studies that preceded the GWAS era; and (d) measurement of trauma, which has been an object of discussion for possibly being inaccurate and responsible for a lack of replication and contradictory results.

Here we focus on limitations inherent to the measurement of trauma, since these variables are pivotal in the identification and replication of GxE interactions. The current typical method for investigating the trauma exposure is a retrospective self-report using validated questionnaires in cross-sectional studies. This method provides a cost-effective and quick assessment that is feasible in a large number of individuals. However, this method has several limitations.

Most importantly, the validity of retrospective questionnaires has been questioned in the past, specifically related to the willingness and capability of individuals to remember and report events and the possibility that individuals may overreport exposure to traumatic events. However, given the stigma and shame associated with many traumatic experiences, especially those that occur in childhood, research suggests individuals are much more likely to under-report these experiences.[82] The potential bias of retrospective assessments also includes the selection of certain events due to the social desirability of a certain answer, misclassification, and uncertainties with regard to temporal relationships. Longitudinal studies, especially those that assess individuals before and after abuse occurs, will address these limitations.

Structured or semi-structured interviews administrated through trained experts provide an alternative to self-reports, reducing the limitations mentioned. However, these interviews are lengthy to complete and may prevent their feasibility in large-scale studies. Other alternatives to self-reported exposure are third-party reports providing to some extent a more objective measurement of exposure, which can include governmental or health insurance records. In an ideal situation, environmental factors would be measured in a prospective study with a large enough sample. A selection of individuals at risk for exposure might also reduce the overall need for a large sample size. Moreover, a prospective assessment can provide longitudinal data using measurements before, during, and after a particular exposure. This is crucial, in particular for causal relationships that are impossible to determine in retrospective cross-sectional studies. However, longitudinal prospective studies are complex and in some cases unethical to perform.

CONCLUSIONS

Although there is a general consensus on the importance of GxE studies, the state of the literature remains too preliminary to make substantive conclusions on how GxE factors affect PTSD. Since one of the major concerns about the feasibility of such studies is sample size, it is believed that Consortia efforts for large-scale GWAS such as the one led by the Psychiatric Genetics Consortium PTSD Working Group will be an important step forward in this process. Furthermore, the integration of common variants with neurobiological data derived from related experiments on the transcriptome and epigenome of PTSD may further our understanding of the functional relevance of GxE association results. Environmental factors influencing risk or resilience toward disease development are accessible to preventive but also therapeutic approaches, thus implying an outstanding potential to influence mental health outcomes.

REFERENCES

1. Hunter DJ. Gene-environment interactions in human diseases. *Nature Reviews Genetics* 2005; 6(4): 287–298.
2. Rutter M. Environmentally mediated risks for psychopathology: Research strategies and findings. *Journal of the American Academy of Child and Adolescent Psychiatry* 2005; 44(1): 3–18.
3. Forresi B, Caffo E, Battaglia M. Gene environment interplays: Why PTSD makes a good case for gene–environment interaction studies and how adding a developmental approach can help. In: Martin C, Preedy V, Patel V (eds.). *Comprehensive guide to post-traumatic stress disorders*. New York: Springer; 2016, pp. 1053–1067.
4. Thomas D. Gene-environment-wide association studies: Emerging approaches. *Nature Reviews Genetics* 2010; 11(4): 259–272.
5. Yang Q, Khoury MJ. Evolving methods in genetic epidemiology. III. Gene-environment interaction in epidemiologic research. *Epidemiologic Reviews* 1997; 19(1): 33–43.
6. Dempfle A, Scherag A, Hein R, Beckmann L, Chang-Claude J, Schafer H. Gene-environment interactions for complex traits: Definitions, methodological requirements and challenges. *European Journal of Human Genetics* 2008; 16(10): 1164–1172.
7. Binder EB, Bradley RG, Liu W, Epstein MP, Deveau TC, Mercer KB, et al. Association of FKBP5 polymorphisms and childhood abuse with risk of posttraumatic stress disorder symptoms in adults. *JAMA* 2008; 299(11): 1291–1305.
8. Koenen KC, Aiello AE, Bakshis E, Amstadter AB, Ruggiero KJ, Acierno R, et al. Modification of the association between serotonin transporter genotype and risk of posttraumatic stress disorder in adults by county-level social environment. *American Journal of Epidemiology* 2009; 169(6): 704–711.
9. American Psychiatric Association. *Diagnostic and statistical manual of mental disorders* (5th ed.). Washington, DC: American Psychiatric Publishing; 2013.
10. Dorahy MJ, Brand BL, Sar V, Kruger C, Stavropoulos P, Martinez-Taboas A, et al. Dissociative identity disorder: An empirical overview. *The Australian and New Zealand Journal of Psychiatry* 2014; 48(5): 402–417.
11. Miller EK, Cohen JD. An integrative theory of prefrontal cortex function. *Annual Review of Neuroscience* 2001; 24: 167–202.
12. Davidson RJ. Anxiety and affective style: Role of prefrontal cortex and amygdala. *Biological Psychiatry* 2002; 51(1): 68–80.
13. Sergerie K, Chochol C, Armony JL. The role of the amygdala in emotional processing: A quantitative meta-analysis of functional neuroimaging studies. *Neuroscience and Biobehavioral Reviews* 2008; 32(4): 811–830.
14. Craig AD. Interoception: The sense of the physiological condition of the body. *Current Opinion in Neurobiology* 2003; 13(4): 500–505.
15. Kim JJ, Diamond DM. The stressed hippocampus, synaptic plasticity and lost memories. *Nature Reviews Neuroscience* 2002; 3(6): 453–462.
16. Squire LR. Memory and the hippocampus: A synthesis from findings with rats, monkeys,

and humans. *Psychological Review* 1992; 99(2): 195–231.
17. Kober H, Barrett LF, Joseph J, Bliss-Moreau E, Lindquist K, Wager TD. Functional grouping and cortical-subcortical interactions in emotion: A meta-analysis of neuroimaging studies. *NeuroImage* 2008; 42(2): 998–1031.
18. Pitman RK, Rasmusson AM, Koenen KC, Shin LM, Orr SP, Gilbertson MW, et al. Biological studies of post-traumatic stress disorder. *Nature Reviews Neuroscience* 2012; 13(11): 769–787.
19. Lanius RA, Vermetten E, Loewenstein RJ, Brand B, Schmahl C, Bremner JD, et al. Emotion modulation in PTSD: Clinical and neurobiological evidence for a dissociative subtype. *The American Journal of Psychiatry* 2010; 167(6): 640–647.
20. Lanius RA, Brand B, Vermetten E, Frewen PA, Spiegel D. The dissociative subtype of posttraumatic stress disorder: Rationale, clinical and neurobiological evidence, and implications. *Depression and Anxiety* 2012; 29(8): 701–708.
21. Reinders AA, Willemsen AT. Dissociative identity disorder and fantasy proneness: A positron emission tomography study of authentic and enacted dissociative identity states. In: *PET and SPECT in psychiatry*. New York: Springer, pp. 411–431.
22. Reinders AA, Nijenhuis ER, Quak J, Korf J, Haaksma J, Paans AM, et al. Psychobiological characteristics of dissociative identity disorder: A symptom provocation study. *Biological Psychiatry* 2006; 60(7): 730–740.
23. Kessler RC, Sonnega A, Bromet E, Hughes M, Nelson CB. Posttraumatic stress disorder in the National Comorbidity Survey. *Archives of General Psychiatry* 1995; 52(12): 1048–1060.
24. Nemeroff CB. Paradise lost: the neurobiological and clinical consequences of child abuse and neglect. *Neuron* 2016; 89(5): 892–909.
25. Sar V, Tutkun H, Alyanak B, Bakim B, Baral I. Frequency of dissociative disorders among psychiatric outpatients in Turkey. *Comprehensive Psychiatry* 2000; 41(3): 216–222.
26. Teicher MH, Samson JA, Polcari A, McGreenery CE. Sticks, stones, and hurtful words: Relative effects of various forms of childhood maltreatment. *The American Journal of Psychiatry* 2006; 163(6): 993–1000.
27. Dube SR, Anda RF, Felitti VJ, Chapman DP, Williamson DF, Giles WH. Childhood abuse, household dysfunction, and the risk of attempted suicide throughout the life span: Findings from the Adverse Childhood Experiences Study. *JAMA* 2001; 286(24): 3089–3096.
28. Edwards VJ, Holden GW, Felitti VJ, Anda RF. Relationship between multiple forms of childhood maltreatment and adult mental health in community respondents: Results from the adverse childhood experiences study. *The American Journal of Psychiatry* 2003; 160(8): 1453–1460.
29. Felitti VJ, Anda RF, Nordenberg D, Williamson DF, Spitz AM, Edwards V, et al. Relationship of childhood abuse and household dysfunction to many of the leading causes of death in adults. The Adverse Childhood Experiences (ACE) Study. *American Journal of Preventive Medicine* 1998; 14(4): 245–258.
30. Macfie J, Cicchetti D, Toth SL. Dissociation in maltreated versus nonmaltreated preschool-aged children. *Child Abuse & Neglect* 2001; 25(9): 1253–1267.
31. Kessler RC, McLaughlin KA, Green JG, Gruber MJ, Sampson NA, Zaslavsky AM, et al. Childhood adversities and adult psychopathology in the WHO World Mental Health Surveys. *The British Journal of Psychiatry* 2010; 197(5): 378–385.
32. Pembrey M, Saffery R. Human transgenerational responses to early-life experience: Potential impact on development, health and biomedical research. *Journal of Medical Genetics* 2014; 51(9): 563–572.
33. Klengel T, Binder EB. Epigenetics of stress-related psychiatric disorders and gene x environment interactions. *Neuron* 2015; 86(6): 1343–1357.
34. Heim C, Binder EB. Current research trends in early life stress and depression: Review of human studies on sensitive periods, gene-environment interactions, and epigenetics. *Experimental Neurology* 2012; 233(1): 102–111.
35. Andersen SL, Teicher MH. Stress, sensitive periods and maturational events in adolescent depression. *Trends in Neurosciences* 2008; 31(4): 183–191.
36. Khan A, McCormack HC, Bolger EA, McGreenery CE, Vitaliano G, Polcari A, et al. Childhood maltreatment, depression, and suicidal ideation: Critical importance of parental and peer emotional abuse during developmental sensitive periods in males and females. *Frontiers in Psychiatry* 2015; 6: 42.
37. Belsky J, Pluess M. Beyond risk, resilience, and dysregulation: Phenotypic plasticity and human development. *Development and Psychopathology* 2013; 25(4 Pt 2): 1243–1261.
38. Frans O, Rimmo PA, Aberg L, Fredrikson M. Trauma exposure and post-traumatic stress disorder in the general population. *Acta Psychiatrica Scandinavica* 2005; 111(4): 291–299.
39. Sartor CE, Grant JD, Lynskey MT, McCutcheon VV, Waldron M, Statham DJ, et al. Common heritable contributions to low-risk trauma, high-risk trauma, posttraumatic stress disorder, and major depression. *Archives of General Psychiatry* 2012; 69(3): 293–299.

40. Digangi J, Guffanti G, McLaughlin KA, Koenen KC. Considering trauma exposure in the context of genetics studies of posttraumatic stress disorder: A systematic review. *Biology of Mood & Anxiety Disorders* 2013; 3(1): 2.
41. Xie P, Kranzler HR, Poling J, Stein MB, Anton RF, Brady K, et al. Interactive effect of stressful life events and the serotonin transporter 5-HTTLPR genotype on posttraumatic stress disorder diagnosis in 2 independent populations. *Archives of General Psychiatry* 2009; 66(11): 1201–1209.
42. Kolassa IT, Ertl V, Eckart C, Glockner F, Kolassa S, Papassotiropoulos A, et al. Association study of trauma load and SLC6A4 promoter polymorphism in posttraumatic stress disorder: Evidence from survivors of the Rwandan genocide. *Journal of Clinical Psychiatry* 2010; 71(5): 543–547.
43. Kilpatrick DG, Koenen KC, Ruggiero KJ, Acierno R, Galea S, Resnick HS, et al. The serotonin transporter genotype and social support and moderation of posttraumatic stress disorder and depression in hurricane-exposed adults. *The American Journal of Psychiatry* 2007; 164(11): 1693–1699.
44. Grabe HJ, Spitzer C, Schwahn C, Marcinek A, Frahnow A, Barnow S et al. Serotonin transporter gene (SLC6A4) promoter polymorphisms and the susceptibility to posttraumatic stress disorder in the general population. *The American Journal of Psychiatry* 2009; 166(8): 926–933.
45. Koenen KC, Amstadter AB, Nugent NR. Gene-environment interaction in posttraumatic stress disorder: An update. *Journal of Traumatic Stress* 2009; 22(5): 416–426.
46. Mercer KB, Orcutt HK, Quinn JF, Fitzgerald CA, Conneely KN, Barfield RT, et al. Acute and posttraumatic stress symptoms in a prospective gene x environment study of a university campus shooting. *Archives of General Psychiatry* 2012; 69(1): 89–97.
47. Pietrzak RH, Galea S, Southwick SM, Gelernter J. Examining the relation between the serotonin transporter 5-HTTPLR genotype x trauma exposure interaction on a contemporary phenotypic model of posttraumatic stress symptomatology: A pilot study. *Journal of Affective Disorders* 2013; 148(1): 123–128.
48. Liu Y, Garrett ME, Dennis MF, Green KT, Workgroup VAM-AMR, Ashley-Koch AE, et al. An examination of the association between 5-HTTLPR, combat exposure, and PTSD diagnosis among U.S. veterans. *PloS One* 2015; 10(3): e0119998.
49. Tian Y, Liu H, Guse L, Wong TK, Li J, Bai Y, et al. Association of genetic factors and gene-environment interactions with risk of developing posttraumatic stress disorder in a case-control study. *Biological Research for Nursing* 2015; 17(4): 364–372.
50. Xie P, Kranzler HR, Poling J, Stein MB, Anton RF, Farrer LA, et al. Interaction of FKBP5 with childhood adversity on risk for post-traumatic stress disorder. *Neuropsychopharmacology* 2010; 35(8): 1684–1692.
51. Nelson EC, Agrawal A, Pergadia ML, Lynskey MT, Todorov AA, Wang JC, et al. Association of childhood trauma exposure and GABRA2 polymorphisms with risk of posttraumatic stress disorder in adults. *Molecular Psychiatry* 2009; 14(3): 234–235.
52. Amstadter AB, Koenen KC, Ruggiero KJ, Acierno R, Galea S, Kilpatrick DG, et al. Variant in RGS2 moderates posttraumatic stress symptoms following potentially traumatic event exposure. *Journal of Anxiety Disorders* 2009; 23(3): 369–373.
53. Kolassa IT, Kolassa S, Ertl V, Papassotiropoulos A, De Quervain DJ. The risk of posttraumatic stress disorder after trauma depends on traumatic load and the catechol-o-methyltransferase Val(158) Met polymorphism. *Biological Psychiatry* 2010; 67(4): 304–308.
54. Lyons MJ, Genderson M, Grant MD, Logue M, Zink T, McKenzie R, et al. Gene-environment interaction of ApoE genotype and combat exposure on PTSD. *American Journal of Medical Genetics. Part B, Neuropsychiatric Genetics* 2013; 162B(7): 762–769.
55. Kimbrel NA, Hauser MA, Garrett M, Ashley-Koch A, Liu Y, Dennis MF, et al. Effect of the APOE epsilon4 allele and combat exposure on PTSD among Iraq/Afghanistan-era veterans. *Depression and Anxiety* 2015; 32(5): 307–315.
56. Feldman R, Vengrober A, Ebstein RP. Affiliation buffers stress: Cumulative genetic risk in oxytocin-vasopressin genes combines with early caregiving to predict PTSD in war-exposed young children. *Translational Psychiatry* 2014; 4: e370.
57. Almli LM, Srivastava A, Fani N, Kerley K, Mercer KB, Feng H, et al. Follow-up and extension of a prior genome-wide association study of posttraumatic stress disorder: Gene x environment associations and structural magnetic resonance imaging in a highly traumatized African-American civilian population. *Biological Psychiatry* 2014; 76(4): e3–4.
58. Uddin M, Chang SC, Zhang C, Ressler K, Mercer KB, Galea S, et al. Adcyap1r1 genotype, posttraumatic stress disorder, and depression among women exposed to childhood maltreatment. *Depression and Anxiety* 2013; 30(3): 251–258.
59. Caspi A, Sugden K, Moffitt TE, Taylor A, Craig IW, Harrington H, et al. Influence of life stress

on depression: Moderation by a polymorphism in the 5-HTT gene 109. *Science* 2003; 301(5631): 386–389.
60. Caspi A, McClay J, Moffitt TE, Mill J, Martin J, Craig IW, et al. Role of genotype in the cycle of violence in maltreated children. *Science* 2002; 297(5582): 851–854.
61. Hornung OP, Heim CM. Gene-environment interactions and intermediate phenotypes: early trauma and depression. Frontiers in endocrinology 2014; 5: 14.
62. Lesch KP, Bengel D, Heils A, Sabol SZ, Greenberg BD, Petri S, et al. Association of anxiety-related traits with a polymorphism in the serotonin transporter gene regulatory region 5. *Science* 1996; 274(5292): 1527–1531.
63. Risch N, Herrell R, Lehner T, Liang KY, Eaves L, Hoh J, et al. Interaction between the serotonin transporter gene (5-HTTLPR), stressful life events, and risk of depression: A meta-analysis. *JAMA* 2009; 301(23): 2462–2471.
64. Karg K, Burmeister M, Shedden K, Sen S. The serotonin transporter promoter variant (5-HTTLPR), stress, and depression meta-analysis revisited: Evidence of genetic moderation. *Archives of General Psychiatry* 2011; 68(5): 444–454.
65. Koenen KC, Aiello AE, Bakshis E, Amstadter AB, Ruggiero KJ, Acierno R, et al. Modification of the association between serotonin transporter genotype and risk of posttraumatic stress disorder in adults by county-level social environment. *American Journal of Epidemiology* 2009; 169(6): 704–711.
66. Walsh K, Uddin M, Soliven R, Wildman DE, Bradley B. Associations between the SS variant of 5-HTTLPR and PTSD among adults with histories of childhood emotional abuse: Results from two African American independent samples. *Journal of Affective Disorders* 2014; 161: 91–96.
67. Zannas AS, Binder EB. Gene-environment interactions at the FKBP5 locus: Sensitive periods, mechanisms and pleiotropism. *Genes, Brain and Behavior* 2014; 13(1): 25–37.
68. Klengel T, Mehta D, Anacker C, Rex-Haffner M, Pruessner JC, Pariante CM, et al. Allele-specific FKBP5 DNA demethylation mediates gene-childhood trauma interactions. *Nature Neuroscience* 2013; 16(1): 33–41.
69. Teh AL, Pan H, Chen L, Ong ML, Dogra S, Wong J, et al. The effect of genotype and in utero environment on interindividual variation in neonate DNA methylomes. *Genome Research* 2014; 24(7): 1064–1074.
70. Kraft P, Hunter D. *The challenge of assessing complex gene–gene and gene–environment interactions.* New York: Oxford University Press; 2010.
71. Adkins DE, Clark SL, Aberg K, Hettema JM, Bukszar J, McClay JL, et al. Genome-wide pharmacogenomic study of citalopram-induced side effects in STAR*D. *Translational Psychiatry* 2012; 2: e129.
72. Cherlyn SY, Woon PS, Liu JJ, Ong WY, Tsai GC, Sim K. Genetic association studies of glutamate, GABA and related genes in schizophrenia and bipolar disorder: A decade of advance. *Neuroscience and Biobehavioral Reviews* 2010; 34(6): 958–977.
73. Moya PR, Dodman NH, Timpano KR, Rubenstein LM, Rana Z, Fried RL, et al. Rare missense neuronal cadherin gene (CDH2) variants in specific obsessive-compulsive disorder and Tourette disorder phenotypes. *European Journal of Human Genetics* 2013; 21(8): 850–854.
74. Kraft P, Yen YC, Stram DO, Morrison J, Gauderman WJ. Exploiting gene-environment interaction to detect genetic associations. *Human Heredity* 2007; 63(2): 111–119.
75. Maity A. Testing in semiparametric models with interaction, with applications to gene-environment interactions. *Journal of the Royal Statistical Society, Series B* 2009; 71: 75–96.
76. Hein R, Beckmann L, Chang-Claude J. Sample size requirements for indirect association studies of gene-environment interactions (G x E). *Genetic Epidemiology* 2008; 32(3): 235–245.
77. Wong M, Day N, Luan J, Chan, K. The detection of gene–environment interaction for continuous traits: Should we deal with measurement error by bigger studies or better measurement? *International Journal of Epidemiology* 2003; 32(Pt 1): 51–57.
78. Mukherjee B, Ahn J, Gruber SB, Chatterjee N. Testing gene-environment interaction in large-scale case-control association studies: Possible choices and comparisons. *American Journal of Epidemiology* 2012; 175(3): 177–190.
79. Boonstra PS, Mukherjee B, Gruber SB, Ahn J, Schmit SL, Chatterjee N. Tests for gene-environment interactions and joint effects with exposure misclassification. *American Journal of Epidemiology* 2016; 183(3): 237–247.
80. Keller MC. Gene x environment interaction studies have not properly controlled for potential confounders: The problem and the (simple) solution. *Biological Psychiatry* 2014; 75(1): 18–24.
81. Duncan LE, Keller MC. A critical review of the first 10 years of candidate gene-by-environment interaction research in psychiatry. *The American Journal of Psychiatry* 2011; 168(10): 1041–1049.
82. Brewin CR, Andrews B, Gotlib IH. Psychopathology and early experience: A reappraisal of retrospective reports. *Psychological Bulletin* 1993; 113(1): 82–98.

18

Trauma in the Medical-Surgical Patient

NADIA QUIJIJE

PSYCHIATRY CONSULTATION FOR TRAUMA AND STRESS IN MEDICAL-SURGICAL PATIENTS

Hospitalization is a stressful event which may enhance recovery from illness and enhance patients' resilience or induce psychologic or psychiatric disturbance and worsen the clinical condition of patients who are suffering from medical and surgical comorbidities.[1] Hospitals can elicit significant stress in patients, since they can be very hectic and scary environments, far from home, with rapid influx of unfamiliar faces, venipuncture, insertions of IVs, Foley catheters, infusions of medications and fluids, administration of new medications, imaging and tests, and complex and confusing medical information. [2] This stress is further accentuated when patients are critically ill, with delusions and hallucinations from delirium and requiring invasive and extensive interventions in the intensive care unit (ICU) setting.[3] Prolonged and complex hospitalization can also lead to sequelae of chronic stress and demoralization, from prolonged periods of time being ill, hospitalized, in pain, away from support, or adjusting to new deconditioning or physical limitation.[4] Transitions from hospital to home affect the lives of families in ways that may affect patient outcomes post-discharge.[5] The consultation liaison psychiatrist brings special expertise to medical-surgical settings with knowledge of the neurobiology of trauma- and stressor-related disorders including posttraumatic stress disorder (PTSD), their biopsychosocial foundations,[6,7,8] and the presenting medical-surgical illnesses of hospitalized patients and their treatments. Co-management with a consultation liaison psychiatrist can have beneficial impacts on the length of hospital stays, reduction of stressors and patient stress, and overall patient well-being.[9]

In the outpatient setting, the patient-centered primary care collaborative model of care consisting of medical, surgical, and psychiatric providers, along with case managers and other staff, can favorably prevent or reduce stress, lower readmission rates and emergency room utilization,[10,11] and improve access of outpatient medical and psychiatric care for patients with comorbid medical and psychiatric illness.[12]

ENVIRONMENT AND CIRCUMSTANCES OF PATIENTS IN MEDICAL-SURGICAL SETTINGS

Diaphoretic, with difficulty breathing, and feeling so weak speech can barely be uttered, a mild levitation is felt and then a thump into a hard surface. Awakening to beeps, cold fluid entering the arms, and two unknown faces appearing from above you calling out your name. You look around to note more unfamiliar walls, ceiling, and suddenly feel a cold round metal appearing object over your chest. Afraid and confused, you began pushing this cold thing away and try to get up, only to be held by more unfamiliar faces, and suddenly feel more fluid running into your arms and fall back asleep.

According to the 2012 National Health Care Expenses in the U.S. Civilian Noninstitutionalized Population, there were 36.5 million hospital stays in the United States, with an average cost of $10,400 per stay,[13] and stays may be extended due to patient stress or stressful experiences interfering with recovery. The cost makes the need to properly evaluate, diagnose, and treat such individuals a major public health mandate and priority to assure appropriate use of fiscal resources. Psychosomatic medicine, or consultation liaison psychiatry, focuses on the diagnosis and treatment of psychiatric disorders and symptoms in complex medically and surgically ill patients in inpatient and outpatient settings.

Specialists in psychosomatic medicine help patients and their care providers with comorbid psychiatric and physical conditions, most of which include severe stress either before the episode of illness, as a result of it, or both.[14]

Case Example
Adjustment Disorder Secondary to Crohn's Disease

A 23-year-old female with recent a diagnosis of Crohn's disease is referred to psychiatry by her gastroenterologist for noncompliance with her immune modulators and concern for a depressive disorder contributing. On evaluation, the patient describes frustration with having to take medications at such a young age, disliking her dietary limitations, and embarrassment of frequent trips to the bathroom. She denies any symptoms consistent with a major depressive disorder but rather complains of low mood, tearfulness, and intermittent hopelessness secondary to the diagnosis of a chronic medical illness and dramatic lifestyle change. This is causing her marked distress and impacting her social functioning.

Comment: This case is an example of a patient having an adjustment disorder directly related to her gastrointestinal (GI) disease, as well as social and psychological sequelae of having a chronic GI disease such as Crohn's.

Additional examples of cases encountered by psychosomatic physicians include treatment of major depressive disorder in an elderly male after a myocardial infarction who is not participating in cardiac rehabilitation; opioid withdrawal in a young pregnant female; panic symptoms in an elderly male with chronic obstructive pulmonary disease (COPD) who just received news of permanently needing supplemental oxygen; catatonia in a middle-aged female with breast cancer complicated by paraneoplastic syndrome; delirium tremens in a young male with multiple orthopedic fractures status post-motor vehicle accident; comanagement of a young female with HIV and antiretroviral noncompliance in the outpatient setting; or psychotic adverse effects from initiation of dopamine agonist in a patient with Parkinson's disease. Psychosomatic physicians work in primary care and outpatient specialty clinics (such as infectious disease or transplant clinics), inpatient medical surgical floors, and ICUs.

The literature suggests that health professionals in nonpsychiatric settings find the complex care of these patients challenging, and consequently the patient's experience of care can be poor.[15,16] Early detection and treatment of psychological distress and psychiatric disorders, including trauma- and stressor-related disorders in individuals with a comorbid medical and surgical disorder, are known to reduce health care costs significantly.[17] Consultation liaison psychiatrists are specially trained to have an extensive clinical understanding of medical-surgical disorders and their relation to abnormal illness behavior and able to develop an effective treatment plan. [18] The psychosomatic psychiatrist is also trained to supervise a multidisciplinary team and work in a collaborative fashion with colleagues within the various medical surgical specialties, nurses, social workers, and all members of the patient's team, as well as the patient's support system.[19] Among the goals of collaboration are to manage patients' anxiety and stress and to reduce unnecessary stress.

ACUTE AND PRIOR TRAUMA IN MEDICAL-SURGICAL PATIENTS

Childhood trauma can be associated with poor clinical outcomes.[20] Therefore, early recognition of premorbid trauma- and stressor-related disorders are important to ensure early therapeutic interventions to improve outcomes.[21] PTSD is common in survivors of critical illness and ICU treatment. [22]

Case Example
PTSD Secondary to ICU Survival and Delirium in a Patient with Childhood Trauma

A 57-year-old female with a pertinent history of coronary artery disease status post three vessel coronary artery bypass grafting was referred by her primary care physician for psychiatric evaluation and management of possible PTSD from her recent complex and prolonged ICU experience. The patient describes how, for the past six weeks, she has been experiencing distressing nightmares of being "tied down with a tube in my mouth" that awakens her from sleep with palpitations, diaphoresis, and shortness of breath. She relays that since being discharged from the hospital four weeks prior, she has been feeling "on edge," irritable, and having "flashing memories" of being in restraints, feeling afraid and confused. She expressed embarrassment when her family described some of her behaviors during her prolonged delirious state while hospitalized. Prior this hospitalization, she denies having any of these symptoms but, on thorough evaluation, endorsed a childhood history of witnessing trauma while growing up in a war-torn town in Cambodia.

Comment: This vignette demonstrates the development of stress-related symptoms from a traumatically experienced ICU stay, with additional vulnerability to a stressor-related disorder secondary to historic trauma.

Estimates of PTSD prevalence in critically ill cohorts are reported to be as high as 63%[23] and may be secondary to critical illness being uniquely stressful from factors associated with the ICU, such as awareness during painful procedures, a sense of helplessness, loss of control, and an imminent threat of death. [24] Modifiable risk factors that exist during the patient's ICU stay may include frightening hallucinations, paranoid delusions, and episodes of extreme agitation. Medications administered in the ICU, particularly benzodiazepines, may play a significant role in pathogenesis of post-ICU PTSD, and minimizing sedatives seems to reduce the occurrence of PTSD symptoms without evidence of patient harm. Psychological distress manifested by anxiety and/or acute stress symptoms is an important marker of post-ICU PTSD risk, warranting attention from providers caring for patients who have survived critical illness before they are discharged from the hospital. [25] Risk factors for medically related PTSD are similar to those for PTSD in general: a history of psychiatric illness or trauma, limited or absent social support, early childhood separation from parents, and family history of trauma- or stressor-related disorders. [26]Given the negative impact of PTSD on patients' quality of life, it is important for clinicians to diagnose PTSD in survivors of critical illness so as to ensure that they receive targeted therapies.[27]

STRESS DISORDER SECONDARY TO MEDICAL OR SURGICAL TREATMENT

Modern intensive care medicine has led to increased survival rates even after severe life-threatening medical conditions. Treatment on ICUs is associated with high long-term rates of depressive, anxiety, and posttraumatic stress disorders.[28] Correlations with increased somatic morbidity and mortality, persisting cognitive impairments, and significant deficits in health-related quality of life must also be taken into consideration. A history of premorbid depression, sociodemographic and socioeconomic risk variables, age, female sex, personality traits, the underlying pathophysiological condition requiring ICU treatment, mode of sedation and analgesia, life support measures, such as mechanical ventilation, and multifold traumatic experience during the stay in the ICU are all particularly important risk factors for development of stress-related symptoms.

Several strategies such as optimized sedation and analgesia, special prophylactic medication (i.e., morphine [29,30]) for pain regarding the major risk of traumatic memories, psychological, and psychotherapeutic interventions in states of increased acute stress symptoms and aids for personal memories and reorientation all can reduce aforementioned modifiable risk factors.[31]

Case Example
Patient with Major Depression and Myocardial Infarction Who Experienced PTSD from Cardioversion

A 75-year-old male Vietnam veteran with a history of major depressive disorder, myocardial infarction, atrial fibrillation, congestive heart failure with ICD implant eight months ago is medically admitted for medical stabilization after five consecutive shocks, last in the emergency room. Psychiatry is consulted for insomnia and severe anxiety prompting request to turn off the device. Upon entering the room, he is visibly nervous, sitting on the edge of his bed, appearing to startle on knocking the door. He reports feeling extremely fearful of a repeat shock, having sleep disturbance the past two nights while in the hospital secondary to these fears preventing him from falling sleep, but also awakening from light sleep secondary to a nightmare of his recent shocks. He reports feeling more irritable, edgy, easily startled, and very distressed talking about it (begins crying at this point), and for the past two days having death wishes but no active suicidal ideations or plans. He also feels confused and further distressed by recurring memories of combat while a soldier in Vietnam. He has had no PTSD symptoms in over 20 years.

Comment: This is an example of a patient with premorbid major depressive disorder and PTSD, both remitted, who had an acute traumatic experience from a medical etiology (the electric shock of his ICD), now relaying and demonstrating symptoms of acute stress disorder. His premorbid psychiatric affective and stressor-related disorders placed him at elevated risk for recurrence of his PTSD. He had an excellent response to initiation of Prazosin 1mg po qHS and slow increasing titration (increments of 25mg every week) of sertraline 25mg PO daily to target of 100mg po daily with improved sleep and reduced PTSD and depressive symptoms.

POSTTRAUMATIC AND DEPRESSIVE SYMPTOMS WITH DELIRIUM

PTSD and depression may accompany delirium, which is an acute and usually transient severe neuropsychiatric syndrome associated with significant long-term physical morbidity. A systematic literature search uncovered the prevalence of depressive symptoms was almost three times higher in patients with delirium than in patients without delirium, there was no statistically significant difference between the prevalence of anxiety symptoms between patients with and without delirium, and the prevalence of PTSD symptoms after delirium was inconclusive.[32] In a prospective survey of patients six months status post-discharge from the ICU, 30% of the sample demonstrated depression, and 13% reported symptoms reflective of posttraumatic stress symptoms. Higher posttraumatic stress symptoms scores were independently associated with frightening experiences in ICU, higher stress and depression scores, pain intensity at baseline, and sleep quality at six months.[33]

PTSD WITH PERSONALITY DISORDER IN THE MEDICAL-SURGICAL SETTING

Individuals with a personality disorder display rigid and maladaptive thinking and reacting behaviors that often disrupt their personal, professional, and social lives.[34] These inflexible patterns of managing the world can be disruptive when an individual is admitted to the hospital, causing distress for both the patient who lacks the skills to deal with the expectations of the hospital environment and the treatment team who can feel ill equipped to manage such behavior. Having a personality disorder has implications for an individual's health care outcomes; those with a personality disorder have a life expectancy nearly two decades shorter than the general population for a multitude of reasons, among them trouble interacting with the health care system. Although a diagnosis of a specific personality disorder may be difficult to make on an acute care unit, identification of dysfunctional personality structures can provide opportunity for better management of an individual's medical and psychological needs.[35]

Childhood trauma, especially emotional, is associated with the development of maladaptive personality traits in later childhood and adulthood.[36] A specific relationship between childhood emotional abuse and the occurrence of borderline personality disorder (BPD) may be mediated by anxious adult attachment. [37] This can come into play with this patient population, given how hospitalization can be experienced as a traumatic stress, induced by frequently rotating medical providers, dynamic medical etiologies, and unintentional stripping of independence by the dynamic of the hospital setting. Patients with BPD have increased rates of the use of medical services, including some for deliberate self-harm, which is helpful to bear in mind when caring for this patient population on the medical-surgical floor.[38] Patients admitted for deliberate self-harm, which is correlated with lifetime abuse,[39] provide a challenge for medical, surgical, and psychological management. In a retrospective review over 11 years, Conlin et al. discovered that patients who have suffered deliberate self-harm by burning have more severe burn injuries and require longer, resource-intensive hospital stays.[40] It is, therefore, important to keep in mind and optimize management of potential stressor-related and other psychiatric disorders that may be premorbid or ensue in this population.

ADJUSTMENT DISORDER

Adjustment disorders, as defined in Chapter 2, that develop secondary to coping difficulties with acute or chronic medical/surgical traumatic stressors, or social/psychological sequelae of organic etiologies, can further impair medical/surgical care in the hospital and after discharge. In a multisite, cohort study of injured patients assessed during hospitalization and at 3 and 12 months postinjury, the prevalence of adjustment disorder was 19% at 3 months and 16% at 12 months, indicating its chronicity. Participants with adjustment disorder reported worse outcomes relative to those with no psychiatric diagnosis but better outcomes compared with those diagnosed with other psychiatric disorders. Participants with adjustment disorder at 3 months postinjury were significantly more likely to meet criteria for a psychiatric disorder at 12 months.[41]

Case Example
Adjustment Disorder to Diagnosis of Metastatic Cancer

A 38-year-old female with no prior medical or psychiatric history presented to the emergency room with unremitting shortness of breath and palpitations and was found to have a pulmonary embolus and incidental pulmonary nodules on CT scan. After her medical work-up, she was found to have stage IV breast cancer with metastasis to the lungs. Despite excellent support from family, friends, and meetings with chaplain, she was intermittently found by nurses on the floor to be crying and expressing hopelessness. Psychiatry was consulted for assessment of emotional dysregulation during which she endorsed feeling very sad, worried about being away from her two children ages 10 and 8, anger that she had this disease despite leading a healthy lifestyle, difficulty falling asleep and frequent interrupted sleep, hopelessness, and feeling trapped and overwhelmed. Psychiatry and social work met with the patient twice per week for supportive therapy, which appeared to ameliorate her symptoms.

Comment: This patient is endorsing acute onset emotional symptoms (sad, worried, angry, insomnia, overwhelmed) temporally correlated with identifiable stressor, diagnosis of metastatic cancer. Given the aforementioned was causing a significant level of subjective distress, the patient meets criteria for an adjustment disorder with mixed anxious and depressed mood. The treatment is supportive therapy while the external stressor continues and monitoring of symptoms to assure the condition does not advance to syndromal depressive or anxiety disorder. Psychotropics such as selective serotonin reuptake inhibitors are not indicated in an adjustment disorder.

MANAGEMENT OF TRAUMA- AND STRESSOR-RELATED DISORDERS IN INPATIENT AND OUTPATIENT SETTINGS

As already described, there are many different forms of trauma experienced by the medical surgical patient, and this is particularly accentuated in the burns and trauma surgery population. Unique issues of traumatic brain injury (TBI), spinal cord injury, pain, amputations, body image, substance use disorders, and violence are some of the additional stressors that this patient population faces which are optimally comanaged by a psychiatrist.[42] Collaborative care interventions that incorporate evidence-based motivational interviewing targeting alcohol use, as well as pharmacotherapy and psychotherapy targeting PTSD, may reduce both alcohol and PTSD symptoms among injured trauma surgery patients, including adolescents.[43,44]

Case Example
Patient with Prior PTSD, Substance Abuse and Withdrawal, and Multiple Traumatic Injuries after a Suicide Attempt

A 23-year-old female with no pertinent medical or surgical history, a psychiatric history of opioid use disorder, PTSD, and self-injurious behaviors (superficial cutting) is admitted after she was seen jumping off a third-story balcony, resulting in polytrauma injuries of pelvic fracture, right ankle fracture, right rib fractures, and right frontal subdural hematoma. Toxicology was positive for opiates, benzodiazepines, and cannabis. Psychiatry was consulted for management of potential opiate and sedative hypnotic withdrawal, management of agitation needing physical restraints, and safety assessment given her presenting state.

Comment: This case with multiple psychiatric disorders potentially leading to severe posttraumatic sequelae illustrates the need for a multimodal approach, first targeting pressing etiologies such as opiate and other drug withdrawal and acute agitation. Then recurrence of prior psychiatric disorders, especially stressor-related disorders, must be kept in mind in order to screen for new onset stressor-related (given higher risk for developing acute stress disorder as previously described) symptoms. Additionally, careful assessment for and acute treatment of any severe psychiatric disorder (affective or psychotic disorders) which may have been the precursor to her critical presentation must be done since there is an association of patients presenting with violence or suicide attempt (as in this case) and increased morbidity and mortality after discharge.

PTSD and Severe Psychiatric Disorders in Inpatient Medical Settings

Severity of affective and psychotic disorders has been associated with hospital-related PTSD symptoms and overall development of stress related syndromes.[45,46] Additionally, a recent study by Zatzick et al. demonstrated association between comorbid psychiatric, substance use, and general medical disorders/TBI with violent events or suicide attempts, and postinjury outcomes of recurrent hospitalization and death.[47]

In a retrospective cohort study conducted at San Francisco General Hospital, 70% of those who committed suicide had a traumatic mechanism of death. During the same two-year period, 2% of the trauma patients admitted to San Francisco General Hospital sustained intentional self-inflicted wounds and 18% of patients with intentional self-inflicted injury died after arrival.[48] Some risk factors found to be associated with repeat suicide attempts were younger age, prior attempts, family history of suicide, and schizophrenia. Identifying patients with these risk factors and ensuring that they receive evaluation for PTSD, substance abuse treatment,[49] and connection with sustained psychiatric treatment may prevent repeat suicide attempts.[50]

Secondary PTSD in Health Care Workers

An increased focus is emerging on PTSD and trauma- and stressor- related disorders, or secondary traumatic stress[51,52] among providers who care for trauma injured patients. A recent system-wide survey was applied to prehospital and in-hospital care providers including paramedics, nurses, trauma surgeons, emergency medicine physicians, and residents. High proportions of health care workers were found to be at risk for secondary traumatic stress and PTSD across all professional groups. Therefore, psychiatrists caring for trauma-injured patients should also keep in mind the extreme stress experienced by colleagues and staff comanaging trauma patients, facilitating referrals of staff when needed.[53,54]

Violence, Social Stressors, and Legal Issues

Violence, social stressors, and legal issues are also unique characteristics found on the burns and trauma surgery patient population. Social determinants of health are identifiable root causes of medical problems[55] and also stress-related disorders. Historical trauma is a collective trauma inflicted on a group of people who share an identity or affiliation and is often characterized by the transgenerational legacy of traumatic experiences, especially in situations of political and social violence and expressed through various psychological and social responses.[56]Traumatic events are ubiquitous exposures that interact with life course events to increase risk of acute psychopathology and alter mental health trajectories. While the majority of people exposed to trauma experience mild to moderate psychological distress followed by a return to pretrauma health, some people experience significant distress that lasts for several years. Trauma-related psychopathology involves the interplay of genetics, neurobiology, individual psychology, and social determinants.[57]

PTSD, Pain, and Addiction

Undertreatment of pain in the acute medical surgical setting with children of all ages and with adults can contribute to psychiatric and physical morbidity in the acute medical surgical setting,[58] since early opiate treatment of pain is associated with reduced PTSD at follow-up.[59] Undertreatment is particularly challenging in patients with comorbid opioid use disorder who will have a higher tolerance for opiates and will need higher than usual doses of opiates as well as adjunctive forms of analgesia.[60] Additionally, patients with substance use disorders commonly have history of childhood trauma, which will increase the risk of this patient population developing a stress-related disorder to their acute trauma, therefore screening and acute treatment is crucial.[61,62] However, continuation of prescribed opiates and other analgesics contribute significantly to substance abuse and addiction.[63,64] Grant et al.[65] identified significant comorbidity of substance use disorders and PTSD, mood, anxiety, and personality disorders. The neurobiology of stress and addiction overlap, especially the stress of withdrawal. In 2012 approximately 2.1 million people in the United States had substance use disorders related to prescription opioid pain relievers, and 467,000 were addicted to heroin. The age of first use of heroin is decreasing, and in 2009, 250,000 US high school students, or 1.2%, had used heroin at least once.[66,67] Lessons learned from the Joint Commission's Pain Standards which increased opiate prescribing[68] are influencing a call to end the opioid epidemic in the United States with improved evaluation and treatment of pain and improved monitoring for and treatment of addiction.[69]

PTSD with Traumatic Brain Injury

Acute neuropsychiatric disturbances including PTSD[70] associated with brain injury can disrupt acute necessary medical treatment and rehabilitation therapies and contribute to functional impairment if they are not appropriately treated.

Behavioral problems in particular are challenging; therefore, in an effort to assure necessary comprehensive treatment, while keeping patients and staff safe, a multidisciplinary approach including psychiatric management is recommended in patients with brain injury.[71] Major depressive disorder and PTSD are prevalent after TBI.[72] Multiple psychiatric, substance use, and chronic general medical disorders are prevalent among injury survivors with and without TBI. Zatzick et al. studied patients hospitalized for an injury and assessed associations between comorbid psychiatric, substance use, and general medical disorders, TBI, and violent events or suicide attempts and the postinjury outcomes of recurrent hospitalization and death. They found increasing cumulative burden of disorders was associated with greater postinjury risk of recurrent hospitalization and death. Screening and intervention procedures that target this spectrum of comorbidities, therefore, is pertinent to decrease post-injury morbidity and mortality.[73]

Amputations

Amputations can provoke psychological trauma, especially PTSD secondary to their cosmetic and functional impacts, often causing disfigurement and disability. Psychiatric and psychological issues of grief, denial, depression, PTSD, and other stressor-related disorders, and pain (including phantom limb pain) may arise.[74,75,76] Multiple studies document high rates of PTSD and posttraumatic symptomatology in children and adults who have had hand or limb amputations, with rates varying from 25% to 52% with full syndrome PTSD, more with posttraumatic stress symptoms, and with posttraumatic symptoms being severe and persistent for up to 10 years in as many as 30% of those with PTSD.[77,78,79] Few are referred to mental health professionals.[80]

PTSD and Burns

While the majority of patients with burn injuries have good clinical outcomes and demonstrate resilience with modern treatment,[81] the presence of psychiatric disorders is associated with poor clinical outcomes and longer hospitalization, decreased survival, and increased complication rates. Premorbid psychopathology, substance abuse, and age were associated with a higher incidence of acute psychiatric disorder after burn than was the severity of the burn wound itself. Routine screening for psychological symptoms of acute psychiatric disorder should be performed in all burn patients to avoid increased rates of short- and long-term morbidity and mortality.[82] In a longitudinal study of psychopathology among burns patient, it was found that posttraumatic, depression, and anxiety symptoms showed a general decreasing tendency across time. At six months, 20% of patients showed clinically significant PTSD symptoms, as assessed with the MINI Neuropsychiatric Interview, somewhat lower than in other studies of burns and other injuries.[83,84] Within this group of patients, anxiety, depression, and hyperarousal increased at 30 days, and avoidance 90 days after injury.[85] Considering the aforementioned facts, preventive interventions, acute treatment, and adequate psychiatric follow-up is warranted to minimize the psychological consequences of burns, but this is provided in only a minority of burn centers.[86]

Body Image

In medical patients, body image, both self-perception and physical functioning, is affected, often for the better, by general medical care and subspecialty care in neurology, general internal medicine, cardiology, pulmonary medicine, gastroenterology, pediatrics, women's medicine, urology, and physical medicine (physiatry). In surgical patients, body image including self-perception and physical functioning is affected by many types of surgery including pediatric surgery, general surgery, obstetrics and gynecology, urology, orthopedics, ophthalmology, otolaryngology, head and neck surgery, cardiac and pulmonary surgeries, trauma surgery, cosmetic and plastic surgery, and subspecialities. For patients with visible or invisible body changes, such as burns, amputation, or disfiguring traumas, body image dissatisfaction may be socially and functionally impairing.[87,88] Social skills training, cognitive behavioral interventions,[89] and psychotherapeutic groups[90] in conjunction with cosmetic and surgical interventions can be beneficial in improving self-image and resulting quality of life.[91] In breast cancer, mastectomy and breast reconstruction treatment can sometimes lead to mutilation and destruction of breast shape with negative effects on body image and self-esteem.[92] Reconstructive and oncoplastic breast surgery is used to satisfy patients and significantly improves their quality of life as well as psychosocial well-being and physical functioning.[93]

Management

Psychotherapeutic Management

Injured patients presenting to acute care medical settings have high rates of PTSD and comorbidities, such as depression and substance use disorders, with population-based surveys demonstrating rates between 62% and 92% with depressive disorders, substance use disorders, and anxiety disorders consistently emerging as common PTSD comorbidities.[94,95] Integrating behavioral interventions that target symptoms of PTSD, such as cognitive behavioral therapy, has been shown to be feasible and acceptable in post-injury care.[96] For transplant patients who have experienced organ loss, group supportive psychotherapy has been shown to increase levels of hope and self-care. This intervention assisted patients in understanding their own problems and take corrective actions so that they could be accepted by others by exchanging their feelings, thoughts, opinions, and experiences through confrontation and self-exploration both individually and in a group.[97] In hospitalized patients with elevated levels of distress or those expressing a wish for psychosocial support, counseling is offered by a psychotherapist and a social worker within the framework of a liaison service.[98] Supportive psychotherapy in chronically medically ill patients is founded upon the instability of the adaptive processes following the manifestation of chronic disease and patients' frustrations of being ill.[99]

The therapist engages in a fully emotional, encouraging, and supportive relationship with the patient as a method of improving healthy coping skills, especially in the context of acute medical-surgical stressors.

Pharmacological Management in the Hospital Setting

Medications can provide quick relief of impairing symptoms of stress-related disorders that cause distress and can impair participation in medical interventions and rehabilitative services.

Antiadrenergic agents such as prazosin and clonidine can aide in quickly dampening intrusive symptoms such as posttraumatic nightmares and hyperarousal.[100,101] According to one author, atypical antipsychotic medications such as risperidone, quetiapine, and olanzapine have a modest benefit for the treatment of PTSD in medical-surgical care.[102] Evidence is growing to support several psychotherapeutic (as mentioned previously) and pharmacological treatments such as trazodone, mirtazapine, or doxepin to manage the sleep disturbances in PTSD.[103] Mood stabilizers such as topiramate, valproic acid, carbamazepine, and lithium in some patients may be helpful in reducing mood lability and anger outbursts and stabilizing mood.[104]

End-of-Life Care

Trauma- and stressor-related disorders in the patient and among relatives may be prevented by optimal care at the end of life. End-of-life care usually occurs in the midst of varying medical, psychiatric (acute stress, pain, depression, anxiety, coping, delirium), and ethical concerns.[105] Patients, families, physicians, and nurses face stressors and multiple challenges when caring for a dying patient in the hospital but can effectively help a dying patient by ensuring optimal palliative and/or in-hospital hospice care and assisting the family in the dying process. Optimal end-of-life care serves to reduce the likelihood of posttraumatic outcomes in the patient and family at the time of death and afterwards, as well as reduces staff stress.[106] Virdun et al. found particular elements in the end-of-life care that patient's and family describe as most important: effective communication and shared decision-making, respectful and compassionate care, adequate environment for care, family involvement, and attention to financial affairs. Additional family themes were maintenance of patient safety, preparation for death, care extending to the family after the patient's death, and enabling the patient a choice at the end of life.[107,108]

Elizabeth Kubler Ross described the transformational process of dying as stages of denial, anger, bargaining, guilt, and eventual acceptance.[109] Dignity therapy is one type of intervention. It is a short course, usually 30- to 60-minute sessions lasting no more than six months, of psychotherapy that focuses on helping patients with terminal illnesses go over things that are most meaningful to them and document their legacy. This form of therapy has been shown to be feasible to deliver at the bedside and effective in helping patients and their families with comfort care near the end of life and facilitate gaining a sense of meaning and purpose at that time.[110]

CONCLUSION

The Greeks define trauma as a piercing of the skin, a breaking of the bodily envelope. Freud described trauma as a psychic piercing and wounding by events, where the mind is envisioned as a protective shield that is selectively sensitive to external stimuli.[111] Hospitalization itself can induce excess external stimulus that may induce psychologic or psychiatric disturbance and worsen the clinical condition of patients who are suffering from medical and surgical comorbidities. Specialists in psychosomatic medicine help patients and their care providers in managing comorbid psychiatric and physical conditions.[112] Some medical conditions can be related to stress-related disorders indirectly, while others, such as critical illness/ICU treatment or direct physical injury, are likely traumatic stressors that can promote stressor-related disorders. Risk factors for medical illness-related PTSD appear similar to risk factors for PTSD in general: a history of psychiatric illness or of a prior traumatic event, limited social support, early childhood separation from parents, and family history of stress-related disorders.[113] Given the negative impact of stress-related disorders on patients' quality of life, it is important that clinicians in mental health diagnose trauma- and stressor-related disorders in patients with medical and surgical illnesses so as to ensure that they receive the care that they need and deserve. Treatment and management can be provided in multiple forms of psychological therapies and psychopharmacology, and within a multidisciplinary team, particularly for the medical-surgical patient.

Finally, psychiatrists, psychologists, and social workers assist patients with terminal illnesses by optimizing end-of-life care, supporting patients and their families, and encouraging approaches (e.g., dignity therapy, palliative care, or hospice care) to allow the transformative process of dying to be meaningful.

REFERENCES

1. Smith GC. (2009). From consultation-liaison psychiatry to integrated care for multiple and complex needs. *Aust N Z J Psychiatry.* 43(1):1–12. http://dx.doi.org/10.1080/00048670802534358
2. Meister RE, Weber T. (2016). Perception of a hectic hospital environment at admission relates to acute stress disorder symptoms in myocardial infarction patients. *Gen Hosp Psychiatry.* 39:8–14. http://dx.doi.org/10.1016/j.genhosppsych.2015.11.004
3. Morrissey M, Collier E. (2016). Literature review of post-traumatic stress disorder in the critical care population. *J Clin Nurs.* 25(11–12):1501–1514. http://dx.doi.org/10.1111/jocn.13138
4. Clarke DM, Cook KE, Coleman KJ, Smith GC. (2006). A qualitative examination of the experience of "depression" in hospitalized medically ill patients. *Psychopathology.* 39(6):303–312. http://dx.doi.org/10.1159/000095778
5. Solan LG, Beck AF. (2015). The family perspective on hospital to home transitions: A qualitative study. *Pediatrics.* 136(6):e1539–1549. http://dx.doi.org/10.1542/peds.2015-2098.
6. Langeland W, Olff M. (2008). Psychobiology of posttraumatic stress disorder in pediatric injury patients: A review of the literature. *Neurosci Biobehav Rev.* 32:161–174. http://dx.doi.org/10.1016/j.neubiorev.2007.07.002
7. Yehuda R, Hoge CW, McFarlane AC. (2015). Post-traumatic stress disorder. *Nature Rev Dis Primer.* 1(8):1–22. http://dx.doi.org/10.1038/nrdp.2015.57
8. Ross DA, Arbuckle MR, Travis MJ. (2017). An integrated neuroscience perspective on formulation and treatment planning for posttraumatic stress disorder: An educational review. *JAMA Psychiatry.* 74(4):407–415. http://dx.doi.org/10.1001/jamapsychiatry.2016.3325
9. Mays N, Pope C, Popay J. (2005). Systematically reviewing qualitative and quantitative evidence to inform management and policy-making in the health field. *J Health Serv Res Policy.* 10(Suppl 1):6–20. http://dx.doi.org/10.1258/1355819054308576
10. Zatzick D, Rivara F, Jurkovich D. (2011). Enhancing the population impact of collaborative care interventions: Mixed method development and implementation of stepped care targeting posttraumatic stress disorder and related comorbidities after acute trauma. *Gen Hosp Psychiatr.* 33(2):123–134. http://dx.doi.org/10.1016/j.genhosppsych.2011.01.001
11. Newman RJ, Bikowski R. (2017). Outcomes of embedded care management in a family medicine residency patient-centered medical home. *Fam Med.* 49(1):46–51.
12. Krupski A, West II, Scharf D, et al. (2016). Integrating primary care into community mental health centers: Impact on utilization and costs of health care. *Psychiatr Serv.* 67(11):1233–1239. http://dx.doi.org/10.1176/appi.ps.201500424
13. Gonzalez JM. (2013). *National health care expenses in the U.S. civilian noninstitutionalized population, 2011* (MEPS Statistical Brief No. 425). Rockville, MD: Agency for Healthcare Research and Quality. https://meps.ahrq.gov/data_files/publications/st425/stat425
14. Stern T, Fricchione G. (2010). Beginnings: Psychosomatic medicine and consultation psychiatry. In: *Massachusetts General Hospital handbook of general hospital psychiatry*, 6th ed. Philadelphia: Saunders/Elsevier, pp. 1–3.
15. Pope WS. (2011). Another face of health care disparity: Stigma of mental illness. *J Psychosoc Nurs Ment Health Serv.* 49(9):27–31. http://dx.doi.org/10.3928/02793695-20110802-01
16. Zolnierek CD. (2009). Non-psychiatric hospitalization of people with mental illness: Systematic review. *J Adv Nurs.* 65(8):1570–1583. http://dx.doi.org/10.1111/j.1365-2648.2009.05044.x
17. Kishi Y, Meller WH, Kathol RG, Swigart SE. (2004). Factors affecting the relationship between the timing of psychiatric consultation and general hospital length of stay. *Psychosomatics.*

45(6):470–476. http://dx.doi.org/10.1176/appi.psy.45.6.470
18. Stoddard FJ, Sheridan R, Selter L. (2015). General surgery: Basic principles. In: B.S. Fogel & D.B. Greenberg, eds. *Psychiatric care of the medical patient*, 3rd ed. New York: Oxford University Press, pp. 1367–1388.
19. Bronheim H, Fulop G. (1998). Practice guidelines for psychiatric consultation in the general medical setting. *Psychosomatics*. 39:S8–S30. http://www.apm.org/prac-gui/psy39-s8.shtml
20. Stoddard FJ, Saxe G. (2001). Ten-year research review of physical injuries. *J Am Acad Child Adolesc Psychiatry*. 40(10):1128–1145.
21. Parsaik AK, Abdelgawad N. (2017). Early-life trauma in hospitalized patients with mood disorders and its association with clinical outcomes. *J Psychiatr Pract*. 23(1):36–43. http://dx.doi.org/10.1097/PRA.0000000000000202
22. Bienvenu OJ, Neufeld KJ. (2011). Post-traumatic stress disorder in medical settings: Focus on the critically ill. *Curr Psychiatry Rep*. 13(1):3–9. http://dx.doi.org/10.1007/s11920-010-0166-y
23. Schelling G, Briegel J. (2001). The effect of stress doses of hydrocortisone during septic shock on posttraumatic stress disorder in survivors. *Biol Psychiatry*. 50(12):978–985.
24. James C, Hart R. (2007). Post-traumatic stress disorder and post-traumatic stress symptoms following critical illness in medical intensive care unit patients: Assessing the magnitude of the problem. *Crit Care*. 11(1):215–217. http://www.scielo.br/pdf/rbti/v22n1/en_a13v22n1.pdf
25. Long A, Kross E. (2014). Posttraumatic stress disorder among survivors of critical illness: Creation of a conceptual model addressing identification, prevention, and management. *Inten Care Med*. 40(6): 820–829. http://dx.doi.org/10.1007/s00134-015-3689-1
26. Stern T, Herman J. (2004). *Massachusetts General Hospital psychiatry update and board preparation*, 2nd ed. Boston: MGH Psychiatry Academy Publishing.
27. Shalev AY, Schreiber S. (1993). Post-traumatic stress disorder following medical events. *Br J Clin Psychol*. 32(Pt 2):247–253.
28. Kapfhammer HP. (2016). Depressive, anxiety and posttraumatic stress disorders as long-term sequelae of intensive care treatment. *Nervenarzt*. 87(3):253–263. http://dx.doi.org/10.1007/s00115-016-0070-8
29. Szczytkowski-Thomson JL. (2013). Morphine prevents the development of stress-enhanced fear learning. *Pharmacol Biochem Behav*. 103(3):672–677. http://dx.doi.org/10.1016/j.pbb.2012.10.013
30. Roque AP.(2015). Pharmacotherapy as prophylactic treatment of post-traumatic stress disorder: A review of the literature. *Issues Ment Health Nurs*. 36(9):740–751. http://dx.doi.org/10.3109/01612840.2015.1057785
31. Samuel F. Sears, J. (2011). Posttraumatic stress and the implantable cardioverter-defibrillator patient: What the electrophysiologist needs to know. *Cir Arrhythm Electrophysiol*. 4:242–250. http://dx.doi.org/10.1161/CIRCEP.110.957670
32. Langan C, Sarode DP. (2017). Psychiatric symptomatology after delirium: A systematic review. *Psychogeriatrics*. 17(5):327–335. http://dx.doi.org/10.1111/psyg.12240
33. Elliott R. (2016). Posttraumatic stress symptoms in intensive care patients: An exploration of associated factors *Rehabil Psychol*. 61(2):141–150. http://dx.doi.org/10.1037/rep0000074
34. American Psychiatric Association. (2013). *Diagnostic and statistical manual of mental disorders*, 5th ed. Washington, DC: American Psychiatric Publishing.
35. Riddle M, Meeks T. (2016). When personality is the problem: Managing patients with difficult personalities on the acute care unit. *J Hosp Med*. 11(12):873–878. http://dx.doi.org/10.1002/jhm.2643
36. de Carvalho HW, Pereira R. (2015). Childhood trauma is associated with maladaptive personality traits. *Child Abuse Negl*. 44:18–25. http://dx.doi.org/10.1016/j.chiabu.2014.10.013
37. Frias A. (2016). Anxious adult attachment may mediate the relationship between childhood emotional abuse and borderline personality disorder. *Personal Ment Health*. 10(4):274–284. http://dx.doi.org/10.1002/pmh.1348
38. Cailhol L, Francois M. (2016). Is borderline personality disorder only a mental health problem? *Personal Ment Health*. 10(4):328–336. http://dx.doi.org/10.1002/pmh.1350
39. O'Hare T, Shen C. (2016). Lifetime physical and sexual abuse and self-harm in women with severe mental illness. *Violence Against Women*. 22(10):1211–1227. http://dx.doi.org/10.1177/1077801215622576
40. Conlin S, Littlechild J. (2016). Surgical and psychiatric profile of patients who self-harm by burning in a regional burn unit over an 11-year period. *Scott Med J*. 61(1):17–25. http://dx.doi.org/10.1177/0036933015619312
41. O'Donnell ML, Alkemade N. (2016). A longitudinal study of adjustment disorder after trauma exposure. *Am J Psychiatry*. Dec 1;173(12):1231–1238. http://dx.doi.org/10.1176/appi.ajp.2016.16010071
42. Findley JK, Sanders KB. (2003). The role of psychiatry in the management of acute trauma surgery patients. *Prim Care Companion J Clin Psychiatry*. Oct;5(5):195–200. http://dx.doi.org/PMC419297

43. Megan P, Douglas Z. (2010). Collaborative care interventions in general trauma patients. *Oral Maxillofac Surg Clin North Am.* May; 22(2):261–267. http://dx.doi.org/10.1016/j.coms.2010.01.002
44. Zatzick D, Russo J, Lord SP. (2014). Collaborative care intervention targeting violence risk behaviors, substance use, and posttraumatic stress and depressive symptoms in injured adolescents: A randomized clinical trial. *JAMA Pediatrics.* Jun;168(6):532–539. http://dx.doi.org/10.1001/jamapediatrics.2013.4784
45. Berry K, Ford S. (2015). Trauma in relation to psychosis and hospital experiences: The role of past trauma and attachment. *Psychol Psychother.* Sep;88(3):227–239. http://dx.doi.org/10.1111/papt.12035
46. Quarantini L, Netto LR. (2009). Comorbid mood and anxiety disorders in victims of violence with posttraumatic stress disorder. *Rev Bras Psiquiatr.* Oct;31(Suppl 2):S66–S76.
47. Zatzick DF. (2017). The cumulative burden of mental, substance use, and general medical disorders and rehospitalization and mortality after an injury. *Psychiatr Serv.* Feb 1:68(6):596–602. http://dx.doi.org/10.1176/appi.ps.201600311
48. Schecter WP, Klassen C. (2005). Suicide: The unmet challenge of the trauma system. *Arch Surg.* Sep;140(9):902–904.
49. Darnell D, Dunn C, Atkins D. (2016). A randomized evaluation of motivational interviewing training for mandated implementation of alcohol screening and brief intervention in trauma centers. *J Subst Abuse Treat.* Jan;60:36–44. http://dx.doi.org/10.1016/j.jsat.2015.05.010
50. van Aalst JA, Shotts SD. (1992). Long-term follow-up of unsuccessful violent suicide attempts: Risk factors for subsequent attempts. *J Trauma.* Sep;33(3):457–464.
51. Figley CR. (1995). Compassion fatigue as secondary stress disorder: An overview. In: CR Figley, Ed. *Compassion fatigue: Coping with secondary traumatic stress disorder in those who treat the traumatized* (Routledge Psychosocial Stress Series). New York: Routledge, pp. 1–20.
52. Merlino JP. (2011). Rescuing ourselves: Self care in the disaster response community. In: FJ Stoddard, A Pandya, CL Katz, Eds. *Disaster psychiatry: Readiness, evaluation and treatment.* Washington, DC: American Psychiatric Publishing, pp. 35–48.
53. Luftman K, Aydelotte. (2017). PTSD in those who care for the injured. *J Injury.* Feb;48(2):293–296. http://dx.doi.org/10.1016/j.injury.2016.11.001
54. Cocker F, Joss N. (2016). Compassion fatigue among healthcare, emergency and community service workers: A systematic review. *Int J Environ Res Public Health.* Jun 22;13(6). http://dx.doi.org/10.3390/ijerph13060618
55. Chung EK, Siegel BS. (2016). Screening for social determinants of health among children and families living in poverty: A guide for clinicians. *Curr Probl Pediatr Adolesc Health Care.* May;46(5):135–153. http://dx.doi.org/10.1016/j.cppeds.2016.02.004
56. Borda Bohigas JP, Carrillo JO. (2015). Historical trauma: Systematic review of a different approach to armed conflict. *Rev Colomb Psiquiatr.* Jan-Mar;44(1):41–49. http://dx.doi.org/10.1016/j.rcp.2014.09.005
57. Fink DS, Galea S. (2015). Life course epidemiology of trauma and related psychopathology in civilian populations. *Curr Psychiatry Rep.* May;17(5):31. http://dx.doi.org/10.1007/s11920-015-0566-0
58. Stoddard FJ, Sheridan RL, Martyn JAJ., Czarnik JE Deal VT. (2011). *Pain management.* In: Ritchie EC, Ed. *Combat and operational behavioral health* (The Textbooks of Military Medicine). Washington, DC: Department of the Army, Office of the Surgeon General, Borden Institute; 2011, pp. 339–358.
59. Holbrook TL, Galarneau MR, Dye JL. (2010). Morphine use after combat injury in Iraq and posttraumatic stress disorder. *N Engl J Med.* 362:110–117. http://dx.doi.org/10.1056/NEJMoa0903326
60. Seddon S, Kenneth K. (2008). Challenges in using opioids to treat pain in persons with substance use disorders. *Addict Sci Clin Pract.* Jun;4(2): 4–25. http://dx.doi.org/PMC2797112
61. Holl J, Wolff S. (2016). Substance use to regulate intense posttraumatic shame in individuals with childhood abuse and neglect. *Dev Psychopathol.* Jun 13:1–13. http://dx.doi.org/10.1017/S0954579416000432
62. Binder EB, Bradley RG. (2008). Association of FKBP5 polymorphisms and childhood abuse with risk of posttraumatic stress disorder symptoms in adults. *JAMA.* Mar 19;299(11):1291–1305. http://dx.doi.org/10.1001/jama.299.11.1291
63. Walwyn W, Miotto K. (2010). Opioid pharmaceuticals and addiction: The issues, and research directions seeking solutions. *Drug Alcohol Depend.* May 1; 108(3):156–165. http://dx.doi.org/10.1016/j.drugalcdep.2010.01.001
64. Toth AR, Possidente CJ. (2016). National and northern New England opioid prescribing patterns, 2013–2014. *Pain Med.* Oct 29;18(9): 1706–1714. http://dx.doi.org/10.1093/pm/pnw231
65. Grant BF, Chou SP, Saha TD. (2017). Prevalence of 12-Month Alcohol Use, High-Risk Drinking,

and DSM-IV Alcohol Use Disorder in the United States, 2001-2002 to 2012-2013: Results From the National Epidemiologic Survey on Alcohol and Related Conditions. *JAMA Psychiatry.* 74(9):911–923. https://doi.org/10.1001/jamapsychiatry.2017.2161
66. Sharma B, Bruner A, Barnett G. (2016). Opioid use disorders. *Child Adol Psychiatric Clin N Am.* 25:473–487. http://dx.doi.org/10.1016/j.chc.2016.03.002
67. Martins SS, Segura LE, Santaella-Tenorio J, et al. (2017). Prescription opioid use disorder and heroin use among 12–34 year-olds in the United States from 2002–2014. *Addict Behav* 65:236–241. http://dx.doi.org/10.1016/j.addbeh.2016.08.033
68. Baker D. (2017). History of the Joint Commission's Pain Standards: Lessons for today's prescription opioid epidemic. *JAMA.* Mar 21;317(11):1117–1118. doi:10.1001/jama.2017.0935
69. Murthy V. (2016). Ending the opioid epidemic—a call to action. *N Engl J Med.* Dec 22;375(25):2413–2415. http://dx.doi.org/10.1056/NEJMp1612578
70. Truss K, Godfrey C, Takagi M, et al. (2017). Trajectories and risk-factors for posttraumatic stress symptoms following pediatric concussion. *J Neurotrauma.* Mar 15;34(14):2272–2279. http://dx.doi.org/10.1089/neu.2016.4842
71. Volkow ND. (2014, April 29). Prescription opioid and heroin abuse. Testimony to the House Committee on Energy and Commerce Subcommittee on Oversight and Investigations. https;//www.drugabuse.gov/about-nida/legislative-activities/testimony-to-congress/2016/prescription-opioid-heroin-abuse
72. Cnossen MC. (2017). Predictors of major depression and posttraumatic stress disorder following traumatic brain injury: A systematic review and meta-analysis. *J Neuropsychiatr Clin Neurosci.* Feb;14:2272–2279 http://dx.doi.org/10.1176/appi.neuropsych.16090165
73. Zatzick DF, Rowhani-Rahbar A, Wang J, et al. (2017). The cumulative burden of mental, substance use, and general medical disorders and rehospitalization and mortality after an injury. *Psychiatr Serv.* 68(6):596-602. http://dx.doi.org/10.1176/appi.ps.201600311
74. Harwood DD, Hanumanthu S. (1992). Pathophysiology and management of phantom limb pain. *Gen Hosp Psychiatry.* Mar;14(2):107–118.
75. Lundberg SG, Guggenheim FG. (1986). Sequelae of limb amputation. *Adv Psychosom Med.* 15:199–210.
76. Stoddard FJ, Sheridan R, Selter L., Greenberg D. (2015). General surgery: Basic principles. In: B.S. Fogel and D.B. Greenberg, Eds. *Psychiatric care of the medical patient*, 3rd ed. New York: Oxford University Press, pp. 1367–1388.
77. Hemmati, MA, Shokoohi H, Masoumi M. (2015). Mental health disorders in child and adolescent survivors of post-war landmine explosions. *Mil. Med. Res.* Nov 13;2:30. http://dx.doi.org/10.1186/s40779-015-0052-3
78. Bhatnagar V, Richard E, Melcer T. (2015). Lower limb amputation and effect of posttraumatic stress disorder on Department of Veterans Affairs outpatient cost trends. *J Rehab Res Devel.* 52(6):827–838. http://www.rehab.research.va.gov/jour/2015/527/pdf/jrrd-2014-11-0288.pdf
79. Ladds E, Redgrave N. (2017). Systematic review: Predicting adverse psychological outcomes after hand trauma. *J Hand Ther.* 30(4):407–419. http://dx.doi.org/10.1016/j.jht.2016.11.006
80. Bolduc A, Hwang B, Hogan, C. (2015). Identification and referral of patients at risk for post-traumatic stress disorder: A literature review and retrospective analysis. *Ann Surg.* 81(9):904–908.
81. Stoddard FJ, Schneider JC, Ryan CM. (2015). Physical and psychiatric recovery from burns. In: *Surgical clinics of North America.* Philadelphia: Elsevier, pp. 863–878.
82. Mahendraraj K, Durgan DM, Chamberlain RS (2016). Acute mental disorders and short and long term morbidity in patients with third degree flame burn: A population-based outcome study of 96,451 patients from the Nationwide Inpatient Sample (NIS) database (2001–2011). *Burns.* Dec;42(8):1766–1773. http://dx.doi.org/10.1016/j.burns.2016.06.001
83. Fauerbach JA, Lawrence JW, Schmidt CW. (2000). Personality predictors of injury-related posttraumatic stress disorder. *J Nerv Ment Dis.* 188:510–517. http://dx.doi.org/10.1016/j.burns.2005.11.005
84. Kassam-Adams N, Winston FK. (2004). Predicting child PTSD: The relationship between acute stress disorder and PTSD in injured children. *J Am Acad Child Adolesc Psychiatry.* 43:403–411. http://dx.doi.org/10.1097/01.chi.0000181045.13960.67
85. Fidel-Kinori SG, Eiroa-Orosa FJ. (2016). The Fenix II study: A longitudinal study of psychopathology among burn patients. *Burns.* Sep;42(6):1201–1211. http://dx.doi.org/10.1016/j.burns.2016.01.026
86. Glass SP, Nejad SH, Fricchione GL, Stoddard FJ. (2017). The burn patient. In: TA Stern, O Freudenreich, FA Smith, GL Fricchione, and JF Rosenbaum, Eds. *Massachusetts General Hospital handbook of general hospital psychiatry,* 7th ed. Philadelphia: Mosby, pp. 359–374.
87. Dahl O, Wickman M. (2016). Early assessment and identification of posttraumatic stress disorder,

satisfaction with appearance and coping in patients with burns. *Burns.* Dec;42(8):1678–1685. http://dx.doi.org/10.1016/j.burns.2016.09.012
88. Wasiak J, Lee SJ. (2017). Female patients display poorer burn-specific quality of life 12 months after a burn injury. *Injury.* Jan;48(1):87–93. http://dx.doi.org/10.1016/j.injury.2016.07.032
89. Tagkalakis P, Demiri E. (2009). A fear avoidance model in facial burn body image disturbance. *Ann Burns Fire Disasters.* Dec 31;22(4):203–207. PMCID:PMC3188186
90. Vanderplate C. (1982). A personal adaptation group for burn injured hospital patients. *Int J Psychiatry Med.* 12(3):237–242.
91. Nicoletti G, Sasso A. (2014). The role of rehabilitative camouflage after cervicofacial reconstructive surgery: A preliminary study. *Clin Cosmet Investig Dermatol.* Jan 30;7:43–49. http://dx.doi.org/10.2147/CCID.S55296
92. Fogel B, Greenburg, D. (2015). *Psychiatric care of the medical patient,* 3rd ed. New York: Oxford University Press.
93. Shekhawat L, Busheri L. (2015). Patient-reported outcomes following breast reconstruction surgery and therapeutic mammoplasty: Prospective evaluation 1 year post-surgery with BREAST-Q Questionnaire. *Indian J Surg Oncol.* Dec;6(4):356–362. http://dx.doi.org/10.1007/s13193-015-0432-x
94. Brady KT. (2000). Comorbidity of psychiatric disorders and posttraumatic stress disorder. *J Clin Psychiatry.* 61(Suppl 7):22–32.
95. Galatzer-Levy I, Nickerson A. (2013). Patterns of lifetime PTSD comorbidity: A latent class analysis. *Depress Anxiety.* 30:489–496. http://dx.doi.org/10.1002/da.22048
96. Darnell D, O'Connor S. (2017). Enhancing the reach of cognitive-behavioral therapy targeting posttraumatic stress in acute care medical settings. *Psychiatr Serv.* 68(3):258–263. http://dx.doi.org/10.1176/appi.ps.201500458
97. Ruchiwit M. (2012). The effect of the one-to-one interaction process with group supportive psychotherapy on the levels of hope, anxiety and self-care practice for patients that have experienced organ loss: An alternative nursing care model. *Int J Nurs Pract.* Aug;18(4):363–372. http://dx.doi.org/10.1111/j.1440-172X.2012.02053.x
98. Söllner W, Maislinger S. (2004). Providing psychosocial support for breast cancer patients based on screening for distress within a consultation-liaison service. *Psychooncology.* Dec;13(12):893–897. http://dx.doi.org/10.1002/pon.867
99. Freyberger H, Freyberger HJ. (1994). Supportive psychotherapy. *Psychother Psychosom.* 61(3–4): 132–142.
100. Kung S, Espinel Z. (2012). Treatment of nightmares with prazosin: A systematic review. *Mayo Clin Proc.* Sep; 87(9):890–900. http://dx.doi.org/10.1016/j.mayocp.2012.05.015
101. Aurora N, Zak N. (2010) Best practice guide for the treatment of nightmare disorder in adults. *J Clin Sleep Med.* Aug 15;6(4):389–401. PMCID:PMC2919672
102. Ahearn EP, Juergens T. (2011). A review of atypical antipsychotic medications for posttraumatic stress disorder. *Int Clin Psychopharmacol.* Jul;26(4):193–200. http://dx.doi.org/10.1097/YIC.0b013e3283473738
103. Brownlow JA, Harb GC. (2015). Treatment of sleep disturbances in post-traumatic stress disorder: A review of the literature. *Curr Psychiatry Rep.* Jun;17(6):41. http://dx.doi.org/10.1007/s11920-015-0587-8
104. Katzman M, Bleau P. (2014). Canadian clinical practice guidelines for the management of anxiety, posttraumatic stress and obsessive-compulsive disorders. *BMC Psychiatry.* 14(Suppl 1):S1. http://dx.doi.org/10.1186/1471-244X-14-S1-S1
105. Gawande A. (2014). *Being mortal: Medicine and what matters at the end.* New York: Henry Holt.
106. Detering K, Hancock A. (2010). The impact of advance care planning on end of life care in elderly patients: Randomised controlled trial. *BMJ.* 340: c1345. https://doi.org/10.1136/bmj.c1345
107. Virdun C, Luckett T. (2016). Dying in the hospital setting: A meta-synthesis identifying the elements of end-of-life care that patients and their families describe as being important. *Palliat Med.* 31(7):587–601. https://doi.org/10.1177/0269216316673547
108. Razmaria A. (2016). End-of-life care. *JAMA.* Jul 5;316(1):115. https://doi.org/10.1001/jama.2016.2440
109. Kubler-Ross E. (2014). *On death and dying: What the dying have to teach doctors, nurses, clergy and their own families.* New York: Scribner.
110. Hall S, Edmonds P. (2009). Assessing the feasibility, acceptability and potential effectiveness of Dignity Therapy for people with advanced cancer referred to a hospital-based palliative care team: Study protocol. *BMC Palliat Care.* May 16;8:5. https://doi.org/10.1186/1472-684X-8-5
111. Garland C. (1998). *Understanding trauma: A psychoanalytic approach,* 2nd ed. London: Karnac.
112. Bronheim H, Fulop G. (1998). Practice guidelines for psychiatric consultation in the general medical setting. *Psychosomatics.* 39:S8–S30.
113. Stern T, Herman J. (2012). Trauma and post traumatic stress disorder. In: *Massachusetts General Hospital psychiatry update and board preparation,* 3rd ed. Boston: MGH Psychiatry Academy Publishing, pp. 127–135.

19

Susceptibility, Resilience, and Trajectories

JACK TSAI, NATALIE JONES, ROBERT H. PIETRZAK,
ILAN HARPAZ-ROTEM, AND STEVEN M. SOUTHWICK

INTRODUCTION

Nearly every person experiences a highly stressful or traumatic event during their lifetime. However, individual responses to such events vary widely from person to person. Some people respond with symptoms of anxiety, depression, acute stress, or posttraumatic stress disorder (PTSD). Yet others experience minimal or no psychiatric symptoms after trauma. What makes one person more susceptible and another person more resilient to the negative effects of trauma? What are the different adaptive trajectories of trauma survivors and what determines their trajectory? These are some of the questions that are examined in this chapter, which focuses on what is currently known about resilience to stress.

This chapter is divided into five sections: (1) definition, prevalence, and measurement of resilience; (2) longitudinal studies on trajectories after trauma exposures; (3) research on factors that are predictive of resilience and different trajectories; (4) interventions that have been developed to increase resilience; and (5) discussion about future directions for research on resilience.

DEFINITION

The complex nature of resilience makes it challenging to construct a definition that is universally accepted. The American Psychological Association (2014) defined resilience as "the process of adapting well in the face of adversity, trauma, tragedy, threats or even significant sources of threat . . . 'bouncing back' from difficult experiences" (para. 4). Others have defined resilience as a stable trajectory of healthy functioning after a highly adverse event, the capacity to adapt successfully to events that disrupt homeostasis, the ability to harness resources to sustain well-being, or enhanced psychobiological capacity to modulate the stress response (Krystal, 2008; Southwick, Bonanno, Masten, Panter-Brick, & Yehuda, 2014).

Resilience is a complex construct that has been viewed as a trait, set of characteristics, a process, or an outcome. In addition, resilience is multifaceted. An individual may be more or less resilient in some domains of his or her life (e.g., work life) but not in others (e.g., personal or family life; Southwick et al., 2014). While resilience is sometimes described as either present or absent, it is best understood on a continuum being present to varying degrees across multiple domains of life (Pietrzak & Southwick, 2011). Resilience is generally spoken of in terms of protective factors that promote positive outcomes (Bonanno, 2004; Luthar, Cicchetti, & Becker, 2000). A resilient individual may experience mild, temporary disturbances to his or her normal functioning but often does not exhibit threshold clinical symptoms (Bonanno, 2004).

Resilience should also be differentiated from posttraumatic growth, which is defined as positive psychological changes that occur as a result of trauma (Tsai, Mota, Southwick, & Pietrzak, 2016) Posttraumatic growth generally requires individuals to experience the negative effects of PTSD and related symptoms, and it is from their negative experience that growth may occur, whereas individuals who are resilient mostly do not experience the negative effects of trauma. Levels of posttraumatic growth in the same individuals can also change over time (Tsai et al., 2016), and resilience is conceptualized as a more stable characteristic. Emerging research suggests that posttraumatic growth may also help promote resilience to future trauma (Tsai et al., 2016).

PREVALENCE

Much of the current knowledge base on how people cope with trauma or loss has been derived from studies that have sampled treatment-seeking individuals, many of whom have pronounced psychological problems. Because of this, resilience has often, mistakenly, assumed to only occur in rare, remarkably healthy individuals (Bonanno, 2004). In actuality, most people cope well with traumatic events or losses and do not experience major disruptions to their work and close relationships (Bonanno, 2004).

For example, recent studies on first responders have shown that most individuals in this line of work are able to maintain stability and well-being (Norris et al., 2002; Norris, Tracy, & Galea, 2009; Van der Velden et al., 2006). Studies on the September 11th terrorist attacks in New York City revealed similar findings. A study examining a large sample of individuals in or near New York City during the event found only 7.5% met criteria for PTSD one month after, and only 6% met criteria for PTSD six months after (Galea et al., 2003). Further, a study with a more highly exposed sample of people who had been in or within close proximity to the World Trade Center found that more than one-third of the individuals had few or no PTSD symptoms (Bonanno, Rennicke, & Dekel, 2005). In concordance with these findings, a longitudinal study on 268 Hurricane Ike survivors measured hurricane-related PTSD symptoms after this natural disaster and only 6.9% to 2.5% exhibited symptoms, which decreased over time. Much like the other studies mentioned, the vast majority of the trauma-exposed sample "bounced back" after the event (Pietrzak et al., 2012).

Because there have been varying definitions of resilience, it is difficult to describe the point-prevalence or the lifetime prevalence of resilience. However, as many studies have shown, the majority of individuals who experience potentially traumatic events do not experience the dysfunction and psychopathology associated with PTSD and related disorders. Nonetheless, this highlights the importance of assessing and studying what factors differentiate those who are resilience and those who are not.

ASSESSMENT

Resilience has been primarily assessed through self-report, although corroborating reports from significant others have also been used (Shakespeare-Finch & Enders, 2008). Some of the most commonly used self-report measures of resilience and related constructs are described next.

Connor-Davidson Resilience Scale

The Connor-Davidson Resilience Scale (CD-RISC) is a 25-item self-report measure that assesses resilience to stressful events (Connor & Davidson, 2003). Respondents are asked to rate items on a 5-point scale from 0 ("Not true at all") to 4 ("True nearly all of the time") based on how they felt over the past month. Sample items are "I am able to adapt when changes occur," and "I tend to bounce back after illness, injury, or other hardships." Five subscales of the CD-RISC have been identified (Connor & Davidson, 2003), which assess personal competence and tenacity, trust in one's instincts and tolerance of negative affect, positive acceptance of chance and secure relationships, control, and spiritual influences. Other variations of subscales for the CD-RISC, derived from factor analysis, have also been used (Karaırmak, 2010; Pietrzak, Russo, Ling, & Southwick, 2010; Yu & Zhang, 2007). Overall, studies have shown the CD-RISC has good internal consistency, test–retest reliability, convergent validity, discriminant validity, and factorial stability (Connor & Davidson, 2003; Tsai, Harpaz-Rotem, Pietrzak, & Southwick, 2012). Developers of the CD-RISC have established two reference samples of PTSD patients (Connor & Davidson, 2003) that generated total scores of 47.8 (SD = 19.5) and 52.8 (SD = 20.4). Abbreviated versions of the CD-RISC have also been developed, including a 10-item (Campbell-Sills & Stein, 2007) and a 2-item version (Vaishnavi, Connor, & Davidson, 2007).

Response to Stressful Experience Scale

The Response to Stressful Experience Scale (RSES) is a 22-item self-report measure that assesses a broad range of behaviors, thoughts, and actions in response to stress, adversity, or trauma (Johnson et al., 2011). The RSES was developed by the Department of Veterans Affairs' National Center for PTSD. Respondents are asked to rate how well statements on the RSES describe them during and after their most stressful life events on a 5-point scale from 0 ("Not at all like me") to 4 ("Exactly like me"). Sample items include "take action to fix things" and "see it as a challenge that will make me better." The RSES consists of a total summed score and six subscales, including Active Coping, Meaning-making, Cognitive Flexibility, Spirituality, Self-efficacy, and Restoration. The RSES has good internal consistency, test–retest reliability, factor stability, and criterion validity (Johnson et al., 2011).

Dispositional Resilience Scale

The Dispositional Resilience Scale (DRS) is a 45-item self-report instrument that provides a measure of hardiness and has been used in military and occupational settings (Bartone, Ursano, Wright, & Ingraham, 1989). Respondents are asked to rate how much they think each item is true in general from a scale from 0 ("Not at all true") to 3 ("Completely true"). Sample items include "Most of my life gets spent doing things that are worthwhile" and "I often wake up eager to take up my life wherever it left off." Factor analyses have identified three subscales for the DRS, labeled Commitment, Challenge, and Control. The DRS and its subscales have shown good internal consistency, factorial stability, and criterion validity (Bartone et al., 1989). A brief 15-item version of the DRS called the Dispositional Resilience Scale-15 has shown to have good construct validity, internal consistency, and test-retest reliability (Bartone, 2007).

Resilience Scale

The Resilience Scale (RS) is a 25-item scale developed to identify degree of individual resilience as it relates to adaptation (Wagnild & Young, 1993). Respondents are asked to rate the degree to which they agree or disagree with each item on a 7-point scale from 1 ("Disagree") to 7 ("Agree"). Sample items include "I usually manage one way or another," and "My life has meaning." Factor analyses of the RS have found two major factors labeled Acceptance of Self and Life, and Individual Competence (Wagnild & Young, 1993). The RS has shown good internal consistency and test–retest reliability, as well as construct and concurrent validity among a wide age range of participants (Wagnild, 2009).

Resilience Scales for Children and Adolescents

The Resilience Scales for Children and Adolescents (RSCA) is a 64-item measure that assess resilience-related attributes of children and adolescents and has been used to screen for psychological vulnerability (Prince-Embury, 2008). The RSCA is written at a third-grade reading level and respondents are asked to rate how they feel about items on a 5-point scale from 0 ("Never") to 4 ("Almost always"). Samples items are "I can make up with friends after a fight" and "No matter what happens things will be all right." The RSCA consists of three separate global scales: Sense of Mastery, Sense of Relatedness, and Emotional Reactivity. Each global scale comprises 20 to 24 questions, and there are 10 subscales. The RSCA has good internal consistency, test–retest reliability, and convergent and discriminant validity (Prince-Embury, 2008).

CAVEAT ABOUT ASSESSMENTS

Given our broad understanding of resilience, caution should be used when attempting to determine whether an individual is resilient strictly on the basis of the aforementioned assessment instruments. As discussed earlier in this chapter, an individual may exhibit resilience in one domain of his or her life but not in others. For example, in a study of 79 mothers with a history of childhood abuse, current resilience was measured across intrapersonal, interpersonal, and intrafamilial domains. While 81.9% of mothers reported significant strength and positive adaptation in at least one domain, only 20.5% noted positive adaptation and strength in all life domains (Wright, Fopma-Loy, & Fischer, 2005). Variations in rates of resilience may also be influenced by sampling methods assessment measures, and other aspects of the study design (Van Voorhees et al., 2012). Further, as is discussed in the next section, resilience is often conceptualized as a stable trajectory of no/minimal psychological symptoms and high functioning after trauma, stress, or adversity; thus cross-sectional self-report assessments of resilience may not fully capture the dynamic nature of this phenomenon.

TRAJECTORIES

Maladaptive and adaptive responses to trauma follows heterogeneous courses over time (Bonanno et al., 2012; Halevi, Djalovski, Vengrober, & Feldman, 2016; Pietrzak et al., 2014). Different individuals and the same individuals at different times may have different responses to trauma. Researchers have tracked responses to trauma over periods of several months to several years after individuals have experienced traumatic events and have attempted to define the various ways that PTSD and related symptoms such as depression evolve over time.

Research on trajectories of PTSD symptoms after trauma exposure, which are identified using latent growth mixture modeling, have commonly revealed four predominant courses of symptoms over time: resistance or resilience (minimal or no symptoms over time), chronic (chronically elevated symptoms over time), recovering (decreasing symptoms over time), and delayed onset (increasing symptoms over time) (Norris et al., 2009; Pietrzak et al., 2014).

Trajectories of PTSD symptoms were examined in a longitudinal study of World Trade Center responders (n = 10,835). World Trade Center-related PTSD symptoms were measured at 3, 6, and 8 years after the 9/11 attacks. The majority of both police responder and nontraditional responders exhibited resistant or resilient trajectories (77.8% of police responders, 58% of nontraditional responders). Other trajectories seen in police responders were delayed onset (8.5%), recovering (8.4%), and chronic (5.3%) as illustrated in Figure 19.1. Other trajectories seen in nontraditional responders were recovering (12.3%), severe chronic (9.5%), subsyndromal increasing (7.3%), delayed onset (6.7%), and moderate chronic trajectories (Pietrzak et al., 2014). In line with these findings, a study that assessed trauma responses among US military service members at predeployment, and at two different time-points (spaced 3 years apart) postdeployment, found five different trajectories of PTSD symptoms. The most common trajectory was resilience (83.1% of those deployed once, 84.9% of those deployed more than once). Other trajectories found were moderate-improving (8.0% of single deployers, 8.5% of multiple deployers), worsening-chronic (6.7% of single deployers, 4.5% of multiple deployers), high-stable (2.2% of multiple deployers only), and high-improving (2.2% of multiple deployers only) (Bonanno et al., 2012). Together, these findings demonstrate the varied trajectories of PTSD symptoms that individuals may experience after trauma. They further highlight the high prevalence of resilience, particularly among individuals who have received professional training in responding to traumatic events, such as police officers and military personnel.

In addition to latent growth mixture modeling, some researchers have used cluster analysis to identify different groups of individuals on the basis of trauma exposure history and psychological symptoms. For example, a recent prospective cohort study of 2,157 veterans from the National Health and Resilience in Veterans Study identified three groups based on their lifetime trauma exposure (i.e., number of lifetime traumatic event types experienced) and current psychological stress (i.e., composite measure of PTSD, depression, and generalized anxiety symptoms): a low trauma exposure group (59.5%), a resilient group (27.4%), and a distressed group (13.1%) (Isaacs et al., 2016). The low trauma exposure group had low collective lifetime trauma exposure and minimal current psychological distress. The resilient group had high cumulative trauma exposure and minimal current psychological distress. The distressed group had high cumulative trauma exposure and significant current distress. The findings of this study revealed that more than half of trauma-exposed veterans (67.7%) were psychologically

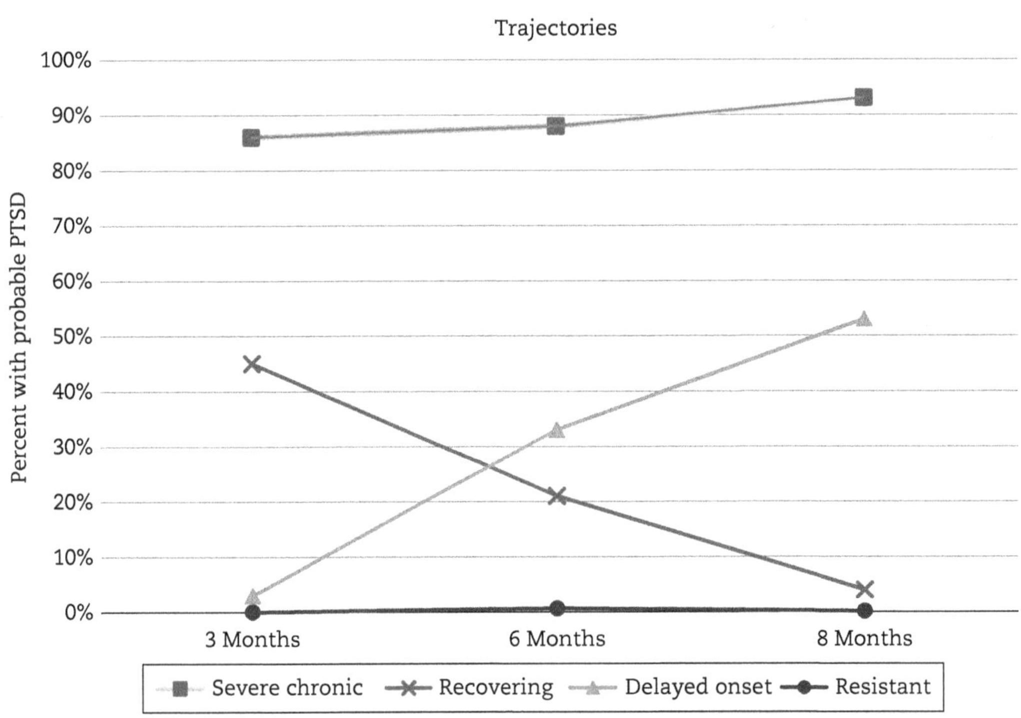

FIGURE 19.1. Trajectories of police responders after the September 11, 2001, events. (See front matter.)

resilient. Factors that were found to be associated with resilience (vs. distress) included emotional stability, extraversion, dispositional gratitude, purpose in life, altruism, and low levels of openness to experiences.

FACTORS ASSOCIATED WITH RESILIENCE

Numerous genetic, developmental, neurobiological, psychological, and social protective factors have been identified in the traumatic stress research literature. In this brief review, we discuss some of these factors, which are summarized in Box 19.1. Among development factors, we describe some early life influences on resilience. Among psychosocial factors, we focus on optimism, social support, and physical fitness. Other psychological factors that have been repeatedly identified in the resilience literature include the ability to regulate emotion, commitment to a meaningful purpose and mission, altruism, support from spirituality and religion, and attention to healthy lifestyle habits (Southwick & Charney, 2012).

Developmental Factors

The environment in which children grow up has an enormous impact on how their brain and neurobiological stress systems develop and on their level of resilience as adults. Animal and human studies have clearly shown that repeated exposure to stress early in life that is uncontrollable and unmanageable (e.g., child abuse, neglect, maternal separation) can lead to exaggerated emotional, behavioral, and neurobiological responses to future stressors during adulthood (Anacker, O'Donnell, & Meaney, 2014; Turecki & Meaney, 2016). On the other hand repeated exposure to stress that the young animal or child can control or master is known to have an inoculating or "steeling" effect on subsequent stress reactivity (Haglund, Nestadt, Cooper, Southwick, & Charney, 2007). Stress-inoculated animals and humans tend to react to future stress with emotional, behavioral, and neurobiological responses that are better modulated and more appropriately matched to the specific challenge at hand than those who have been exposed to repeated uncontrollable stress, or even than those who have been exposed to little or no stress. That is, stress that can be successfully mastered tends to promote resilience while stress that is overwhelming tends be toxic (Brockhurst, Cheleuitte-Nieves, Buckmaster, Schatzberg, & Lyons, 2015; Lyons, Parker, & Schatzberg, 2010).

In studies on hospitalization stress among pediatric inpatients, children with previous periods of "positive separation" from parents, such as staying with their grandparents, experienced reduced stress during hospital stays (Stacey, Dearden, & Pill, 1970). Consistent with these findings, adolescents who have been exposed to

BOX 19.1. FACTORS RELATED TO RESILIENCE

1. Developmental factors
   - Stress that young child can master can have positive "steeling" effect
   - Early secure attachment predicts resilience in later life
2. Positive emotions and optimism
   - Positive emotions are associated with higher levels of resilience
   - Optimism is linked with positive physical and mental health
3. Social support
   - Social support buffers negative effects of stress
   - High social support is associated with enhanced sense of control and mastery, active problem-focused coping
4. Physical fitness
   - Regular physical activity suppresses cortisol and increase neurotrophic factors
   - Aerobic exercise may be as effective as cognitive-behavioral therapy
5. Neurobiological factors
   - Resilience is associated with activation of sympathetic nervous system and HPA axis
   - Quick return to baseline following stress response may be regulated by neuropeptide Y, dehydroepiandrosterone, and galanin

mild stress during childhood were found to have decreased blood pressure and heart rate in response to stress-inducing laboratory tests (Boyce & Chesterman, 1990). Of note, researchers emphasize that response to stress is highly variable from one person to the next and that it is important to consider characteristics such as age, culture, family functioning, and genetic inheritance when evaluating stress reactivity. (Masten & Narayan, 2012).

Perhaps the most significant early life influence on later resilience is the attachment formed between child and caregiver. A loving parenting style in which the caregiver protects the child from overwhelming stress while still allowing the child to explore and master new challenges tends to foster secure attachments and a secure attachment style. Secure attachments with caregivers lay the foundation for a host of important life skills: self-control, delayed gratification, problem-solving under stress, emotional regulation, and the ability to form and maintain supportive relationships founded on love and trust (Masten, Monn, & Supkoff, 2011). Studies have shown that emotionally responsive parenting, greater discipline consistency, more positive expectations for the child's future, and positive parent mental health predict resiliency in at-risk children and that competent parenting partly mediates that relationship (Wyman et al., 1999). In contrast, an unstable parenting style, in which caregivers are neglectful, abusive, inconsistent in their behaviors toward the child, unresponsive to the child's needs, or overly intrusive, tends to foster insecure attachment between caregiver and child. Insecure attachments hold children back from reaping the resilience-promoting benefits of healthy, trusting relationships because children learn to view relationships as unstable and unreliable, and as a result children fear building close ties to others (Berkman, 1995).

Positive Emotion and Optimism

The "Broaden-and-Build" model of positive emotion reduce physiological arousal and broaden visual focus, thoughts, and behaviors. Such broadening tends to result in more inclusive, flexible, creative, and integrative thinking, as well as increased capacity to solve problems (Fredrickson, 2013). The broadening of resources has been associated with a number of healthy coping strategies such as positive appraisal of challenging situations, imbuing ordinary events with meaning, and problem-focused coping (Fredrickson, 2001). The model also posits that negative emotions such as anger, disgust, and fear tend to increase activation of the sympathetic nervous system with an increase in physiological arousal and a narrowing of focus, attention, and behaviors (Fredrickson, 2001; Southwick & Charney, 2012).

Optimism repeatedly has been linked with positive physical and mental health. A number of studies have found that optimism is associated with physical well-being and with feeling psychologically healthy and satisfied with life (Carver & Scheier, 2014; DuBois et al., 2015). Optimists, compared to pessimists, reported greater pursuit of goals, better health, stronger social relationships, and more successful working careers. In addition, in the Women's Health Initiative study that followed 95,000 women over eight years, optimists were less likely to develop coronary artery disease or to die from any cause (Tindle et al., 2009).

The relationship between optimism and resilience has also been studied in working settings. For example, Meneghel, Salanova, and Martinez (2016) used the Broaden and Build hypothesis to examine the relationship between resilience, positive emotion, and performance in 216 teams of employees across 40 companies. Five collective positive emotions were measured: enthusiasm, optimism, satisfaction, comfort, and relaxation. Teams with higher levels of positive emotion exhibited higher levels of resilience as measured by a scale based on principles of resilience in organizations (Mallak, 1998). In addition, results found that collective positive emotions helped foster team resilience, which in turn enhanced team performance.

Twin studies have estimated that approximately 30% to 50% of personality traits, like optimism, are genetically transmitted. The other 50% to 70% depends on environment. It is likely that many genes and gene variants are related to optimism and that they each contribute a small amount to the expression of optimism (Rana et al., 2014). A number of brain regions, systems, and circuits, including the amygdala, ventral striatum, and prefrontal cortex, play a central role in the expression of positive emotions. In a competitive game, resilient individuals, unlike controls, maintained activation of reward circuitry during trials in which they lost money as well as during trials in which they won money. This suggests that resilient individuals may be better able to maintain positive emotions and optimism, despite loss or perhaps adversity (Vythilingam et al., 2009). Positive emotions have been associated with high activity of the left prefrontal cortex and more prolonged engagement of the ventral striatal reward system, which is associated with the ability to sustain positive mood (Davidson, 2000).

Social Support

The effects of social support are far-reaching. High levels of social support have long been associated with positive psychological and physical health (Cobb, 1976; Kaplan, Cassel, & Gore, 1977). In the mid-1980s, Cohen and Wills (1985) published a systematic literature review and concluded that social support has both a direct beneficial effect, as well as a buffering effect, in which it mediates the relationship between stress and health/well-being. Since that time, high social support has been associated with reduced levels of depression in patients with multiple sclerosis, cardiac illness, and cancer; lower rates of obesity in adult children of obese mothers; better psychological outcome after severe traumas such as child sexual abuse; reduced risk of death after a heart attack; and overall reduced mortality (Berkman, 1995; Berkman, Leo-Summers, & Horwitz, 1992; Garay-Sevilla et al., 1995; Gonzalez et al., 2004). On the other hand, low levels of social support has been associated with greater likelihood of developing PTSD after serving in a war zone, increased risk of coronary artery disease, elevated heart rate and blood pressure, impaired immune function (Berkman & Syme, 1979; Southwick, Ozbay, Charney, & McEwen, 2008; Tsai et al., 2012; Uchino, Cacioppo, & Kiecolt-Glaser, 1996), and reduced life expectancy that may be equivalent to the effects of hypertension, cigarette smoking, low level of activity, or obesity (Holt-Lunstad, Smith, & Layton, 2010).

A number of psychological, behavioral, and neurobiological mechanisms may help explain the relationship between social support, resilience, and well-being. High social support has been associated with enhanced sense of control and mastery, appraisal of negative or stressful events as less threatening, active problem-focused coping, motivation to adopt healthy and less risky behaviors, increased medication adherence, and increased self-esteem (DiMatteo, 2004; Garay-Sevilla et al., 1995; Gonzalez et al., 2004; Kelly et al., 1993; Milkulincer & Shaver, 2007). In addition, positive social support has been shown to inhibit fear-related neurobiological systems, to enhance processing of safety cues, and to stimulate the release of oxytocin (Lin et al., 2015; Wald et al., 2016). Oxytocin is known to have anxiolytic effects and to facilitate social cognition, accurate identification of facial affect, and social approach and perceptions of trustworthiness (Feldman, 2017; Naim et al., 2015; Wald et al., 2016).

Physical Fitness

The benefits of physical health on mental health are well-known (Penedo & Dahn, 2005), and there may be specific benefits in terms of resilience. For one, exercise increases concentrations of compounds that affect mood, such as dopamine and serotonin (Erickson et al., 2011), which can enhance one's ability to respond to stress. Regular physical activity and exercise can also protect against the negative effects of stress by suppressing cortisol and increasing the production of neurotrophic factors (Silverman & Deuster, 2014). These neurotropic factors promote the repair and growth of neurons. There may also be protective effects on cognitions as studies have found that aerobic exercise can lead to improved memory, increased brain-derived neurotropic factor, and an increase in hippocampal volume (Erickson et al., 2011). Several studies have found that aerobic exercise is as effective as cognitive behavioral therapy in reducing depression and anxiety (Asmundson et al., 2013). So, clearly, exercise and physical fitness can enhance physical and emotional resilience through various neurobiological mechanisms that can dampen the stress response and protect against the effects of trauma and chronic stress.

Neurobiological Factors

The neurobiology of resilience is characterized by the complex interplay of genes, epigenetic alterations in gene expression, endocrine and neurotransmitter systems, and the neural circuitry that underlies the regulation of vital processes such as attention, learning, memory, and emotion. Animal and human research has led to a variety of neurobiological hypotheses regarding resilience and how it contrasts with stress vulnerability. It has been proposed that resilience is associated with activation of the sympathetic nervous system and hypothalamic-pituitary-adrenal (HPA) axis in response to stress but a relatively quick return to baseline following modulation by regulators such as neuropeptide Y, dehydroepiandrosterone (DHEA), and galanin. It has been argued that hippocampal activity sufficiently dampens the HPA axis and differentiates dangerous from safe environments; specifically, that prefrontal cortical functioning regulates limbic, behavioral, and emotional responses to stress. These processes are suggested to be involved in the mesocorticolimbic dopaminergic reward system, which can maintain a positive outlook in the context of danger and chronic stress (Feder, Charney, & Collins, 2011; Horn, Charney, & Feder, 2016). Additionally, it has been proposed that resilient individuals are less likely than those who are stress vulnerable to overconsolidate emotional memories and/or overgeneralize specific conditioned stimuli to a broader context, as well as better able to extinguish traumatic memories and to reorganize these memories (Charney, 2004; Horn et al., 2016).

Although a full review of neurobiological factors associated with resilience is beyond the scope of this review, we next focus briefly on the sympathetic nervous system (SNS) and the HPA axis. The SNS is one of the main systems that dictate our stress response. In response to stress the SNS releases epinephrine and norepinephrine (NE), which constricts blood vessels, elevates heart rate and blood pressure, and slows digestion (Guidances & Watch, 2007). While a robust SNS response to stress and danger is critical for survival, if this response persists relatively "unchecked," it may contribute to chronic anxiety, cardiovascular disease, and trauma-related symptoms such as hypervigilance and intrusive memories (Southwick et al., 1999). One neuropeptide that helps to maintain SNS activity within an optimal range or "window" is neuropeptide Y. Neuropeptide Y is a 36 amino acid peptide that is co-localized with a variety of neurotransmitters, including NE. It is released with NE when the SNS is strongly activated and helps inhibit further release of NE so that the SNS does not "overshoot." In military veterans with PTSD, cerebrospinal fluid, plasma resting, and stress-provoked plasma levels of NPY have been reported as significantly lower than normal (Rasmusson et al., 2000). In contrast, Morgan et al. (2002, 2000) found high levels of plasma NPY among elite resilient Special Forces soldiers during intense survival training. NPY levels were positively associated with performance and negatively associated with stress-induced dissociation. Overall, animal and human studies point to NPY as a neurobiological resilience factor that serves to maintain the SNS within an optimal level of activation.

The HPA axis plays a critical role in coordinating the stress response. Activation of the HPA axis begins with the release of corticotropin-releasing factor, which then activates adrenocorticotropic hormone (ACTH). ACTH, in turn, triggers the release of cortisol. Cortisol mobilizes energy stores and increases vigilance, selective attention, arousal, and consolidation of memory. Cortisol also helps to contain the immune response and inhibit growth (Yehuda, 2002). Although cortisol is critical for survival, chronic overstimulation of the HPA axis and cortisol can have toxic effects, including damage to neurons in the hippocampus (McEwen, 2007). In contrast, DHEA, which is secreted with cortisol from the adrenal glands, promotes neurogenesis and helps to protect against the neurotoxic effects of cortisol (Charney, 2004). In studies of Special Forces and Navy Seal trainees, DHEA and DHEA/cortisol ratios have been associated with resilience, and among military veterans receiving treatment, DHEA responses have been positively related to recovery (Morgan et al., 2004; Yehuda et al., 2014).

Clearly, there are other endocrine and neurotransmitter systems and neurobiological markers found to be associated with resilience to stress. Readers are referred to more comprehensive reviews on the topic (Feder, Nestler, & Charney, 2009; Russo, Murrough, Han, Charney, & Nestler, 2012; Southwick, Vythilingam, & Charney, 2005).

RESILIENCE INTERVENTIONS

Training to increase resilience can take many forms. Some interventions address individual factors that have been associated with resilience. Examples include learned optimism, a cognitive behavioral therapy designed to increase optimistic explanatory style; exercise regimens geared toward improving physical fitness; meaning and purpose-based interventions, such as Viktor Frankl's logotherapy, that help individuals embrace their own meaning, purpose and mission (Frankl, 1992; Seligman, 2011). Additional approaches designed to modify appraisals of potential threat include learning to control where one directs one's attention (e.g., attention modification therapy and mindfulness), as well as learning to appraise or reappraise adverse and negative events in a more positive light. It is also likely that resilience can be enhanced in some people through a number of neurobiological interventions, such as the use of antidepressants to enhance neurogenesis and the use of the NPY to help regulate SNS and HPA axis activity.

Other approaches to enhance resilience address multiple resilience factors as part of an overall intervention. For example, resilience-enhancing skills are typically taught as part of training programs for professions who deal with stress and trauma on a regular basis, such as police, firefighters, and soldiers. Pretrauma resilience training for these professions often involves learning specific job-related skills (e.g., self-defense for police academy trainees), as well as more general stress management skills (e.g., breathing techniques, relaxation training). These trainings are designed to increase task-specific skill level, confidence, self-efficacy, and the capacity to regulate emotional responses to stress. A primary goal of such training is to provide the skills needed for the individual to approach future stressors/traumas as challenges (i.e., the belief that one has the tools necessary to deal with the stressor). Although there are numerous types of training for resilience, scenario-based training appears to be particularly effective for professions that involve danger. Scenario-based training includes highly realistic situations where trainees learn by doing and then receive constructive feedback (Adler, Bliese, McGurk, Hoge, & Castro, 2009). Ideally, such training helps the individual to assess future traumas as challenges that they believe they have the tools to handle rather than threats that they believe they cannot master.

Research on interventions for resilience is a developing but burgeoning field. Several promising psychological interventions have been created, which are discussed in this section.

Stress Inoculation Training

The Department of Veterans Affairs/Department of Defense Practice Guideline for management of PTSD has identified stress inoculation therapy as an effective psychotherapy intervention for treatment of PTSD (U.S. Department of Veterans Affairs & U.S. Department of Defense, 2010). Stress inoculation training, based on a transactional model of stress (Lazarus & Folkman, 1984), occurs in three stages (Meichenbaum & Cameron, 1989). In the first stage, a partnership between therapist and patient is established and patients are coached on how to recognize various responses to stress-related triggers and self-monitor the emotions, behaviors, physiological changes, and thoughts they have in response to stress cues. In the second phase, patients learn new coping mechanisms and work with therapists to identify skills they already have. In the third phase, patients are told to practice the skills they have learned in phase 1 and 2. Patients practice these skills through reenactment, role playing, imagery rehearsal, and behavioral rehearsal. Individuals begin with the lesser of their most stressful situations, and, once mastered, they move onto their next most stressful situation, and so on, until the patient masters all of his or her most stressful situations (Southwick, Pietrzak, & White, 2011). When stress inoculation training was tested on a group of rape victims, researchers observed significant improvements in PTSD symptoms, with decreases in rape-related distress, generalized anxiety, and depressive symptoms. Furthermore, those who went through stress inoculation training saw more improvement than those in a supportive counseling group and a prolonged exposure group (Foa, Rothbaum, Riggs, & Murdock, 1991).

Hardiness Training

Hardiness can be conceived of as a set of three attitudes (the 3Cs)—commitment, control, and challenge—that together promote the turning of stressful experiences into opportunities for growth. The 3Cs can be seen as a cognitive/emotional amalgam comprising a learned, growth-oriented, personality buffer (Maddi, 2006, 2012). If one has the Challenge attitude, one understands and accepts that stress is a natural part of life. That person views stressful experiences as opportunities to learn through attempting to turn the stressful changes to his or her favor. If a person has the Commitment attitude, he or she continues to participate in what is going on no matter how challenging things get. When things get hard, they stay involved and do not sink away into patterns of detachment and alienation. People who have the Control attitude think they need to keep trying to turn adverse situations into opportunities for growth, no matter how hard things may become.

Hardiness training consists of teaching individuals to better manage stress through building the three Cs. Training teaches individuals how to find dual-directional supportive relationships, where individuals both provide and accept encouragement and assistance from others. Hardiness training has been found to lead to enhanced ability to cope with difficult situations, elevated job performance and job satisfaction, and well as decreased stress, depression, and anxiety levels in adults (Southwick & Charney, 2012; Southwick, Litz, Charney, & Friedman, 2011). Studies have even found that psychological hardiness predicts neuroimmunological responses to stress (Sandvik et al., 2013). The training has been shown to be beneficial for college students, military personnel, and health care professionals (Bartone, Eid, & Hystad, 2016; Southwick, Litz, et al., 2011).

Well-Being Therapy

Well-being therapy is a short-term psychotherapeutic strategy that extends over 8 to 12 sessions (Fava, Rafanelli, Cazzaro, Conti, & Grandi, 1998).

The therapy is based on Ryff and Singer's (1996) six dimensions of psychological well-being, including self-acceptance, positive relations with others, autonomy, environmental mastery, purpose in life, and personal growth. Well-being therapy focuses on these six aspects of healthy psychological functioning and emphasizes self-observation. Self-observation is carried out through interactions between the therapist and individual, as well as structured diary keeping. In initial sessions, individuals are asked to keep a log of the circumstances encircling their episodes of well-being. Individuals are told to rate situations on a scale of 0 to 100, with zero being an absence of well-being and 100 being the highest possible level of well-being. This initial phase generally lasts a couple sessions but is dependent upon therapy compliance (Fava & Ruini, 2003). In later sessions, after the individual has successfully identified instances of well-being, therapists work with individuals to determine their thoughts and beliefs that result in interrupted development of well-being. In this phase, the therapist may challenge an individual's thoughts that are identified by asking particular probing questions. The therapist may also promote the individual to participate in activities that are likely to help build well-being (Fava & Ruini, 2003). Several rigorous studies have found that well-being therapy for several clinical populations results in symptom reduction and improvements in psychological well-being (Fava et al., 1998; Fava et al., 2004).

Battlemind Training

The term "battlemind" has been described as "the soldier's inner strength to face fear and adversity in combat with courage" (Adler et al., 2009, p. 230). Battlemind training consists of several components, including predeployment training and postdeployment training (Castro, Hoge, & Cox, 2006). Predeployment Battlemind training is designed to build soldier resilience by developing his or her confidence and mental toughness. The training focuses on soldiers' strengths, identifying specific actions that soldiers can engage in to meet the challenges of combat. Postdeployment Battlemind training includes psychological debriefing, developing social support, and addressing barriers to seeking help. While there has been limited study of predeployment training, randomized trials of postdeployment Battlemind training have found that soldiers who were trained had fewer stress-related symptoms and were less likely to report alcohol abuse problems than soldiers who only received stress education (Adler et al., 2009; Mulligan et al., 2012).

FUTURE DIRECTIONS

Considerable work has been done to define and assess resilience, identify factors related to resilience, and develop interventions to promote resilience. However, more work is needed in these areas as the trauma field progresses. Given the various ways resilience has been defined, it may be useful for the field to move toward developing a more unified and perhaps operational definition of resilience so that different studies can be compared and synthesized (e.g., meta-analysis). For example, Bonanno (2012) has proposed criteria for conducting methodologically sound studies of resilience, which include the following: (1) the temporal boarders of the event are explicitly operationally defined, and (2) resilience is clearly categorized as a stable pattern of healthy adjustment after the event, which (a) involves something more than simply the absence of diagnosable pathology, (b) is based on measurements collected at several different points in time, and (c) has an initial measurement of outcome collected relatively close in time to the occurrence of the event. Consideration of these criteria may be useful as the study of resilience develops. Certainly, further study on the relation between resilience and other different but important constructs, such as recovery and posttraumatic growth, may also be important.

While several self-report measures of resilience have been developed, some of which were described in this chapter, multidimensional measures of resilience that assess resilience across various life domains may be useful. Objective or biological-based measures of resilience should also be explored. The field of neurobiology is rapidly advancing, and there is much promising but preliminary research on neurobiological and genetic factors related to resilience and PTSD. Studies linking neurobiology to psychosocial outcomes are important to bridging the larger body of psychosocial studies on resilience with more biologically based studies and developing more comprehensive biopsychosocial models of resilience.

In addition to neurobiology, other ways of studying resilience should also be encouraged. Moving beyond traditional research methods, some have argued that transdisciplinary and mixed methods research should be utilized more often (Luthar & Brown, 2007). Further, the generalizability of findings and contextual and cultural variations in resilience should be examined (Ungar, 2013).

In terms of interventions, we are moving into an era of precision medicine where the goal is to individualize care and tailor interventions to conditions and settings. The same approach may be argued in efforts to promote and foster resilience. Developing interventions that build on individual strengths may be worth exploring instead of a one-size-fits all approach. Training programs that incorporate a range of resilience building mechanisms and intervention approaches (cognitive, emotional, and psychological) may be most efficient in promoting resilience in the greatest number of people (Adler, 2013). Resilience training should also be incorporated in standard training for high-risk careers, such as the in the military, police, and first responders. Given the importance of social support, future efforts to develop interventions should focus on ways to mobilize social resources and harness the benefits of social support to improve resilience. As trauma is a common experience in human life, it is incumbent on us to learn how to tap internal and external resources to overcome adversity and live healthy and fulfilling lives.

REFERENCES

Adler, A. B. (2013). Resilience in a military occupational health context: Directions for future research. In R. R. Sinclair and T.W. Britt (Eds.). *Building Psychological Resilience in Military Personnel: Theory and Practice* (pp. 223–235). American Psychological Association: Washington, DC.

Adler, A. B., Bliese, P. D., McGurk, D., Hoge, C. W., & Castro, C. A. (2009). Battlemind debriefing and battlemind training as early interventions with soldiers returning from Iraq: Randomization by platoon. *Journal of Consulting and Clinical Psychology*, *77*(5), 928–940. doi:10.1037/a0016877

American Psychological Association. (2014). The road to resilience. Retrieved from http://www.apa.org/helpcenter/road-resilience.aspx

Anacker, C., O'Donnell, K. J., & Meaney, M. J. (2014). Early life adversity and the epigenetic programming of hypothalamic-pituitary-adrenal function. *Dialogues in Clinical Neuroscience*, *16*(3), 321–333.

Asmundson, G. J., Fetzner, M. G., DeBoer, L. B., Powers, M. B., Otto, M. W., & Smits, J. A. (2013). Let's get physical: A contemporary review of the anxiolytic effects of exercise for anxiety and its disorders. *Depression and Anxiety*, *30*(4), 362–373.

Bartone, P. T. (2007). Test-retest reliability of the dispositional resilience scale-15: A brief hardiness scale. *Psychological Reports*, *101*(3), 943–944.

Bartone, P. T., Eid, J., & Hystad, S. W. (2016). Training hardiness for stress resilience. In N. Maheshwari & V. V. Kumar (Eds.), *Military psychology: Concepts, trends and interventions* (pp. 231–248). Greater Noida, India: SAGE.

Bartone, P. T., Ursano, R. J., Wright, K. M., & Ingraham, L. H. (1989). The impact of a military air disaster on the health of assistance workers: A prospective study. *Journal of Nervous and Mental Disease*, *177*(6), 317–328.

Berkman, L. F. (1995). The role of social relations in health promotion. *Psychosomatic Medicine*, *57*(3), 245–254.

Berkman, L. F., Leo-Summers, L., & Horwitz, R. I. (1992). Emotional support and survival after myocardial infarction: A prospective, population-based study of the elderly. *Annals of Internal Medicine*, *117*(12), 1003–1009.

Berkman, L. F., & Syme, S. L. (1979). Social networks, host resistance, and mortality: A nine-year follow-up study of Alameda County residents. *American Journal of Epidemiology*, *109*(2), 186–204.

Bonanno, G. A. (2004). Loss, trauma, and human resilience: Have we underestimated the human capacity to thrive after extremely aversive events? *American Psychologist*, *59*(1), 20.

Bonanno, G. A. (2012). Uses and abuses of the resilience construct: Loss, trauma, and health-related adversities. *Social Science & Medicine*, *74*(5), 753–756.

Bonanno, G. A., Mancini, A. D., Horton, J. L., Powell, T. M., LeardMann, C. A., Boyko, E. J., . . . Smith, T. C. (2012). Trajectories of trauma symptoms and resilience in deployed US military service members: Prospective cohort study. *The British Journal of Psychiatry*, *200*(4), 317–323.

Bonanno, G. A., Rennicke, C., & Dekel, S. (2005). Self-enhancement among high-exposure survivors of the September 11th terrorist attack: Resilience or social maladjustment? *Journal of Personality and Social Psychology*, *88*(6), 984.

Boyce, W. T., & Chesterman, E. (1990). Life events, social support, and cardiovascular reactivity in adolescence. *Journal of Developmental & Behavioral Pediatrics*, *11*(3), 105–111.

Brockhurst, J., Cheleuitte-Nieves, C., Buckmaster, C. L., Schatzberg, A. F., & Lyons, D. M. (2015). Stress inoculation modeled in mice. *Translational Psychiatry*, *5*, e537. doi:10.1038/tp.2015.34

Campbell-Sills, L., & Stein, M. B. (2007). Psychometric analysis and refinement of the Connor–Davidson resilience scale (CD-RISC): Validation of a 10-item measure of resilience. *Journal of Traumatic Stress*, *20*(6), 1019–1028.

Carver, C. S., & Scheier, M. F. (2014). Dispositional optimism. *Trends in Cognitive Sciences, 18*(6), 293–299.

Castro, C. A., Hoge, C. W., & Cox, A. L. (2006). *Battlemind training: Building soldier resiliency*. Retrieved from http://www.dtic.mil/dtic/tr/fulltext/u2/a472734.pdf.

Charney, D. S. (2004). Psychobiological mechanisms of resilience and vulnerability. *Focus, 2*(3):368–391.

Cobb, S. (1976). Social support as a moderator of life stress. *Psychosomatic Medicine, 38*(5), 300–314.

Cohen, S., & Wills, T. A. (1985). Stress, social support, and the buffering hypothesis. *Psychological Bulletin, 98*(2), 310.

Connor, K. M., & Davidson, J. R. (2003). Development of a new resilience scale: the Connor-Davidson Resilience Scale (CD-RISC). *Depression and Anxiety, 18*(2), 76–82. doi:10.1002/da.10113

Davidson, R. J. (2000). Affective style, psychopathology, and resilience: Brain mechanisms and plasticity. *American Psychologist, 55*(11), 1196–1214.

DiMatteo, M. R. (2004). Social support and patient adherence to medical treatment: A meta-analysis. *Health Psychology, 23*(2), 207–218. doi:10.1037/0278-6133.23.2.207

DuBois, C. M., Lopez, O. V., Beale, E. E., Healy, B. C., Boehm, J. K., & Huffman, J. C. (2015). Relationships between positive psychological constructs and health outcomes in patients with cardiovascular disease: A systematic review *International Journal of Cardiology, 195*, 265–280.

Erickson, K. I., Voss, M. W., Prakash, R. S., Basak, C., Szabo, A., Chaddock, L., . . . White, S. M. (2011). Exercise training increases size of hippocampus and improves memory. *Proceedings of the National Academy of Sciences, 108*(7), 3017–3022.

Fava, G. A., Rafanelli, C., Cazzaro, M., Conti, S., & Grandi, S. (1998). Well-being therapy: A novel psychotherapeutic approach for residual symptoms of affective disorders. *Psychological Medicine, 28*(2), 475–480.

Fava, G. A., & Ruini, C. (2003). Development and characteristics of a well-being enhancing psychotherapeutic strategy: Well-being therapy. *Journal of Behavior Therapy and Experimental Psychiatry, 34*(1), 45–63.

Fava, G. A., Ruini, C., Rafanelli, C., Finos, L., Salmaso, L., Mangelli, L., & Sirigatti, S. (2004). Well-being therapy of generalized anxiety disorder. *Psychotherapy and Psychosomatics, 74*(1), 26–30.

Feder, A., Charney, D., & Collins, K. (2011). Neurobiology of resilience. In S. M. Southwick, B. T. Litz, D. Charney, & M. J. Friedman (Eds.), *Resilience and mental health: Challenges across the lifespan* (pp. 1–29). New York: Cambridge University Press.

Feder, A., Nestler, E. J., & Charney, D. S. (2009). Psychobiology and molecular genetics of resilience. *Nature Reviews Neuroscience, 10*(6), 446–457.

Feldman, R. (2017). The Neurobiology of Human Attachments. *Trends in Cognitive Science, 21*(2), 80–99. doi:10.1016/j.tics.2016.11.007

Foa, E. B., Rothbaum, B. O., Riggs, D. S., & Murdock, T. B. (1991). Treatment of posttraumatic stress disorder in rape victims: A comparison between cognitive-behavioral procedures and counseling. *Journal of Consulting and Clinical Psychology, 59*(5), 715–723.

Frankl, V. E. (1992). *Man's search for meaning: An introduction to logotherapy* (4th ed.). Boston: Beacon Press.

Fredrickson, B. L. (2001). The role of positive emotions in positive psychology: The broaden-and-build theory of positive emotions. *American Physiology, 56*.

Fredrickson, B. L. (2013). Positive emotions broaden and build. *Advances in Experimental Social Psychology, 47*(1), 53.

Galea, S., Vlahov, D., Resnick, H. S., Ahern, J., Susser, E., Gold, J., . . . Kilpatrick, D. (2003). Trends of probable post-traumatic stress disorder in New York City after the September 11 terrorist attacks. *American Journal of Epidemiology, 158*(6), 514–524.

Garay-Sevilla, M., Nava, L. E., Malacara, J. M., Huerta, R., de León, J. D., Mena, A., & Fajardo, M. E. (1995). Adherence to treatment and social support in patients with non-insulin dependent diabetes mellitus. *Journal of Diabetes and its Complications, 9*(2), 81–86.

Gonzalez, J. S., Penedo, F. J., Antoni, M. H., Durán, R. E., McPherson-Baker, S., Ironson, G., . . . Schneiderman, N. (2004). Social support, positive states of mind, and HIV treatment adherence in men and women living with HIV/AIDS. *Health Psychology, 23*(4), 413.

Guidances, C., & Watch, T. (2007). Social support and resilience to stress: From neurobiology to clinical practice. *Psychiatry, 4*(5), 35–40.

Haglund, M. E., Nestadt, P. S., Cooper, N. S., Southwick, S. M., & Charney, D. (2007). Psychobiological mechanisms of resilience: Relevance to prevention and treatment of stress-related psychopathology. *Developmental Psychopathology, 19*(3), 889–920. doi:10.1017/S0954579407000430

Halevi, G., Djalovski, A., Vengrober, A., & Feldman, R. (2016). Risk and resilience trajectories in war-exposed children across the first decade of life.

Journal of Child Psychology and Psychiatry, 57(10), 1183–1193.

Holt-Lunstad, J., Smith, T. B., & Layton, J. B. (2010). Social relationships and mortality risk: A meta-analytic review. *PLoS Medicine, 7*(7), e1000316.

Horn, S. R., Charney, D. S., & Feder, A. (2016). Understanding resilience: New approaches for preventing and treating PTSD. *Experimental Neurology, 284*(Pt B), 119–132. doi:10.1016/j.expneurol.2016.07.002

Isaacs, K., Mota, N. P., Tsai, J., Harpaz-Rotem, I., Cook, J. M., Kirwin, P. D., . . . Pietrzak, R. H. (2016). Psychological resilience in U.S. military veterans: A 2-year, nationally representative prospective cohort study. *Journal of Psychiatric Research, 84*, 301–309. doi:10.1016/j.jpsychires.2016.10.017

Johnson, D. C., Polusny, M. A., Erbes, C. R., King, D., King, L., Litz, B. T., . . . Southwick, S. M. (2011). Development and initial validation of the Response to Stressful Experiences Scale. *Military Medicine, 176*(2), 161–169.

Kaplan, B. H., Cassel, J. C., & Gore, S. (1977). Social support and health. *Medical Care, 15*(5), 47–58.

Karaırmak, Ö. (2010). Establishing the psychometric qualities of the Connor–Davidson Resilience Scale (CD-RISC) using exploratory and confirmatory factor analysis in a trauma survivor sample. *Psychiatry Research, 179*(3), 350–356.

Kelly, J. A., Murphy, D. A., Bahr, G. R., Koob, J. J., Morgan, M. G., Kalichman, S. C., . . . St Lawrence, J. S. (1993). Factors associated with severity of depression and high-risk sexual behavior among persons diagnosed with human immunodeficiency virus (HIV) infection. *Health Psychology, 12*(3), 215–219.

Krystal, H. (2008). Resilience: Accommodation and recovery. In H. Parens, H. P. Blum, & S. Akhtar (Eds.), *The unbroken soul: Tragedy, trauma, and human resilience* (pp. pp. 47–64). Lanham, MD: Jason Aronson.

Lazarus, R. S., & Folkman, S. (1984). *Stress, appraisal, and coping*: New York: Springer.

Lin, T., Vaisvaser, S., Fruchter, E., Admon, R., Wald, I., Pine, D., . . . Hendler, T. (2015). A neurobehavioral account for individual differences in resilience to chronic military stress. *Psychological Medicine, 45*(5), 1011–1023.

Luthar, S. S., & Brown, P. J. (2007). Maximizing resilience through diverse levels of inquiry: Prevailing paradigms, possibilities, and priorities for the future. *Developmental Psychopathology, 19*. doi:10.1017/s0954579407000454

Luthar, S. S., Cicchetti, D., & Becker, B. (2000). The construct of resilience: A critical evaluation and guidelines for future work. *Child Development, 71*. doi:10.1111/1467-8624.00164

Lyons, D. M., Parker, K. J., & Schatzberg, A. F. (2010). Animal models of early life stress: Implications for understanding resilience. *Developmental Psychobiology, 52*(7), 616–624.

Maddi, S. R. (2006). Hardiness: The courage to grow from stresses. *The Journal of Positive Psychology, 1*(3), 160–168.

Maddi, S. R. (2012). *Hardiness: Turning stressful circumstances into resilient growth*: New York: Springer Science & Business Media.

Mallak, L. (1998). Putting organizational resilience to work. *Industrial Management, 40*(6), 8–13.

Masten, A. S., Monn, A. R., & Supkoff, L. M. (2011). Resilience in children and adolescents. In In S. M. Southwick, B. T. Litz, D. Charney, & M. J. Friedman (Eds.), *Resilience and mental health: Challenges across the lifespan* (pp. 103–119). Cambridge, UK: Cambridge University Press.

Masten, A. S., & Narayan, A. (2012). Child development in the context of disaster, war, and terrorism: Pathways of risk and resilience. *Psychology, 63*, 227–257.

McEwen, B. S. (2007). Physiology and neurobiology of stress and adaptation: Central role of the brain. *Physiological Reviews, 87*(3), 873–904.

Meichenbaum, D., & Cameron, R. (1989). Stress inoculation training. In by M. Jaremko & Donald Meichenbaum (Eds.), *Stress reduction and prevention* (pp. 115–154). New York: Springer.

Meneghel, I., Salanova, M., & Martínez, I. M. (2016). Feeling good makes us stronger: How team resilience mediates the effect of positive emotions on team performance. *Journal of Happiness Studies, 17*(1), 239–255.

Milkulincer, M., & Shaver, P. R. (2007). *Attachment in adulthood: Structure, dynamics, and change.* New York: Guilford Press.

Morgan, C. A., Rasmusson, A., Wang, S., Hoyt, G., Hauger, R. L., & Hazlett, G. (2002). Neuropeptide-Y, cortisol, and subjective distress in humans exposed to acute stress: Replication and extension of previous report. *Biological Psychiatry, 52*(2), 136–142.

Morgan, C. A., Southwick, S., Hazlett, G., Rasmusson, A., Hoyt, G., Zimolo, Z., & Charney, D. (2004). Relationships among plasma dehydroepiandrosterone sulfate and cortisol levels, symptoms of dissociation, and objective performance in humans exposed to acute stress. *Archives of General Psychiatry, 61*(8), 819–825.

Morgan, C. A., Wang, S., Southwick, S. M., Rasmusson, A., Hazlett, G., Hauger, R. L., & Charney, D. S. (2000). Plasma neuropeptide-Y concentrations in humans exposed to military survival training. *Biological Psychiatry*, *47*(10), 902–909.

Mulligan, K., Fear, N. T., Jones, N., Alvarez, H., Hull, L., Naumann, U., . . . Greenberg, N. (2012). Postdeployment Battlemind training for the UK armed forces: A cluster randomized controlled trial. *Journal of Consulting and Clinical Psychology*, *80*(3), 331–341.

Naim, R., Abend, R., Wald, I., Eldar, S., Levi, O., Fruchter, E., . . . Adler, A. B. (2015). Threat-related attention bias variability and posttraumatic stress. *American Journal of Psychiatry*, *172*(12), 1242–1250.

Norris, F. H., Friedman, M. J., Watson, P. J., Byrne, C. M., Diaz, E., & Kaniasty, K. (2002). 60,000 disaster victims speak: Part I. An empirical review of the empirical literature, 1981–2001. *Psychiatry*, *65*(3), 207–239.

Norris, F. H., Tracy, M., & Galea, S. (2009). Looking for resilience: Understanding the longitudinal trajectories of responses to stress. *Social Science & Medicine*, *68*(12), 2190–2198.

Penedo, F. J., & Dahn, J. R. (2005). Exercise and well-being: A review of mental and physical health benefits associated with physical activity. *Current Opinion in Psychiatry*, *18*(2), 189–193.

Pietrzak, R. H., Feder, A., Singh, R., Schechter, C. B., Bromet, E. J., Katz, C. L., . . . Crane, M. (2014). Trajectories of PTSD risk and resilience in World Trade Center responders: An 8-year prospective cohort study. *Psychological Medicine*, *44*(1), 205–219.

Pietrzak, R. H., Russo, A. R., Ling, Q., & Southwick, S. M. (2010). Suicidal ideation in treatment-seeking veterans of Operations Enduring Freedom and Iraqi Freedom: The role of coping strategies, resilience, and social support. *Journal of Psychiatric Research*, *123*(1–3), 102–107.

Pietrzak, R. H., & Southwick, S. M. (2011). Psychological resilience in OEF–OIF veterans: Application of a novel classification approach and examination of demographic and psychosocial correlates. *Journal of Affective Disorders*, *133*(3), 560–568.

Pietrzak, R. H., Tracy, M., Galea, S., Kilpatrick, D. G., Ruggiero, K. J., Hamblen, J. L., . . . Norris, F. H. (2012). Resilience in the face of disaster: Prevalence and longitudinal course of mental disorders following Hurricane Ike. *PLoS One*, *7*(6), e38964. doi:10.1371/journal.pone.0038964

Prince-Embury, S. (2008). The resiliency scales for children and adolescents, psychological symptoms, and clinical status in adolescents. *Canadian Journal of School Psychology*, *23*(1), 41–56.

Rana, B. K., Darst, B. F., Bloss, C., Shih, P. A., Depp, C., Nievergelt, C. M., . . . Jeste, D. V. (2014). Candidate SNP associations of optimism and resilience in older adults: Exploratory study of 935 community-dwelling adults. *American Journal of Geriatric Psychiatry*, *22*(10), 997–1006 e1005. doi:10.1016/j.jagp.2014.03.009

Rasmusson, A. M., Hauger, R. L., Morgan, C. A., Bremner, J. D., Charney, D. S., & Southwick, S. M. (2000). Low baseline and yohimbine-stimulated plasma neuropeptide Y (NPY) levels in combat-related PTSD. *Biological Psychiatry*, *47*(6), 526–539.

Russo, S. J., Murrough, J. W., Han, M. H., Charney, D., & Nestler, E. J. (2012). Neurobiology of resilience. *Nature Neuroscience*, *15*(11), 1475–1484.

Ryff, C. D., & Singer, B. (1996). Psychological well-being: meaning, measurement, and implications for psychotherapy research. *Psychotherapy and Psychosomatics*, *65*(1), 14–23.

Sandvik, A. M., Bartone, P. T., Hystad, S. W., Phillips, T. M., Thayer, J. F., & Johnsen, B. H. (2013). Psychological hardiness predicts neuroimmunological responses to stress. *Psychology, Health & Medicine*, *18*(6), 705–713.

Seligman, M. E. P. (2011). *Learned optimism: How to change your mind and your life*. New York: Vintage Books.

Shakespeare-Finch, J., & Enders, T. (2008). Corroborating evidence of posttraumatic growth. *Journal of Traumatic Stress*, *21*(4), 421–424.

Silverman, M. N., & Deuster, P. A. (2014). Biological mechanisms underlying the role of physical fitness in health and resilience. *Interface Focus*, *4*(5), 20140040.

Southwick, S. M., Bremner, J. D., Rasmusson, A., Morgan, C. A., Arnsten, A., & Charney, D. S. (1999). Role of norepinephrine in the pathophysiology and treatment of posttraumatic stress disorder. *Biological Psychiatry*, *46*(9), 1192–1204.

Southwick, S. M., Bonanno, G. A., Masten, A. S., Panter-Brick, C., & Yehuda, R. (2014). Resilience definitions, theory, and challenges: interdisciplinary perspectives. *European Journal of Psychotraumatology*, *5*. doi:10.3402/ejpt.v5.25338

Southwick, S. M., & Charney, D. S. (2012). The science of resilience: Implications for the prevention and treatment of depression. *Science*, *338*(6103), 79–82.

Southwick, S. M., Litz, B. T., Charney, D., & Friedman, M. J. (Eds.). (2011). *Resilience and mental health: Challenges across the lifespan.* New York: Cambridge University Press.

Southwick, S. M., Ozbay, F., Charney, D., & McEwen, B. (2008). Adaptation to stress and psychobiological mechanisms of resilience. In V. Tepe & B. J. Lukey (Eds.), *Biobehavioral resilience to stress* (pp. 91–116). London: Taylor & Francis.

Southwick, S. M., Pietrzak, R. H., & White, G. (2011). Interventions to enhance resilience and resilience-related constructs in adults. In S. M. Southwick, B. T. Litz, D. Charney, & M. J. Friedman (Eds.), *Resilience and mental health: Challenges across the lifespan* (pp. 289–306). New York: Cambridge University Press.

Southwick, S. M., Vythilingam, M., & Charney, D. S. (2005). The psychobiology of depression and resilience to stress: Implications for prevention and treatment. *Annual Review of Clinical Psychology, 1*, 255–291.

Stacey, M., Dearden, R., & Pill, R. (1970). *Hospitals, children and their families: The report of a pilot study.* London: Routledge & Kegan Paul.

Tindle, H. A., Chang, Y. F., Kuller, L. H., Manson, J. E., Robinson, J. G., Rosal, M. C., . . . Matthews, K. A. (2009). Optimism, cynical hostility, and incident coronary heart disease and mortality in the Women's Health Initiative. *Circulation, 120*(8), 656–662. doi:10.1161/CIRCULATIONAHA.108.827642

Tsai, J., Harpaz-Rotem, I., Pietrzak, R. H., & Southwick, S. M. (2012). The role of coping, resilience, and social support in mediating the relation between PTSD and social functioning in veterans returning from Iraq and Afghanistan. *Psychiatry: Interpersonal and Biological Processes, 75*(2), 133–148.

Tsai, J., Mota, N. P., Southwick, S. M., & Pietrzak, R. H. (2016). What doesn't kill you makes you stronger: A national study of U.S. military veterans. *Journal of Affective Disorders, 189*, 269–271. doi:10.1016/j.jad.2015.08.076

Turecki, G., & Meaney, M. J. (2016). Effects of the social environment and stress on glucocorticoid receptor gene methylation: A systematic review. *Biological Psychiatry, 79*(2), 87–96. doi:10.1016/j.biopsych.2014.11.022

U.S. Department of Veterans Affairs, & U.S. Department of Defense. (2010). *VA/DoD clinical practice guideline for management of post-traumatic stress.* Retrieved from http://www.healthquality.va.gov/guidelines/MH/ptsd/cpgPTSDFULL201011612c.pdf

Uchino, B. N., Cacioppo, J. T., & Kiecolt-Glaser, J. K. (1996). The relationship between social support and physiological processes: A review with emphasis on underlying mechanisms and implications for health. *Psychological Bulletin, 119*(3), 488.

Ungar, M. (2013). Resilience, trauma, context, and culture. *Trauma, Violence, & Abuse, 14*(3), 255–266. doi:10.1177/1524838013487805

Vaishnavi, S., Connor, K., & Davidson, J. R. T. (2007). An abbreviated version of the Connor-Davidson Resilience Scale (CD-RISC), the CD-RISC2: Psychometric properties and applications in psychopharmacological trials. *Psychiatry Research, 152*(2), 293–297.

Van der Velden, P. G., Christiaanse, B., Kleber, R. J., Marcelissen, F. G., Dorresteijn, S. A., Drogendijk, A. N., . . . Olff, M. (2006). The effects of disaster exposure and post-disaster critical incidents on intrusions, avoidance reactions and health problems among firefighters: A comparative study. *Stress, Trauma, and Crisis, 9*(2), 73–93.

Van Voorhees, E. E., Dedert, E. A., Calhoun, P. S., Brancu, M., Runnals, J., VA Mid-Atlantic MIRECC Workgroup, & Beckham, J. C. (2012). Childhood trauma exposure in Iraq and Afghanistan war era veterans: Implications for posttraumatic stress disorder symptoms and adult functional social support. *Child Abuse & Neglect, 36*(5), 423–432.

Vythilingam, M., Nelson, E. E., Scaramozza, M., Waldeck, T., Hazlett, G., Southwick, S. M., . . . Ernst, M. (2009). Reward circuitry in resilience to severe trauma: An fMRI investigation of resilient special forces soldiers. *Psychiatry Research, 172*(1), 75–77. doi:10.1016/j.pscychresns.2008.06.008

Wagnild, G. M. (2009). A review of the resilience scale. *Journal of Nursing Measurement, 17*(2), 105–113.

Wagnild, G. M., & Young, H. M. (1993). Development and psychometric evaluation of the Resilience Scale. *Journal of Nursing Measurement, 1*(2), 165–178.

Wald, I., Fruchter, E., Ginat, K., Stolin, E., Dagan, D., Bliese, P., . . . Bar-Haim, Y. (2016). Selective prevention of combat-related post-traumatic stress disorder using attention bias modification training: A randomized controlled trial. *Psychological Medicine, 46*(12), 2627–2636.

Wright, M., Fopma-Loy, J., & Fischer, S. (2005). Multidimensional assessment of resilience in mothers who are child sexual abuse survivors. *Child Abuse & Neglect, 29*(10), 1173–1193.

Wyman, P. A., Cowen, E. L., Work, W. C., Hoyt-Meyers, L., Magnus, K. B., & Fagen, D. B. (1999). Caregiving and developmental factors differentiating young at-risk urban children showing resilient versus stress-affected outcomes: A replication and extension. *Child Development*, *70*(3), 645–659.

Yehuda, R. (2002). Current status of cortisol findings in post-traumatic stress disorder. *Psychiatric Clinics of North America*, *25*(2), 341–368, vii.

Yehuda, R., Pratchett, L. C., Elmes, M. W., Lehrner, A., Daskalakis, N. P., Koch, E., . . . Bierer, L. M. (2014). Glucocorticoid-related predictors and correlates of post-traumatic stress disorder treatment response in combat veterans. *Interface Focus*, *4*(5), 20140048. doi:10.1098/rsfs.2014.0048

Yu, X., & Zhang, J. (2007). Factor analysis and psychometric evaluation of the Connor-Davidson Resilience Scale (CD-RISC) with Chinese people. *Social Behavior and Personality*, *35*(1), 19–30.

20

Evidence-Based Psychotherapies for Adults with PTSD

JULIETTE M. HARIK, JESSICA L. HAMBLEN, SONYA B. NORMAN, AND PAULA P. SCHNURR*

INTRODUCTION

The evidence-based practice movement originated in the 1980s, with the goal of incorporating relevant empirical evidence into all aspects of clinical practice, including assessment, diagnosis, and treatment (Rousseau & Gunia, 2016). Since then, the emphasis on using scientific research results to inform patient care has evolved into a global movement that has influenced numerous health care domains, including mental health care (Tanenbaum, 2005). Generally, the term *evidence-based treatment* (or alternatively, *empirically supported treatment*) is used to denote interventions for which there is consistent scientific evidence of efficacy or effectiveness. There is, however, a lack of consensus regarding the amount and quality of research support necessary for a treatment to be considered evidence-based (Chambless & Ollendick, 2001).

Consistent with the larger evidence-based practice movement, clinicians and policymakers within the field of posttraumatic stress disorder (PTSD) have increasingly looked to the research literature to guide decisions about care for patients with PTSD. The existing foundation of empirical evidence—consisting of more than 400 randomized controlled trials—shows that PTSD can be targeted effectively with a number of evidence-based treatments. In this chapter, we focus specifically on evidence-based psychotherapies (EBPs) for PTSD in adults (evidence-based psychotherapies for child traumatic stress are reviewed in Chapter 21, and evidence-based pharmacotherapies for adults with PTSD are reviewed in Chapter 22). We define EBPs for PTSD as those that have received the strongest possible recommendation in any of the current clinical practice guidelines for the treatment of PTSD.

One approach to promoting evidence-based practice for PTSD has been through the development of treatment guidelines. Current PTSD treatment guidelines for adults include those published by the following national and international organizations:

- The United Kingdom's National Institute for Health and Clinical Excellence (2005)
- Phoenix Australia (2013; formerly the Australian National Health and Medical Research Council)
- International Society for Traumatic Stress Studies (ISTSS; 2008)
- American Psychological Association (APA; 2017)
- Department of Veterans Affairs/ Department of Defense (VA/DoD; 2017)

Each organization rated the strength of the evidence for the efficacy of various PTSD treatments and, in doing so, identified treatments with the strongest evidence (i.e., treatments with first-level ratings, see Table 20.1). The guidelines used diverse methodologies and differ, for example, with respect to the level of evidence required for a treatment to receive a first-level rating and the relative weight given to statistical results versus expert consensus (for a review, see Forbes et al.,

* Corresponding author: National Center for PTSD, White River Junction VA Medical Center (116D), 215 North Main Street, White River Junction, VT 05009. Phone: 802-295-9363, ext. 5621. Fax: 802-295-5135. Email: Juliette.Harik@va.gov

TABLE 20.1. PSYCHOTHERAPIES WITH FIRST-LEVEL RATINGS IN PTSD CLINICAL PRACTICE GUIDELINES

Guidelines	Year	First-Level Rating
VA/DoD	2017	Trauma-focused psychotherapy with primary components of exposure, cognitive restructuring, or eye movements
ISTSS	2008	Exposure, Cognitive Processing Therapy, cognitive therapy, stress inoculation training, EMDR
NICE	2005	TF-CBT, EMDR
Phoenix Australia	2013	TF-CBT, EMDR
American Psychological Association	2017	TF-CBT

Note: EMDR = Eye Movement Desensitization and Teprocessing; ISTSS = International Society for Traumatic Stress Studies; NICE = United Kingdom's National Institute for Health and Clinical Excellence; PTSD = posttraumatic stress disorder; TF-CBT = trauma-focused cognitive-behavioral therapy; VA/DoD = Department of Veterans Affairs/Department of Defense.

2010). Given that these guidelines were published across a span of over ten years, they also differ in the body of included studies.

Despite having used different approaches, the guidelines consistently have given a first-level rating to trauma-focused cognitive behavioral therapy (TF-CBT) as a collective group, or to specific types of TF-CBT (e.g., the ISTSS guideline gave separate first-level ratings to exposure and Cognitive Processing Therapy, both of which are considered TF-CBT.) Eye Movement Desensitization and Reprocessing (EMDR) also has received a first-level rating in four of the five guidelines. This chapter provides an overview of these psychotherapies, including a review of the theory, techniques, and empirical support for each.

EVIDENCE-BASED PSYCHOTHERAPIES: COMMON GROUND AND UNIQUE DIFFERENCES

The current evidence-based psychotherapies for PTSD (as defined previously) are arguably more similar than they are different. All are manualized interventions, meaning that there is a structured protocol for administration. Although the treatment manuals identify the specific tasks and topics to be covered at each session, therapists can exercise clinical judgement within these protocols to tailor treatment to the individual, and a strong working alliance is an important component of administering these psychotherapies. Each of the EBPs for PTSD involves regular meetings with a therapist—usually weekly or twice weekly—so the time commitment associated with attending scheduled sessions is similar across interventions. Psychoeducation is a key element of all EBPs, and none require that a patient receive concurrent pharmacotherapy. Although current EBPs for PTSD share common elements, it is important to note that none of these elements has proven to be an essential element of EBP. Indeed, future research may indeed identify alternative EBPs for PTSD that include techniques with little or no overlap with the psychotherapies currently identified as evidence-based.

Despite some similarities, there are important differences among individual EBPs for PTSD. The treatments have diverse theoretical underpinnings and therefore vary with respect to the tasks or exercises that the patient is asked to complete. Although all EBPs for PTSD can be delivered in individual format, only some have been adapted for group formats. See Table 20.2 for a comparison of some of the key features of the various treatments. In the next section, we provide a detailed description of each EBP for PTSD and a brief overview the body of research that supports its effectiveness.

TRAUMA-FOCUSED COGNITIVE BEHAVIORAL THERAPY

Trauma-focused cognitive behavioral therapy (TF-CBT) is a broad term that refers to several specific types of psychotherapy for PTSD. *Trauma-focused* means that the treatment focuses on the memory of the traumatic event and its meaning. *Cognitive behavioral therapy* refers to a type of psychotherapy that focuses on identifying and changing certain patterns of thinking or behaving that are maintaining symptoms.

PTSD treatment guidelines differ in their approach to classifying TF-CBT treatments, with some evaluating separately the strength of the evidence for individual TF-CBT interventions and others evaluating all TF-CBT interventions collectively. In

TABLE 20.2. CHARACTERISTICS OF EVIDENCE-BASED PSYCHOTHERAPIES FOR PTSD

	Trauma-Focused CBT			Eye Movement Desensitization and Reprocessing
	Primarily Cognitive	Primarily Exposure	Mixed Cognitive-Exposure	
How does it work?	Teaches patients to identify negative thinking patterns and consider other perspectives	Helps patients gradually confront and emotionally process trauma reminders and memories	Uses a combination of techniques and exercises from primarily exposure and primary cognitive treatments	Helps patients process their memory of the trauma
What will the patient be asked to do in session?	Talk and write about how their thoughts about themselves and others have changed since the trauma	Repeatedly recount the details of the trauma and approach safe situations they have been avoiding		Think about the trauma and associated thoughts/feelings while focusing their eyes on a back-and-forth movement
What will the patient do between sessions?	Complete writing assignments and worksheets	Read or listen to their description of the trauma and/or practice activities they have avoided		No between-session homework
Is it a group or individual treatment?	Either	Usually individual	Usually individual	Individual

Note: CBT = cognitive-behavioral therapy; PTSD = posttraumatic stress disorder.

this chapter, we split TF-CBT treatments into three groups: (a) TF-CBT interventions that use primarily exposure techniques, (b) TF-CBT interventions that use primarily cognitive techniques, and (c) TF-CBT interventions that use mixed cognitive and exposure techniques.

Primarily Exposure

Exposure therapy is one of the most widely studied treatments for PTSD. The goal of exposure is to reduce distress related to trauma reminders and promote emotional processing of the trauma through gradual and repeated exposure to safe but distress-evoking memories and cues (Foa, Hembree, & Rothbaum, 2007).

Theory

The theoretical foundation for exposure therapy is emotional processing theory (Foa & Kozak, 1985). This theory posits that PTSD symptoms develop when trauma survivors form a mental model about danger (i.e., a fear network) in which they associate safe or neutral stimuli with a fear response. For example, the fear network of a person with combat-related PTSD may link stimuli such as fireworks (by association with mortar rounds) or roadside garbage (by association with explosive devices) with a fear response. Emotional processing theory holds that successful PTSD treatment involves activating the fear network and presenting new information that challenges the mistaken association. Toward this end, patients in exposure therapy are encouraged to think and talk systematically about the trauma, engage with trauma-related feelings, and/or approach safe reminders of the trauma in daily life.

Techniques

Exposure therapy for PTSD includes the use of imaginal exposure, which involves repeatedly retelling the account of the traumatic experience, and/or in-vivo exposure, which involves repeatedly engaging in safe activities or behaviors that the patient avoids because of the trauma. These techniques are used until the patient habituates to the traumatic memory or to the feared situation, meaning that the anxiety associated with these cues has decreased.

Exposure therapy protocols vary in the extent to which they use imaginal versus in-vivo exposure, the sequencing of these exposure components, and the degree to which they incorporate other treatment elements such as breathing retraining or relaxation. The method by which patients engage in imaginal or in-vivo exposure also varies across protocols. For example, imaginal exposure can be accomplished by having patients verbally recount the trauma aloud, as in Prolonged Exposure (PE; Foa et al., 2007; see Box 20.1) or write a detailed trauma account (as in Written Exposure Therapy; Sloan, Marx, & Resick, 2016). In-vivo exposure may involve approaching avoided situations in real life (e.g., visiting a crowded stadium) or can be conducted with the assistance of virtual reality technology that uses real-time computer graphics and body-tracking devices to create a computer-generated environment (Rizzo et al., 2010). There are currently insufficient data to suggest that any one method of exposure therapy is superior to another.

Research Evidence

A large body of scientific literature supports the effectiveness of exposure therapy for PTSD. A meta-analysis included 27 randomized controlled trials evaluating exposure therapy (10 of which examined PE). On average, exposure therapies had a meta-analytic effect size of 1.08 (considered a large effect) when compared to control conditions, such as another PTSD treatment or a waitlist (Watts et al., 2013). There is also evidence that patients who receive exposure therapy in routine clinical care experience clinically meaningful decreases in PTSD symptoms (e.g., Eftekhari et al., 2013; Goodson, Lefkowitz, Helstrom, & Gawrysiak, 2013). In addition, the benefits of PE have been found to

BOX 20.1. PROLONGED EXPOSURE

One of the most common exposure therapy protocols for PTSD is Prolonged Exposure (Foa et al., 2007). Prolonged Exposure is a 9- to 12-session manualized treatment that consists of four primary components:

PSYCHOEDUCATION

During the initial sessions, the therapist explains the rationale for exposure therapy. The therapist and patient discuss common reactions to trauma, which provides a framework for understanding PTSD symptoms.

BREATHING RETRAINING

The therapist introduces a relaxation skill called *breathing retraining*. Patients are encouraged to use this skill to help manage immediate distress.

IN-VIVO EXPOSURE

In-vivo exposure begins in session 2 with the construction of a hierarchy of feared situations. Beginning with a situation that is expected to cause moderate distress, the patient gradually confronts situations on the hierarchy. In-vivo exercises are practiced by the patient between sessions, though progress is reviewed at each session.

IMAGINAL EXPOSURE

Beginning in session 3, the patient recounts the details of the trauma aloud in session (approximately 40 minutes). This is followed by 15 to 20 minutes of *processing*, which involves discussing reactions to the exercise. Imaginal exposure is repeated at every subsequent session and patients listen to a audio recordings of the imaginal exposure each day.

extend beyond PTSD symptoms to symptoms of depression, physical health, and social functioning (Foa et al., 2013; Rauch et al., 2009). The sizeable body of research supporting the efficacy and tolerability of exposure therapy has served to assuage early concerns about its safety in the treatment of PTSD (e.g., Kilpatrick & Best, 1984). Although some patients experience a temporary worsening of PTSD symptoms during exposure therapy, most do not (Jayawickreme et al., 2014; Larsen et al., 2016). Moreover, patients who do experience temporary symptom increases are equally likely to complete treatment and benefit from it as those who do not experience a spike in symptoms (Foa et al., 2002). There is also growing evidence that exposure is safe and effective for PTSD patients with a wide variety of comorbid conditions, including alcohol dependence (Foa et al., 2013), borderline personality disorder (Harned, Korslund, Foa, & Linehan, 2012), psychosis (van den Berg et al., 2015), and a history of traumatic brain injury (Sripada et al., 2013).

Primarily Cognitive

Several TF-CBT protocols use primarily cognitive techniques to treat PTSD (e.g., Ehlers, Clark, Hackmann, McManus, & Fennell, 2005; Resick, Monson, & Chard, 2016). These interventions target PTSD symptoms by modifying faulty thoughts or beliefs related to the traumatic event.

Theory

Theoretical models underpinning cognitive therapy for PTSD suggest that people with PTSD develop negative and inaccurate beliefs about the trauma or its meaning that prevent natural recovery (Resick et al., 2016) and create a persistent state of perceived threat (Ehlers & Clark, 2000). These beliefs can focus on the self (*I deserve what happened to me*), others (*no one can be trusted*), or the world (*the world is a very dangerous place*). These beliefs can lead to feelings of fear, anger, sadness, shame, and guilt. Cognitive therapy aims to assist patients in identifying balanced thoughts about the meaning of the trauma, thereby allowing the patient to accept the reality of the trauma without adopting extreme negative beliefs. The cognitive model assumes that thoughts are related to feelings and that by changing negative thoughts, patients can reduce emotional distress.

Techniques

A major focus of primarily cognitive therapies is the identification of maladaptive trauma-related thoughts.[†] Throughout treatment, patients learn and practice a multistep process to evaluate and change these thoughts, called cognitive restructuring. Although each protocol has a unique approach to this process (i.e., protocols have different names for this process and break the process into different steps), we provide a general overview here. First, the patient identifies the maladaptive thought and the associated emotion. This is an important step given that many negative trauma-related thoughts occur automatically, without the patient's awareness. Next, the patient considers evidence for and against the thought. During this phase, the therapist uses gentle, probing, and clarifying questions to help the patient evaluate the accuracy of firmly held negative beliefs. For example, if a patient identifies the belief that "I am to blame for the car accident" the therapist may encourage him to consider other factors that may have contributed to the accident, such as road conditions and the actions of other drivers on the road. After considering the evidence, the patient can choose to identify a new, more balanced thought. Patient worksheets, used both in and outside session, are integral to this process. Often, complexity of the worksheets increases as treatment progresses.

It is common for cognitive therapies to include additional techniques to aid in or augment cognitive restructuring. For example, the cognitive therapy protocol developed by Ehlers and colleagues (2005) uses behavioral experiments to demonstrate that efforts to suppress or avoid unhelpful thoughts are often ineffective. The original protocol for Cognitive Processing Therapy (CPT; see Box 20.2) included a trauma narrative (though, notably, a more recent alternate version of CPT omits the trauma narrative given a dismantling study that showed the narrative did not enhance effectiveness; Resick et al., 2008; Resick et al., 2016); this written narrative is not needed for habitation but rather to allow cognitive interpretations and emotions related to trauma memory to be expressed and modified (Resick et al., 2008).

[†] Different protocols use various terms to describe these thoughts, including maladaptive beliefs, stuck points, and faulty cognitions.

BOX 20.2. COGNITIVE PROCESSING THERAPY

One widely used cognitive therapy protocol for PTSD is cognitive processing therapy (CPT; Resick, Monson, & Chard, 2016). CPT typically takes approximately 12 sessions, but this can vary from person to person. CPT has four main parts:

PSYCHOEDUCATION

CPT starts with education about trauma and PTSD. The therapist explains how thoughts about the trauma can influence emotions. The therapist also explains how CPT works and talks with the patient about treatment goals.

PROCESSING THE TRAUMA

Patients write an *impact statement* about how the trauma has changed their beliefs about themselves, others, and the word. Depending on the type of CPT, the patient may also be asked to write a description of the trauma, called a *trauma account*. Writing and rereading this trauma account helps patients feel their feelings related to the trauma and identify negative trauma-related beliefs.

LEARNING TO CHALLENGE THOUGHTS ABOUT THE TRAUMA

Patients learn a skill to identify and examine negative thoughts that are getting in the way of recovery. The therapist introduces a series of worksheets to aid in this process. Patients complete worksheets in session and at home.

TRAUMA THEMES

The last several sessions of CPT focus on five themes: safety, trust, power and control, esteem, and intimacy. Often, people with PTSD have problems in one or more of these areas. The patient completes worksheets to evaluate any negative beliefs related to these themes.

Research Evidence

There have been more than 20 well-controlled trials evaluating trauma-focused cognitive therapies for PTSD. Taken together, these trials provide robust support for the effectiveness of these interventions (Hedges' $g = 1.63$; Watts et al., 2013). Cognitive therapy has demonstrated effectiveness in patients exposed to a broad range of trauma types, including combat veterans (Monson et al., 2006), male and female survivors of abuse (Galovski, Blain, Mott, Elwood, & Houle, 2012), and military sexual trauma survivors (Surís, Link-Malcom, Chard, Ahn, & North, 2013). There is also evidence that trauma-focused cognitive therapy is effective with patients who present with a variety of comorbidities and clinical complexities, including chronic PTSD (Ehlers et al., 2005), serious mental illness (Mueser et al., 2008), suicidal ideation (Gradus, Suvak, Wisco, Marx & Resick, 2013), and alcohol dependence (Kaysen et al., 2014).

Some cognitive therapies for PTSD, such as CPT, can be offered as either group or individual treatments. However, trials evaluating group therapy tend to produce smaller treatment effects (Barrera, Mott, Hofstein, & Teng, 2013; Sloan, Feinstein, Gallagher, Beck, & Keane, 2013). A study of CPT in routine care (Jeffreys et al., 2014) and a randomized controlled trial comparing group and individual CPT (Resick et al., 2016) suggest that cognitive therapy delivered individually has an advantage over group delivery.

Mixed Cognitive Exposure

A smaller number of trauma-focused CBT protocols combine cognitive and exposure techniques without prioritizing one over the other. Several of these mixed cognitive-exposure protocols were developed to test the hypothesis that adding cognitive restructuring to an exposure protocol (or, conversely, adding exposure to a cognitive protocol) would enhance outcomes.

Research Evidence

Trials evaluating the effectiveness of mixed treatments have met with inconsistent results. Two studies found that augmenting exposure therapy with cognitive restructuring demonstrated no advantage over exposure therapy alone (Foa et al., 2005; Paunovic & Öst, 2001). Similarly, a third study comparing cognitive restructuring, PE, and their combination found that all three conditions similarly improved PTSD symptoms (Marks et al., 1998). To explain these findings, some researchers have proposed that when cognitive and exposure techniques are combined in a single protocol, patients may receive a smaller dose of each technique, which may in turn attenuate the effectiveness of the technique (Foa et al., 2005). Other studies, however, have reported that adding cognitive restructuring to an exposure protocol enhanced treatment gains (Bryant, Moulds, Guthrie, Dang, & Nixon, 2003; Bryant et al., 2008; see Box 20.3 for an overview of this protocol). Overall, the evidence to date suggests that mixed cognitive-exposure treatments are effective for PTSD, but uncertainty remains about the effectiveness of these protocols relative to primarily cognitive or primarily exposure treatments.

EYE MOVEMENT DESENSITIZATION AND REPROCESSING

EMDR is designed to alleviate the distress associated with traumatic memories (Shapiro, 1989). The goal of EMDR is to assist patients in accessing and processing traumatic memories in order to bring these memories to an adaptive resolution.

Theory

EMDR is based on adaptive information processing theory, which was proposed as a working hypothesis to describe EMDR's mechanism (Soloman & Shapiro, 2008). The theory posits that PTSD symptoms reflect dysfunctionally stored memories and that EMDR helps patients successfully process these memories within larger adaptive networks. Concentrating on internal emotional, cognitive, and physical experiences while simultaneously focusing the eyes on external rhythmic stimulus is said to assist with memory processing and reconsolidation. Specifically, the dual focus on internal and external stimuli is thought to activate the brain to naturally process information.

BOX 20.3. COGNITIVE RESTRUCTURING PLUS IMAGINAL EXPOSURE

This protocol combines both cognitive and exposure elements delivered in approximately eight weekly 90-minute sessions. The initial session is devoted to education about PTSD and cognitive restructuring. Patients learn about cognitive restructuring prior to imaginal exposure (which begins in session 2) so they understand how to monitor and challenge distressing thoughts that may arise during exposures. Future sessions are split between cognitive restructuring and imaginal exposure.

COGNITIVE RESTRUCTURING

Approximately 25 minutes of each session are devoted to cognitive restructuring. Patients learn to identify unrealistic thoughts about the trauma, themselves, and the future. They engage in daily monitoring of thoughts and feelings and learn to modify unrealistic thoughts with evidence-based thinking.

IMAGINAL EXPOSURE

Beginning in session 2, approximately 45 minutes of each session are devoted to imaginal exposure. Patients provide a verbal narrative of the trauma by reciting it in the present tense. During the narrative, patients are instructed to focus on any sensations or emotions that arise. Exposures are not audiotaped, but patients rehearse the exposure for daily homework.

During the final session, the patients and therapy discuss relapse prevention strategies, including the use of both exposure and cognitive restructuring techniques.

Techniques

In EMDR, the patient and therapist collaborate to identify a disturbing image that represents the worst part of the trauma, called a target. The patient holds this image in mind while focusing on any physical sensations or negative thoughts or emotions associated with the image. The patient simultaneously tracks the therapist's fingers, which move back and forth in the patient's visual field (i.e., saccadic eye movements), or on another form of bilateral stimulation (e.g., a tone that rings in one ear and then the next). Each eye movement set lasts approximately 20 seconds. In successive eye-movement episodes, the patient concentrates on any changes or new associations that have occurred. Eye movement episodes are repeated until negative affect has decreased and there are no new associations. The patient then tracks the therapist's finger while rehearsing a new, positive belief. This sequence is repeated until the new belief feels true.

Research Evidence

EMDR has been evaluated in at least 15 randomized controlled trials (Cusack et al., 2016). Like other EBPs for PTSD, a recent meta-analysis suggests that EMDR produces large treatment effects (Hedges' $g = 1.01$; Watts et al., 2013). The empirical support for EMDR has been a source of controversy, in part due to the limited methodological quality of several early EMDR trials. Indeed, some reviews and meta-analytic studies have excluded more than half of the published EMDR trials from analyses because these studies used methods that put them at a high risk for biased results (e.g., Cusack et al., 2016).

Although alternating eye movements are part of the classic EMDR technique, there is disagreement regarding the extent to which eye movements add to the effectiveness of EMDR. Two prior meta-analyses found no incremental effect for the eye movement component of EMDR (Davidson & Parker, 2001; Devilly, 2002). A more recent meta-analysis (Lee & Cuijpers, 2013), showed support for the effectiveness of eye movements for subjective distress but not for PTSD symptoms. The precise mechanisms of effectiveness in EMDR have yet to be determined, and there are differing perspectives on the extent to which the mechanism of effectiveness in EMDR may overlap with that of TF-CBT interventions. The VA/DoD Clinical Practice Guideline (2010), for example, suggests that the mechanisms of EMDR are likely similar to that of other exposure and cognitive therapies for PTSD whereas others suggest that EMDR's mechanisms are unique (Rogers & Silva, 2002).

SUMMARY AND FUTURE DIRECTIONS

PTSD treatment guidelines have identified a number of first-line psychotherapies for PTSD, including TF-CBT, and EMDR. Each of these treatments has been tested in a variety of patient samples and demonstrates effectiveness for patients who vary with respect to trauma type, comorbidities, gender, and age. Although there is a menu of effective psychotherapies, the field of PTSD continues to grow and investigate how these effective treatments compare to one another in terms of benefits and risks (in general and for specific patients), to explore various methods to enhance existing treatments, and to evaluate the effectiveness of other novel psychotherapies for PTSD.

Comparative Effectiveness

No single psychotherapy has emerged as most effective for PTSD. A recent review and meta-analysis of PTSD treatments conducted by the Agency for Healthcare Research and Quality concluded that there is insufficient head-to-head evidence to determine whether any one EBP is superior to another (Cusack et al., 2016). The EBPs for PTSD also appear to be similarly well tolerated (Jayawickreme et al., 2014), given that they report comparable attrition (Hembree et al., 2003; Imel et al., 2013). Research on prescriptive factors that predict which patients may fare better in one EBP versus another is nascent. Currently, there is little evidence to suggest that any EBPs are more effective for patients with a particular trauma type or of a particular gender or age (Cusack et al., 2016), although ongoing comparative effectiveness research will help to fill this gap (e.g., Schnurr et al., 2015). The lack of empirical guidance for patient-treatment matching highlights the importance of considering patient preferences when selecting a course of treatment (VA/DoD, 2017).

Enhancing Evidence-Based Psychotherapies

Although existing EBPs have consistently demonstrated effectiveness, there is room for improvement. Widespread efforts to disseminate EBP for PTSD are making inroads, yet it appears that a relatively small proportion of patients with PTSD receive an EBP (Karlin & Cross, 2014); among those who do initiate EBP, roughly 20% to 30% do not complete treatment (Imel et al.,

2013). A portion of patients who complete the full treatment will not respond or will show only modest gains. To address these limitations, researchers are increasingly exploring how to best enhance the effectiveness, efficiency, and accessibility of existing treatments. Several studies, for example, have evaluated whether augmenting psychotherapy with certain pharmacological agents—such as D-cycloserine or hydrocortisone—may lead to improved outcomes, though results have been mixed (for a review, see McGuire et al., 2017). Others have assessed whether combining an EBP with an intervention that targets, for example, emotion regulation (Cloitre et al., 2010) or sleep impairment (Galovski et al., 2016) may enhance patient response. Innovations targeting improved access have evaluated the delivery of EBP via video-teleconferencing and has shown encouraging results (e.g., Morland et al., 2015). To improve efficiency, other researchers have examined modifications to session length or frequency. In some cases, providers may be able to decrease the session length (Nacasch et al., 2015) or the number of sessions delivered (Galovski et al., 2012) without negatively impacting outcomes. Likewise, it appears that massed delivery in which patients received an entire course of TF-CBT in two weeks or less (Blount et al., 2014; Ehlers et al., 2014) may hold promise.

Emerging Psychotherapies

There is also ongoing research examining emerging psychotherapies for PTSD. In the past five years, researchers have added to the field of PTSD with numerous randomized trials evaluating novel interventions. The VA/DoD Guideline for PTSD that were revised in 2017 recommended several additional trauma focused treatments, including Brief Eclectic Psychotherapy (Nijdam, Gersons, Reitsma, de Jongh, & Olff, 2012), Narrative Exposure Therapy (Ertl, Pfeiffer, Schauer, Elbert, & Neuner, 2011) and written exposure therapy (e.g., Sloan et al., 2012).—Some treatments, such as Acceptance and Commitment Therapy, have met with little research support (Lang et al., 2017). Others—including Present Centered Therapy (initially developed to control for the nonspecific benefits of psychotherapy; Schnurr et al., 2005), Interpersonal Psychotherapy (Markowitz et al., 2015), and mindfulness-based stress reduction (Polusny et al., 2015), have shown more promising results. At this time, however, none of these interventions have received first-level ratings in current PTSD treatment guidelines, though it is possible that future revisions of the guidelines will expand the list of evidence-based psychotherapies for PTSD.

SUMMARY

Adults with PTSD can select from a number of evidence-based psychotherapy options. These interventions are effective in reducing PTSD and related distress in a range of complex patients. TF-CBT and EMDR have the most support. Comparative effectiveness studies are needed to determine which treatments work best for which types of patients. Given that there are a number of effective options, we encourage providers to engage patients in the treatment selection process to identify the specific treatment for PTSD that is most consistent with the patient's values and goals.

REFERENCES

American Psychological Association (2017). Clinical Practice Guideline for the Treatment of PTSD. Retrieved from http://www.apa.org/ptsd-guideline/ptsd.pdf on 01/21/2018.

Barrera, T. L., Mott, J. M., Hofstein, R. F., & Teng, E. J. (2013). A meta-analytic review of exposure in group cognitive behavioral therapy for posttraumatic stress disorder. *Clinical Psychology Review*, *33*, 24–32. doi:10.1016/j.cpr.2012.09.005

Blount, T. H., Cigrang, J. A., Foa, E. B., Ford, H. L., & Peterson, A. L. (2014). Intensive outpatient Prolonged Exposure for combat-related PTSD: A case study. *Cognitive and Behavioral Practice*, *21*, 89–96. doi:10.1016/j.cbpra.2013.05.004

Bryant, R. A., Moulds, M. L., Guthrie, R. M., Dang, S. T., Mastrodomenico, J., Nixon, R. D., . . . Creamer, M. (2008). A randomized controlled trial of exposure therapy and cognitive restructuring for posttraumatic stress disorder. *Journal of Consulting and Clinical Psychology*, *76*, 695–703. doi:10.1037/a0012616

Bryant, R. A., Moulds, M. L., Guthrie, R. M., Dang, S. T., & Nixon, R. D. (2003). Imaginal exposure alone and imaginal exposure with cognitive restructuring in treatment of posttraumatic stress disorder. *Journal of Consulting and Clinical Psychology*, *71*, 706–712. doi:10.1037/0022-006X.71.4.706

Chambless, D. L., & Ollendick, T. H. (2001). Empirically supported psychological interventions: Controversies and evidence. *Annual Review of Psychology*, *52*, 685–716. doi:10.1146/annurev.psych.52.1.685

Chemtob, C. M., Novaco, R. W., Hamada, R. S., & Gross, D. M. (1997). Cognitive-behavioral treatment for severe anger in posttraumatic stress disorder. *Journal of Consulting and Clinical Psychology*, *65*, 184–189. doi:10.1037/0022-006X.65.1.184

Cloitre, M., Stovall-McClough, K. C., Nooner, K., Zorbas, P., Cherry, S., Jackson, C. L., . . . Petkova, E. (2010). Treatment for PTSD related to childhood abuse: A randomized controlled trial. *American Journal of Psychiatry, 167*, 915–924 doi:10.1176/appi.ajp.2010.09081247

Cusack, K., Jonas, D. E., Forneris, C. A., Wines, C., Sonis, J., Middleton, J. C., . . . Weil, A. (2016). Psychological treatments for adults with posttraumatic stress disorder: A systematic review and meta-analysis. *Clinical Psychology Review, 43*, 128–141. doi:10.1016/j.cpr.2015.10.003

Davidson, P. R., & Parker, K. C. H. (2001). Eye movement desensitization and reprocessing (EMDR): A meta-analysis. *Journal of Consulting and Clinical Psychology, 69*, 305–316. doi:10.1037//0022-006X.69.2.305

Department of Veterans Affairs, & Department of Defense. (2017). *VA/DoD clinical practice guideline for the management of post-traumatic stress*. Retrieved from https://www.healthquality.va.gov/guidelines/MH/ptsd/VADoDPTSDCPGFinal012418.pdf

Devilly, G. J. (2002). Eye movement desensitization and reprocessing: A chronology of its development and scientific standing. *The Scientific Review of Mental Health Practice, 1*, 113–138. Retrieved from http://www.srmhp.org/

Eftekhari, A., Ruzek, J. I., Crowley, J. J., Rosen, C. S., Greenbaum, M. A., & Karlin, B. E. (2013). Effectiveness of national implementation of Prolonged Exposure therapy in Veterans Affairs care. *JAMA Psychiatry, 70*, 949–955. doi:10.1001/jamapsychiatry.2013.36

Ehlers, A., & Clark, D. M. (2000). A cognitive model of posttraumatic stress disorder. *Behaviour Research and Therapy, 38*, 319–345. doi:10.1016/S0005-7967(99)00123-0

Ehlers, A., Clark, D. M., Hackmann, A., McManus, F., & Fennell, M. (2005). Cognitive therapy for post-traumatic stress disorder: Development and evaluation. *Behaviour Research and Therapy, 43*, 413–431. doi:10.1016/j.brat.2004.03.006

Ehlers, A., Hackmann, A., Grey, N., Wild, J., Liness, S., Albert, I., . . . Clark, D. M. (2014). A randomized controlled trial of 7-day intensive and standard weekly cognitive therapy for PTSD and emotion-focused supportive therapy. *American Journal of Psychiatry, 171*, 294–304. doi:10.1176/appi.ajp.2013.13040552

Ertl, V., Pfeiffer, A., Schauer, E., Elbert, T., & Neuner, F. (2011). Community-implemented trauma treatment for former child soldiers in northern uganda: A randomized controlled trial. *Journal of the American Medical Association, 306*, 503–512. http://dx.doi.org/10.1001/jama.2011.1060

Foa, E. B., Dancu, C. V., Hembree E. A., Jaycox, L. H., Meadows, E. A., & Street, G. P. (1999). A comparison of exposure therapy, stress inoculation training, and their combination for reducing posttraumatic stress disorder in female assault victims. *Journal of Consulting and Clinical Psychology, 67*, 194–200. doi:10.1037/0022-006X.67.2.194

Foa, E. B., Hembree, E. A., Cahill, S. P., Rauch, S. A. M., Riggs, D. S., Feeny, N. C., & Yadin, E. (2005). Randomized trial of Prolonged Exposure for posttraumatic stress disorder with and without cognitive restructuring: Outcome at academic and community clinics. *Journal of Consulting and Clinical Psychology, 73*, 953–964. doi:10.1037/0022-006X.73.5.953

Foa, E. B., Hembree, E. A., & Rothbaum, B. O. (2007). *Prolonged exposure therapy for PTSD: Emotional processing of traumatic experiences: Therapist guide*. New York: Oxford University Press.

Foa, E. B., Keane, T. M., Friedman, M. J., & Cohen, J. A. (2008). *Effective treatments for PTSD: Practice guidelines of the International Society for Traumatic Stress Studies* (2nd ed.,). New York: Guilford Press.

Foa, E. B., & Kozak, M. J. (1985). Treatment of anxiety disorders: Implications for psychopathology. In A. H. Tuma & J. D. Maser (Eds.), *Anxiety and the anxiety disorders* (pp. 421–452). Hillsdale, NJ: Erlbaum.

Foa, E. B., Rothbaum, B. O., Riggs, D. S., & Murdock, T. B. (1991). Treatment of posttraumatic stress disorder in rape victims: A comparison between cognitive-behavioral procedures and counseling. *Journal of Consulting and Clinical Psychology, 59*, 715–723. doi:10.1037/0022-006X.59.5.715

Foa, E. B., Yusko, D. A., McLean, C. P., Suvak, M. K., Bux, D. A., Oslin, D., . . . Volpicelli, J. (2013). Concurrent naltrexone and Prolonged Exposure therapy for patients with comorbid alcohol dependence and PTSD: A randomized clinical trial. *JAMA, 310*, 488–495. doi:10.1001/jama.2013.8268

Foa, E. B., Zoellner, L. A., Feeny, N. C., Hembree, E. A., & Alvarez-Conrad, J. (2002). Does imaginal exposure exacerbate PTSD symptoms? *Journal of Consulting and Clinical Psychology, 70*, 1022–1028. doi:10.1037/0022-006X.70.4.1022

Foley, F. W., Bedell, J. R., LaRocca, N. G., Scheinberg, L. C., & Reznikoff, M. (1987). Efficacy of stress-inoculation training in coping with multiple sclerosis. *Journal of Consulting and Clinical Psychology, 55*, 919–922. doi:10.1037/0022-006X.55.6.919

Forbes, D., Creamer, M., Bisson, J. I., Cohen, J. A., Crow, B. E., Foa, E. B., . . . Ursano, R. J. (2010). A guide to guidelines for the treatment of PTSD and related conditions. *Journal of Traumatic Stress, 23*, 537–552. doi:10.1002/jts.20565

Galovski, T.E., Harik, J. M., Blain, L.M., Elwood, L.S., Gloth, C., & Fletcher, T. (2016). Augmenting cognitive processing therapy to improve sleep impairment in PTSD: A randomized controlled trial. *Journal of Consulting and Clinical Psychology, 84*, 167–177. doi:10.1037.ccp0000059

Galovski, T. E., Blain, L. M., Mott, J. M., Elwood, L., & Houle, T. (2012). Manualized therapy for PTSD: Flexing the structure of cognitive processing therapy. *Journal of Consulting and Clinical Psychology, 80*, 968–981. doi:10.1037/a0030600

Goodson, J. T., Lefkowitz, C. M., Helstrom, A. W., & Gawrysiak, M. J. (2013). Outcomes of Prolonged Exposure therapy for veterans with posttraumatic stress disorder. *Journal of Traumatic Stress, 26*, 419–425. doi:10.1002/jts.21830

Gradus, J. L., Suvak, M. K., Wisco, B. E., Marx, B. P., & Resick, P. A. (2013). Treatment of posttraumatic stress disorder reduces suicidal ideation. *Depression and Anxiety, 30*, 1046–1053. doi:10.1002/da.22117

Harned, M. S., Korslund, K. E., Foa, E. B., & Linehan, M. M. (2012). Treating PTSD in suicidal and self-injuring women with borderline personality disorder: Development and preliminary evaluation of a dialectical behavior therapy Prolonged Exposure protocol. *Behaviour Research and Therapy, 50*, 381–386. doi:10.1016/j.brat.2012.02.011

Hembree, E. A., Foa, E. B., Dorfan, N. M., Street, G. P., Kowalski, J., & Tu, X. (2003). Do patients drop out prematurely from exposure therapy for PTSD? *Journal of Traumatic Stress, 16*, 555–562. doi:10.1023/B:JOTS.0000004078.93012.7d

Hensel-Dittmann, D., Schauer, M., Ruf, M., Catani, C., Odenwald, M., Elbert, T., & Neuner, F. (2011). Treatment of traumatized victims of war and torture: A randomized controlled comparison of narrative exposure therapy and stress inoculation training. *Psychotherapy and Psychosomatics, 80*, 345–352. doi:10.1159/000327253

Imel, Z. E., Laska, K., Jakupcak, M., & Simpson, T. L. (2013). Meta-analysis of dropout in treatments for posttraumatic stress disorder. *Journal of Consulting and Clinical Psychology, 81*, 394–404. doi:10.1037/a0031474

Jayawickreme, N., Cahill, S. P., Riggs, D. S., Rauch, S. A., Resick, P. A., Rothbaum, B. O., & Foa, E. B. (2014). D. *Depression and Anxiety, 31*, 412–419. doi:10.1002/da.22225

Jeffreys, M. D., Reinfeld, C., Nair, P. V., Garcia, H. A., Mata-Galan, E., & Rentz, T. O. (2014). Evaluating treatment of posttraumatic stress disorder with cognitive processing therapy and Prolonged Exposure therapy in a VHA specialty clinic. *Journal of Anxiety Disorders, 28*, 108–114. doi:10.1016/j.janxdis.2013.04.010

Karlin, B. E., & Cross, G. (2014). From the laboratory to the therapy room: National dissemination and implementation of evidence-based psychotherapies in the US Department of Veterans Affairs Health Care System. *American Psychologist, 69*, 19–33. doi:10.1037/a0033888

Kaysen, D., Schumm, J., Pedersen, E. R., Seim, R. W., Bedard-Gilligan, M., & Chard, K. (2014). Cognitive processing therapy for veterans with comorbid PTSD and alcohol use disorders. *Addictive Behaviors, 39*, 420–427. doi:10.1016/j.addbeh.2013.08.016

Kilpatrick, D. G., & Best, C. L. (1984). Some cautionary remarks in treating sexual abuse victims with implosion. *Behavior Therapy, 15*, 421–423. doi:10.1016/S0005-7894(84)80011-8

Kilpatrick, D. G., Veronen, L. J., & Resick, P.E. (1982). Psychological sequelea to rape: Assessment and treatment strategies. In D. M. Dolays & R. L. Meredith (Eds.), *Behavioral medicine: Assessment and treatment strategies* (pp. 473–497). New York: Plenum Press. doi:10.1007/978-1-4684-4070-6_19

Lang, A. J., Schnurr, P. P., Jain, S., He, F., Walser, R. D., Bolton, E., . . . Strauss, J. (2017). Randomized controlled trial of acceptance and commitment therapy for distress and impairment in OEF/OIF/OND veterans. *Psychological Trauma: Theory, Research, Practice, and Policy, 9*(Suppl. 1), 74–84. doi:10.1037/tra0000127

Larsen, S. E., Stirman, S. W., Smith, B. N., & Resick, P. A. (2016). Symptom exacerbations in trauma-focused treatments: Associations with treatment outcome and non-completion. *Behaviour Research and Therapy, 77*, 68–77. doi:10.1016/j.brat.2015.12.009

Lee, C. W., & Cuijpers, P. (2013). A meta-analysis of the contribution of eye movements in processing emotional memories. *Journal of Behavior Therapy and Experimental Psychiatry, 44*, 231–239. doi:10.1016/j.jbtep.2012.11.001

Lee DJ, Schnitzlein CW, Wolf JP, Vythilingam M, Rasmusson AM, & Hoge CW. (2016). Psychotherapy versus pharmacotherapy for posttraumatic stress disorder: Systemic re view and meta-analyses to determine first-line treatments. *Depression and Anxiety, 33, 92-806.*

Markowitz, J. C., Petkova, E., Neria, Y., Van Meter, P. E., Zhao, Y., Hembree, E., . . . Marshall, R. D. (2015). Is exposure necessary? A randomized clinical trial of interpersonal psychotherapy for PTSD. *American Journal of Psychiatry, 172*, 430–440. doi:10.1176/appi.ajp.2014.14070908

Marks, I., Lovell, K., Noshirvani, H., Livanou, M., & Thrasher, S. (1998). Treatment of posttraumatic stress disorder by exposure and/or cognitive restructuring: A controlled study. *Archives of General Psychiatry, 55*, 317–325. doi:10.1001/archpsyc.55.4.317

McGuire, J. F., Wu, M. S., Piacentini, J., McCracken, J. T., & Storch, E. A. (2017). A meta-analysis of d-cycloserine in exposure-based treatment: Moderators of treatment efficacy, response, and diagnostic remission. *The Journal of Clinical Psychiatry, 78*(2), 196–206. doi:10.4088/JCP.15r10334

Meichenbaum, D. (1974). *Cognitive-behavior modification.* Morristown, NJ: General Learning Press.

Monson, C. M., Schnurr, P. P., Resick, P. A., Friedman, M. J., Young-Xu, Y., & Stevens, S. P. (2006). Cognitive processing therapy for veterans with military-related posttraumatic stress disorder. *Journal of Consulting and Clinical Psychology, 74*, 898–907. doi:10.1037/0022-006X.74.5.898

Morland, L. A., Mackintosh, M. A., Rosen, C. S., Willis, E., Resick, P., Chard, K., & Frueh, B. C. (2015). Telemedicine versus in-person delivery of cognitive processing therapy for women with posttraumatic stress disorder: A randomized noninferiority trial. *Depression and Anxiety, 32*, 811–820. doi:10.1002/da.22397

Mueser, K. T., Rosenberg, S. D., Xie, H., Jankowski, M. K., Bolton, E. E., Lu, W., . . . Wolfe, R. (2008). A randomized controlled trial of cognitive-behavioral treatment for posttraumatic stress disorder in severe mental illness. *Journal of Consulting and Clinical Psychology, 76*, 259–271. doi:10.1037/0022-006X.76.2.259

Nacasch, N., Huppert, J. D., Su, Y. J., Kivity, Y., Dinshtein, Y., Yeh, R., & Foa, E. B. (2015). Are 60-minute Prolonged Exposure sessions with 20-minute imaginal exposure to traumatic memories sufficient to successfully treat PTSD? A randomized noninferiority clinical trial. *Behavior Therapy, 46*, 328–341. doi:10.1016/j.beth.2014.12.002

National Institute for Health and Care Excellence. (2005). *Post-traumatic stress disorder: Management* (NICE Clinical Guideline No. 26). Retrieved from https://www.nice.org.uk/guidance/cg26

Nijdam, M. J., Gersons, B. P., Reitsma, J. B., de Jongh, A., & Olff, M. (2012). Brief eclectic psychotherapy v. eye movement desensitisation and reprocessing therapy for post-traumatic stress disorder: Randomised controlled trial. *The British Journal of Psychiatry, 200*, 224–231. doi:10.1192/bjp.bp.111.099234

Paunovic, N., & Öst, L. G. (2001). Cognitive-behavior therapy vs exposure therapy in the treatment of PTSD in refugees. *Behaviour Research and Therapy, 39*, 1183–1197. doi:10.1016/S0005-7967(00)00093-0

Phoenix Australia, Centre for Posttraumatic Mental Health. (2013). *Australian guidelines for the treatment of acute stress disorder and posttraumatic stress disorder.* Retrieved from http://phoenixaustralia.org/wp-content/uploads/2015/03/Phoenix-ASD-PTSD-Guidelines.pdf

Polusny, M. A., Erbes, C. R., Thuras, P., Moran, A., Lamberty, G. J., Collins, R. C., . . . Lim, K. O. (2015). Mindfulness-based stress reduction for posttraumatic stress disorder among veterans: A randomized clinical trial. *JAMA, 314*, 456–465. doi:10.1001/jama.2015.8361

Rauch, S. A. M., Grunfeld, T. E. E., Yadin, E., Cahill, S. P., Hembree, E., & Foa, E. B. (2009). Changes in reported physical health symptoms and social function with Prolonged Exposure therapy for chronic posttraumatic stress disorder. *Depression and Anxiety, 26*, 732–738. doi:10.1002/da.20518

Resick, P. A., Galovski, T. E., Uhlmansiek, M. O. B., Scher, C. D., Clum, G. A., & Young-Xu, Y. (2008). A randomized clinical trial to dismantle components of cognitive processing therapy for posttraumatic stress disorder in female victims of interpersonal violence. *Journal of Consulting and Clinical Psychology, 76*, 243–258. doi:10.1037/0022-006X.76.2.243

Resick, P. A., Monson, C. M., & Chard, K. M. (2016). *Cognitive processing therapy for PTSD: A comprehensive manual.* New York: Guilford.

Resick, P. A., Wachen, J. S., Dondanville, K. A., et al., (2017). Effect of Group vs Individual Cognitive Processing Therapy in Active-Duty Military Seeking Treatment for Posttraumatic Stress Disorder: A Randomized Clinical Trial. *JAMA Psychiatry, 74, 28-36.* doi: 10.1001/jamapsychiatry.2016.2729.

Rizzo, A., Difede, J., Rothbaum, B. O., Reger, G., Spitalnick, J., Cukor, J., & Mclay, R. (2010). Development and early evaluation of the virtual Iraq/Afghanistan exposure therapy system for combat-related PTSD. *Annals of the New York Academy of Sciences, 1208*, 114–125. doi:10.1111/j.1749-6632.2010.05755.x

Rogers, S., & Silver, S. M. (2002). Is EMDR an exposure therapy? A review of trauma protocols. *Journal of Clinical Psychology, 58*, 43–59. doi:10.1002/jclp.1128

Rousseau, D. M., & Gunia, B. C. (2016). Evidence-based practice: The psychology of EBP implementation. *Annual Review of Psychology, 67*, 667–692. doi:10.1146/annurev-psych-122414-033336

Schnurr, P. P., Chard, K. M., Ruzek, J. I., Chow, B. K., Shih, M. C., Resick, P. A., . . . Lu, Y. (2015). Design of VA Cooperative Study #591: CERV-PTSD, comparative effectiveness research in veterans with PTSD. *Contemporary Clinical Trials, 41,* 75–84. doi:10.1016/j.cct.2014.11.017

Schnurr, P. P., Friedman, M. J., Engel, C. C., Foa, E. B., Shea, M. T., Resick, P. M., . . . Chow, B. K. (2005). Issues in the design of multisite clinical trials of psychotherapy: VA Cooperative Study No. 494 as an example. *Contemporary Clinical Trials, 26,* 626–636. doi:10.1016/j.cct.2005.09.001

Shapiro, F. (1989). Eye movement desensitization: A new treatment for post-traumatic stress disorder. *Journal of Behavior Therapy and Experimental Psychiatry, 20,* 211–217. doi:10.1016/0005-7916(89)90025-6

Sloan, D. M., Feinstein, B. A., Gallagher, M. W., Beck, J. G., & Keane, T. M. (2013). Efficacy of group treatment for posttraumatic stress disorder symptoms: A meta-analysis. *Psychological Trauma: Theory, Research, Practice, and Policy, 5,* 176.

Sloan, D. M., Marx, B. P., & Resick, P. A. (2016). Brief treatment for PTSD: A non-inferiority trial. *Contemporary Clinical Trials, 48,* 76–82. doi:10.1016/j.cct.2016.04.003

Sloan, D. M., Marx, B. P., Bovin, M. J., Feinstein, B. A., & Gallagher, M. W. (2012). Written exposure as an intervention for PTSD: A randomized clinical trial with motor vehicle accident survivors. *Behavior Research and Therary, 50,* 627–635.

Solomon, R. M., & Shapiro, F. (2008). EMDR and the adaptive information processing model potential mechanisms of change. *Journal of EMDR Practice and Research, 2,* 315–325. doi:10.1891/1933-3196.2.4.315

Sripada, R. K., Rauch, S. A. M., Tuerk, P. W., Smith, E., Defever, A. M., Mayer, R. A., . . . Venners, M. (2013). Mild traumatic brain injury and treatment response in Prolonged Exposure for PTSD. *Journal of Traumatic Stress, 26,* 369–375. doi:10.1002/jts.21813

Surís, A., Link-Malcolm, J., Chard, K., Ahn, C., & North, C. (2013). A randomized clinical trial of cognitive processing therapy for veterans with PTSD related to military sexual trauma: Randomized trial of CPT for MST-related PTSD. *Journal of Traumatic Stress, 26,* 28–37. doi:10.1002/jts.21765

Tanenbaum, S. J. (2005). Evidence-based practice as mental health policy: Three controversies and a caveat. *Health Affairs, 24,* 163–173. doi:10.1377/hlthaff.24.1.163

Taylor, S., Thordarson, D. S., Maxfield, L., Fedoroff, I. C., Lovell, K., & Ogrodniczuk, J. (2003). Comparative efficacy, speed, and adverse effects of three PTSD treatments: Exposure therapy, EMDR, and relaxation training. *Journal of Consulting and Clinical Psychology, 71,* 330–338. doi:10.1037/0022-006X.71.2.330

van den Berg, D. P. G., de Bont, P. A. J. M., van der Vleugel, B. M., de Roos, C., de Jongh, A., Van Minnen, A., & van der Gaag, M. (2015). Prolonged exposure vs eye movement desensitization and reprocessing vs waiting list for posttraumatic stress disorder in patients with a psychotic disorder: A randomized clinical trial. *JAMA Psychiatry, 72,* 259–267. doi:10.1001/jamapsychiatry.2014.2637

Watts, B. V., Schnurr, P. P., Mayo, L., Young-Xu, Y., Weeks, W. B., & Friedman, M. J. (2013). Meta-analysis of the efficacy of treatments for posttraumatic stress disorder. *Journal of Clinical Psychiatry, 74,* 541–550. doi:10.4088/JCP.12r08225

21

Psychosocial Interventions for Child Traumatic Stress

GLENN N. SAXE, HANNAH GARTNER, AND ADAM D. BROWN

INTRODUCTION

As detailed in previous chapters of this volume, trauma exposure is common in childhood, and a significant minority of traumatized children may develop deleterious psychiatric responses that have considerable consequences for healthy development and functioning. Thus a great many traumatized children are in need of effective intervention. Fortunately, a variety of interventions have been developed for child traumatic stress over the past two decades and for a variety of purposes. This chapter reviews the array of psychosocial interventions available for the treatment of child traumatic stress and the specific qualities of these interventions for addressing the needs of traumatized children and their families. The literature supporting the efficacy or effectiveness of these interventions is reviewed in detail. Unlike other reviews of the literature on this topic—which largely focus on highlighting the interventions with the highest level of empirical evidence from clinical trials—this chapter emphasizes the information that clinicians and their agencies will need in selecting interventions for traumatized children and families and the available evidence supporting such interventions. Accordingly, this chapter also highlights the gaps in our empirical knowledge that will be necessary to address in order to ensure that the interventions we provide can be effective, take root, and achieve acceptable scale in the settings where traumatized children typically receive care.

There is a growing consensus that many of the interventions with demonstrated efficacy or effectiveness in clinical trials have not been able to penetrate routine clinical practice and accordingly have not been able to improve the lives of the children and families who most need them (Beidas et al., 2015; Hoagwood & Olin, 2002; Kendall & Beidas, 2007; Saxe & Acri, 2017; Torrey et al., 2001). Interventions aimed to help traumatized children and families must be able to address their complex needs, the complex needs of the clinicians who deliver these interventions, and those of the agencies in which these interventions are delivered for the interventions to fully take root and achieve scale. In the next section, we detail these complex needs and their relevance for psychosocial interventions that have a meaningful impact on children with traumatic stress. Then we review the literature on psychosocial interventions with these complexities in mind.

THE COMPLEXITIES OF CARE FOR CHILDREN WITH TRAUMATIC STRESS

For a psychosocial intervention to have impact in the settings where children with traumatic stress typically receive care, the intervention must adequately address a host of complexities related to the children that need care, the realities of the social environments in which these children live, the needs of the agencies in which they receive care, and the challenges imposed by the service delivery system in which these agencies must operate. If the interventions that would be delivered miss these sorts of complexities, it is very unlikely that they will prove effective in the real world. These problems highlight four types of complexity that must be addressed:

1. *The complexity of the child*: A host of factors may affect a child's response to trauma and the child's engagement in—and response to—treatment, including the child's age, sex, cultural/religious/racial background, and medical/health status and the type of trauma experienced (e.g., sexual abuse, physical abuse, disasters) and its chronicity over development. Moreover, children have a wide variety of individual strengths and vulnerabilities that also affect

their response to trauma and engagement in treatment. Information related to this diversity should be integrated within a clinical approach for interventions to fully address a child's needs. The symptoms and developmental functional impact of trauma is not homogeneous and must be carefully assessed and addressed in treatment. The most common psychiatric disorder associated with trauma is posttraumatic stress disorder (PTSD). However, many disorders are commonly associated with PTSD such as depression, attention deficit hyperactivity disorder, substance abuse, and conduct disorder (Ackerman, Newton, McPherson, Jones, & Dykman, 1998; De Bellis et al., 2001; Famularo, Fenton, Kinscherff, & Augustyn, 1996; Greeson et al., 2014; Kilpatrick et al., 2003; Scheeringa & Zeanah, 2008), and so comorbidities are not unusual. Further, exposure to interpersonal trauma at an early age, repeated over time, can lead to more pervasive consequences for child development including impact on a child's capacity to regulate emotion, maintain stable relationships, and form a healthy sense of self. These pervasive developmental consequences have been called "complex traumatic stress" or "developmental traumatic stress" (Cook et al., 2005; D'Andrea, Ford, Stolbach, Spinazzola, & van der Kolk, 2012; van der Kolk & D'Andrea, 2010; van der Kolk, 2009; Wamser-Nanney & Vandenberg, 2013). Occasionally, symptoms related to child traumatic stress reach a level of acuity in which the child is at risk of harming him or herself or others. Accordingly, interventions must be able to provide clinical guidance for the ubiquitous problems of comorbidity, pervasive impact on development, and acuity of symptoms that will commonly be encountered in typical care settings. It is worth noting that the information that comes to the field from clinical trials primarily concerns the efficacy or effectiveness of an intervention to diminish PTSD symptoms with little information about impact on comorbidities, pervasiveness of developmental responses, or risk of harm.

2. *The complexity of social environment*: For too many children with traumatic stress, the response to the events of concern is not fully posttraumatic. Children may be exposed to ongoing maltreatment, witness ongoing family violence, or be exposed to the consequences of parental substance and/or severe mental illness in a continuing way. Often, reminders of traumatic events are omnipresent in children's environments. Again, the information that comes to the field about interventions validated in clinical trials is frequently silent about how providers should manage these problems or about their impact on engagement of families in treatment. Often children who live in such unstable environments are excluded from clinical trials.
3. *The complexity of care setting*: Interventions are delivered within care settings comprised of clinical and nonclinical staff and organizational leadership who use established organizational processes to manage the care delivered, and this care must be aligned with organizational policy and financial constraints. Providers responsible for delivering interventions may vary widely in their training and clinical skill. Organizational leadership may vary widely in their motivation to support the implementation of an intervention, and the organizational budget may provide significant constraints on the time and effort that can be allocated to deliver an intervention to a child. All of these factors influence the way in which a specified intervention can be delivered within a given clinical setting. Such factors may have considerable impact on whether an intervention evaluated with a defined fidelity standard can be delivered at anything close to its fidelity standard within a given setting. Notably, it is extremely rare for fidelity to be assessed when interventions are delivered in typical care settings.
4. *The complexity of service delivery systems*: Children with traumatic stress often receive services outside of the mental health system including the special education system, the child welfare system, and the juvenile justice system. Within the mental health system, children with traumatic stress may transition between different levels of care including outpatient, inpatient,

> residential, and emergency/crisis care. Sometimes interventions/services a child with traumatic stress receives will be fully complementary to the mental health intervention the child receives. Sometimes these interventions/services will work at cross-purposes or even undermine the child's trauma-informed mental health intervention. Accordingly, it is often critical for providers of interventions for traumatized children to collaborate with providers from other service systems, to inform services delivered in other service systems, and to advocate for needed services. This sort of coordination, collaboration, communication, and advocacy may be the most important driver of impact for interventions that are delivered to traumatized children and their families but are frequently considered as a peripheral part of care within many interventions evaluated in clinical trials.

The interventions available to treat children with traumatic stress vary widely in their guidance to clinicians for addressing each of these areas of complexity and in terms of the outcomes they aim to address. Many existing interventions—particularly those with the highest level of clinical evidence from clinical trials—mainly target PTSD outcomes exclusively. Some interventions have been developed to better address the complexity of the child's response to trauma. More recently, there has been an acknowledgment that interventions need to integrate specific approaches for addressing the complexities of the child's social environment, clinical care setting, and services system, and newer interventions have been developed to address these areas.

Next, we review available psychosocial interventions for child traumatic stress related to their empirical evidence base and their capacity to address the aforementioned complexities. For readers interested in more comprehensive reviews of interventions evaluated in clinical trials, there are several excellent articles that have recently been published (e.g., Dorsey et al., 2017; Gillies, Taylor, Gray, O'Brien, & D'Abrew, 2013; Leenarts, Diehle, Doreleijers, Jansma, & Lindauer, 2013). Our aim is not to repeat these reviews but to describe the breadth of psychosocial interventions available for specific purposes and to detail their strengths and weaknesses for addressing the four areas of complexity critical for usual clinical practice. The empirical literature supporting the respective interventions will be reviewed in this context.

THE ARRAY OF AVAILABLE PSYCHOSOCIAL INTERVENTIONS

There is now a wide array of available psychosocial treatments for a range of problems experienced by children with traumatic stress. Although there are a great many points of intersection between many of these treatments they can—broadly—be divided into four categories:

1. Behavioral/exposure-based interventions
2. Cognitive behavioral interventions
3. Developmental/relational interventions
4. Systems interventions

Next, we review interventions in each of these categories with the understanding of the overlap between categories (e.g., developmental/relational interventions can often contain both cognitive behavioral and systems components; systems interventions can contain both developmental/relational and cognitive behavioral components). Accordingly, interventions are placed in categories related to their primary focus, but interventions will commonly have secondary or tertiary areas of focus that cross into other categories. This review primarily focuses on psychosocial interventions for children with traumatic stress who are school aged and older as another chapter in this book is focused on younger children. This review is also focused on interventions designed to treat traumatic stress and not on those designed to prevent it.

Behavioral/Exposure-Based Interventions

Exposure-based interventions serve to provide a safe and therapeutic environment for structured exposure of the child to stimuli reminiscent of the trauma in order to extinguish the traumatic stress response. There are several models of therapeutic exposure that have been implemented with children. In gradual exposure, the child is encouraged to verbally recount aspects of the trauma to which he or she was exposed while the therapist assists the child in processing general or minor elements of the traumatic event (Catani et al., 2009; Foa, McLean, Capaldi, & Rosenfield, 2013; Gilboa-Schechtman et al., 2010; Ruf et al., 2010). As gradual exposure therapy progresses, the treatment works to reduce the child's distress surrounding the trauma and its reminders through various media, including writing stories, drawing pictures, talking into a tape recorder, and playing out aspects of the traumatic experience. As memories of the trauma become less activating, the therapist encourages the child to access, discuss, and process increasingly anxiety-provoking traumatic memories in the context of the safe therapeutic environment. In contrast to gradual exposure therapy, in imaginal flooding therapy, children imagine specific details of the traumatic event while the therapist continually monitors the child's subjective ratings of emotional distress (Saigh, Yule, & Inamdar, 1996). The theory underlying exposure therapy techniques suggests that if children re-experience aspects of the traumatic event in a controlled and safe environment, the memories associated with the trauma will no longer be connected to distressing physiological and emotional reactions. Unpairing traumatic memories and disturbing affect can result in increased habituation and decreased avoidance symptoms.

Exposure therapy techniques have long been empirically supported for the treatment of PTSD symptoms in adults (Foa et al., 1999; Foa, Rothbaum, Riggs, & Murdock, 1991) and have been extended to treat children with histories of trauma exposure (Catani et al., 2009; Deblinger & Heflin, 1996; Deblinger, Lippmann, & Steer, 1996; Foa et al., 2013; Gilboa-Schechtman et al., 2010; Ruf et al., 2010). Several randomized controlled trials (RCTs) from the past decade have demonstrated the efficacy of Prolonged Exposure therapy for treating PTSD symptoms in children and adolescents. Foa and colleagues (2013) found that Prolonged Exposure therapy was significantly more effective than supportive counseling in reducing sexual abuse–related PTSD symptoms in adolescent girls. Gilboa-Schectman and colleagues (2010) similarly found that Prolonged Exposure therapy was more effective than time-limited dynamic therapy in decreasing PTSD symptoms in adolescent victims of single-event traumas. Ruf et al. (2010) and Catani et al. (2009) both demonstrated evidence that KIDNET— a narrative exposure therapy for children—significantly improved PTSD symptoms and overall functioning in refugee children traumatized by organized violence and natural disasters.

The results of these studies indicate that exposure treatments have proven efficacious for PTSD in some groups of traumatized children. Further research is needed on the impact of exposure therapy for traumatized children with more diagnostic complexity (i.e., comorbidities, pervasive developmental responses, self-destructive/aggressive symptoms) and across ages and cultural groups. Exposure therapy may be particularly problematic for children who live in environments with ongoing exposure to adversities/traumas. In these children, the events are not in the child's past and therefore not subject to extinction through therapeutic exposure to past traumas: they are part of the child's day-to-day life. If exposure-based therapy is to be considered for a child, the complexity of the child's social environment must be carefully assessed.

Cognitive Behavioral Interventions

Generally, cognitive interventions can serve to challenge thoughts that maintain traumatic stress responses (Resick & Schnicke, 1992). These techniques are useful when employed to correct cognitive errors and equip children with more adaptive coping skills. Children with traumatic stress histories often demonstrate cognitive distortions, including thoughts of a foreshortened future, self-blame, survivor guilt, and overgeneralization of the traumatic event.

Cognitive coping is a specific cognitive intervention that has been modified by Deblinger and Heflin (1996) from Beck's (1976) cognitive treatment for depression. Cognitive coping has been adapted specifically for the treatment of traumatized children and teaches patients about the relationship between maladaptive automatic thoughts, negative emotional states, and dysfunctional behaviors. Through cognitive coping, children learn emotion regulation skills by simultaneously altering negative cognitions and assessing the impact on behavior.

The integration of cognitive therapy approaches with exposure-based approaches—as used in cognitive behavior therapy (CBT)—is now the most extensively studied intervention approach for childhood traumatic stress. The most extensively studied version of CBT for traumatized children is trauma-focused cognitive behavioral therapy (TF-CBT; Cohen, Mannarino, & Deblinger, 2006, 2017). TF-CBT is a 12- to 25-session intervention model with eight therapeutic elements anchored by the PRACTICE acronym: (a) **P**sychoeducation and parenting skills, (b) **R**elaxation, (c) **A**ffective expression and regulation, (d) **C**ognitive coping, (e) **T**rauma narrative development and processing, (f) **I**n vivo gradual exposure, (g) **C**onjoint parent-child sessions, and (h) **E**nhancing safety and future development.

There are many variants of CBT models, but they generally include several distinct components, including psychoeducation, cognitive coping, stress management, cognitive processing, exposure-based exercises, and relapse prevention. Additionally, most efficacious CBT treatments include cognitive and behavioral parental components (de Arellano et al., 2014). The parent elements of treatment offer an opportunity for parents to express and process their own feelings regarding their child's traumatic experience and related behaviors and emotions. Parents may learn stress management skills to facilitate their own coping (Cohen, Mannarino, Berliner, & Deblinger, 2000; Cohen & Mannarino, 1993). Some variants to CBT models emphasize grief and loss as a part of traumatic stress (Kaplow, Layne, Saltzman, Cozza, & Pynoos, 2013; Layne et al., 2001; Saltzman et al., 2017).

In addition to individual CBT, the efficacy of group CBT interventions for childhood traumatic stress have demonstrated promising results (Jaycox et al., 2010; Kataoka et al., 2003; McMullen, O'Callaghan, Shannon, Black, & Eakin, 2013; O'Callaghan, McMullen, Shannon, Rafferty, & Black, 2013; Runyon, Deblinger, & Steer, 2010; Stein et al., 2003). Similar to individual CBT interventions, group CBT interventions implement cognitive and behavioral exercises, including psychoeducation, cognitive therapy, exposure-based behavior therapy, and relapse prevention. The specific goal of group trauma-focused CBT is for children to integrate traumatic memories within their self-concept through group-based exposures and cognitive exercises. The unique strength of group treatments lies in their ability to provide treatment to greater numbers of children representing underserved populations (Deblinger, Pollio, & Dorsey, 2016). Group CBT has also been adapted for specific use in schools. Cognitive Behavioral Intervention for Trauma in Schools (CBITS) is a group-based treatment designed for delivery in schools that focuses on psychoeducation about trauma, relaxation training, cognitive therapy, exposure therapy, and social problem-solving (Jaycox, Kataoka, Stein, Langley, & Wong, 2012).

Eye Movement Desensitization and Reprocessing

We include eye movement desensitization and reprocessing (EMDR) under the category of CBT-oriented treatments because—even though there is a unique component of the intervention involving specific eye movements or bilateral stimulation using other sensory modalities—that part of the intervention is implemented in the service of enabling the child to have greater access to trauma memories for cognitive processing and extinction of traumatic stress responses. Based on Adaptive Information Processing Theory, EMDR suggests that traumatic memories can be processed neurophysiologically using dual attention tasks (Shapiro, Kaslow, & Maxfield, 2011). Key components of treatment include psychoeducation about the trauma and therapy, preparation of the target traumatic memory, desensitization of the memory, identification and processing of body sensations, and re-evaluation of the target memory (Diehle, Opmeer, Boer, Mannarino, & Lindauer, 2015). During the desensitization phase, the EMDR therapist induces rapid eye movements (or other types of bilateral stimulation) in the child, who is guided simultaneously through imaginal exposure of a traumatic memory. The child reports images, thoughts, and feelings that arise as a result of each set of eye movements. The therapist continues guiding eye movements (or other types of bilateral stimulation) in conjunction with imaginal exposure and cognitive restructuring until the target memory no longer induces distress (Diehle et al., 2015).

Clinical trials of CBT interventions (and variants) have been extensive with approximately 22 RCTs having been conducted to date (de Arellano et al., 2014; Deblinger et al., 2016; Dorsey et al., 2017). Meta-analyses of CBT interventions for trauma have also been published documenting their efficacy and effectiveness across the cohorts studied (Kowalik, Weller, Venter, & Drachman, 2011; Lenz & Hollenbaugh, 2015). CBT-oriented interventions have been extensively studied across trauma types, subject ages, and populations. These treatments have mainly been tested for PTSD outcomes, but outcomes such as anxiety disorders and depression have also been studied. RCTs have demonstrated effectiveness of individual CBT in children with histories of sexual abuse (Cohen & Mannarino, 1996; Cohen & Mannarino, 1998; Cohen et al., 2000; Cohen, Mannarino, Perel, & Staron, 2007; Cohen, Mannarino, & Rogal, 2001; Cohen, Mannarino, & Knudsen, 2005; Deblinger et al., 1996; Deblinger, Mannarino, Cohen, Runyon, & Steer, 2011; King et al., 2000), domestic violence (Cohen, Mannarino, & Iyengar, 2011; Smith et al., 2007), childhood traumatic grief (Cohen et al., 2006), single-incident trauma (Smith et al., 2007), multiple traumatic experiences (Jensen et al., 2014), and heterogeneous types of trauma (Goldbeck, Muche, Sachser,

Tutus, & Rosner, 2016; Murray et al., 2015; Nixon, Vandervord, Sterk, & Pearce, 2012; Smith et al., 2007; Weiner, Schneider, & Lyons, 2009). RCTs of individual TF-CBT from the past decade are briefly described here:

Goldbeck and colleagues (2016) examined the effectiveness of TF-CBT for children and adolescents with a wide range of different trauma types in eight German mental health clinics. Compared with children in the waitlist control condition, children receiving TF-CBT experienced significantly greater remission of posttraumatic stress symptoms, dysfunctional trauma-related cognitions, PTSD diagnoses, depression, anxiety, and other internalizing and externalizing symptoms.

Murray et al. (2015) compared lay counselor–provided TF-CBT with treatment as usual (TAU) in 257 traumatized orphans and vulnerable children at community sites in Lusaka, Zambia. Children in the TF-CBT group showed significantly greater improvements in PTSD symptoms and overall functioning than their counterparts in the TAU condition, providing evidence that TF-CBT can be effective even when administered by lay counselors in an underresourced community.

In a study of 156 multiply-traumatized adolescents (participants reported being exposed to an average of 3.6 different traumatic events), Jensen and colleagues (2014) compared TF-CBT to TAU in community clinics in Norway. They found that TF-CBT was significantly more effective than TAU in reducing symptom levels on all measures of posttraumatic stress, depression, and general mental health.

Smith et al. (2007) demonstrated that for children who had experienced single-incident trauma (including motor-vehicle accidents, interpersonal violence, and domestic violence), 10 sessions of TF-CBT was significantly more effective than the waitlist condition in improving PTSD symptoms, depression, anxiety, and overall functioning.

Cohen and colleagues (2007) compared the effects of TF-CBT + placebo with TF-CBT + a selective serotonin reuptake inhibitor (sertraline) in children with histories of sexual abuse. Both groups showed significant improvement in PTSD symptoms, with no significant differences between the groups, providing further evidence for the effectiveness of TF-CBT alone.

Cohen, Mannarino, and Iyengar (2011) evaluated the efficacy of an abbreviated course of TF-CBT (eight sessions) for children who had been exposed to intimate partner violence directed at the child's mother. This study compared eight sessions of TF-CBT with child-centered therapy at a women's shelter/intimate partner violence center and found that abbreviated TF-CBT was significantly more effective than child-centered therapy in reducing PTSD symptoms, providing evidence that TF-CBT may be effective in briefer doses.

Several studies have examined whether TF-CBT can be effective without the trauma exposure component. Deblinger et al. (2011) examined the differential effects of TF-CBT with or without the trauma narrative component in 8 versus 16 sessions in a sample of 210 sexually abused children. They found that regardless of the number of sessions or the inclusion of the trauma narrative component, TF-CBT was effective in improving symptomology as well as parenting skills and children's personal safety skills. This study provides further evidence that TF-CBT can be effective in briefer doses and also indicates that TF-CBT may not require a trauma narrative component. Nixon and colleagues (2012) further examined this question by comparing the efficacy of traditional TF-CBT with trauma-focused cognitive therapy *without exposure* in youth who had experienced single-incident trauma. They found that both interventions significantly reduced the severity of PTSD, depression, and general anxiety. A follow-up study reported that both groups maintained these posttreatment gains at one-year follow-up, concluding that PTSD following single-incident trauma can be successfully treated with trauma-focused cognitive behavioral interventions with or without the use of exposure techniques (Nixon, Sterk, Pearce, & Weber, 2016).

CBT-oriented interventions have also been tested with demonstrated effectiveness in group formats (Jaycox et al., 2010; Kataoka et al., 2003; McMullen et al., 2013; O'Callaghan et al., 2013; Runyon, Deblinger, & Steer, 2010; Stein et al., 2003). Two RCTs in the Democratic Republic of Congo demonstrated that group-based TF-CBT was significantly more effective than the waitlist control in reducing trauma symptoms as well as overall psychosocial distress, depression, anxiety, and conduct problems in former child soldiers (McMullen et al., 2013) and sexually exploited and war-affected girls (O'Callaghan et al., 2013). Runyon and colleagues compared the efficacy of group-based combined parent-child CBT with group-based parent only CBT for children who had been physically abused and their offending or at-risk parent. Runyon et al. found that children and parents in the combined parent-child CBT group demonstrated greater improvements in total posttraumatic stress symptoms and positive parenting skills compared with those who participated in the parent-only CBT group. Two RCTs to date have demonstrated evidence for CBITS (Stein et al., 2003; Kataoka et al., 2003). In a study of students exposed to violence, Stein and colleagues found that students in the CBITS group experienced significantly greater reductions in PTSD symptoms than those in the waitlist control group. Kataoka and colleagues evaluated CBITS for Latino immigrant students who had been exposed to community violence and found that students in the intervention group showed significantly greater improvement in PTSD and depressive symptoms compared with those on the waitlist at three-month follow-up. In a more recent quasi-experimental study of New Orleans schoolchildren following Hurricane Katrina, Jaycox and colleagues found that CBITS led to significant reductions in PTSD symptoms.

EMDR has shown effectiveness in children with histories of disaster-related trauma (Chemtob, Nakashima, & Carlson, 2002; de Roos et al., 2011) and heterogeneous types of trauma (Ahmad, Larsson, & Sundelin-Wahlsten, 2007; Diehle et al., 2015; Farkas, Cyr, Lebeau, & Lemay, 2010). In the first empirical study of EMDR with traumatized children, Chemtob et al. evaluated the use of EMDR to treat disaster-related PTSD symptoms in 32 children whose symptoms had not improved 3.5 years following exposure to a hurricane and one year after receiving a school counselor-administered treatment. Children were randomly assigned to a three-session early or delayed EMDR intervention, and participants reported significantly reduced symptoms of PTSD, depression, and anxiety. These improvements were maintained at six-month follow-up. Ahmad et al. compared the efficacy of EMDR with a waiting list control group in a sample of 33 children meeting criteria for PTSD and also having grown up with a family member with criminality, substance abuse, chronic illness, handicap, or a history of being physically or mentally unavailable for the child. Children who received eight weekly EMDR sessions showed significantly more improvement in PTSD and PTSD-related symptoms than those in the control group, with the biggest difference between groups being the improvement in re-experiencing symptoms for children in the EMDR condition. Farkas and colleagues compared the efficacy of a new treatment—Motivation-Adaptive Skills-Trauma Resolution (MASTR)/EMDR—with a routine care condition for maltreated adolescents who were in the charge of youth protective services and were exhibiting conduct problems and internalizing and externalizing behaviors. MASTR/EMDR is a treatment that combines EMDR with MASTR—a treatment that incorporates empirically validated strategies for youth with conduct problems. Adolescents in the EMDR/MASTR group showed significantly greater improvements in their trauma symptoms and behavioral problems than those in the control group, and these effects were maintained at three-month follow-up. Several RCTs have found that EMDR can be just as effective as CBT in treating traumatic stress symptoms (de Roos et al., 2011; Diehle et al., 2015; Jaberghaderi, Greenwald, Rubin, Zand, & Dolatabadi, 2004). Jaberghaderi and colleagues compared CBT and EMDR interventions in 12- and 13-year-old sexually abused Iranian girls. Youth in both treatments showed significant improvements on levels of PTSD symptoms, with no differences between the groups. EMDR was, however, more efficient, with patients in the EMDR group completing the treatment in fewer sessions than those in the CBT group. De Roos and colleagues (2011) also compared the efficacy of CBT with EMDR, but with 52 children exposed to a factory explosion. This study also found that EMDR was equally effective as CBT, with both treatments producing significant and lasting improvements on measures of PTSD symptoms, depression, anxiety, and behavior problems. Treatment gains of EMDR were reached in fewer sessions than in CBT, replicating the finding of Jaberghaderi and colleagues. In a more recent study, Diehle and colleagues compared the efficacy of EMDR with TF-CBT in a sample of 48 traumatized youth in Amsterdam, finding that both treatments were equally effective in reducing PTSD symptoms.

Although the empirical literature supporting CBT (and variants) for PTSD and several other outcomes is extensive and impressive for children with a variety of trauma types, the literature is not nearly as extensive on the impact of CBT for children with acute levels of risk and with more pervasive developmental responses to trauma. Moreover, these treatments do not provide much guidance to providers for the ongoing management of psychiatric risk or about risk to the child from ongoing trauma/abuse. These are frequently concerns of clinicians providing care to traumatized children. CBT approaches also do not provide specific guidance about fit for the treatment within the organizations that would implement it, or the integration of the treatment with other interventions in the services system. These concerns will often limit an interventions' capacity to take root or scale within the setting in which it is implemented.

Developmental/Relational Interventions

Interventions in this category were developed from a growing recognition that the focus of most behavioral and cognitive behavioral interventions misses the complexity of the impact of repetitive interpersonal trauma on child development. A conceptualization of the complexity of the child's response has been called complex trauma or developmental trauma (Cook et al., 2005; D'Andrea et al., 2012; van der Kolk & D'Andrea, 2010; van der Kolk, 2009; Wamser-Nanney & Vandenberg, 2013) and is primarily related to the child's experience of chronic interpersonal trauma/maltreatment. Accordingly, several interventions have been developed to address these problems based on the more pervasive developmental responses that come from chronic interpersonal trauma. Although not formally included in the *Diagnostic and Statistical Manual of Mental Disorders* (fifth edition), this approach to traumatized children has gained much ground in the field, and many providers find such an approach clinically useful. The initiative to define complex or developmental trauma conceptualized the comorbidities commonly diagnosed in children exposed to repetitive interpersonal trauma as a part of a unified clinical picture. Complex/developmental trauma focused on such critical developmental and relational consequences of chronic interpersonal trauma as emotional regulation (including self-destruction/aggression), self-development, and stability of relationships. Treatments developed for complex/developmental trauma are designed to specifically address these problems and tend to provide more emphasis than behavioral or cognitive behavioral interventions on such critical elements of treatment as the safety in the therapeutic relationship and how enactments of previous interpersonal trauma can occur in the therapeutic relationship.

Treatments in this category include

Trauma Affect Regulation: Guide for Education and Therapy (TARGET): TARGET is an intervention for children over the age of 10 and contains three key components: The first key component of TARGET is psychoeducation about the biological and behavioral reactions to trauma. The second key component is the instruction and guided practice of a seven-skill sequence for managing traumatic stress symptoms, summarized by the acronym FREEDOM: **F**ocus, **R**ecognize triggers, **E**motion self-check, **E**valuate thoughts, **D**efine goals, **O**ptions, and **M**ake a contribution. These skills are aimed toward mental focusing, self-regulation skills, information/emotion processing, executive functioning, mindfulness, and interpersonal engagement/interaction. The third and final key component in TARGET is the development of an autobiographical narrative that incorporates the trauma. TARGET is frequently used with single parent families and children in foster, residential, or juvenile justice placements and is typically delivered in 10 to 12 group or individual sessions (Ford & Russo, 2006).

Structured Psychotherapy for Adolescents Responding to Chronic Stress (SPARCS): SPARCS is a group-based, present-focused intervention designed to address the needs of chronically stressed adolescents who may *still* be living with ongoing stress in their environment and are experiencing problems in several areas of functioning including difficulties with affect regulation, impulsivity, self-perception, relationships, somatization, dissociation, numbing, avoidance, struggles with their own purpose and meaning in life, and negative worldviews that impede their ability to envision a future for themselves. The treatment has been implemented with at-risk youth in a variety of settings including schools, juvenile justice, foster care (Weiner, Schneider, & Lyons, 2009), and residential treatment centers (Habib, Labruna, & Newman 2013). The intervention is typically delivered in 16-hour-long group sessions and key components of treatment include psychoeducation about traumatic stress and triggers, mindfulness practice, distress tolerance, problem-solving, relationship-building/communication skills, and meaning making (DeRosa & Pelcovitz, 2008). This intervention is designed to be culture-specific, and practitioners are expected to engage group members in discussions around the meaning of their traumas in the context of their respective cultures.

Attachment, Self-Regulation, and Competency (ARC): ARC is an intervention framework for youth of all ages (2–21) and their families. The intervention was specifically designed to address the needs of children and adolescents who have experienced multiple, chronic and of often ongoing stressors, including early childhood trauma. The approach is based in attachment theory and focuses on making a child's entire care-giving system more trauma-informed. ARC is not a manualized standard protocol but rather a flexible framework employing multiple modalities including individual, group, and family treatment; parent workshops; milieu/systems intervention; and home-based prevention programs. ARC identifies three core domains frequently impaired in chronically traumatized youth—(a) attachment, (b) self-regulation, and (c) competency. Within those domains, 10 key components of trauma-informed treatment and service are identified for assessment and intervention (Blaustein & Kinniburgh, 2017).

Integrative Treatment of Complex Trauma (ITCT): ITCT is for the treatment of children and adolescents of all ages (2–21) and was developed to address the needs of inner-city, culturally diverse, and often economically disadvantaged youth and families that have experienced multiple types of traumas. Recognizing the wide range of needs and resources of this population, ITCT is somewhat flexible in that it allows for shorter or longer-term therapy (average length of treatment is 16 to 36 sessions) and allows for the use of multiple modalities including individual, collateral, group, and family interventions. ITCT utilizes aspects of the self-trauma model (Briere, 2002), as well as cognitive models, and integrates both relational and cognitive behavioral approaches to addressing complex trauma. Key components of treatment include building safety, affect regulation training, emotional and cognitive processing of trauma, and improving attachment/relationships. Treatment also targets other complex/developmental trauma issues as they arise including chronic negative relational schema, identify-related issues, and substance abuse (Lanktree & Briere, 2015).

Skills Training in Affective and Interpersonal Functioning (STAIR): STAIR is an intervention approach for providing improved affect regulation and interpersonal/social skills to trauma survivors and has also been used to provide these skills for nontraumatized populations as well. It can be provided either individually or in groups. STAIR uses a "flexible toolkit" approach to provide psychoeducation, emotion regulation skills, interpersonal skills, and cognitive reappraisals, in the service of building mastery. A specific version, STAIR-A, has been developed to meet the developmental needs of adolescents (Levitt & Cloitre, 2005).

Real Life Heroes (RLH): RLH is an approach for addressing childhood trauma involving both youth and caregivers. Primary goals of treatment include improving emotion regulation and interpersonal relationships. It is a manualized approach which includes materials and activities for practitioners to use in sequenced child and family sessions. Examples of these include creating and sharing a life story book, creative arts activities, mindfulness exercises, and psychoeducation. RLH has been used in residential, education, and outpatient mental health settings (Kagan, 2016).

Although the focus of this chapter is on psychosocial interventions for school-age and older children, two interventions for younger children would fit within the developmental/relational intervention category: Child Parent Psychotherapy (CPP), a treatment for children under 6 and their primary caregivers based on psychodynamic principles and attachment theory (Lieberman, Van Horn & Ghosh Ippen, 2005), and Attachment and Biobehavioral Catch-Up (ABC), an attachment-based intervention which attempts to improve the child-caregiver relationship and thereby improve children's emotional regulation (Dozier et al., 2009).

Psychodynamic Approaches

Although psychodynamic approaches are not typically considered within the category of treatments for complex/developmental trauma, they share many characteristics with the interventions previously described in this category. Psychodynamic approaches are included in this category because they share an emphasis on understanding the impact of trauma through a developmental lens and, particularly, on the complexity of the individual child's response based on the interpersonal nature of the trauma. Psychodynamic therapy—like the models previously described focus on how dysregulation occurs in an interpersonal context related to the child's experience of caregiving particularly in early childhood. Psychodynamic approaches particularly emphasize the expression of dysregulated emotional states in response to the therapist and the information this provides for understanding the child's emotional life as expressed within his or her set of interpersonal relationships. Psychodynamic approaches, like the previously described approaches, also emphasize the impact of trauma—and the consequential pattern of dysregulated emotional states in relationships—on the child's developing sense-of-self. Psychodynamic approaches particularly emphasize the expression of these problems symbolically through displacement via therapeutic means such as play, art, and stories. These approaches tend to be less structured than other approaches in this category and often use more sessions over a longer period of time.

The developmental/relational interventions described in this category have the advantage of addressing the complexity of the child's response, as described previously. They are highly focused on addressing the pervasive developmental impact of interpersonal trauma and thus have a real advantage over treatments that focus on a much more narrow range of problems such as PTSD. They also have a much more integrated way of understanding psychopathology related to trauma as not a separate set of disconnected comorbidities but as an array of interconnected problems related to interpersonal trauma, as such events impact development. These interventions also tend to be delivered to children and families who live in adverse environments and often provide guidance on helping clinicians manage the social environmental complexities described previously. They are often delivered within front-line service delivery settings such as inner-city clinics, residential programs, and juvenile justice facilities and so they often include some guidance related to the complexity of clinical care setting and the complexity of services delivery system, but this guidance tends not to be as specific as the system interventions that is discussed next.

There is a growing empirical literature supporting the effectiveness of many of the developmental/relational interventions described in this section. This literature is not, however, nearly as extensive as the literature supporting the behavioral or the cognitive behavioral interventions. In a RCT, Ford, Steinberg, Hawke, Levine, and Zhang (2012). Ford and colleagues (2012) compared TARGET with relational supportive therapy in 59 delinquent adolescent girls. Girls in the TARGET condition showed significantly greater decreases in anxiety, depression, and trauma-related cognitions as compared with those in the supportive therapy group. A study of adolescents across three juvenile justice programs showed that early implementation of TARGET was associated with decreases in disciplinary incidents the use of seclusion and recidivism (Ford & Hawke, 2012). In a pilot study of SPARCS in residential treatment facilities by Habib, Labruna, and Newman (2013), 24 adolescents with histories of interpersonal trauma participated in SPARCS groups for 16 to 20 weeks. Following the SPARCS intervention, adolescents showed significant improvements in PTSD symptoms, as well as somatic complaints, intrapersonal distress, interpersonal relations, and behavioral dysfunction. Weiner, Schneider, and Lyons (2009) found that SPARCS was just as effective as TF-CBT in reducing trauma stress symptoms in children in foster care. The organizational implementation of the ARC model was evaluated in two residential treatment centers where it was integrated into both clinical and direct care practices (Hodgdon, Kinniburgh, Gabowitz, Blaustein, & Spinazzola, 2013). Findings indicate improvements in PTSD symptoms, reduced externalizing and internalizing behaviors, and decreased use of physical restraints. A study of ARC for use in outpatient settings with 481 adopted children with complex trauma demonstrated significant improvement in both child symptoms and caregiver stress following treatment and at 12-month follow-up (Hodgdon, Blaustein, Kinniburgh, Peterson, & Spinazzola, 2016). Lanktree and colleagues (2012) evaluated the efficacy of ITCT in a study of 121 traumatized children living in underserved settings and found that children that completed the ITCT intervention showed significant improvements in a variety of mental health domains, including PTSD and sexualized problems. In an early RCT evaluating the efficacy of STAIR, Cloitre and colleagues (2010) randomized 104 women with PTSD related to child abuse to one of three treatment conditions: (a) STAIR followed by exposure (STAIR/exposure), (b) supportive counseling followed by exposure (support/exposure), and (c) skills training followed by supportive counseling (STAIR/support). Findings demonstrated that the STAIR/exposure group was more likely to achieve sustained and full PTSD remission relative to the other groups. A study of the development and implementation of a brief adaptation of STAIR-A designed for adolescent inpatient settings looked at 38 adolescents participating in STAIR-A groups in an inpatient psychiatric unit in a public city hospital and found significant reductions in PTSD symptoms (Gudiño et al., 2014). RLH was evaluated in a pilot study of 41 children with traumatic stress (Kagan, Douglas, Hornik, & Kratz, 2008). Children who underwent RLH treatment showed significant reductions in trauma symptoms and problem behaviors. In a more recent study, Kagan and colleagues (2014) found that RLH led to significant decreases in internalizing and externalizing behaviors and PTSD symptoms in a sample of 117 traumatized youth across seven service settings. Currently, there is only an emerging clinical trial literature supporting the effectiveness of less structured psychodynamic treatments (Lieberman, Ippen & Marans, 2009). One RCT (Trowell et al., 2002) compared individual psychoanalytic treatment with group psychoeducation-focused treatment for 58 girls who were sexually abused. Although both treatments resulted in improved functioning, it was found that girls receiving individual psychoanalytic treatment showed greater reduction in PTSD symptoms both at one and two years posttreatment compared with those in the group therapy condition. This study is an important contribution to the childhood PTSD treatment literature, as it is the first RCT to compare individual psychoanalytic psychotherapy with a nonspecific group intervention in the treatment of sexually abused children.

Systems Interventions

Systems interventions largely developed because of observed gaps in the clinical and empirical literature for three of the four types of complexity described at the beginning of this chapter. The developmental/relational interventions primarily emphasize areas of the complexity of child's response to trauma based on its pervasive impact on development. The developmental/relational interventions usually contain more emphasis on the complexities of the child's social environment, the clinical care setting (and the providers), and/or the need for integrated care in the services system than the behavioral and cognitive behavioral interventions, but this emphasis tends not to be as specific as what is found within the systems interventions. Accordingly, systems interventions tend to emphasize approaches for understanding how the child's social environment influences his or her clinical presentation and provides guidance on how to intervene based on this understanding. Systems interventions also tends to provide more specific approaches for adjusting the model to the care setting that uses it and the integration of care across systems. There also tends to be a greater emphasis within the systems interventions on the creation and support of teams of providers to deliver trauma-informed care and the alignment of the values of a trauma-informed culture within the organization that supports this work.

Two intervention approaches are included in this category:

The Sanctuary Model: The Sanctuary Model is primarily an organizational approach to create a trauma-informed culture within agencies that treat traumatized children and families. This approach seeks to understand all aspects of the agency and to work to instill a set of values known to be important for trauma-informed care as the organization seeks to establish a safe and productive environment for people to heal from trauma. The Sanctuary Model also includes an endorsed clinical approach that is consistent with those specified in the developmental/relational category of interventions but contains less specificity about the conduct of the clinical interventions than those defined within that category. The Sanctuary Model has four key components. The first is to develop knowledge about trauma, adversity, and attachment in all providers of care within the organization. The second is the organization's adoption of shared values, organized around "The Seven Sanctuary Commitments." These include commitments to nonviolence, emotional intelligence, social learning, open communication, democracy, social responsibility, and growth and change. The third key component is the development of a shared and accessible language among administration, staff, and clients around four key domains of trauma healing identified by the model. These four domains are summarized by the acronym SELF and include **S**afety (attaining safety in the self, relationships, and the environment), **E**motional management (identifying and regulating emotions in response to memories, persons, and events), Loss (feeling grief and dealing with personal losses), and Future (trying out new roles and ways of relating as a "survivor" to maintain personal safety and help others). The fourth key component of the Sanctuary Model is a set of practical instructions, called the Sanctuary Toolkit, for creating and maintaining a "Sanctuary Culture." These include instructions on using the SELF framework to drive psychoeducation, service planning, and team meetings. It also provides instruction on how best to conduct community meetings, red flag reviews, and self-care planning for providers (Bloom, 2013; Esaki, Hopson, & Middleton, 2014).

Trauma Systems Therapy (TST): TST is a systems-oriented clinical intervention within a defined organizational framework. The systems-oriented approach defines a "Trauma System" based on two interacting dimensions: (a) the child's difficulty regulating survival-laden emotional states and (b) the incapacity of those around the child to help her or him to regulate emotional states and/or protect the child from threats/trauma reminders in the environment. TST integrates a defined assessment process to evaluate the child's mental health problems related to these two dimensions of the trauma system and—based on the results of this assessment—interventions are delivered to help the child become more regulated in the face of defined trauma triggers and to help those around the child to be more equipped to help the child regulate emotion and to protect the child from ongoing threats. Depending on the ability of existing caregivers to help the child manage emotion and protect the child from threat—and the child's capacity to safely manage emotional states—the child (and those around him or her) is placed in one of three phases of intervention: (a) *safety focused* treatment defines intensive home and community-based interventions to make sure those around the child can keep the child safe from threat and keep the child safe from dangerous impulses, (b) *regulation-focused* treatment defines an intervention approach dedicated to helping the child to regulate emotional states and building the capacity of those around the child to help him or her maintain regulation, and (c) *beyond trauma* treatment is provided when the environment is stable/safe enough and the child has sufficient capacity to regulate emotion. In this phase, children are provided with therapeutic opportunities to process the traumatic events using cognitive behavioral approaches, to create meaningful rituals about the event, and to work to plan for a future in which children feel the trauma is in their past. TST creates an organizational framework for the creation of a TST program that specifies details about program operations defined in collaboration with organizational leaders and key stakeholders. Such a framework defines how the organization's programs and staffing will be integrated, how the program will be financed for sustainability, relevant interagency agreements, interface within the services system, and training/supervision needs of staff allocated to the program. TST intervention is always managed within a multidisciplinary treatment team that oversees the quality of the interventions provided and the process for supporting team members. TST has been adapted for—and implemented within—mental health clinics, foster care programs, child welfare prevention units, substance abuse programs, refugee programs, shelters for unaccompanied refugee minors, residential treatment programs, and medical units (Saxe, Ellis, & Kaplow, 2007; Saxe, Ellis, & Brown, 2015; Brown, McCauley, Navalta, & Saxe, 2013).

The systems interventions defined within this category place greater emphasis on the organizational and services systems aspects of care than the interventions found in other categories. Their approach to the complexity of the child's problems is most consistent with the developmental/relational interventions. Sanctuary defines this through their SELF protocol and TST defines this through how the child's survival-laden emotional states tend to become evoked, in the context of interpersonal triggers that evoke memories of prior interpersonal trauma. TST has a particular focus on addressing social environmental complexity with specific interventions that help protect the child from threats including processes to advocate for the child's placement in a safe-enough environment, if necessary.

Like the developmental/relational interventions, the systems interventions have had less extensive evaluation in clinical trials than the behavioral or cognitive behavioral interventions. An important reason is that these systems interventions include a specific organizational framework as an integral part of the model that cannot be unpacked from the clinical elements of the model. As such, they tend to be disseminated organization-wide, and this leads to challenges in finding appropriate comparison groups (and "matching" between organizations leads to considerable methodologic challenges). Nevertheless, the Sanctuary Model has several published studies looking at youth outcomes and organizational implementation factors. Findings from a preliminary study in an adolescent residential center implementing the Sanctuary Model indicate that youth showed increased coping skills and an "improved sense of control over their own lives." In addition, improvement was seen on several domains of an organizational scale measuring program environment on units implementing the model versus those that were not (Rivard, Bloom, McCorkle, & Abramovitz, 2005). A more recent exploratory study of the implementation of the Sanctuary Model explores the perspectives of indirect care staff in a child welfare agency. Indirect care staff reported, on average, moderate openness to change and modest success in implementing the Sanctuary Model. An analysis of organizational factors found an association between organizational readiness for systems change and staff members perceptions of success (Esaki, Hopson, & Middleton, 2014). TST was initially evaluated in an open trial of cohorts in an inner-city outpatient psychiatry clinic and a rural child welfare prevention program with positive results for diminishing traumatic stress symptoms and increasing emotional regulation and stability of the social environment (Saxe, Ellis, Fogler, Hansen, & Sorkin, 2005). A 15-month extension of this study for the child welfare cohort demonstrated continuing improvements in children's symptoms and environmental stability (Ellis et al., 2012). This study also reported on significant cost saving to the child welfare agency for implementing TST. A report on the termination of a RCT of TST was published documenting the dramatically different attrition rates within an inner-city outpatient clinic between the usual care control group (90%) and the TST group (10%) (Saxe, Ellis, Folger, & Navalta, 2011). This report highlighted TST's effective treatment engagement approach. A large study of TST for 1,500 foster children using a unique quasi-experimental design was recently published documenting the impact of providing TST with fidelity on this cohort of children (Murphy, Moore, Redd, & Malm, 2017). Children's emotional and behavioral regulation—and the stability of the child's foster care placement—improved with higher levels of fidelity to the model. This study also documented that improvements in outcome were greatest with consistent fidelity delivered by all those that participated in care (i.e., clinicians, case workers, supervisors, foster parents).

CONCLUSIONS

There are a wide variety of available psychosocial interventions developed to address specific facets of the problem of child traumatic stress. There is also a growing empirical literature supporting the efficacy and effectiveness of many of these interventions. Cumulatively, the success of these interventions will be observed to the degree that they are able to impact the diversity of clinical problems experienced by traumatized children and families amongst a meaningful proportion of the children and families with these problems. This chapter documented four areas of complexity that will strongly influence the capacity of the psychosocial interventions to achieve this impact and described available psychosocial interventions based on their (relative) emphasis on specific areas of this complexity. This chapter also documented the empirical literature supporting the efficacy or effectiveness of these interventions within these categories. There is a great amount of empirical evidence supporting interventions that cover a relatively narrow range of the complexities detailed in this chapter. The success of the field of psychosocial interventions for child traumatic stress will be dependent on the growth of empirical knowledge about how interventions can most effectively address known areas of complexity that strongly determine a child's recovery from traumatic stress.

REFERENCES

Ackerman, P. T., Newton, J. E. O., McPherson, W. B., Jones, J. G., & Dykman, R. A. (1998). Prevalence of posttraumatic stress disorder and other psychiatric diagnoses in three groups of abused children (sexual, physical, and both). *Child Abuse & Neglect*, *22*(8), 759–774. https://doi.org/10.1016/S0145-2134(98)00062-3

Ahmad, A., Larsson, B., & Sundelin-Wahlsten, V. (2007). EMDR treatment for children with

PTSD: Results of a randomized controlled trial. *Nordic Journal of Psychiatry, 61*(5), 349–354. https://doi.org/10.1080/08039480701643464

Beck, A. T. (1976). *Cognitive therapy and the emotional disorders.* New York: International Universities Press.

Beidas, R. S., Marcus, S., Aarons, G. A., Hoagwood, K. E., Schoenwald, S., Evans, A. C., . . . Mandell, D. S. (2015). Predictors of community therapists' use of therapy techniques in a large public mental health system. *JAMA Pediatrics, 169*(4), 374–382. https://doi.org/10.1001/jamapediatrics.2014.3736

Blaustein, M. E., & Kinniburgh, K. M. (2017). Attachment, self-regulation, and competency (ARC). In M. A. Landolt, M. Cloitre, & U. Schnyder (Eds.), *Evidence-based treatments for trauma related disorders in children and adolescents* (pp. 299–319). New York: Springer. https://doi.org/10.1007/978-3-319-46138-0_14

Bloom, S. L. (2013). The sanctuary model. In J. D. Ford & C. A. Courtois (Eds.), *Treating complex traumatic stress disorders in children and adolescents: Scientific foundations and therapeutic models* (pp. 277–294). New York: Guilford Press.

Briere, J. (2002). Treating adult survivors of severe childhood. In J. E. B. Myers (Ed.), *The APSAC handbook on child maltreatment* (pp. 175–203). Thousand Oaks, CA: SAGE.

Brown, A. D., McCauley, K., Navalta, C. P., & Saxe, G. N. (2013). Trauma systems therapy in residential settings: Improving emotion regulation and the social environment of traumatized children and youth in congregate care. *Journal of Family Violence, 28*(7), 693–703. https://doi.org/10.1007/s10896-013-9542-9

Catani, C., Kohiladevy, M., Ruf, M., Schauer, E., Elbert, T., & Neuner, F. (2009). Treating children traumatized by war and tsunami: A comparison between exposure therapy and meditation-relaxation in North-East Sri Lanka. *BMC Psychiatry, 9*(1). https://pub.uni-bielefeld.de/publication/1783191

Chemtob, C. M., Nakashima, J., & Carlson, J. G. (2002). Brief treatment for elementary school children with disaster-related posttraumatic stress disorder: A field study. *Journal of Clinical Psychology, 58*(1), 99–112.

Cloitre, M., Stovall-McClough, K. C., Nooner, K., Zorbas, P., Cherry, S., Jackson, C. L., & Petkova, E. (2010). Treatment for PTSD related to childhood abuse: A randomized controlled trial. *American Journal of Psychiatry, 167*(8), 915–924. https://doi.org/10.1176/appi.ajp.2010.09081247

Cohen, J. A., & Mannarino, A. (1993). A treatment model for sexually abused preschoolers. *Journal of Interpersonal Violence, 8*(1), 115–131. https://doi.org/10.1177/088626093008001009

Cohen, J. A., & Mannarino, A. P. (1998). Interventions for sexually abused children: Initial treatment outcome findings. *Child Maltreatment, 3*(1), 17–26. https://doi.org/10.1177/1077559598003001002

Cohen, J. A., Mannarino, A. P., & Deblinger, E. (2006). *Treating trauma and traumatic grief in children and adolescents* (1st ed.). New York: Guilford Press.

Cohen, J. A., Mannarino, A. P., & Iyengar, S. (2011). Community treatment of posttraumatic stress disorder for children exposed to intimate partner violence: A randomized controlled trial. *Archives of Pediatrics & Adolescent Medicine, 165*(1), 16–21. https://doi.org/10.1001/archpediatrics.2010.247

Cohen, J. A., Mannarino, A. P., & Knudsen, K. (2005). Treating sexually abused children: 1 year follow-up of a randomized controlled trial. *Child Abuse & Neglect, 29*(2), 135–145. https://doi.org/10.1016/j.chiabu.2004.12.005

Cohen, J. A., Mannarino, A. P., & Rogal, S. (2001). Treatment practices for childhood posttraumatic stress disorder. *Child Abuse & Neglect, 25*(1), 123–135. https://doi.org/10.1016/S0145-2134(00)00226-X

Cohen, J., & Mannarino, A. (1996). A treatment outcome study for sexually abused preschool children: Initial findings. *Journal of the American Academy of Child & Adolescent Psychiatry, 35*(1), 42–50. https://doi.org/10.1097/00004583-199601000-00011

Cohen, J., Mannarino, A., Berliner, L., & Deblinger, E. (2000). Trauma-focused cognitive behavioral therapy for children and adolescents: An empirical update. *Journal of Interpersonal Violence, 15*(11), 1202–1223. https://doi.org/10.1177/088626000015011007

Cohen, J., Mannarino, A., & Deblinger, E. (2017). *Treating trauma and traumatic grief in children and adolescents* (2nd ed.). New York: Guilford Press.

Cohen, J., Mannarino, A., Perel, J., & Staron, V. (2007). A pilot randomized controlled trial of combined trauma-focused CBT and sertraline for childhood PTSD symptoms. *Journal of the American Academy of Child & Adolescent Psychiatry, 46*(7), 811–819. https://doi.org/10.1097/chi.0b013e3180547105

Cook, A., Ford, J., Lanktree, C., Blaustein, M., Cloitre, M., & Van der Kolk. (2005). Complex trauma. *Psychiatric Annals, 35*(5), 390–398.

D'Andrea, W., Ford, J., Stolbach, B., Spinazzola, J., & van der Kolk, B. A. (2012). Understanding interpersonal trauma in children: Why we need a developmentally appropriate trauma diagnosis. *American Journal of Orthopsychiatry, 82*(2), 187–200. https://doi.org/10.1111/j.1939-0025.2012.01154.x

de Arellano, M. A. R., Lyman, D. R., Jobe-Shields, L., George, P., Dougherty, R. H., Daniels, A. S., . . . Delphin-Rittmon, M. E. (2014). Trauma-focused cognitive-behavioral therapy for children and adolescents: Assessing the evidence.

Psychiatric Services, *65*(5), 591–602. https://doi.org/10.1176/appi.ps.201300255

De Bellis, M. D., Broussard, E. R., Herring, D. J., Wexler, S., Moritz, G., & Benitez, J. G. (2001). Psychiatric co-morbidity in caregivers and children involved in maltreatment: A pilot research study with policy implications. *Child Abuse & Neglect*, *25*(7), 923–944. https://doi.org/10.1016/S0145-2134(01)00247-2

de Roos, C., Greenwald, R., den Hollander-Gijsman, M., Noorthoorn, E., van Buuren, S., & de Jongh, A. (2011). A randomised comparison of cognitive behavioural therapy (CBT) and eye movement desensitisation and reprocessing (EMDR) in disaster-exposed children. *European Journal of Psychotraumatology*, *2*. https://doi.org/10.3402/ejpt.v2i0.5694

Deblinger, E., & Heflin, A. H. (1996). *Treating sexually abused children and their nonoffending parents: A cognitive behavioral approach* (Vol. XV). Thousand Oaks, CA: SAGE.

Deblinger, E., Lippmann, J., & Steer, R. (1996). Sexually abused children suffering posttraumatic stress symptoms: Initial treatment outcome findings. *Child Maltreatment*, *1*(4), 310–321. https://doi.org/10.1177/1077559596001004003

Deblinger, E., Mannarino, A. P., Cohen, J. A., Runyon, M. K., & Steer, R. A. (2011). Trauma-focused cognitive behavioral therapy for children: Impact of the trauma narrative and treatment length. *Depression and Anxiety*, *28*(1), 67–75. https://doi.org/10.1002/da.20744

Deblinger, E., Pollio, E., & Dorsey, S. (2016). Applying trauma-focused cognitive–behavioral therapy in group format. *Child Maltreatment*, *21*(1), 59–73. https://doi.org/10.1177/1077559515620668

DeRosa, R., & Pelcovitz. D. (2008). Igniting SPARCS of change: Structured psychotherapy for adolescents responding to chronic stress. In J. Ford, R. Pat-Horenczyk, & D. Brom (Eds.), *Treating traumatized children: risk, resilience and recovery* (pp. 1–20). New York: Routledge.

Diehle, J., Opmeer, B. C., Boer, F., Mannarino, A. P., & Lindauer, R. J. L. (2015). Trauma-focused cognitive behavioral therapy or eye movement desensitization and reprocessing: What works in children with posttraumatic stress symptoms? A randomized controlled trial. *European Child & Adolescent Psychiatry*, *24*(2), 227–236. https://doi.org/10.1007/s00787-014-0572-5

Dorsey, S., McLaughlin, K. A., Kerns, S. E. U., Harrison, J. P., Lambert, H. K., Briggs, E. C., . . . Amaya-Jackson, L. (2017). Evidence base update for psychosocial treatments for children and adolescents exposed to traumatic events. *Journal of Clinical Child & Adolescent Psychology*, *46*(3), 303–330. https://doi.org/10.1080/15374416.2016.1220309

Dozier, M., Lindhiem, O., Lewis, E., Bick, J., Bernard, K., & Peloso, E. (2009). Effects of a foster parent training program on young children's attachment behaviors: Preliminary evidence from a randomized clinical trial. *Child & Adolescent Social Work Journal: C & A*, *26*(4), 321–332. https://doi.org/10.1007/s10560-009-0165-1

Ellis, B. H., Fogler, J., Hansen, S., Forbes, P., Navalta, C. P., & Saxe, G. N. (2012). Trauma systems therapy: 15-month outcomes and the importance of effecting environmental change. *Psychological Trauma: Theory, Research, Practice, and Policy*, *4*(6), 624–630. https://doi.org/10.1037/a0025192

Esaki, N., Hopson, L., & Middleton, J. (2014). Sanctuary model implementation from the perspective of indirect care staff. *Families in Society: The Journal of Contemporary Social Services*, *95*(4), 261–268. https://doi.org/10.1606/1044-3894.2014.95.31

Famularo, R., Fenton, T., Kinscherff, R., & Augustyn, M. (1996). Psychiatric comorbidity in childhood post traumatic stress disorder. *Child Abuse & Neglect*, *20*(10), 953–961. https://doi.org/10.1016/0145-2134(96)00084-1

Farkas, L., Cyr, M., Lebeau, T. M., & Lemay, J. (2010). Effectiveness of MASTR/EMDR therapy for traumatized adolescents. *Journal of Child & Adolescent Trauma*, *3*(2), 125–142. https://doi.org/10.1080/19361521003761325

Foa, E. B., Dancu, C. V., Hembree, E. A., Jaycox, L. H., Meadows, E. A., & Street, G. P. (1999). A comparison of exposure therapy, stress inoculation training, and their combination for reducing posttraumatic stress disorder in female assault victims. *Journal of Consulting and Clinical Psychology*, *67*(2), 194–200.

Foa, E. B., Rothbaum, B. O., Riggs, D. S., & Murdock, T. B. (1991). Treatment of posttraumatic stress disorder in rape victims: A comparison between cognitive-behavioral procedures and counseling. *Journal of Consulting and Clinical Psychology*, *59*(5), 715–723.

Foa, E. B., McLean, C. P., Capaldi, S., & Rosenfield, D. (2013). Prolonged exposure vs supportive counseling for sexual abuse-related PTSD in adolescent girls: A randomized clinical trial. *JAMA*, *310*(24), 2650–2657. https://doi.org/10.1001/jama.2013.282829

Ford, J. D., & Hawke, J. (2012). Trauma affect regulation psychoeducation group and milieu intervention outcomes in juvenile detention facilities. *Journal of Aggression, Maltreatment & Trauma*, *21*(4), 365–384. https://doi.org/10.1080/10926771.2012.673538

Ford, J. D., & Russo, E. (2006). Trauma-focused, present-centered, emotional self-regulation approach to integrated treatment for posttraumatic stress and addiction: Trauma adaptive recovery group education and therapy (TARGET). *American Journal of Psychotherapy*, *60*(4), 335–355.

Ford, J. D., Steinberg, K. L., Hawke, J., Levine, J., & Zhang, W. (2012). Randomized trial comparison of emotion regulation and relational psychotherapies for PTSD with girls involved in delinquency. *Journal of Clinical Child & Adolescent Psychology*, *41*(1), 27–37. https://doi.org/10.1080/15374416.2012.632343

Gilboa-Schechtman, E., Foa, E., Shafran, N., Aderka, I. M., Powers, M. B., Rachamim, L., . . . Apter, A. (2010). Prolonged exposure vs dynamic therapy for adolescent PTSD: A pilot randomized controlled trial. *Journal of the American Academy of Child & Adolescent Psychiatry*, *49*(10), 1034–1042. https://doi.org/10.1016/j.jaac.2010.07.014

Gillies, D., Taylor, F., Gray, C., O'Brien, L., & D'Abrew, N. (2013). Psychological therapies for the treatment of post-traumatic stress disorder in children and adolescents (Review). *Evidence-Based Child Health: A Cochrane Review Journal*, *8*(3), 1004–1116. https://doi.org/10.1002/ebch.1916

Goldbeck, L., Muche, R., Sachser, C., Tutus, D., & Rosner, R. (2016). Effectiveness of trauma-focused cognitive behavioral therapy for children and adolescents: A randomized controlled trial in eight German mental health clinics. *Psychotherapy and Psychosomatics*, *85*(3), 159–170. https://doi.org/10.1159/000442824

Greeson, J. K. P., Briggs, E. C., Layne, C. M., Belcher, H. M. E., Ostrowski, S. A., Kim, S., . . . Fairbank, J. A. (2014). Traumatic childhood experiences in the 21st century: Broadening and building on the ACE studies with data from the National Child Traumatic Stress Network. *Journal of Interpersonal Violence*, *29*(3), 536–556. https://doi.org/10.1177/0886260513505217

Gudiño, O. G., Weis, J. R., Havens, J. F., Biggs, E. A., Diamond, U. N., Marr, M., . . . Cloitre, M. (2014). Group trauma-informed treatment for adolescent psychiatric inpatients: A preliminary uncontrolled trial. *Journal of Traumatic Stress*, *27*(4), 496–500. https://doi.org/10.1002/jts.21928

Habib, M., Labruna, V., & Newman, J. (2013). Complex histories and complex presentations: Implementation of a manually guided group treatment for traumatized adolescents. *Journal of Family Violence*, *28*(7), 717–728. https://doi.org/10.1007/s10896-013-9532-y

Hoagwood, K., & Olin, S. S. (2002). The NIMH Blueprint for Change Report: Research priorities in child and adolescent mental health. *Journal of the American Academy of Child & Adolescent Psychiatry*, *41*(7), 760–767. https://doi.org/10.1097/00004583-200207000-00006

Hodgdon, H. B., Blaustein, M., Kinniburgh, K., Peterson, M. L., & Spinazzola, J. (2016). Application of the ARC model with adopted children: Supporting resiliency and family well being. *Journal of Child & Adolescent Trauma*, *9*(1), 43–53. https://doi.org/10.1007/s40653-015-0050-3

Hodgdon, H. B., Kinniburgh, K., Gabowitz, D., Blaustein, M. E., & Spinazzola, J. (2013). Development and implementation of trauma-informed programming in youth residential treatment centers using the ARC framework. *Journal of Family Violence*, *28*(7), 679–692. https://doi.org/10.1007/s10896-013-9531-z

Jaberghaderi, N., Greenwald, R., Rubin, A., Zand, S. O., & Dolatabadi, S. (2004). A comparison of CBT and EMDR for sexually abused Iranian girls. *Clinical Psychology & Psychotherapy*, *11*(5), 358–368. https://doi.org/10.1002/cpp.395

Jaycox, L. H., Cohen, J. A., Mannarino, A. P., Walker, D. W., Langley, A. K., Gegenheimer, K. L., . . . Schonlau, M. (2010). Children's mental health care following Hurricane Katrina: A field trial of trauma focused psychotherapies. *Journal of Traumatic Stress*, *23*(2), 223–231. https://doi.org/10.1002/jts.20518

Jaycox, L. H., Kataoka, S. H., Stein, B. D., Langley, A. K., & Wong, M. (2012). Cognitive behavioral intervention for trauma in schools. *Journal of Applied School Psychology*, *28*(3), 239–255. https://doi.org/10.1080/15377903.2012.695766

Jensen, T. K., Holt, T., Ormhaug, S. M., Egeland, K., Granly, L., Hoaas, L. C., & Wentzel-Larsen, T. (2014). A randomized effectiveness study comparing trauma-focused cognitive behavioral therapy with therapy as usual for youth. *Journal of Clinical Child & Adolescent Psychology*, *43*(3), 356–369. https://doi.org/10.1080/15374416.2013.822307

Kagan, R. (2016). *Real life heroes: Toolkit for treating traumatic stress in children and families* (2nd ed.). Boca Raton, FL: Taylor & Francis.

Kagan, R., Douglas, A. N., Hornik, J., & Kratz, S. L. (2008). Real Life Heroes pilot study: Evaluation of a treatment model for children with traumatic stress. *Journal of Child & Adolescent Trauma*, *1*(1), 5–22. https://doi.org/10.1080/19361520801929845

Kagan, R., Henry, J., Richardson, M., Trinkle, J., & LaFrenier, A. (2014). Evaluation of Real Life Heroes treatment for children with complex PTSD. *Psychological Trauma: Theory, Research, Practice, and Policy*, *6*(5), 588–596. https://doi.org/10.1037/a0035879

Kaplow, J. B., Layne, C. M., Saltzman, W. R., Cozza, S. J., & Pynoos, R. S. (2013). Using multidimensional grief theory to explore the effects of deployment, reintegration, and death on military youth and families. *Clinical Child and Family Psychology Review, 16*(3), 322–340. https://doi.org/10.1007/s10567-013-0143-1

Kataoka, S. H., Stein, B.D., Jaycox, L. H., Wong, M., Escudero, P., Tu, W., . . . Fink, A. (2003). A school-based mental health program for traumatized Latino immigrant children. *Journal of the American Academy of Child & Adolescent Psychiatry, 42*(3), 311–318. https://doi.org/10.1097/00004583-200303000-00011

Kendall, P. C., & Beidas, R. S. (2007). Smoothing the trail for dissemination of evidence-based practices for youth: Flexibility within fidelity. *Professional Psychology: Research and Practice, 38*(1), 13–20. https://doi.org/10.1037/0735-7028.38.1.13

Kilpatrick, D. G., Ruggiero, K. J., Acierno, R., Saunders, B. E., Resnick, H. S., & Best, C. L. (2003). Violence and risk of PTSD, major depression, substance abuse/dependence, and comorbidity: Results from the National Survey of Adolescents. *Journal of Consulting and Clinical Psychology, 71*(4), 692–700. https://doi.org/10.1037/0022-006X.71.4.692

King, N., Tongue, B. J., Mullen, P., Myerson, N., Heyne, D., Rollings, S., & Ollendick, T. H. (2000). Treating sexually abused children with posttraumatic stress symptoms: A randomized clinical trial. *Journal of the American Academy of Child & Adolescent Psychiatry, 39*(11), 1347–1355. https://doi.org/10.1097/00004583-200011000-00008

Kowalik, J., Weller, J., Venter, J., & Drachman, D. (2011). Cognitive behavioral therapy for the treatment of pediatric posttraumatic stress disorder: A review and meta-analysis. *Journal of Behavior Therapy and Experimental Psychiatry, 42*(3), 405–413. https://doi.org/10.1016/j.jbtep.2011.02.002

Lanktree, C. B., & Briere, J. N. (2015). *Treating complex trauma in children and their families: An integrative approach*. Thousand Oaks, CA: SAGE.

Lanktree, C. B., Briere, J., Godbout, N., Hodges, M., Chen, K., Trimm, L., & Freed, W. (2012). Treating multitraumatized, socially marginalized children: Results of a naturalistic treatment outcome study. *Journal of Aggression, Maltreatment & Trauma, 21*(8), 813–828. https://doi.org/10.1080/10926771.2012.722588

Layne, C. M., Pynoos, R. S., Saltzman, W. R., Arslanagić, B., Black, M., Savjak, N., & Houston, R. (2001). Trauma/grief-focused group psychotherapy: School-based postwar intervention with traumatized Bosnian adolescents. *Group Dynamics: Theory, Research, and Practice, 5*(4), 277–290. https://doi.org/10.1037/1089-2699.5.4.277

Leenarts, L. E. W., Diehle, J., Doreleijers, T. A. H., Jansma, E. P., & Lindauer, R. J. L. (2013). Evidence-based treatments for children with trauma-related psychopathology as a result of childhood maltreatment: A systematic review. *European Child & Adolescent Psychiatry, 22*(5), 269–283. https://doi.org/10.1007/s00787-012-0367-5

Lenz, A. S., & Hollenbaugh, K. M. (2015). Meta-analysis of trauma-focused cognitive behavioral therapy for treating PTSD and co-occurring depression among children and adolescents. *Counseling Outcome Research and Evaluation, 6*(1), 18–32. https://doi.org/10.1177/2150137815573790

Levitt, J. T., & Cloitre, M. (2005). A clinician's guide to STAIR/MPE: Treatment for PTSD related to childhood abuse. *Cognitive and Behavioral Practice, 12*(1), 40–52. https://doi.org/10.1016/S1077-7229(05)80038-0

Lieberman, A. F., Horn, P. V., & Ippen, C. G. (2005). Toward evidence-based treatment: Child-parent psychotherapy with preschoolers exposed to marital violence. *Journal of the American Academy of Child & Adolescent Psychiatry, 44*(12), 1241–1248. https://doi.org/10.1097/01.chi.0000181047.59702.58

Lieberman, A. F., Ippen, C. G., & Marans, S. (2009). Psychodynamic therapy for child trauma. In E. B. Foa, T. M. Keane, M. J. Friedman, & J. A. Cohen (Eds.), *Effective treatments for PTSD: Practice guidelines from the International Society for Traumatic Stress Studies* (2nd ed., pp. 370–387). New York: Guilford Press.

McMullen, J., O'Callaghan, P., Shannon, C., Black, A., & Eakin, J. (2013). Group trauma-focused cognitive-behavioral therapy with former child soldiers and other war-affected boys in the DR Congo: A randomized controlled trial. *Journal of Child Psychology and Psychiatry, and Allied Disciplines, 54*(11), 1231–1241. https://doi.org/10.1111/jcpp.12094

Murphy, K., Moore, K. A., Redd, Z., & Malm, K. (2017). Trauma-informed child welfare systems and children's well-being: A longitudinal evaluation of KVC's Bridging the Way Home initiative. *Children and Youth Services Review, 75*, 23–34. https://doi.org/10.1016/j.childyouth.2017.02.008

Murray, L. K., Skavenski, S., Kane, J. C., Mayeya, J., Dorsey, S., Cohen, J. A., & Bolton, P. A. (2015). Effectiveness of trauma-focused cognitive behavioral therapy among trauma-affected children in Lusaka, Zambia: A randomized clinical trial. *JAMA Pediatrics, 169*(8), 761–769. https://doi.org/10.1001/jamapediatrics.2015.0580

Nixon, R. D., Sterk, J., Pearce, A., & Weber, N. (2016). A randomized trial of cognitive behavior therapy and cognitive therapy for children with posttraumatic stress disorder following single-incident trauma: Predictors and outcome at 1-year follow-up. *Psychological Trauma: Theory, Research, Practice, and Policy, 9*(4), 471–478. https://doi.org/10.1037/tra0000190

Nixon, R. D., Vandervord, Sterk, J., & Pearce, A. (2012). A randomized trial of cognitive behavior therapy and cognitive therapy for children with posttraumatic stress disorder following single-incident trauma. *Journal of Abnormal Child Psychology, 40*(3), 327–37. https://doi.org/http://dx.doi.org/10.1007/s10802-011-9566-7

O'Callaghan, P., McMullen, J., Shannon, C., Rafferty, H., & Black, A. (2013). A randomized controlled trial of trauma-focused cognitive behavioral therapy for sexually exploited, war-affected Congolese girls. *Journal of the American Academy of Child & Adolescent Psychiatry, 52*(4), 359–369. https://doi.org/10.1016/j.jaac.2013.01.013

Resick, P. A., & Schnicke, M. K. (1992). Cognitive processing therapy for sexual assault victims. *Journal of Consulting and Clinical Psychology, 60*(5), 748–756.

Rivard, J. C., Bloom, S. L., McCorkle, D., & Abramovitz, R. (2005). Preliminary results of a study examining the implementation and effects of a trauma recovery framework for youths in residential treatment. *Therapeutic Community, 26*(1), 83–96.

Ruf, M., Schauer, M., Neuner, F., Catani, C., Schauer, E., & Elbert, T. (2010). Narrative exposure therapy for 7- to 16-year-olds: A randomized controlled trial with traumatized refugee children. *Journal of Traumatic Stress, 23*(4), 437–445. https://doi.org/10.1002/jts.20548

Runyon, M. K., Deblinger, E., & Steer, R. (2010). Group cognitive behavioral treatment for parents and children at-risk for physical abuse: An initial study. *Child & Family Behavior Therapy, 32*(3), 196–218. https://doi.org/10.1080/07317107.2010.500515

Saigh, P. A., Yule, W., & Inamdar, S. C. (1996). Imaginal flooding of traumatized children and adolescents. *Journal of School Psychology, 34*(2), 163–183. https://doi.org/10.1016/0022-4405(96)00005-2

Saltzman, W., Layne, C., Pynoos, R., Olafson, E., Kaplow, J., & Boat, B. (2017). *Trauma and grief component therapy for adolescents: A modular approach to treating traumatized and bereaved youth.* Cambridge, UK: Cambridge University Press.

Saxe, G., & Acri, M. (2017). Democratizing implementation and innovation in mental health care. *Administration and Policy in Mental Health, 44*(2), 155–159. https://doi.org/10.1007/s10488-015-0714-1

Saxe, G. N., Ellis, B. H., & Brown, A. D. (2015). *Trauma systems therapy for children and teens* (2nd ed.). New York: Guilford Press.

Saxe, G. N., Ellis, B. H., Fogler, J., Hansen, S., & Sorkin, B. (2005). Comprehensive care for traumatized children: An open trial examines treatment using trauma systems therapy. *Psychiatric Annals, 35*(5), 443–448.

Saxe, G. N., Ellis, B. H., Fogler, J., & Navalta, C. P. (2011). Innovations in practice: Preliminary evidence for effective family engagement in treatment for child traumatic stress–trauma systems therapy approach to preventing dropout. *Child and Adolescent Mental Health, 17*(1), 58–61. https://doi.org/10.1111/j.1475-3588.2011.00626.x

Saxe, G.N., Ellis, B. H., & Kaplow J. B., (2007). *Collaborative treatment of traumatized children and teens: The trauma systems therapy approach* (1st ed.). New York: Guilford Press.

Scheeringa, M. S., & Zeanah, C. H. (2008). Reconsideration of harm's way: Onsets and comorbidity patterns of disorders in preschool children and their caregivers following Hurricane Katrina. *Journal of Clinical Child and Adolescent Psychology, 37*(3), 508–518. https://doi.org/10.1080/15374410802148178

Shapiro, F., Kaslow, F. W., & Maxfield, L. (2011). *Handbook of EMDR and family therapy processes.* Hoboken, NJ: John Wiley.

Smith, P., Yule, W., Perrin, S., Tranah, T., Dalgleish, T., & Clark, D. M. (2007). Cognitive-behavioral therapy for PTSD in children and adolescents: A preliminary randomized controlled trial. *Journal of the American Academy of Child & Adolescent Psychiatry, 46*(8), 1051–1061. https://doi.org/10.1097/CHI.0b013e318067e288

Stein, B. D., Jaycox, L. H., Kataoka, S. H., Wong, M., Tu, W., Elliott, M. N., & Fink, A. (2003). A mental health intervention for schoolchildren exposed to violence: A randomized controlled trial. *JAMA, 290*(5), 603–611. https://doi.org/10.1001/jama.290.5.603

Torrey, W. C., Drake, R. E., Dixon, L., Burns, B. J., Flynn, L., Rush, A. J., . . . Klatzker, D. (2001). Implementing evidence-based practices for persons with severe mental illnesses. *Psychiatric Services, 52*(1), 45–50. https://doi.org/10.1176/appi.ps.52.1.45

Trowell, J., Kolvin, I., Weeramanthri, T., Sadowski, H., Berelowitz, M., Glasser, D., & Leitch, I. (2002). Psychotherapy for sexually abused girls: Psychopathological outcome findings and patterns of change. *The British Journal of Psychiatry, 180*(3), 234–247 https://doi.org/10.1192/bjp.180.3.234

van der Kolk, B., A. (2009). [Developmental trauma disorder: Towards a rational diagnosis for chronically traumatized children]. *Praxis der Kinderpsychologie und Kinderpsychiatrie, 58*(8), 572–586.

van der Kolk, B. A., & D'Andrea, W. (2010). Towards a developmental trauma disorder diagnosis for childhood interpersonal trauma. In R. A Lanius, E. Vermetten, & C. Pain (Eds.). *The impact of early life trauma on health and disease: The hidden epidemic*(pp. 57–68). Thousand Oaks, CA: SAGE.

Wamser-Nanney, R., & Vandenberg, B. R. (2013). Empirical support for the definition of a complex trauma event in children and adolescents. *Journal of Traumatic Stress*, *26*(6), 671–678. https://doi.org/10.1002/jts.21857

Weiner, D. A., Schneider, A., & Lyons, J. S. (2009). Evidence-based treatments for trauma among culturally diverse foster care youth: Treatment retention and outcomes. *Children and Youth Services Review*, *31*(11), 1199–1205. https://doi.org/10.1016/j.childyouth.2009.08.013

22

Pharmacologic Treatment of Adults with Trauma- and Stressor-Related Disorders

PTSD, ASD, and Adjustment Disorder

DAVID M. BENEDEK AND GARY H. WYNN

INTRODUCTION

In recent years, clinicians have increasingly looked to practice guidelines to inform treatment decisions. Practice guidelines do not define the standard of care as clinical judgment, and informed consent must ultimately drive treatment decisions. Yet guidelines are important tools because they evaluate, synthesize, and summarize research literature to facilitate decision-making. Much of the empirical evidence for the treatment of posttraumatic stress disorder (PTSD) and acute stress disorder (ASD) summarized in such guidelines was developed in the decade before the 2013 conceptualization of trauma and stressor-related disorders (TSRD) in the *Diagnostic and Statistical Manual of Mental Disorders* (fifth edition; DSM-5). In fact, since publication of the DSM-5, there has only been one new guideline published for the treatment of PTSD or ASD—the VA/DoD Clinical Practice Guideline for Management of Post-Traumatic Stress in 2017. The guidelines published in association the fourth edition of the DSM (APA, 2004) reflect much of the evidence pertaining to treatment of core symptoms of PTSD or ASD at the time of publication of this chapter. There is no published practice guideline for adjustment disorder (AD). In fact, neither the typically transient ADs nor the transient by definition ASD have received much attention in the scientific literature with regard to pharmacologic treatment.

In this chapter, evidence-based pharmacological treatments for PTSD, ASD, and AD in adults are reviewed. While emphasis is given to treatments that have received the strongest recommendations from the various published clinical practice guidelines and meta-analyses, mention is also made of pharmacological interventions introduced subsequent to changes in diagnostic definitions or that fall outside the recommendations of one or another of the practice guidelines.

PHARMACOLOGIC TREATMENT OF PTSD

Using varied methodologies and including research conducted over different time spans each PTSD practice guidelines rated the strength of the evidence for the efficacy of various pharmacologic and psychosocial approaches, and each identified specific treatments supported by the strongest evidence (Forbes et al., 2010). The guidelines identified a first-line role for a pharmacologic treatment of PTSD with two exceptions. The Institute of Medicine (IOM) guideline used the most stringent guidelines for selection of randomized controlled trials (RCTs) and excluded studies reviewed in the other analyses. The IOM (2008) did not recommend any pharmacologic agent as first-line therapy for PTSD. Also, the National Institute for Health and Clinical Excellence (NICE; 2005) guideline, utilizing a relatively high cutoff score for effect size of 0.5, did not recognize any medication intervention as first-line treatment for PTSD. However, all other guidelines identified at least one medication as first-line therapy for PTSD (see Tables 22.1 and 22.2). These guidelines along with other reviews have determined additional agents to be helpful to varying degrees as described here:

SSRIs

SSRIs have proven to be effective in treating PTSD and are recommended as first-line agents in all but two of the previously noted treatment guidelines (Forbes et al., 2010). Both sertraline and paroxetine

TABLE 22.1. FREQUENTLY CITED PTSD AND ASD TREATMENT GUIDELINES

American Psychiatric Association (2004a)
United Kingdom's National Institute for Health and Clinical Excellence (2005)
Australian National Health and Medical Research Council (2007)
International Society for Traumatic Stress Studies (Foa et al., 2009)
Institute of Medicine (2008)
Department of Veterans Affairs/Department of Defense (2010)

Note: PTSD = posttraumatic stress disorder; ASD = acute stress disorder.

have Food and Drug Administration approval for PTSD. Over 3,000 patients have participated in studies of paroxetine, sertraline, and fluoxetine. These medications have a broad spectrum of action and have been shown to reduce symptoms of all core PTSD symptom clusters. As a class, they are generally well tolerated.

The Cochrane Collaboration published a review of the evidence regarding pharmacological treatments in PTSD (Stein et al., 2006). This review identified 35 short-term RCTs of PTSD (4,597 participants). Three of these RCTs contained a maintenance component and five were unpublished. The authors concluded that while no clear evidence exists to show that any particular class of medication is more effective or better tolerated than any other, the greatest number of trials showing efficacy to date, as well as the largest studies, were with SSRIs. The review recommends SSRIs as first-line agents in the pharmacotherapy of PTSD and supports their use in long-term treatment.

A meta-analysis of four RCTs comparing SSRIs to placebo without regard to diagnostic criteria, duration, severity, or comorbid diagnoses, reported that treatment favored the drug in all four trials—but only one study (with 183 subjects) reached statistical significance. Two RCTs maintained treatment with an SSRI for 64 weeks and 40 weeks, respectively. One study reported that 50% of patients experienced worsening symptoms when placebo was substituted for active drug, and in the second report, patients on placebo were greater than six times more likely to relapse compared to the drug group. An analysis of large SSRI trials concluded that six of seven studies involving a total of over 2,000 patients found fluoxetine, paroxetine, and sertraline superior to placebo (Stein and Ipser, 2011). While citalopram, escitalopram, and fluvoxamine have been not been studied sufficiently to warrant a recommendation, the common mechanism of action would suggest similar efficacy.

SSRIs and Combat-Related PTSD

Studies of SSRIs specifically for combat-related PTSD have been less consistent—and generally disappointing. A 2002 multisite study of individuals (not necessarily combatants) residing in war-torn regions of Europe, Israel, and South Africa found fluoxetine superior to placebo (Martenyi et al., 2002). However, in a later randomization of 88 war veterans with PTSD, none of those receiving eight weeks of fluoxetine treatment achieved remission as measured by the Clinician Administered PTSD Scale (CAPS) at six-month follow-up (van der Kolk et al., 2007). Negative results had been previously reported in Vietnam War veterans in a smaller placebo controlled RCT of fluoxetine (Hertzberg et al., 2000). Additionally, in a large multicenter trial of 169 veterans randomized to flexibly dosed sertraline versus placebo, Friedman and colleagues (2007) observed no difference between sertraline and placebo. These three negative results stand in contrast to a study of 144 combat veterans of the Balkan Wars recruited at eight sites in Bosnia-Herzegovina and Croatia that randomized participants to fluoxetine (20–80 mg/day) or placebo for both a 12-week acute phase and 24-week relapse prevention phase. In the acute phase, fluoxetine was superior to placebo on all PTSD outcome measures and for depression and anxiety. In the relapse prevention phase, fluoxetine was again superior in sustaining improvement on PTSD measures, and the risk of relapse was significantly greater in the placebo arm (Marteni and Soldatenkova, 2006). The veterans in this study were younger, had been more recently traumatized, and had likely received less treatment for their symptoms prior to study entry. Therefore, chronicity of symptoms at time of study entry may, at least in part, explain the disappointing results in other SSRI studies.

Other Antidepressants

Venlafaxine, a serotonin and norepinephrine reuptake inhibitor, has been shown to have positive results in two trials totaling more than 800 participants with non-combat-related PTSD (Davidson, 2006a, 2006b) and is identified as first-line therapy in several practice guidelines. Duloxetine and desvenlafaxine have not been

TABLE 22.2. PTSD PHARMACOLOGIC TREATMENT FOR ADULTS IN PRACTICE GUIDELINES

	Department of Veterans Affairs/Department of Defense	American Psychiatric Association	National Institute for Health and Clinical Excellence	Australian National Health and Medical Research Council	International Society for Traumatic Stress Studies (adults)	Institute of Medicine
Recommendations: Initiation of pharmacotherapy	Initiate treatment with evidence-based psychotherapy and if not available or not preferred then initiate pharmacotherapy	Initiate treatment with both psychotherapy and pharmacotherapy	Drug treatment should not be used as routine first line in preference to TF psychological therapy (A)	Drug treatment should not be used as routine first line in preference to TF psychological therapy (A)	Medication is a reasonable initial option if CBT is unavailable, not preferred by patient, or in combination with CBT	
Pharmacotherapy for PTSD: 1st level rating	Monotherapy (recommended for): Sertraline, Paroxetine, Fluoxetine, Venlafaxine	SSRIs(I)		SSRIs—General and specialist (B)	Best evidence SSRIs and SNRIs SSRIs—sertraline, paroxetine, fluoxetine (A) SNRI-venlafaxine (A) TCAs (A) Mirtazapine (A) Nefazodone (A) MAOIs: phenelzine (A) Prazosin (A)	NA
Pharmacotherapy for PTSD: 2nd level rating	Monotherapy (suggest for): Nefazodone, Imipramine, Phenelzine	TCAs (II) MAOIs (II)	Paroxetine (B) Mirtazapine (B) general and mental health specialist Amitriptyline (B) Phenelzine (B) mental health specialist	Mirtazapine (B) TCAs (B)	Bupropion (C) Trazodone (C)	
Pharmacotherapy for ASD		SSRIs (II) Other antidepressants		Medication for ASD not recommended		N/A

Note: PTSD = posttraumatic stress disorder; TF = trauma-focused; SSRI = serotonin selective reuptake inhibitors; CBT = cognitive-behavioral therapy; SNRI: serotonin and norepinephrine reuptake inhibitors; TCA = tricyclic antidepressants MAOI = monoamine oxidase inhibitors; ASD = acute stress disorder. Strength of recommendations: American Psychiatric Association: [I] Recommended with substantial clinical confidence. [II] Recommended with moderate clinical confidence. National Institute for Health and Clinical Excellence: [A] At least one randomized controlled trial of overall good quality and consistency addressing the specifying recommendation (Evidence Level I) without extrapolation. [B] Well-conducted clinical studies but no randomized clinical trial (Evidence Levels II or II), or extrapolation from Level I evidence. Australian National Health and Medical Research Council: [A] Body of evidence can be trusted to guide practice. [B] Body of evidence can be trusted to guide practice in most situations [C] Body of evidence provides some support for recommendations; care should be taken in application. International Society for Traumatic Stress Studies: [A] Evidence is based on randomized, well-controlled clinical trials for individuals with PTSD. [B] Evidence is based on well-designed clinical studies, without randomization or placebo comparison for individuals with PTSD. [C] Evidence is based on service and naturalistic clinical studies, combined with clinical observations that are sufficiently compelling to warrant use of the treatment technique or follow the specific recommendation. Institute of Medicine: [1] Evidence is sufficient to conclude efficacy (a qualifier of magnitude may be added if appropriate). [2] Evidence is suggestive but not sufficient to conclude the efficacy. [4] Evidence is suggestive that *X* treatment is ineffective in treating PTSD.
Adapted from Forbes et al. (2010).

studied. In a 24-week comparison trial, venlafaxine performed as well as sertraline in a civilian population (Davidson, 2006b).

Other monotherapy recommendations include mirtazapine, nefazodone, tricyclic antidepressants (TCAs), and monoamine oxidase inhibitors (MAOIs), although these agents have been studied in fewer patients and are not considered first-line treatment options. Of the TCAs, only amitriptyline and imipramine have demonstrated positive outcomes, while data on desipramine and nortriptyline have been negative and from poor-quality studies. Nefazodone has been the subject of several small- to mid-sized RCTs and case-control studies (Davis et al., 2000; Garfield et al., 2001; Gillin et al., 2001; Hertzberg et al., 1998; Hidalgo et al., 1999; Zisook et at., 2000). In all six studies, the drug was helpful in improving scores on the CAPS and Hamilton Depression scale, improving sleep, and reducing anxiety. In a trial of combat- and sexual assault-origin PTSD, nefazodone was more effective than placebo (Davis et al., 2004). Nefazodone has demonstrated efficacy equivalent to sertraline in two trials (McRae et al., 2004; Saygin et al., 2002) although concerns about hepatic toxicity continue to limit its use. Two trials with mirtazapine (Davidson, 2003; Chung, 2004) have demonstrated positive findings. However, in the placebo-controlled trial (Davidson, 2003), both mirtazapine and placebo had large effect sizes. In a trial of military veterans, mirtazapine was as efficacious as sertraline, but there was no placebo comparison arm (Chung, 2004). Of the currently available MOAIs, only phenelzine has been studied. In a placebo comparison trial, Vietnam veterans assigned to phenelzine had significant improvement in the Impact of Events Scale (IES) compared to placebo (Kosten, 1991). Although some studies suggest patients may respond to antidepressants in less than three weeks, others suggest 12 weeks or longer may be necessary to achieve full effect (Martenyi et al., 2002). Such variability in response to pharmacologic interventions is likely in some part explained by individual factors including pharmacokinetic and pharmacodynamics factors.

Atypical Antipsychotics

There have been few RCTs of atypical antipsychotics for PTSD. Of these studies, most fail to distinguish between subjects with and without comorbid psychotic symptoms. Two of three reviews of atypical antipsychotics as monotherapy, one for risperidone (Ahern et al., 2011), and one for quetiapine (Pae et al., 2008), suggested positive results. In the review that distinguished between psychotic symptoms and more typical symptoms of PTSD, the former improved while the latter did not (Ahearn et al., 2011).

The efficacy of atypical antipsychotics as adjunctive treatment to antidepressants has been studied in several small but positive trials. Improvement has generally been observed in hyperarousal and re-experiencing symptom clusters. There have been 10 published RCTs of two different antipsychotics, risperidone and olanzapine. Quetiapine has been studied in one small open-label trial. Olanzapine as an adjunctive treatment improved CAPS scores and sleep quality compared to placebo in a small eight-week trial (Stein et al., 2002). Quetiapine improved both the Positive and Negative Symptom Scale (PANSS) and CAPS scores compared to baseline (Hamner et al., 2003).

Six small trials, of variable design quality, used risperidone as augmentation to other medications, rather than as a primary treatment. Risperidone has been shown to improve psychotic symptoms. One trial addressed risperidone's role in comorbid PTSD. Here, veterans treated with risperidone and placebo both had significant improvement in their CAPS scores. The results of the remaining five trials showed risperidone to have some benefit as adjunct to antidepressants, although only a small net benefit.

The largest clinical trial of an atypical antipsychotic for PTSD conducted by the VA Cooperative Study Group (Krystal et al., 2011), randomized 247 veterans with military-related PTSD deemed antidepressant resistant to risperidone (up to 4 mg/day) or placebo as adjunctive treatment. After six months the changes from baseline in CAPS scores were not significant between the two treatment arms. Changes in CAPS subscale scores for reexperiencing and hyperarousal were statistically significant favoring risperidone but the differences were not considered clinically important. No difference in the symptom scales for anxiety, depression, positive or negative symptoms, sleep, or quality of life were found. The authors concluded that compared to placebo, risperidone did not reduce PTSD symptoms. This is the largest clinical trial of an atypical antipsychotic as a treatment of PTSD to date. The results of this study, when considered with the limitations of those preceding it, led to the authors of the Veterans Administration/Department of Defense (VA-DoD) practice guideline to make no recommendation for atypical antipsychotics as monotherapy or adjunctive therapy for PTSD. Guidelines published earlier suggest utility particularly in cases with comorbid psychosis. No more recent evidence supports the use of atypical antipsychotics in PTSD.

Anticonvulsants

Current evidence does not support the use of anticonvulsants as monotherapy for the management of PTSD core symptoms. Tiagabine has been compared to placebo in two RCTs, with no difference in response (Connor 2006; Davidson 2007). Valproate, as monotherapy, did not differ from placebo in one RCT (Davis et al., 2008). Anticonvulsants are frequently used as adjunctive treatments. A meta-analysis showed benefit in the use of valproate in PTSD (Adamou, 2007). Only topiramate has been studied as adjunctive therapy in veterans, with negative results (Lindley et al., 2007).

Benzodiazepines

Benzodiazepines are widely used for symptomatic control of insomnia, panic/anxiety, and irritability. However, as with anticonvulsants, the evidence that they reduce the core symptoms of PTSD is lacking (Viola et al., 1997). Moreover, benzodiazepines may reduce the effectiveness of exposure therapy (Van Minnen et al., 2012). The evidence to date does not support the use of benzodiazepines in PTSD (VA/DoD, 2017).

In a randomized double-blind cross-over study, alprazolam showed no significant benefit in alleviating PTSD symptoms compared with placebo. A slight reduction in anxiety symptoms was offset by withdrawal effects documented after only five weeks of treatment (Braun et al., 1990). In 2004, a small, single-blind cross-over placebo-controlled study compared clonazepam with placebo for the treatment of sleep dysfunction associated with combat-related PTSD. The study showed no significant difference between the benzodiazepine and placebo treatments (Cates et al., 2004). An early case series described by Risse and colleagues (1990) described typical clinical experience when benzodiazepines were utilized for treating combat-related PTSD. In this study, alprazolam was used to augment treatment of anxiety symptoms in eight combat veterans with chronic PTSD and comorbid conditions (mostly alcohol misuse). Although anxiety initially improved with treatment, as the benzodiazepine was gradually withdrawn patients experienced severe reactions, including anxiety, sleep disturbance, rage, hyperalertness, increased nightmares, and intrusive thoughts; six of the eight veterans developed a level of rage—in some cases with homicidal ideation—that they had never experienced previously.

Antiadrenergic Medications

Among the antiadrenergics, prazosin has, in numerous studies, shown efficacy in improving sleep and reducing nightmares in PTSD studies. In five relatively small studies (Raskind et al., 2002; Raskind et al., 2003; Raskind et al., 2007; Raskind et al., 2013; Taylor et al., 2006; Taylor et al., 2008), prazosin demonstrated efficacy in reducing nightmares and in improving CAPS subscores related to sleep disturbance, as well as clinician assessment and patient self-report scores of overall functioning. Unfortunately, in other studies, less consistent results across the full span of specific PTSD symptoms have been demonstrated (Friedman et al., 2009; Rothbaum et al., 2011). Studies have shown no significant difference between prazosin and hydroxyzine (Ahmadpanah et al., 2014) or behavioral sleep interventions (Germain et al., 2012), minimal difference between prazosin and quetiapine (Byers et al., 2010), and no benefit from use of prazosin for PTSD symptoms in active drinkers (Petrakis et al., 2016).

Guanfacine has been compared to placebo in two trials (Neylan et al. 2006; Davis et al., 2008). There was no differential effect on measures of PTSD symptom severity in the active treatment group in either study.

Other Agents

Buspirone, a non-benzodiazepine anti-anxiety drug, is reported to have "clinical efficacy" in two very small studies (Duffy and Malloy, 1994; Wells et al., 1991). Eszopiclone, in one small study, was shown to have benefits in overall PTSD symptoms and sleep disturbance (Pollack et al., 2011). This randomized, double-blind, placebo-controlled, cross-over study evaluated subjects over a three-week period. Confirmation studies are needed to validate the potential utility of this drug in PTSD. Ketamine has recently been evaluated for use in PTSD. Separately an RCT of ketamine found rapid and significant reduction in PTSD symptoms at 24 hours post-infusion of ketamine compared to midazolam (Feder et al., 2014). However, the permanence of symptom relief after single dosing, the optimal frequency of dosing, and the long-term safety of recurrent dosing strategies remain open questions. There are multiple ongoing trials of ketamine for PTSD which will hopefully shed light on the utility of ketamine for PTSD.

Medication Augmentation of Psychotherapy for PTSD

In clinical practice pharmacologic agents are frequently used concurrent with exposure-based or cognitive therapies to achieve additive effects or potentially facilitate the extinction learning processes of exposure-based psychotherapy. There have been three RCTS of SSRI-augmented Prolonged Exposure (PE) therapy, and results have been mixed. In a 2006 study, Rothbaum and colleagues randomized 88 patients treated with open label sertraline for eight weeks to either continuation of sertraline alone or sertraline + PE. The sertraline +PE group demonstrated further reduction in PTSD symptoms while the sertraline alone group plateaued. In 2008 Simon et al. randomized 23 subjects who first received eight sessions of PE to receive either paroxetine or placebo during continued PE. However, paroxetine failed to boost the response to subsequent sessions of PE compared to placebo (Simon et al., 2008). Finally, in a randomized placebo-controlled study of 37 survivors of the 9/11 World Trade Center attacks concurrent administration of paroxetine and PE for 10 weeks reduced PTSD symptoms more than PE + placebo (Schneier et al., 2012). These studies suggest simultaneous use of PE and SSRI may be more effective than either treatment alone, even if "pretreatment" with SSRI does not appear to boost subsequent response to psychotherapy.

Other adjunctive medications have been proposed and studied in an effort to speed or otherwise boost the effects of psychotherapy. The most well studied of these "cognitive enhancers" is D-cycloserine (DCS), an N-methyl-D-aspartate partial agonist thought to enhance the process of extinction learning and reconsolidation of memories through its modulation of glutamate activity in brain structures associated with these processes. While there is evidence that DCS enhances exposure therapy for anxiety, the two RCTs specifically targeting PTSD demonstrated contradictory results (De Kleine et al., 2012; Litz et al., 2012). One study using doses twice as high as the prior studies (i.e., 100 mg vs. 50 mg) demonstrated positive results (Difede et al., 2014) suggesting higher doses of DCS may enhance psychotherapy. Additional studies of DCS and another potential augmentation agent (hydrocortisone) are presently underway. While there is mounting evidence from animal and preclinical human studies that administration of glucocorticoids, 17B-estradiol, GABAergic neurosteroids or agents that increase their synthesis may facilitate extinction learning, there are as yet no published clinical positive trials in PTSD specifically. In one recently published RCT of intranasal oxytocin administered twice daily for eight days, beginning within 12 days of traumatic exposure there were no significant reduction CAPS scores between placebo and oxytocin groups and those 1.5, 3, or 6 months, although those with the highest CAPS scores at baseline were observed to receive more benefit from oxytocin (van Zuiden et al., 2017).

PHARMACOLOGIC TREATMENT OF ACUTE STRESS DISORDER

According to the DSM-5, ASD is distinguished from PTSD by the fact that the symptom pattern in ASD is restricted to a period of three days to one month after traumatic exposure. Peritraumatic symptoms occurring immediately upon exposure and resolving within two days are considered an acute stress reaction (for which no pharmacologic treatment guidelines have been published). Since ASD does not adequately identify the majority of people who will develop PTSD, identifying and treating persons with ASD cannot be viewed as a mechanism for preventing PTSD. Indeed, there is presently insufficient evidence to support pharmacological intervention for the prevention of ASD or PTSD. The DSM-5 criteria for ASD no longer require the presence of symptoms from each symptom clusters but specify the presence of at least 9 of 14 symptoms persisting for three days to one month after traumatic exposure. Thus persons with ASD will now present with symptoms akin to severe acute (subsyndromal) PTSD, so previously described pharmacological trials for acute PTSD should remain applicable. The treatments for ASD with the strongest evidence are psychotherapeutic approaches (see ASD chapter). Published practice guidelines recommend only brief pharmacologic intervention and then only for severe insomnia, agitation, or psychotic symptoms that may be simultaneously be present even though these symptoms may not represent ASD.

Studies of acute pharmacological intervention in ASD as a means of secondary prevention for PTSD have generally been disappointing. In 2012, Shalev and colleagues published a large and well-controlled study of 242 patients with ASD admitted through an emergency room. These patients were randomized to SSRI (escitalopram), cognitive restructuring therapy, PE therapy, placebo, or waitlist (subsequently randomized to restructuring or exposure therapy). At nine-week follow-up, rates of PTSD were lower in those receiving either type of psychotherapy than in the SSRI or placebo groups (Shalev et al., 2012).

Small case series of adults (Blake et al., 1986) and children (Robert et al., 1999) with ASD have suggested efficacy of brief trials of tricyclic antidepressants while studies of brief trials of benzodiazepines have had contradictory results (Gelpin et al., 1996; Mellman et al., 1998). The positive results of an initial pilot study demonstrating that propranolol administered in the acute aftermath of traumatic exposure resulted in reduced reactivity to traumatic reminders at three months (Cahill et al., 1994) were followed by a positive (but noncontrolled) study demonstrating reduced symptoms of PTSD at two months after exposure (Vaiva et al., 2003). A larger controlled prospective trial and a separate retrospective analysis of traumatically exposed persons receiving propranolol within 48 hours of exposure failed to demonstrate reduced rates of PTSD (Stein et al., 2007; Sharp et al., 2010). Additionally, animal models demonstrating that acquisition and initial consolidation of fear memories may be modulated by glucocorticoids have led to clinical trials targeting this process. An RCT of high-dose hydrocortisone versus placebo administered hours after traumatic exposure resulted in lower rates of ASD symptoms and lower rates of PTSD (Zohar et al., 2011). Case series and naturalistic studies also suggest that morphine administered acutely after trauma results in lower rates of PTSD or PTSD symptoms at longitudinal follow-up (Bryant et al., 2009 Holbrook et al., 2010). Finally, ketamine was assessed in a naturalistic study and found to increase symptoms of dissociation, re-experiencing, hyperarousal, and avoidance three days post-event compared to individuals who had not received ketamine (Schonenberg et al., 2008).

Taken as a whole, these studies suggest the potential for secondary prevention of PTSD via *immediate* post-exposure pharmacologic intervention. However, the evidence is preliminary at best, and studies focused on secondary prevention of PTSD provide little guidance regarding relief of acute symptoms of ASD itself. With the DSM-5's shift of emphasis from ASD as predictor of PTSD to ASD as an identifier of persons in severe distress and in need of clinical attention, new trials specifically targeting relief of acute symptoms—rather than focusing on prevention of subsequent PTSD—are also necessary. There have been no published trials of pharmacologic interventions specifically for ASD as defined in DSM-5. Presently the strongest evidence for treatment of ASD supports psychotherapeutic intervention. The practice guidelines that make recommendations specifically for ASD suggest pharmacologic intervention should be reserved for disabling sleep disturbance or severe and acutely dangerous co-morbid symptoms (VA/DoD, 2017).

PHARMACOLOGIC TREATMENT OF ADJUSTMENT DISORDERS

Like ASD, the ADs are brief generally self-limiting disorders. The DSM-5 specifies that symptoms must not persist more than six months after the stressor or its consequences have terminated (American Psychiatric Association, 2013). While published studies of psychosocial interventions for AD are fairly limited, those addressing pharmacological intervention are even more uncommon. To date, there are no published practice guidelines for the pharmacologic treatment of adults with ADs although a Cochrane Systematic review of RCTs is currently being developed (Casey et al., 2013).

CLINICAL TRIALS

In 1989, De Leo compared placebo, supportive psychotherapy, antidepressant, and benzodiazepine treatment in $n = 85$ patients with AD and found no difference between interventions with all patients improving. The specific subtype of AD was not specified. No other placebo-controlled studies have been published. Other recent studies compared the non-benzodiazepine anxiolytic etifoxine to lorazepam (Nguyen et al., 2006) and to alprazolam (Stein, 2015) in patients with AD with anxiety over 28 days. In both studies symptoms were significantly reduced in both the etifoxine and benzodiazepine groups; however, in both studies, rebound anxiety was more likely to develop in the benzodiazepine groups after withdrawal of treatment. One additional study of AD with anxiety found anxiolytics and antidepressants equally effective (Ansseau et al., 1996), and one small pilot study of AD with anxious and depressed mood found trazodone superior to benzodiazepine (Razavi et al., 1999).

Recently, placebo-controlled studies of several herbal treatments for AD and other complementary and alternative medicine (CAM) interventions have been published. These trials have been small, and often the definition of AD has not been clearly stated. These studies are summarized in chapter 24 of this volume.

Clearly, RCTs for all subtypes of AD are lacking. Given the fact that antidepressants are among the most commonly prescribed medications in the United States and are quite frequently prescribed for ADs (Olfson and Marcus, 2009), more research is necessary to evaluate the efficacy of these agents for AD. This research is needed before any empirically informed guidance may be promulgated for the pharmacological treatment of specific subtypes of AD.

FUTURE DIRECTIONS: PHARMACOLOGIC MANAGEMENT OF PTSD, ASD, AND ADS

In summary, recent decades have seen the emergence of relatively robust evidence for the efficacy of antidepressants and in particular SSRIs as first-line treatment for non-combat PTSD. Considerable evidence has also emerged for prazosin with regard to sleep disturbance in both combat-related and civilian PTSD. Little attention has been devoted to pharmacologic intervention for ASD symptoms. However, its reclassification in DSM-5 to reflect persons who are acutely distressed and in need of clinical attention (i.e., rather than an attempt to identify those at risk for subsequent development of PTSD) suggest that identification of short-term pharmacologic intervention strategies is needed. Since ASD does not adequately predict the development of PTSD, strategies to identify persons who are at highest risk for the development of PTSD will be necessary before preventive pharmacologic interventions can truly be studied.

While ADs have long been recognized in the DSM, their characterization as generally self-limited disorders has likely reduced interest in development of pharmacologic treatment strategies. Still, studies targeting the specific symptoms of specific AD subtypes may be helpful, particularly in light of the recognition that AD symptoms may persist if the precipitating stressors cannot be eliminated. Similarly, studies to date have not identified pharmacologic strategies to target specific symptom-clusters in PTSD. Such studies may help tailor future interventions to symptoms that are either particularly disabling or those that persist after partially effective psychotherapy. Combat-related PTSD appears to be particularly resistant to psychopharmacological intervention strategies identified to date and remains an area requiring further study.

Across the range of TSRD, pharmacologic interventions which may speed or augment psychotherapeutic intervention have not been consistently identified. Likewise, the extent to which pharmacologic intervention may augment emerging technology-delivered therapies (e.g., "virtual reality therapy," computer-delivered CBT, or other Internet-delivered "self-help" programs) has not been explored. Finally, as clinicians increasingly consider—and patients increasingly elect—CAM strategies to address their symptoms, head-to-head comparisons of CAM interventions and traditional medications (and traditional psychotherapies) for PTSD must be explored.

REFERENCES

Adamou, M., Puchalska, S., Plummer, W., Hale, A. S. (2007). Valproate in the treatment of PTSD: Systemic review and meta-analysis. *Current Med Res Opin*. 23:1285–1291.

Ahearn, E. P., Juergens, T., Cordes, T. (2011). A review of atypical antipsychotic medications for posttraumatic stress disorder. *Int Clin Psychopharmacol*. 26(4):193–200.

Ahmadpanah, M. S. P., Hosseini, S. M., Torabian, S., Haghighi, M., Jahangard, L., Bajoghli, H., Holsboer-Trachsler, E., Brand, S. (2014). Comparing the effect of prazosin and hydroxyzine on sleep quality in patients suffering from posttraumatic stress disorder. *Neuropsychobiology*. 69(4):235–242.

American Psychiatric Association. (2004a). *Diagnostic and statistical manual of mental disorders* (4th ed.). Washington, DC: Author.

American Psychiatric Association. (2004b). *Practice guidelines for the treatment of patients with acute stress disorder and posttraumatic stress disorder.* Washington DC: Author.

American Psychiatric Association. (2013). *Diagnostic and statistical manual of mental disorders* (5th ed.). Washington, DC: Author.

Ansseau, M., Bataille, M., Briole, G. (1996). Controlled comparison of tianeptine, alprazolam and mianserin in the treatment of ADs with anxiety and depression. *Hum Psychopharmacol*. 11:293–298.

Blake, D. J. (1986). Treatment of acute posttraumatic stress disorder with tricyclic antidepressants. *South Med J*. 79(2):201–204.

Braun, P., Greenberg, D., Dasberg, H., Lerer, B. (1990). Core symptoms of posttraumatic stress disorder unimproved by alprazolam treatment. *J Clin Psychiatry*. 51(6):236–238.

Bryant, R. A., Creamer, M., O'Donnell, M. (2009). A study of the protective function of acute morphine administration on the subsequent posttraumatic stress disorder. *Biol Psychiatry*. 65(5):438–440.

Byers, M. G., Allison, K. M., Wendel, C. S., Lee J. K. (2010). Prazosin versus quetiapine for nighttime posttraumatic stress disorder symptoms in veterans: An assessment of long-term comparative effectiveness and safety. *J Clin Psychopharmacol.* 30(3):225–229.

Cahill, L., Prins, B., Weber, M. (1994). Beta-adrenergic activation and memory for emotional events. *Nature.* 371(6499):702–704.

Casey, P., Pillay, D., Wilson, L., Maercker, A., Rice, A., Kelly, B. (2013). Pharmacological interventions for adjustment disorders in adults. *Cochrane Database Sys Rev.* doi:10.1002/14651858.CD010530

Cates, M. E., Bishop, M. H., David, L. L., Lowe, J. S., Woolley, T. W. (2004). Clonazepam for treatment of sleep disturbances associated with combat-related posttraumatic stress disorder. *Ann Pharmacother.* 38:1395–1399.

Chung, M. Y., Min, K. H., Jun, Y. J., Kim, S. S., Kim, W. C., Jun, E. M. (2004). Efficacy and tolerability of mirtazaoine and sertraline in Korean veterans with posttraumatic stress disorder: A randomized open label trial. Hum *Psychopharmacology.* 19:489–494.

Connor, K. M., Davidson, J. R., Weisler, R. H., Zhang, W., Abraham, K. (2006). Tiagabine for posttraumatic stress disorder: Effects if open-label and double-blind discontinuation treatment. *Psychopharmacology.* 184:21–25.

Davidson, J., Baldwin, D., Stein, D. J., Kuper, E., Benattia, I., Pedersen, A. S., Musgnung, J. (2006a). Treatment for posttraumatic stress disorder with venlafaxine extended release: A 6-month randomized controlled trial. *Arch Gen Psychiatry.* 63:1158–1165.

Davidson, J., Rothbaum, B. O., Tucker, P., Asnis, G., Benattia, I., Musgnung, J. J. (2006b). Venlafaxine extended release in posttraumatic stress disorder: A sertraline and placebo-controlled study. *J Clin Psychopharmacol.* 26:259–267.

Davidson, J. R., Brady, K., Mellman, T. A., Stein, M. B., Pollack, M. H. (2007). The efficacy and tolerability of tiagabine in adult patients with post-traumatic stress disorder. *J Clin Psychopharmacol.* 27:85–88.

Davidson, J. R., Weisler, R. H., Butterfield, M. I., Casat, C. D., Conner, K. M., Barnett, S., Van Meters, S. (2003). Mirtazapine vs. placebo in posttraumatic stress disorder: A pilot trial. *Biol Psychiatry.* 53:188–191.

Davis, L. L., Davidson, J. R., Ward, L. C., Bartolucci, A, Bowden, C. L., Petty, F. (2008). Divalproex in the treatment of posttraumatic stress disorder: A randomized, double-blind, placebo-controlled trial in a veteran population. *J Clin Psychopharmacol.* 28:84–88.

Davis, L. L., Jewell, M. E., Ambrose, S., Farley, J., English, B., Bartolucci, A., Petty, F. (2004). A placebo-controlled study of nefazodone for the treatment of chronic posttraumatic stress disorder: A preliminary study. *J Clin Psychopharmacol.* 24:291–297.

Davis, L. L., Nugent, A. L., Murray, J., Kramer, G. L., Petty, F. (2000). Nefazodone treatment for chronic posttraumatic stress disorder: an open trial. *J Clin Psychopharmacol.* 20(2):159–164.

De Leo, D. (1989). Treatment of adjustment disorders: A comparative evaluation. *Psychol Rep.* 64(1):51–54.

De Kleine, R. A., Hendriks, G. J., Kusters, W. J., Broekman, T. G., & van Minnen, A. (2012). A randomized placebo-controlled trial of D-cycloserine to enhance exposure therapy for posttraumatic stress disorder. *Biol Psychiatry.* 71(11):962–968.

Department of Veterans Affairs, Department of Defense. (2017). VA/DoD clinical practice guidelines for the management of posttraumatic stress. Retrieved from https://www.healthquality.va.gov/guidelines/MH/ptsd/VADoDPTSDCPGFinal010818.pdf

Difede, J., Cukor, J., Wyka, K., Olden, M., Hoffman, H., Lee, F. S., Altemus, M. (2014) D-cycloserine augmentation of exposure therapy for PTSD: A pilot study, *Neuropsychopharmacology.* 39(5):1052–1058.

Duffy, J. D., & Malloy, P. F. (1994). Efficacy of buspirone in the treatment of posttraumatic stress disorder: an open trial. *Ann Clin Psychiatry.* 6(1):33–37.

Feder, A., Parides, M. K., Murrough, J. W., Perez, A. M., Morgan, J. E., Saxena, S., Kirkwood, K., aan het Rot, M., Lapidus, K. A., Wan, L. B., Iosifescu, D., Charney, D. S. (2014). Efficacy of intravenous ketamine for treatment of chronic posttraumatic stress disorder: A randomized clinical trial. *JAMA Psychiatry.* 71(6):681–688. doi:10.1001/jamapsychiatry.2014.62

Foa, E. B., Keane, T. M., Friedman, M. J., Cohen, J. A., eds. (2009). *Effective treatments for PTSD: Practice guidelines from the International Society for Traumatic Stress Studies,* 2nd ed. New York: Guilford Press.

Forbes, D., Creamer, M., Bisson, J. I., Cohen, J. A., Crow, B. E., Foa, E. B., Ursano, R. J. (2010). A guide to guidelines for the treatment of PTSD and related conditions. *J Trauma Stress.* 23(5):537–552. doi:10.1002/jts.20565

Forbes, D., Creamer, M., Phelps, A., Bryant, R., McFarlane, A., Devilly, G. J., Matthews, L., Raphael, B., Doran, C., Merlin, T., Newton, S. (2007). Australian guidelines for the treatment of adults with acute stress disorder and posttraumatic stress disorder. East Melbourne. Australian National Health and Medical Research Council.

Friedman, M. J., Davidson, J. R. T., Stein, D. J. (2009). Psychopharmacotherapy for adults. In E. B. Foa, T. M. Keane, M. J. Friedman, J. A. Cohen (eds.), *Effective treatments for PTSD: Practice* guidelines from the International Society for Traumatic Stress Studies (2nd ed., pp. 139–222). New York: Guilford Press.

Friedman, M. J., Marmar, C. R., Baker, D. G., Sikes, C. R., Farfel, G. M. (2007). Randomized, double-blind comparison of sertraline and placebo for posttraumatic stress disorder in a Department of Veterans Affairs setting. *J Clin Psychiatry.* 68:711–720.

Garfield, D. A., Fichtner, C. G., Leveroni, C., Mahableshwarkar, A. (2001). Open trial of nefazodone for combat veterans with posttraumatic stress disorder. *J Trauma Stress.* 14(3):453–460.

Gelpin, E., Bonne, O., Peri, T. (1996). Treatment of recent trauma survivors with benzodiazepines: a prospective study. *J Clin Psychiatry.* 57(9):390–394.

Germain A, R., Richardson, R., Moul, D. E., Mammen, O., Haas, G., Forman, S. D., Rode, N., Begley, A., Nofzinger, E. A. (2012). Placebo-controlled comparison of prazosin and cognitive-behavioral treatments for sleep disturbances in US military veterans. *J Psychosom Res.* 72(2):89–96.

Gillin, J. C., Smith-Vaniz, A., Schnierow, B., Rapaport, M. H., Kelsoe, J., Raimo, E., Marler, M. R., Goyette, L. M., Stein, M. B., Zisook, S. (2001). An open-label, 12-week clinical and sleep EEG study of nefazodone in chronic combat related posttraumatic stress disorder. *J Clin Psychiatry.* 62(10):789–796.

Hamner, M. B., Deitsch, S. E., Brodrick, P. S., Ulmer, H. G., Lorberbaum, J. P. (2003b). Quetiapine treatment in patients with posttraumatic stress disorder: An open trial of adjunctive therapy. *J Clin Psychopharmoacol.* 23:15–20.

Hertzberg, M. A., Feldman, M. E., Beckham, J. C. (1998). Open trial of nefazodone for combat-related posttraumatic stress disorder. *J Clin Psychiatry.* 59(9):460–464.

Hertzberg, M. A., Feldman, M. E., Beckham, J. C., Kudler H. S., & Davidson J. R. (2000). Lack of efficacy for fluoxetine in PTSD: a placebo controlled trial in combat veterans. *Ann Clin Psychiatry.* 12(2):101–105.

Holbrook, T. L., Galarneau, M. R., Dye, J. L. (2010). Morphine use after combat injury in Iraq and post-traumatic stress disorder. *N Engl J Med.* 362(2):110–117.

Hidalgo, R., Hertzberg, M. A., Mellman, T. (1999). Nefazodone in post-traumatic stress disorder: Results from six open-label trials. *Int Clin Psychopharmacol.* 14(2):61–68.

Institute of Medicine. (2008). *Treatment of PTSD: An assessment of evidence.* Washington, DC: National Academics Press.

Kosten, T. R., Frank, J. B., Dan, E. (1991). Pharmacotherapy for posttraumatic stress disorder using phenelzine or imipramine. *J Nerv Ment Dis.* 179(6):366–370.

Krystal, J. H., Rosenheck, R. A., Cramer, J. A. (2011). Adjunctive risperidone treatment for antidepressant-resistant symptoms of chronic military service-related PTSD: A randomized trial. *JAMA* 306(5):4930502

Lindley, S. E., Carlson, E. B., Hill, K. (2007). A randomized, double-blind, placebo-controlled trail of augmentation topiramate for chronic combat-related posttraumatic stress disorder. *J Clin Psychopharmacol.* 27:677–681.

Martenyi, F., Soldatenkova, V. (2006). Fluoxetine in the acute treatment and relapse prevention of combat-related post-traumatic stress disorder. Analysis of the veteran group of placebo-controlled, randomized clinical trial. *Eur Neuropsychopharmacol.* 16:340–349.

Martenyi, F., Brown, E. B., Zhang, H., et al. (2002). Fluoxetine versus placebo in posttraumatic stress disorder. *J Clin Psychol.* 63:199–206.

McRae, A. L., Brady, K. T., Mellman, T. A., Sonne, S. C., Killeen, T. K., Timmerman, M. A., Bayles-Dazet, W. (2004). Comparison of nefazodone and sertraline for the treatment of posttraumatic stress disorder. *Depress Anxiety.* 19:190–196.

Mellman, T. A., Byers, P. M., Augenstein, J. S. (1998). Pilot evaluation of hypnotic medication during acute traumatic stress response. *J Trauma Stress.* 11(3):563–569.

National Institute for Clinical Excellence. (2005). *Post-traumatic stress disorder: The management of post traumatic stress disorder in primary and secondary care.* London: Author.

Neylan, T., Lenoci, M., Samuelson, K., Metzler, T., Henn-Haase, C., Hierholzer, R., Lindley, S., Otte, C., Schoenfeld, F., Yesavage, J., Marmar, C. (2006). No improvement of posttraumatic stress disorder symptoms with guanfacine treatment. *Am J Psychiatry.* 163:2186–2188.

Olfson, M., Marcus, S. (2009). National patterns in antidepressant medication treatment. *Arch Gen Psychiatry.* 66:848.

Nguyen, N., Fakra, E., Pradel, V. (2006). Efficacy of etifoxine compared to lorazepam monotherapy in the treatment of patients with adjustment disorders with anxiety: A double-blind controlled study in general practice. *Human Psychopharmacol.* 21(3):139–49.

Pae, C. U., Lim, H. K., Peindl, K. (2008). The atypical antipsychotics olanzapine and risperidone in the treatment of posttraumatic stress disorder: A meta-analysis of randomized, double-blind, placebo-controlled clinical trials. *Int Clin Psychopharmacol.* 23(1):1–8.

Petrakis, I. L, Desai, N., Gueorguieva, R., Arias, A., O'Brien, E., Jane, J. S., Sevarino, K., Southwick, S., Ralevski, E. (2016). Prazosin for veterans with posttraumatic stress disorder and comorbid alcohol dependence: A clinical trial. *Alcohol Clin Exp Res*, 40(1):178–186.

Pollack, M. H., Hoge, G. A., Worthington, J. J., Moshier, S. J., Wechsler, R. S., Brandes, M., Simon, N. M. (2011). Eszopiclone for the treatment of posttraumatic stress disorder and associated insomnia: A randomized, double-blind, placebo-controlled trial. *Journal of Clinical Psychiatry*, *72*(7), 892–897.

Raskind, M. A., Peskind, E. R., Hoff, D. J., Hart, K. L., Holmes, H. A., Warren, D., Shofer, J., O'Connell, J., Taylor, F., Gross, C., Rohde, K., McFall, M. E. (2007). A parallel group placebo controlled study of prazosin for trauma nightmares and sleep disturbance in combat veterans with post-traumatic stress disorder. *Biol Psychiatry*. 61:928–934.

Raskind, M. A., Peskind, E. R., Kanter, E.D., Petrie, E. C., Radant, A., Thompson, C. E., Dobie, D. J., Hoff, D., Rein, R. J., Straits-Troster, K., Thomas, R. G., McFall, M. M. (2003). Reduction of nightmares and other PTSD symptoms in combat veterans by prazosin: A placebo-controlled study. *Am J Psychiatry*. 160:371–373.

Raskind, M. A., Peterson, K., Williams, T., Hoff, D. J., Hart, K., Holmes, H., Peskind, E. R. (2013). A trail of prazosin for combat trauma PTSD with nightmares in active duty soldiers returned from Iraq and Afghanistan. *Am J Psychiatry*. 170(9):1003–1010. http://dx.doi.org/10.1176/appi.ajp.2013.12081133

Raskind, M. A., Thompson, C., Petrie, E. C., Dobie, D. J., Rein, R. J., Hoff, D. J., McFall, M. E., Peskind, E. R. (2002). Prazosin reduces nightmares in combat veterans with posttraumatic stress disorder. *J Clin Psychiatry*. 63:565–568.

Razavi, D., Kormoss, N., Collard, A. (1999). Comparative study of the efficacy and safety of trazodone versus clorazepate in the treatment of adjustment disorders in cancer patients: A pilot study. *J Int Med Res*. 27:264–272.

Robert, R., Blakeney, P. E., Villareal, C., Rosenberg, L., & Meyer, W. J. III. (1999). Imipramine treatment in pediatric burn patients with symptoms of acute stress disorder: a pilot study. *J Am Acad Child Adolesc Psychiatry*. 38(7):873–882.

Risse, S. C., Whitters, A., Burke, J., Chen, S., Scurfield, R. M., Raskind, M. A. (1990). Severe withdrawal symptoms after discontinuation of alprazolam in eight patients with combat-induced post-traumatic stress disorder. *J Clin Psychiatry*. 51:206–209.

Rothbaum, B. O., Cahill, S. P., Foa, E. B. (2006). Augmentation of sertraline with prolonged exposure in treatment of posttraumatic stress disorder. *J Trauma Stress*. 19:625–638.

Rothbaum, B. O., Gerardi, M., Bradley, B. (2011). Evidence based treatments for PTSD in OEF/OIF military personnel. In *Caring for veterans with deployment-related stress disorders* (pp. 215–239). Washington, DC: American Psychological Association.

Saygin, M. Z., Sungar, M. Z., Sabol, E. U., Cetinkaya, P. (2002). Nefazodone versus sertraline in treatment of posttraumatic stress disorder. *Klinik Psikofarmakoloji Bulteni*. 12:1–5.

Schneier, F. R., Neria, Y., Pavicova, M., Hembree, E., Suh, E. J., Amsel, L., Marshall, R. D. (2012). Combined prolonged exposure therapy and paroxetine for PTSD related to the World Trade Center attack: A randomized controlled trial. *Am J Psychiatry* 169 (1):80–88. doi:10.1176/appi.ajp.2011.11020321

Schonenberg, M., Reichwald, U., Domes, G., Badke, A., Hautzinger, M. (2008). Ketamine aggravates symptoms of acute stress disorder in a naturalistic sample of accident victims. *J Psychopharmcol.* 22(5):493–497.

Shalev, A. Y., Ankri, Y., Israeli-Shalev, Y. (2012). Prevention of posttraumatic stress disorder by early treatment: Results from Jerusalem Trauma Outreach and Prevention. *Arch Gen Psychiatry*. 96(2):166–176.

Sharp, S., Thomas, C., Rosenberg, L., Rosenberg, M., Meyer, W. (2010). Propranolol does not reduce risk for acute stress disorder in pediatric burn trauma. *J Trauma-Inj Infect Crit Care*: 68(1):193–197.

Simon, N. M., Conner, K. M., Lang, A. J. (2008) Paroxetine CR augmentation for posttraumatic stress disorder refractory to prolonged exposure therapy. *J Clin Psychiatry*. 69:400–405.

Stein, D. J. (2015). Etifoxine versus alprazolam for the treatment of adjustment disorder with anxiety: A randomized controlled trial. *Adv Therapy*. 32:57–68.

Stein M. B., Kline, N. A., Matloff, J. L. (2002). Adjunctive olanzapine for SSRI-resistant combat-related PTSD: A double-blind, placebo-controlled study. *Am J Psychiatry*. 159:1777–1779.

Stein, D. J., Ipser, J. C. Pharmacotherapy of PTSD. In Post-Traumatic Stress Disorder. pp 149–162. Edited by Stein, D.J., Friedman, M.J., Blanco, C. New York: Wiley, 2011.

Stein, D. J., Ipser, J. C., Seedat, S. (2006). Pharmacotherapy for post-traumatic stress disorder (PTSD). *Cochrane Database Sys Rev.* 1:CD002795.

Stein, M. B., Kerridge, C., Dimsdale, J. E. (2007). Pharmacotherapy to prevent PTSD: Results from a randomized controlled proof-of-concept trial in physically injured patients. *J Trauma Stress.* 20(6):923–932.

Taylor, F. B., Lowe, K., Thompson, C., McFall, M. M., Peskind, E. R., Kanter, E. D., Allison, N, Williams, J., Martin, P., Raskind, M. A. (2006). Daytime prazosin reduces psychological distress to trauma specific cues in civilian trauma posttraumatic stress disorder. *Biol Psychiatry.* 59:577–581.

Taylor, F. B., Martin, P., Thompson, C. (2008). Prazosin effects on objective sleep measures and clinical symptoms in civilian trauma posttraumatic stress disorder: A placebo-controlled study. *Biol Psychiatry.* 63:629–632.

Vaiva, G., Ducrocq, F., Jezequel, K. (2003). Immediate treatment with propranolol decreases posttraumatic stress disorder two months after trauma. *Biol Psychiatry.* 54(9):947–949.

Viola, J., Ditzler, T., Batzer, W., Harazin, J., Adama, D., Lettich, L., Berigan, T. (1997). Pharmacological management of posttraumatic stress disorder: Clinical summary of a five-year retrospective study, 1990–1995. *Military Med.* 162(9):616–619.

van der Kolk, B. A., Spinazzola, J., Blaustein, M. E. (2007). A randomized clinical trial of eye movement desensitization and reprocessing (EMDR), fluoxetine, and pill placebo in the treatment of posttraumatic stress disorder: Treatment effects and long-term maintenance. *J Clin Psychiatry.* 68:37–46.

van Minnen, A., Harned, M. S., Zoellner, L., Mills, K. (2012). Examining potential contraindications for prolonged exposure therapy for PTSD. *Eur J Psychotraumatol.* doi: 10.3402/ejpt.v3i0.18805

van Zuiden, M., Frijling, J. L., Nawijn, L., Koch, S. B., Goslings, J. C., Luitse, J. S., Biesheuval, T. H., Honig, A., Veltman, D. G., Olff, M. (2017) Intranasal oxytocin to prevent posttraumatic stress disorder symptoms: A randomized controlled trial in emergency department patients. *Biol Psychiatry.* 81(12): 1030–1040. doi: 101016/j.biopsych.2016.11.012

Wells, B. G., Chu, C. C., Johnson, R., Nasdahl, C., Ayubi, M. A., Sewell, E., & Statham, P. (1991). Buspirone in the treatment of posttraumatic stress disorder. *Pharmacotherapy.* 11(4):340–343.

Zisook, S., Chentsova-Dutton, Y. E., Smith-Vaniz, A., Kline, N. A., Ellenor, G. L., Kodsi, A. B., & Gillin, J. C. (2000). Nefazodone in patients with treatment-refractory posttraumatic stress disorder. *J Clin Psychiatry.* 61(3):203–208.

Zohar, J., Yahalom, H., Kozlovsky, N. (2011). High does hydrocortisone immediately after trauma may alter the trajectory of PTSD: Interplay between clinical and animal studies. *Eur Neuropsychopharmacol.* 21(11):796–809.

23

Pharmacologic Treatment of Children with Trauma- and Stressor-Related Disorders

SUNI JANI, RYAN HERRINGA, AND DEREK HURSEY

INTRODUCTION

Psychopharmacological clinical guidelines for treatment of conditions in children, particularly with regard to trauma- and stressor-related disorders (TSRD), are difficult to establish due to the variability in trauma- and stressor-related symptomatic presentations within children and adolescents as well as the paucity of randomized control trials (RCTs) using psychopharmacology in this population. This population requires strong multidisciplinary treatment and has established evidence-based psychotherapeutic treatments including trauma-focused cognitive behavioral therapy (TF-CBT), prolonged exposure, and eye movement desensitization and reprocessing (Cohen et al., 2016; Foa et al., 2013). When the illness is of significant severity and functionally impairing, carefully monitored psychopharmacological interventions may be indicated, particularly for comorbid conditions.

TSRD are common in children with varied and complex presentations which can lead to persisting functional impairment if the condition is not identified and treated in a timely and evidence-based manner. As discussed in other chapters, children 6 years and older share the diagnostic criteria for posttraumatic stress disorder (PTSD) including direct experiencing, witnessing, discovering, or repeatedly experiencing actual or threatened death, serious injury, or sexual violence. While children and adults share symptoms of PTSD such as persistence avoidance of stimuli associated with the trauma, negative alterations in cognitions and mood, hyperreactivity, and avoidance, there are key differences in the symptomatic presentation that should be noted. Children older than 6 may demonstrate repetitive or re-enactment play with themes or aspects of traumatic events instead of explicitly reporting distressing intrusive memories or dissociative symptoms which are more commonly reported in adults. Children may also report frightening dreams without recognizable content in lieu of nightmares related to the trauma. Children younger than 6 years are discussed in Chapter 8 and require fewer symptoms for diagnosis of PTSD to meet full criteria for a *Diagnostic and Statistical Manual of Mental Disorders* (DSM) diagnosis. These same criteria apply to acute stress disorder (ASD), a condition lasting three days to one month occurring after exposure to severe traumatic stress (American Psychiatric Association [APA], 2013)

A new diagnosis of note for TSRDs is adjustment disorders (ADs). Unlike PTSD or ASD, the criteria for AD do not include specific diagnostic considerations for children which can further complicate their psychopharmacological management. Since 1952, AD diagnoses have undergone numerous classification changes despite an unchanging name. In the fifth edition of the DSM (DSM-5), they were placed under the TSRD category for the first time; however, it remains complex to distinguish them from normal stress reactions, particularly as they lack specific diagnostic criteria for symptom numbers or combinations. Given its diagnostic evolution, prevalence studies of AD, particularly in children, are rare and research into its pharmacological treatment is even scarcer. However, as part of the TSRD group, it is an important diagnostic consideration to understand their prognosis, particularly as ADs can be associated with suicidality in adolescents (Casey, 2014; Pelkonen et al., 2005).

This chapter will also discuss emerging psychopharmacological treatments and theories of TSRDs common to childhood, reactive attachment disorder (RAD), and disinhibited social engagement disorder (DSED). Briefly, RAD is usually manifested in children before the age of 5 as a consistent pattern of inhibited, emotionally withdrawn behavior toward adult caregivers with minimal social responsiveness to others. This is thought to stem from frequent changes in caregivers or neglect, reflecting deprivation from normal parental care in a key developmental period. This same early neglect is also thought to lead to DSED, a disorder manifesting with inappropriate familiarity and lack of caution for their developmental age (APA, 2013). Treatment of these attachment disorders is critical as they are crucially linked to the development of adult psychopathology (Lehmann et al., 2016).

Regardless of meeting criteria for TSRDs, most traumatized children require integrated multidisciplinary systems of care from psychopharmacologists, psychotherapists, school, and family (Briere, 2001). Pharmacotherapy is an adjunct intervention for treatment of TSRDs, but there is limited literature on its role in this area, in part due to a lack of RCTs and also the stigma of treating children with psychotropic medications (Rothenberger & Rothenberger, 2013). However, the American Academy of Child and Adolescent Psychiatry (AACAP) acknowledges α- and β-adrenergic blocking agents, novel antipsychotic agents, selective serotonin reuptake inhibitor (SSRI) antidepressants such as tricyclic antidepressants (TCAs), and mood-stabilizing agents may be effective for children based on several open clinical trials (Cohen, 2010) which are discussed in this chapter in addition to existing promising clinical trials. At the same time, any medication consideration in children must take into account potential side effects, medication interactions, and black box warnings as they specifically apply to the pediatric population. We review these areas more in depth in the following sections.

PRINCIPLES OF PHARMACOLOGIC TREATMENT IN CHILDREN AND ADOLESCENTS

Prescribing medications to children is a complex matter often mired in legal, ethical, and biological factors that vary across experience and research. Lakhan and colleagues (2007) noted several myths practitioners often fall privy to, believing medicating children is analogous to adults as they are "little adults" or have similar presentation of psychiatric conditions to adults and require lower dosing of the same medication. Some practitioners may believe children do not have reasons to develop or experience depression or anxiety, and opposing prescribers may feel medications are the most successful option for treating children with mental illnesses. Children are as vulnerable to mental illness as adults, but they are ultimately developing adults who experience neural change at a faster rate than adults, rendering it difficult for psychotropics approved for adults to work predictably in children. Societal and academic reluctance to enroll children in clinical trials of psychotropic drugs has often increased their vulnerability as a population which in turn creates difficulties in developing clinical practice guidelines (Lakhan et al. 2007).

Psychotropic drugs for various disorders commonly used by child and adolescent psychiatrists include stimulants, nonstimulants, anxiolytics, antidepressants, and antipsychotics, albeit with limited Food and Drug Administration (FDA) approval and black box warnings on antidepressants (O'Brien, 2017). The scientific basis for psychotropic use is limited, particularly in young children (Gleason et al., 2007). In addition to complexities of consent, study design, and diagnostic clarification, psychopharmacology in children has numerous genetic, pharmacokinetic, pharmacodynamics, metabolic, and elimination factors that require particular sophistication in justifying the use of medications that are traditionally prescribed to adults or approved for other, non-trauma related diagnoses in youth (Clein & Riddle, 1995). Furthermore, the delineation of developmental neurobiology from infancy through childhood has created an increasing area of study that could influence future practice with regard to diagnosis and treatment. Notably, an improved understanding of the role of neurotransmitter systems in neurodevelopment (glutaminergic, endorphin, g-aminobutyric acid [GABA]-ergic, dopaminergic, serotonergic, and cholinergic) could allow more rationale choices in psychopharmacological treatment in children (Drury & Cuthbert, 2015; Stoddard et al., 2006).

PHARMACOLOGIC TREATMENT OF PTSD IN CHILDREN AND ADOLESCENTS

While certain SSRIs such as fluoxetine and escitalopram have limited FDA approval for treating children and adolescents with depression and obsessive-compulsive disorder (OCD), there are no FDA-approved medications for the treatment of TSRD in children (FDA, 2014). Unfortunately few RCTs exist in this population, perhaps due to difficulty in recruitment for studies as well as physiological differences from adults in medication response, concern of side effects creating risks that outweigh benefits, and established and effective evidence-based psychotherapeutic interventions (Cohen, 2010).

Internationally, the United Kingdom–based National Institute for Healthcare and Excellence discourages routine use of medications for pediatric PTSD but notes comorbid conditions such as attention deficit hyperactivity disorder (ADHD) or generalized anxiety may require a psychotropic intervention (National Institute for Health and Care Excellence, 2005). The World Health Organization (WHO) has guidelines that state benzodiazepines and antidepressants should not be given to children experiencing significant daily functional impairment from acute traumatic stress symptoms. The WHO offers a mental health global access program (mhGAP) recommendation for psychological first aid to children who have been recently exposed to potentially traumatic events (WHO, 2013).

Presently, the AACAP encourages trauma-focused psychotherapies as first-line treatment for children and adolescents with PTSD with the addition of SSRIs if there is no improvement with first-line treatment. The AACAP notes in its practice parameters that antidepressant studies in children with PTSD historically found placebo effects responsible for improvements (Birmaher et al., 1996) and cautions child psychiatrists about basing treatment decisions on the outcomes of adult studies. The AACAP's rationale is consistent with findings from 2008, when the National Center for PTSD published psychopharmacological research highlights on the treatment of PTSD. This is illustrated in a study that compared TF-CBT with and without sertraline in 24 sexually abused children ages 10 to 17 years old and did not find a statistically significant difference in outcomes, but this was attributed to a low sample size (Cohen et al., 2007; Cohen, 2008). The consensus from this study as well as the history of placebo effect improvements is responsible for the AACAP's present stance on psychopharmacology as an adjunct or second-line treatment if symptom severity or lack of improvement persists (Cohen, 2010).

Furthermore, TSRDs in children can become chronic and are frequently comorbid with other chronic conditions such as anxiety and mood disorders. Children with multiple chronic conditions can have more mental and physical health problems and result in increased school absences, decreased peer relationships and quality of life, and increased health services compared to other children (Newacheck & Stoddard, 1994). Despite risks of using medications with children, this significant morbidity of chronicity may require medication as they are effective for some individuals including those with more severe and complex presentations. These treatment options should always be made in consultation with the young persons and their families (Hetrick et al., 2010).

Overall, the use of antidepressants in prepubertal children is a controversial issue, and current research findings have not supported consistent efficacy (Garland et al., 2009); however, it is still an important aspect of PTSD treatment that requires careful consideration of existing literature to make informed future clinical decisions.

PHARMACOLOGIC INTERVENTIONS

Selective Serotonin Reuptake Inhibitors

Overall, SSRIs have long replaced TCAs as preferred agents for the treatment of childhood depression, PTSD, OCD, and generalized anxiety disorder because of their lower side-effect profile and reduced drug-drug interactions which contributes to their comparative safety in the event of overdose compared with TCAs (Leonard et al., 1997). A more recent Cochrane review has demonstrated that SSRIs are effective in reducing core symptoms of pediatric OCD (Ipser et al. 2009). SSRIs have minimal anticholinergic, metabolic, and cardiovascular effects compared to TCAs due to their low affinity for histamine, alpha-1, and muscarinic receptors. For complex patients with medical comorbidities who have also been prescribed other medications, prescribers should note SSRIs may impair platelet aggregation. Clinicians prescribing SSRIs concurrently with agents that have antiplatelet or anticoagulant effects should be monitored appropriately. Additionally, epistaxis has been reported in the literature (Lake et al. 2000). Despite the black box warning for suicidality, fluoxetine retains FDA approval for pediatric depression (Nathan & Gorman, 2015), and citalopram, sertraline, and other SSRIs remain commonly used in child and adolescent psychiatry (Stoddard et al., 2006; Bushnell et al., 2015).

Despite suggesting caution with the use of SSRIs, the AACAP's practice parameters for childhood PTSD do note promise from certain SSRI studies. Seedat et al. (2002) found comparable improvement in an open label study of 24 children and 14 adult subjects who received doses of citalopram between 20 and 40 mg per day.

A Turkish open trial of 7 to 20 mg of fluoxetine showed effectiveness in improving earthquake-related PTSD symptoms in 26 participants 7 to 17 years old (Yorbik et al., 2001). Nefazodone and cyproheptadine, also serotonergic agents, have been used in adolescents, but safety data are lacking (Domon et al., 2000; Gupta et al., 1998). The aforementioned study showed negligible improvement with the addition of sertraline to TF-CBT. More recently in 2015, Martsenkovsky and colleagues (2015) conducted a 12-week double-blind placebo -controlled study of 110 Ukranian children aged 12 to 18 years that found 20 to 40 mg of fluoxetine demonstrated improved scores in the Clinician-Administrated PTSD Scale for DSM-5.

Regardless, risks associated with SSRI use are likely to outweigh any modest benefits for PTSD specifically. Side effects such as akathisia, irritability, insomnia, gastrointestinal side effects, or inattention can exacerbate hyperarousal and may be contraindicated for children presenting predominantly with these symptoms (Mitka, 2003; Hammad, 2004). There was also a consideration that SSRIs may be beneficial in comorbid cases where patients also have anxiety disorders, depression, or OCD, but so far the only TF-CBT study with sertraline noted more than 60% of the participants had comorbid major depressive disorder and still did not produce demonstrable improvement in PTSD or depression scores above and beyond TF-CBT itself (Cohen et al., 2007; Robb et al., 2008).

Since October 2003, SSRIs carry an advisory from the FDA reporting suicidal ideation and attempts from clinical trials of various antidepressant drugs in pediatric patients (Mitka, 2003). This advisory remains despite the fact suicidality could not be definitively linked to SSRIs because it occurred in both treated and untreated patients with major depression. Furthermore, no links between SSRIs and suicidality were found in a study of more than 65,000 children and adults treated for depression between 1992 and 2002. Instead, this study found a decrease in suicide risk with antidepressant use (Scheeringa et al., 2003). However, in 2006, Olfson and colleagues conducted a case-control study of Medicaid beneficiaries in America of all ages who carried a diagnosis of depression and had been hospitalized. They evaluated patients who attempted suicide following their hospitalization and had filled prescriptions for antidepressants of any class, not only SSRIs. The study found children on antidepressants were 1.52 times more likely to attempt suicide whereas there was no difference in attempts between treated and untreated adults. Olfson and colleagues found the highest risk of suicide with the serotonin-norepinephrine reuptake inhibitor (SNRI) venlafaxine which resulted in a 2.3 times higher risk of suicide attempts than no treatment. Apart from sertraline, the study did not find SSRIs to be a significant predictor of youth suicide attempts. The authors hypothesized the results may have occurred as they evaluated the most clinically unstable population who had been recently been hospitalized and youths in the general population may have benefitted from antidepressant prescribing (Olfson et al., 2006). This assertion was partly because their 2003 study from a pharmaceutical database of 588 children aged 10 to 19 prescribed antidepressants from 1990 to 2000 that found a decrease of adolescent suicides as prescribing rates of antidepressants increased (Olfson et al., 2003). In 2014, Miller and colleagues conducted a propensity score–matched cohort study of the link between antidepressant dosing and suicidal ideation using population-based health care utilization data from 162, 625 US residents aged 10 to 64 years and diagnosed with depression. The authors found the rate of deliberate self-harm among children, adolescents, and young adults aged 24 or younger was higher on average in youth who received high doses of SSRIs (citalopram 40 mg, sertraline 200 mg, or fluoxetine 80 mg) though these doses did not impact adult rates of suicidality or self-harm (Miller et al. 2014). In 2015, a Danish study found the risk for suicide attempts in adults in their early 20s was highest in the first three months after redeeming their first prescription for an SSRI, especially if they had fewer risk factors (Christiansen et al., 2016).

However, there are variations in the studies evaluating adolescent suicidality with antidepressants. Following the implementation of the FDA warning, Gibbons and colleagues (2007) evaluated prescription rates in the United States and the Netherlands for SSRIs from 2003 to 2005 in children and adolescents up to age 19 along with suicide rates through 2004 in the United States and through 2005 in the Netherlands. The study found a decrease of prescription rates for SSRIs by about 22% in both the United States and the Netherlands after the black box warnings were issued. The study found youth suicide rate increased inversely in response to decreased SSRI prescription in both the Netherlands and the United States. The Netherlands had an increase of youth suicides by 49% between 2003 and 2005, and United States youth suicide rates increased by

14% between 2003 and 2004. The authors noted the change in the United States was the largest since 1979 when the Centers for Disease Control and Prevention began collecting suicide data (Gibbons et al., 2007).

There are significant methodological limitations with many studies examining the relationship of dose and treatment response. In addition, there are studies that show that blood concentration, rather than dose of SSRI antidepressants, such as fluoxetine and citalopram, may be related to eventual antidepressant response in depressed adolescent and adult patients (Sakolsky et al. 2011). While it seems that most individuals treated with SSRIs will actually have serotonin reuptake inhibition at a blood level considered to be necessary for response, individual differences in drug metabolism could necessitate a higher dose in some patients to attain adequate blood level and receptor binding to result in response. As a result, while SSRIs may sometimes be considered for treatment of pediatric TSRDs, they should be dosed cautiously and monitored closely in youth (Brent & Gibbons, 2014).

A summary of SSRIs and their use in pediatric populations can be found in Table 23.1. (Janicak et al., 2010).

Opioids

Pain management in acutely burned hospitalized children with PTSD also found a linear association between early morphine dosage and a six-month reduction in PTSD symptoms in children aged 6 to 16 (Saxe et al., 2001), and preliminary findings confirm this in children aged 0 to 4 (Stoddard et al, 2009). Stoddard and colleagues evaluated seventy 12- to 48-month-old children with acute burns during their hospitalization and at one-, three-, and six-month follow-up times after discharge. The study found higher early doses of morphine were associated with decreased arousal symptoms months after the major trauma may be associated with a decreasing number of PTSD symptoms, especially those of arousal, in the months after major trauma. Adult studies with injured soldiers, and with adult burn patients, also found associations of early morphine administration postinjury with reduced PTSD symptomatology (Holbrook et al., 2010).

Antiadrenergic Agents

The Practice Guideline of the AACAP does note antiadrenergic agents, specifically α2- and β-adrenergic antagonists such as clonidine and propranolol, respectively, may be useful in decreasing sympathetic hyperarousal, impulsivity, and re-experiencing symptoms, particularly as there is evidence of increased adrenergic tone in children with PTSD (Famularo et al., 1988; Perry, 1994; Harmon & Riggs, 1996; De Bellis et al., 2001; Strawn & Geracioti, 2008). Unfortunately, there are no RCTs examining adrenergic antagonists in pediatric TRSDs.

Clonidine is a medication approved by the FDA to treat essential hypertension in children. The extended release formulation of clonidine known as Kapvay has FDA approval to treat ADHD in children aged 6 and older. Clonidine has been previously used in the acute setting for managing neonatal opioid withdrawal and helping with sedation in the critically ill (Hudak & Tan, 2012; Wang et al. 2015). In a case study, clonidine treatment resulted in improved sleep and increased neural integrity of the anterior cingulate (DeBellis et al., 2001) An additional two open-label trials of clonidine, one with oral clonidine given in doses of 0.05 to 0.1 mg per day (Perry et al., 1994) and another with 0.1 to 0.2 mg per day (Harmon et al., 1996) of clonidine transdermal patches, noted a reduction in anxiety, arousal, insomnia, and impulsive and aggressive behavior in children with PTSD. Clonidine does have a side effect of drowsiness, hypotension, lethargy, sedation, and headache with rare risks for anxiety and depression. Clonidine should not be taken with other medications that might cause drowsiness such as muscle relaxants, antihistamines, or medications for insomnia. They may interact with SSRIs as well (Lexicomp, 2017).

Propranolol is a peripheral nonselective beta-adrenergic antagonist resulting in decreased chronotropic, inotropic, and vasodilator responses to beta-adrenergic stimulation thereby lowering blood pressure. It has FDA approval for tremors, angina hypertension, and arrhythmia in adults and infantile hemangioma (Lexicomp, 2017). Abused children aged 8 to 10 with PTSD had a reduction in intrusion and arousal symptoms with five weeks of propranolol (Famularo et al., 1988). Children who take propranolol most commonly experience side effects of insomnia, irritability, restlessness, dry mouth, hyperventilation, mucoid cough, breathing difficulties, and chest tightness (Lexicomp, 2017).

Guanfacine is a selective alpha-2A adrenergic agonist approved for children and adolescents with ADHD (Lexicomp 2017); however, it has been used in treatment of childhood TSRDs as well. Guanfacine has been effective in reducing nightmares in a case study (Horrigan,

TABLE 23.1. SSRIS STUDIED IN THE TREATMENT OF PEDIATRIC TSRDS

SSRIs	FDA Approval in Pediatric Populations	Metabolic Pathway	Pharmacokinetics	Clinical Considerations
Fluoxetine	Approved by FDA for treatment of depression in children aged 8 and older as well as obsessive-compulsive disorder in children	Inhibits the serotonin transporter protein and is a weak norepinephrine reuptake inhibitor (effect increases with higher doses). Also an antagonist at 5HT2C receptors	Metabolized in the liver by isoenzymes of the cytochrome P450 system, including CYP2D6	Fluoxetine has a half-life of 2 to 5 days in healthy young adults and its active metabolite norfluoxetine has a half-life of 7 to 9 days. Due to the half-life, a washout period is needed when coadministering a drug that has MAOI-like potential like Linezolid. Although not an absolute contraindication, clinicians should be aware of this.
Sertraline	Approved by FDA for treatment of obsessive-compulsive disorder in children	Inhibition of CNS neuronal uptake of serotonin (5HT)	Sertraline is metabolized by multiple cytochrome 450 isoforms: CYP2D6, CYP2C9, CYP2B6, CYP2C19 and CYP3A4.	Sertraline is a moderate inhibitor of CYP2D6 and CYP2B6 in vitro. It can cause increased blood levels of CYP2D6 substrates such as metoprolol, dextromethorphan, desipramine, imipramine and nortriptyline, as well as the CYP3A4/CYP2D6 substrate haloperidol. Like fluoxetine, interaction between sertraline and the MAOIs isocarboxazid and tranylcypromine may cause serotonin syndrome.
Citalopram	No FDA approval for pediatric populations	Potentiation of serotonergic activity in the CNS resulting from its inhibition of CNS neuronal reuptake of serotonin (5-HT)	Metabolized in the liver mostly by CYP2C19, but also by CYP3A4 and CYP2D6	The half-life of citalopram is about 35 hours. Approximately 80% is cleared by the liver and 20% by the kidneys. With once-daily dosing, steady plasma concentrations are achieved in about a week. Potent inhibitors of CYP2C19 and 3A4 might decrease citalopram clearance.

Note: SSRI = selective serotonin reuptake inhibitors; FDA = Food and Drug Administration; TSRD = trauma- and stress-related disorder; MAOI = monoamine oxidase inhibitors; CNS = central nervous system.

1996) as well as an eight-week open-label study of 19 children aged 6 to 18 (Connor et al. 2013). Guanfacine's most common side effects are somnolence, sedation, abdominal pain, dizziness, hypotension/decreased blood pressure, dry mouth, and constipation (Lexicomp, 2017).

Another agent with potential use of treating PTSD symptoms is prazosin, a medication that has received FDA approval for hypertension in adults but no approval in children (Lexicomp, 2017). A systematic review found prazosin has been effective in children to reduce nightmares and improve sleep for children with PTSD. The review's rationale for prazosin's effectiveness is linked to noradrenergic and hypothalamic-pituitary-adrenal (HPA) systems. Evidence suggests PTSD arousal symptoms such as intrusiveness, hyperarousal, and nightmares occur due to changes to the prefrontal cortex area of the brain resulting in increased noradrenergic responsiveness. The prefrontal cortex reduces stress response through projections in the norepinephrine system that inhibit the locus ceruleus from firing. The HPA axis regulates neuroendocrine response to stress. In PTSD, the adrenergic modification following trauma can result in an exaggerated increase in cardiovascular response following intrusion and hyperarousal symptoms. Due to its centrally acting alpha-1 receptor antagonism, prazosin may be effective in reducing this PTSD-linked noradrenergic response. The review of prazosin also noted that it was well tolerated in all six case reports with no reported adverse effect except for weight gain and increased body mass index in a 7-year-old boy after 11 months of therapy. (Akinsanya et al., 2017). The most common side effects of prazosin are dizziness, syncope, orthostatic hypotension, and drowsiness with less common risks of palpitations, lower extremity edema, and urinary incontinence. Prescribers should be aware of environmental allergies with prazosin due to its norepinephrine response reduction that may compromise adequate immune response to pollen (Lexicomp, 2017).

Anticonvulsants

Anticonvulsants may show promise for treating PTSD symptoms other than avoidance (Cohen, 2010), particularly carbamazepine which has demonstrated promise in small open-label studies of children and adolescents with chronic PTSD. However, carbamazepine has potentially serious systemic side effects and toxicity including toxic epidermal necrolysis, Stevens-Johnson syndrome, aplastic anemia, agranulocytosis, thromboembolism, and myocardial infarction which are also contraindications (Center for Drug Evaluation and Research, 2013). In this study, 22 out of 28 children treated with carbamazepine dosed between 300 to 1200 mg per day with serum levels of 10 to 11.5 experienced remission. The remaining six children continued to experience nightmares but felt other PTSD symptoms improved moderately. This study cautioned that there were limitations of carbamazepine's effectiveness in children with comorbid conditions such as depression, ADHD, substance use, or oppositionality. The study results were limited by the fact that the children were on concomitant treatments for other diagnoses and a variety of them took imipramine, fluoxetine, sertraline, clonidine, or methylphenidate, all medications that have demonstrated some efficacy in the treatment of TSRD in children (Loof et al., 1995). Clinicians should be aware carbamazepine has significant interactions as a CYP3A4 substrate and inducer, particularly a very unique auto induction in which the drug can induce itself and lead to elevated drug levels. The pharmacokinctics of this drug arc a major limitation in the use of the drug (Lexicomp, 2017).

Benzodiazepines

Benzodiazepines lack sufficient evidence in reducing the treatment of PTSD symptoms in adults despite their indication to treat severe anxiety. In practice, they are commonly prescribed in children for anxiety symptoms, including those of PTSD and other TSRDs. However, the WHO (2013) and AACAP Guidelines (2010) state they should not be used to treat PTSD in children due to concerns for oversedation, potential for tolerance and addiction, and risk of long-term cognitive slowing (Foa et al. 2008; Cohen, 2010). Adult practice guidelines (e.g., from the Veterans Administration) discourage their use due to animal studies finding that they increase PTSD symptoms. In 2008, Colville and colleagues interviewed 102 consecutive children aged between 7 and 17 years about their pediatric intensive care unit experience three months after their discharge using the ICU Memory Tool (a checklist of intensive care memories) and an abbreviated version of the Impact of Event Scale (a screen for PTSD). This study found delusional memories were reported by almost one-third of children and were associated both with the duration of opiates/benzodiazepines and risk of TSRDs (Colville et al. 2008).

Dopamine Antagonists (Antipsychotics)

Excess dopaminergic activity is thought to have partial involvement in TSRD symptoms, and several antipsychotics have been used in the treatment of PTSD (De Bellis et al., 1999). Children have increased sensitivity to adverse effects such as tardive dyskinesia and caution should be utilized, particularly for traumatized children (Correll et al., 2009; Fraguas et al., 2011). The long-term risk for incident type 2 diabetes mellitus is increased among youths initiating second-generation antipsychotics, particularly in those who use antidepressants concomitantly (Rubin et al., 2015).

In an open trial, 13 out of 18 children with chronic PTSD treated with risperidone experienced symptom remission. However, 85% had comorbid ADHD and 35% had comorbid bipolar disorder, making it difficult to confirm if PTSD symptom remission was a reduction of mood disorder–related symptoms (Horrigan & Horrigan, 1999). Risperidone has a higher incidence of diabetes mellitus compared to other antipsychotics (Rubin et al. 2015). Quetiapine is an atypical antipsychotic that has been used in different psychotic and nonpsychotic disorders in children and adolescents in RCTs, open-label studies and chart reviews. Controlled studies support quetiapine's short-term efficacy in treating psychosis, mania, and aggression, but its long-term efficacy and benefits are not established. Though quetiapine's extrapyramidal and hyperprolactinemia side effects are low compared to risperidone, weight gain, and alterations in lipid changes need to be closely monitored (Masi et al., 2015). In 2005, Stathis and colleagues noted the high volume of PTSD in the youth juvenile justice system and reported case series on six individuals within a youth detention center aged 15 to 17 years. Using the Traumatic Symptom Checklist in Children, the researchers noted that the patients who received quetiapine ranging in dose from 50 to 200 mg per day demonstrated significant improvements in symptoms of depression, anger, and dissociation over six weeks. The patients did not report or exhibit persisting side effects beyond nighttime sedation, which was considered beneficial; however, no metabolic monitoring was performed (Stathis et al. 2005). Second-generation antipsychotics should be used with caution in children and adolescents as they are associated with a high liability to experience cardiometabolic and endocrine side-effects such as QTc prolongation, dystonias, dyskinesias, and arrhythmias weight gain and hyperprolactinemia within a month (De Hert et al., 2011). Though promising, both studies cannot justify an evidence base for the use of antipsychotics in children with TSRDs. Future evaluations of the use of antipsychotics in treatment will require larger studies with blinding in order to form a more robust evidence base for clinical use.

ADJUSTMENT DISORDER

Quantifying the prevalence of AD in child and adolescent populations is difficult, due to changes in the diagnostic criteria over time (Casey, 2014). However, monitoring, treating, and identifying them is crucial in this population as they are at higher risk of developing morbidity and persisting psychiatric illness from a lack of treatment (Steinhausen & Erdin, 1991; Kovacs & Pollock, 1995). Furthermore, numerous studies have identified suicidal behaviors as prominent sequelae of AD in patients of all ages. (Greenberg et al., 1995; Kryzhanovskaya & Canterbury, 2001; Mitrev, 1996; Polyakova et al., 1998). A variety of studies have estimated between one-fifth and one-half of adolescents with diagnoses of AD have attempted suicide or reported suicidal thoughts (Marttunen et al., 1993; Marttunen et al., 1994; Greenberg et al., 1995; Kovacs et al., 1994; Spalletta et al., 1996). In 1998, Goldston and colleagues noted a predominant dysphoric mood in adolescents with AD who had attempted suicide, and in 2003 Gould and colleagues noted "subthreshold" depressive disorders, including AD, were a risk for suicidal behavior. The persistence of depressive mood in AD remains a significant factor in continued suicidal ideation and suicide attempts in adolescents (Spirito et al., 2003), but additional studies also noted the role of psychomotor restlessness and impulsivity as an indicator of externalized anxiety and hyperarousal which were also associated with suicidality in AD (Ohring et al., 1995; Stein et al., 1998). These characteristics were also associated with suicidal adult patients (Kryzhanovskaya et al., 2001). These findings suggest not only significance in assessing the wide spectrum of AD symptoms of intolerable negative affect arousal such as anger, irritability, impulsivity, and dysphoria, (Pelkonen et al., 2005) but to consider the role of psychopharmacology in addressing mortality from suicide due to significant valence of pathophysiological emotions.

A review of the literature yielded no psychopharmacological interventions or guidance for children and adolescents with AD, but given existing studies demonstrating promise of the reduction of hyperarousal, irritability, and impulsivity with adrenergic agents, future research should consider a physiological treatment of these symptoms of youth AD in order to prevent suicide attempts.

ACUTE STRESS DISORDER AND PREVENTIVE PSYCHOPHARMACOLOGY FOR TSRD

Though previous studies suggest ASD in children may not develop into PTSD (Kassam-Adams &

Winston, 2004), more recent literature has shown ASD is strongly predictive of PTSD. Meiser-Stedman and colleagues (2017) found ASD at two weeks following a trauma was associated with PTSD at week 9 though about 30% of eventual PTSD cases did not have ASD at week 2, suggesting ASD may not capture all clinically significant traumatic stress in the acute phase and is only moderately sensitive for later PTSD. ASD is a clinically significant, functionally impairing, and distressing condition that may benefit from amelioration of select clinically distressing symptoms, particularly as it can interfere with recovery from other conditions (Sharp et al., 2010). However, a review of ASD treatment emphasizes a role for preventive psychopharmacology in the acute trauma phase rather than treatment once ASD criteria are met (Sijbrandij, 2015).

There are several studies evaluating psychopharmacological treatment of children following acute trauma. In 1988, Famularo and colleagues evaluated four boys and seven girls with a mean age of 8.5 diagnosed with the DSM (third edition) criteria for PTSD. The 11 children received propranolol dosed at 0.8 mg/kg per day three times a day and gradually increased over a two-week period to about 2.5 mg/kg per day. The researchers noted significant reductions in hypervigilance and hyperarousal, though one child experienced excessive sedation and another two had drops in blood pressure and heart rate though no hypotension or bradycardia was noted. Following cessation of the use of propranolol in the setting, some children reported a resurgence of these symptoms which the researchers noted could be attributed to propranolol, but a confounding factor was the ongoing interactions with mental health personnel (Famularo et al., 1988).

Propranolol was revisited in 2010 as a preventive measure for the development of ASD symptoms. In a 2010 study by Nugent and colleagues, 29 injury patients between the ages of 10 and 18 who were determined to be at risk of PTSD were randomized to a double-blind 10-day trial of propranolol or placebo that they received within 12 hours postadmission. Following the hospitalization, trauma symptoms and heart rate were assessed in six weeks. The researchers found girls receiving propranolol reported more PTSD symptoms relative to girls receiving placebo and boys receiving propranolol showed a nonsignificant trend toward fewer PTSD symptoms than boys receiving placebo (Nugent et al. 2010). Given the report of propranolol's potential benefit with PTSD in children, Sharp and colleagues (2010) evaluated its potential for ASD. They hypothesized that individuals who were administered propranolol acutely would be less likely to develop ASD than those who were not. The researchers evaluated 363 pediatric burn patients (232 boys, 131 girls) of which 22 had previously been diagnosed and treated for ASD and 341 were in a non-ASD group in a blinded RCT trial. The study found no statistically significant difference in the development of ASD in children who received propranolol or placebo in the first 30 days of recovery following their trauma (Sharp et al. 2010).

In an investigation early postinjury administration of sertraline to prevent PTSD symptoms, Stoddard and colleagues (2011) assessed 26 children aged 6 to 20 in a 24-week double-blind, placebo-controlled design in a pediatric burn center, where they received between 25 and 150 mg of sertraline a day or placebo. The final sample included 17 participants assigned to the treatment group and 9 participants assigned to the control group who were evaluated 24 weeks after the initiation of medication. Though the placebo group had a significant decrease in depressive and PTSD symptoms compared to the baseline, their original depressive symptom scores were higher. On the other hand, parent-rated child PTSD symptoms were reduced in the sertraline group compared to the placebo group (Stoddard et al., 2011). Since it was not a treatment study, this RCT to prevent PTSD cannot be compared to the TF-CBT and sertraline treatment study. The study did not prove potential benefit from the early use of sertraline for postinjury prevention of PTSD symptoms in children, although a subgroup may benefit.

Robert and colleagues (1999) conducted a RCT that found imipramine, a TCA, was superior to chloral hydrate, a sedative, in reducing symptoms of ASD in 2- to 19-year-old acute care burn unit patients six months later. Concerns about imipramine causing potentially serious cardiac conduction delays prevent the widespread use of this medication on an outpatient basis, and it is not recommended as a first-line treatment for PTSD in children (Robert et al., 1999).

Two studies of propranolol in acute stages of trauma indicate it is not helpful in preventing the development of trauma-related symptoms which conflates its usage in active PTSD where it has been found to reduce hyperarousal symptoms. The equivocal outcomes of the preliminary antidepressant studies suggests prevention of ASD in youths may not require an adrenergic focus but would benefit from further evaluation of serotonergic systems in the prevention of developing ASD.

PSYCHOPHARMACOLOGICAL CONSIDERATIONS FOR THE TREATMENT OF CHILDREN WITH TSRDS

A summary of the current medications used in the psychopharmacological treatment of TSRDs in children and adolescents can be found in Table 23.2. It is important to note that none of the medications have undergone appropriate evaluations that would allow them to be first-line recommendations for TSRDs; however, the benefit they have demonstrated in small studies could be extrapolated for future cases where significant psychosocial intervention and therapeutic treatments have not alleviated suffering or functional impairment. The quality of evidence was determined utilizing standard criteria from the GRADE system with most studies scoring a B for moderate quality or C for low quality. Data determined to have moderate quality implies further research is likely to have an important impact on our confidence in the estimate of effect and may change the estimate. Low-quality data requires a significantly increased number of high-quality studies and research in order to impact clinical practices and current knowledge (Guyatt et al., 2008).

CASE 1: 11-YEAR-OLD

FJ is an 11-year-old boy with a diagnosis of PTSD and ADHD. He had a full-term birth with no developmental issues but he was raised in a home with parents who had a history of drug abuse, incarceration, and violence. His mother was incarcerated for most of his life, but he would see her periodically. Their specific diagnoses were unknown. FJ denied ever experiencing physical, emotional, or sexual abuse from his parents, recounting their time together fondly despite other family members expressing concern to him that he may have been neglected.

FJ was 5 years old when his father overdosed and passed away. FJ and his brother wandered the streets of a nearby city for several days looking for help as he was wondering why his father would not wake up. A police officer found FJ and his brother and as no relatives could be identified he was placed in foster care for a month. He was placed in his grandmother's custody after she returned from an out-of-town trip. When interviewed as a 10-year-old, FJ denies ever feeling his life was in danger and continues to note he wondered why his father was sleeping so much.

FJ's grandmother noted after he was placed with her that he had become physically aggressive toward family and peers, wake up frequently from sleep due to nightmares of his grandmother dying, and cry immediately if left alone in a room without an adult. He also had ongoing difficulty sitting still and completing tasks and would often speak out of turn.

FJ would often refer to himself as a "bad kid," particularly following a fight with his grandmother or siblings. After four years of play therapy moderately improved his ability to remain in a room alone and connect with peers, his escalating aggression and poor school performance prompted his grandmother to seek a medication evaluation when he was 10 years old.

At this visit FJ's symptoms were felt to be consistent with ADHD, as well as PTSD related to his father's overdose. He was prescribed guanfacine 1 mg for treatment of his inattention and impulsivity as a first-line psychotropic. His grandmother noted it seemed to reduce the intensity and frequency of his rage episodes when provoked but felt it continued to impair his function and the sense of safety in his household. After the medication was increased to 2 mg for one month, his grandmother did not notice any improvement in his aggression or impact on his nightmares. Due to concern for the severity of his aggression, he was started on risperidone 0.25 mg at bedtime that was gradually titrated to 0.25 mg twice a day after one month and 0.5 mg twice a day at two months. His grandmother reported a dramatic difference with the addition of risperidone, stating he did not attempt to hit when agitated and while he would become annoyed during disagreements, he no longer screamed or threatened.

FJ began TF-CBT after he was moderately stabilized on medications. He and his grandmother reported a reduction in nightmares as well as an improved sense of self. He began relating better to classmates and making friends, and he developed an interest in his coursework.

Comment: This case illustrates a child with who required treatment of TSRD symptoms as well as ADHD. This case is notable for its use of an antipsychotic shortly after initiation of guanfacine, a common though ill-advised scenario due to the high side effect burden. While his symptoms did reduce with risperidone, given the patient's age and existing diagnosis of ADHD, ideally the dose of guanfacine would have been increased before switching to or adding a different adrenergic agent such as clonidine or prazosin. A stimulant such as methylphenidate or amphetamine

TABLE 23.2. SUMMARY OF MEDICATIONS EVALUATED FOR TREATMENT OF TSRD IN CHILDREN AND ADOLESCENTS

Medication	Dose Studied	Grading of Recommendations Assessment, Development and Evaluation	Mechanism of Action	Side Effects	Outcome in TSRD Studies
			SSRIs		
Citalopram	20 to 40 mg per day	C	Potentiation of serotonergic activity in the CNS resulting from its inhibition of CNS neuronal reuptake of serotonin (5-HT)	Gastrointestinal symptoms, anorgasmia, sedation, insomnia, increased lacrimation or urination, appetite changes FDA Black box warning for suicidality in adolescents.	Improved PTSD symptoms
Fluoxetine	20 or 40 mg per day	B	Inhibits the serotonin transporter protein and is a weak norepinephrine reuptake inhibitor (effect increases with higher doses). Also an antagonist at 5HT2C receptors.	Gastrointestinal symptoms, anorgasmia, sedation, insomnia, increased lacrimation or urination, increased appetite, worsening anxiety, palpitations. FDA Black box warning for suicidality in adolescents.	Reduction of PTSD symptoms following exposure to earthquake
Sertraline	50 to 150 mg per day	C	Inhibition of CNS neuronal uptake of serotonin (5HT)	Gastrointestinal symptoms, anorgasmia, sedation, insomnia, increased lacrimation or urination, increased appetite, worsening anxiety, palpitations, tremors FDA Black box warning for suicidality in adolescents.	No effect on prevention of ASD in pediatric burn patients. There was a lack of benefit beyond TF-CBT for PTSD.

(*continued*)

TABLE 23.2. CONTINUED

Medication	Dose Studied	Grading of Recommendations Assessment, Development and Evaluation	Mechanism of Action	Side Effects	Outcome in TSRD Studies
			Non-SSRI Antidepressants		
Imipramine	1 mg per kg; max dose of 100 mg	C	Inhibition of neuronal reuptake of norepinephrine and serotonin by binding the sodium-dependent serotonin transporter and sodium-dependent norepinephrine transporter. Also causes down-regulation of cerebral cortical beta-adrenergic receptors and sensitization of post-synaptic serotonergic receptors with chronic use. This leads to enhanced serotonergic transmission.	Dry mouth, blurred vision, headache, drowsiness, dizziness, constipation, nausea, vomiting, loss of appetite, diarrhea, stomach cramps, weight gain/loss, and increased sweating. Serious concern of cardiac conduction delay	Reduction of PTSD symptoms in pediatric burn patients compared to chloral hydrate which could maintain or worsen symptoms
Nefazodone	200 mg BID to 600 mg per day	C	Occupies central 5-HT2 receptors at nanomolar concentrations, and acts as an antagonist at this receptor. Antagonizes alpha1-adrenergic receptors, a property which may be associated with postural hypotension	Somnolence, nausea, postural hypotension, and vomiting at higher doses.	Reduction in anger, aggression, restlessness, insomnia, and improved concentration
			Anti-Adrenergic Agents		
Propranolol	0.8 mg/kg to 2.5 mg/kg	C	Blocks the action of epinephrine (adrenaline) and norepinephrine (noradrenaline) at both β1- and β2-adrenergic receptors.	Mucoid cough in children, anxiety, dry mouth, hyperventilation, hypotension, irritability, restlessness, oversedation, unusual dreams, insomnia	Reduction in hyperarousal in active PTSD but no preventive benefit for ASD

Prazosin	1 to 4 mg per day	B	Selective alpha 1-adrenergic blocking agent that produces vasodilation and reduces peripheral resistance but generally has little effect on cardiac output.	Drowsiness, dry mouth, dizziness, hypotension	Reduction in nightmares, intrusive thoughts, and hyperarousal
Guanfacine	1 to 4 mg	C	Centrally acting selective alpha-2 adrenergic agonist.	Drowsiness, dizziness, constipation, fatigue, nausea, headache, weight gain, irritability, hallucinations	Reduction in intrusive symptoms
Clonidine	0.05 to 0.2 mg per day	B	Centrally acting selective alpha-2 adrenergic agonist with specificity towards the presynaptic α2 receptors in the vasomotor center in the brainstem.	Drowsiness, dizziness, constipation, diarrhea, fatigue, nausea, impotence, insomnia, nightmares, fever, impotence, anorgasmia	Reduction in anxiety, arousal, insomnia, and impulsive and aggressive behavior
			Anti-Histaminic Agents		
Cyproheptadine	4 to 12 mg	C	SERT, NET, serotonin, muscarinic, dopaminergic, and histaminic antagonist	Drowsiness, dizziness, blurred vision, constipation, diarrhea, nausea, weight gain, lacrimation, increased urination, dry mouth or throat, hallucinations, tremor, arrhythmia	Reduction in intrusive symptoms
			Dopamine Antagonists (Antipsychotics)		
Risperidone	0.5 mg to 2 mg	C	D2, 5HT2A, alpha-1, alpha-2, and H1 antagonist	Drowsiness, dizziness, blurred vision, constipation, diarrhea, nausea, weight gain, akathisia, dyskinesia, parkinsonism, hyperprolactinemia	Reduction in intrusive thoughts and hyperarousal

(*continued*)

TABLE 23.2. CONTINUED

Medication	Dose Studied	Grading of Recommendations Assessment, Development and Evaluation	Mechanism of Action	Side Effects	Outcome in TSRD Studies
Quetiapine	50 mg to 200 mg	C	5HT2A and D2 antagonism, 5HT1A partial agonism, alpha-1 and H1 antagonism	Asthenia, constipation, dizziness, drowsiness, headache, sedation, increased serum cholesterol, increased serum triglycerides, increased thyroid stimulating hormone level, and xerostomia.	Reduction in anxiety, depression, and anger
			Anticonvulsants		
Carbamazepine	300 to 1200 mg per day	C	Use-dependant blocker of voltage-gated sodium channel and GABA receptor agonist	Toxic epidermal necrolysis, Stevens-Johnson syndrome, aplastic anemia, agranulocytosis, thromboembolism, and myocardial infarction	Reduction in hyperarousal, anxiety, and insomnia but no change in nightmares

Note: TSRD = trauma- and stress-related disorder; CNS = central nervous system; FDA = Food and Drug Administration; PTSD = posttraumatic stress disorder; ASD = acute stress disorder; TF-CBT = trauma-focused cognitive-behavioral therapy; SERT = NET =

TABLE 23.3. COMMON INTERACTIONS OF PSYCHOTROPIC MEDICATIONS USED IN THE TREATMENT OF TSRDS

Medications	SSRIs	TCAs	Alpha Agonist	Beta Blocker	Anti-Histaminergic	Antipsychotics	Anticonvulsants
SSRIs	Risk of serotonin syndrome with combined SSRIs	Increased plasma concentrations of TCA causing increased adverse effects. Serotonin syndrome possible, especially with clomipramine		Increased beta-blocking effects, Bradycardia with propranolol by affecting 2D6	Fluoxetine and sertraline increases and cyproheptadine decreases serotonin levels. Cyproheptadine decreases effects of citalopram by pharmacodynamic antagonism	SSRIs can increase the level or effect of risperidone or quetiapine by affecting hepatic enzyme CYP2D6 metabolism and may affect QTc interval.	Increased plasma concentrations of carbamazepine and phenytoin with fluoxetine and sertraline. Carbamazepine decreases levels of citalopram by affecting hepatic/intestinal enzyme CYP3A4 metabolism.
TCAs	Increased plasma concentrations of TCA causing increased adverse effects. Serotonin syndrome possible, especially with clomipramine	Polypharmacy may result in toxicity	Antihypertensive effects of alpha agonists are reduced or abolished		Imipramine increases and cyproheptadine decreases serotonin levels. Both may cause oversedation.	Increased sedation, additive anticholinergic effects Plasma concentrations of phenothiazines and/or the TCA may be increased	TCA levels are generally reduced with induction of antiepileptic drugs (i.e., carbamazepine, phenytoin, phenobarbital, and primidone). Valproic acid inhibits TCA metabolism and, therefore, may increase TCA serum levels.
Alpha Agonist		Antihypertensive effects of alpha agonists are reduced or abolished		Non selective beta blocker administration during withdrawal from centrally acting alpha agonists may result in rebound hypertension.		Additive hypotensive effects of clonidine and risperidone which may cause potential delirium.	Carbamazepine will decrease the level or effect of guanfacine by affecting hepatic/intestinal enzyme CYP3A4 metabolism
Beta Blocker	Increased beta-blocking effects, Bradycardia with propranolol by affecting 2D6		Non selective beta blocker administration during withdrawal from centrally acting alpha agonists may result in rebound hypertension				

(continued)

TABLE 23.3. CONTINUED

Medications	SSRIs	TCAs	Alpha Agonist	Beta Blocker	Anti-Histaminergic	Antipsychotics	Anticonvulsants
Anti-Histaminergic	Fluoxetine and sertraline increases and cyproheptadine decreases serotonin levels. Cyproheptadine decreases effects of citalopram by pharmacodynamic antagonism	Imipramine increases and cyproheptadine decreases serotonin levels. Both may cause oversedation.				Cyproheptadine and risperidone or quetiapine both increase sedation	
Antipsychotic	SSRIs can increase the level or effect of risperidone or quetiapine by affecting hepatic enzyme CYP2D6 metabolism and may affect QTc interval.	Increased sedation, additive anticholinergic effects Plasma concentrations of phenothiazines and/or the TCA may be increased	Additive hypotensive effects of clondine and risperidone which may cause potential delirium.		Cyproheptadine and risperidone or quetiapine both increase sedation	Together, quetiapine and risperidone both increase sedation, QTc, and antidopaminergic effects, including extrapyramidal symptoms and neuroleptic malignant syndrome.	Carbamazepine decreases levels of risperidone by increasing metabolism. Carbamazepine will decrease the level or effect of quetiapine by affecting hepatic/ intestinal enzyme CYP3A4 metabolism while quetiapine may increase the level or effect of carbamazepine by decreasing metabolism.
Anticonvulsant	Increased plasma concentrations of carbamazepine and phenytoin with fluoxetine and sertraline. Carbamazepine decreases levels of citalopram by affecting hepatic/ intestinal enzyme CYP3A4 metabolism.	TCA levels are generally reduced with induction of carbamazepine	Carbamazepine will decrease the level or effect of guanfacine by affecting hepatic/ intestinal enzyme CYP3A4 metabolism			Carbamazepine decreases levels of risperidone by increasing metabolism. Carbamazepine will decrease the level or effect of quetiapine by affecting hepatic/intestinal enzyme CYP3A4 metabolism while quetiapine may increase the level or effect of carbamazepine by decreasing metabolism.	

Note: TSRD = trauma- and stress-related disorder; SSRI = selective serotonin reuptake inhibitors; TCA = tricyclic antidepressants.

would have also been a reasonable intervention to address the hyperactivity. In an ideal scenario, prior to any medication intervention, the patient's PTSD would have been identified sooner and he would have been enrolled in TF-CBT immediately. Clinicians should retain a high index of suspicion for PTSD when evaluating a child with agitation, aggression, and sleep difficulties.

It is notable that many practitioners may recommend these medications in conjunction but should be aware of potential interactions illustrated in Table 23.2. While many interactions noted in the table have been established (Janicak et al., 2010), a particularly notable interaction and long-term effect is the interaction between SSRIs and stimulants. Steiner and colleagues (2014) found youths who receive a stimulant such as methylphenidate along with SSRIs have significant gene regulations resulting in neuroadaptations in the dopamine pathways and their projection targets, particularly the nucleus accumbens, ventral tegmental area, and striatum. These changes mimic long-term effects of drugs such as cocaine which presents as dysregulated mood and motivation enduring into adulthood (Steiner et al. 2014).

SPECIAL POPULATIONS

Preschool

Symptoms of TSRD can be present in children as young as 3 years old, but there is less empirical evidence validating and characterizing presentations or treatment in this group (Scheeringa et al., 2001; Scheeringa et al., 2004; Scheeringa et al., 2005). Play therapy and psychosocial interventions are indicated prior to the initiation of psychopharmacologic treatments (Luby, 2013). The Preschool Psychopharmacology Working Group, developed to review existing literature on psychopharmacology use in preschoolers, notes significant biological, practice, and research limitations to creating evidence-based psychopharmacological recommendations for treatment of any preschoolers with psychiatric illness (Gleason et al., 2007). There are almost no controlled studies to guide the use of very early medication interventions in traumatized children (Cohen, 2008). Apart from a study of school-aged children with burn-related PTSD in acute care finding that adequate pain management with morphine reduces long-term symptoms of PTSD (Saxe et al., 2001), there are only case reports on alternative medications for preschool children. One case report investigated the tolerability and efficacy of fluoxetine in preschool-age children with anxiety disorders which included TSRD prior to the DSM-5 reclassification. One study used a retrospective chart review to investigate fluoxetine for the treatment of preschool anxiety and depressive disorders (Zuckerman et al., 2007) and noted behavioral activation concerns that were similar to those previously noted in children aged 6 to 17. The significant differences in neurotransmitter symptoms targeted by SSRIs as well as metabolic differences in preschool children are thought to be responsible for higher rates of adverse events in this group (Wagner et al., 2004). Based on the high risk-to-benefit ratio as well as the lack of controlled testing of the efficacy and safety of medication in preschoolers, there is no adequate evidence base for a psychopharmacological recommendation to treat preschoolers.

CASE 2: FOUR-YEAR-OLD

SD is a 4-year-old girl who was brought to clinic as she had difficulty sitting still, would often impulsively run around the room, had difficulty completing tasks such as coloring or while at play, and eventually began bumping her head into different objects due to her inability to sit still.

SD was born full term and met all developmental milestones on time. She was raised by both her parents who described her as energetic but did not note the behavioral problems until she was in nursery school. SD's medical history was significant for a month-long hospitalization as an infant due to smoke inhalation when her father's house and car were set on fire by gangs in the area. Her parents report staying with her during the hospitalization and denied seeing any irritability, aggression, or significant behavioral changes following this experience. On further evaluation, SD's mother revealed her own trauma history from sexual abuse but stated her symptoms were well controlled following a trial of medication with therapy.

When SD began school, she initially made friends, but they would quickly exclude her as she would rapidly get angry when she felt games did not go the way she wanted them to. Her parents noted she began sleeping less at night, and she told them about different frightening monsters, people, or images but they had no reason to believe she had been abused in any way. She was diagnosed with ADHD and started on dextroamphetamine 2.5 mg which her parents noted appeared to give her more energy and palpitations; she was later switched to methylphenidate 2.5 mg which appeared to help her sit still longer though she continued to struggle with impulsivity and poor sleep.

Eventually, she was started on clonidine 0.1 mg at bedtime. Her parents noted her nightmares reduced significantly and she was able to sleep through the night. She also began waiting her turn to speak and was able to relate with her peers in a more developmentally appropriate manner. After several weeks of gradual improvement, she had an intense crying tantrum in school at which point it appeared her symptoms had recurred since she began running around the classroom and banging into things. Collateral information from her teacher revealed her symptoms appeared shortly after she smelled burnt lunch from the school cafeteria's kitchen. While she did not meet full criteria for a TSRD, given the extent of her hyperreactivity and history of significant hospitalization, she was referred for psychotherapy and her clonidine was increased to 0.2 mg at bedtime. At one-month follow-up, she continued to sustain therapeutic gains and had improved behavioral and emotional control.

Comment: As seen in many preschool-aged children, the patient in this case did not meet full criteria for a TSRD. Clonidine served a dual purpose in managing her hyperreactivity as well as her overlapping ADHD symptoms, though she would have benefitted from a therapy referral from the outset. As in all comprehensive treatment plans for TSRDs in this age group, psychopharmacological interventions are adjunctive to psychotherapy.

Reactive Attachment Disorder and Disinhibited Social Engagement Disorder (see also Chapter 2)

It is important to acknowledge the varied presentation of TSRD in children to include RAD and DSED (Zeanah et al., 2015; Goldbeck & Jensen, 2017) Though linked to similar neurochemical processes as traditional TSRDs such as PTSD or ASD through the HPA axis (Corbin, 2007), RAD and DSED differ in primary symptomatic presentations related to intrusive thoughts, hyperarousal, sleep difficulties, or significant anger or anxiety symptoms (American Psychiatric Association, 2013). The AACAP reports no recommended psychopharmacological treatments for RAD or DSED, noting limitations in data on short-term and long-term effects on children making it difficult to recommend an appropriate medication regimen, particularly in preschool-aged children (Zeanah et al., 2016). A 2010 paper reported two cases of sertraline use in RAD improving irritability and depressive symptoms as early childhood maltreatment alters development corticolimbic circuits and serotonenergic they did not feel the behavioral and attachment issues were specifically addressed by SSRIs (Weinberg, 2010).

PRESCRIBING TO CHILDREN INVOLVED IN THE WELFARE SYSTEM

Parents or guardians of children and adolescents must be closely involved in prescribing medication to a child, particularly as they provide consent and are instrumental in ensuring adherence and follow-up appointments. Understanding the authority that consents for children is particularly important for children in the welfare system who are more likely to have experienced forms of abuse, neglect, and trauma. As there is no FDA approval for medications in the treatment of childhood TSRD, correct consent and assent is critical in all pediatric populations. Clinicians should be aware that parents, child welfare agencies, courts, or another state-supported agencies with expertise in mental health treatment and psychopharmacology may be sources of consent. However, after becoming familiar with local laws and standards of children in the welfare system and prior to prescribing, the clinician should obtain youth assent by discussing assessment findings, the role of medication in the treatment of symptoms along with possible side effects, and alternative treatment options. It is particularly important to prioritize the youth, regardless of their ability to consent, as children and adolescents in the welfare system experience limited decision-making ability or control in welfare decisions. Involving all children in the medication-prescribing decision enhances treatment engagement and adherence. For children and adolescents with agitation or aggression as major presenting symptoms of their TSRD, authority agencies, parents, or guardians may emergently request psychiatric medications, but clinicians are encouraged to elicit sufficient information to support psychiatric evaluation and treatment planning. Psychotropics are appropriate for youths who have appropriate levels of structure, supervision, and stability that are integrated with psychosocial interventions as unsupervised prescribing may lead to polypharmacy. In transient welfare placements, foster parents or kinship caregivers might be less likely to participate in parent skills training which makes prescribing less of a priority than advancing psychosocial treatments (Lee et al., 2015).

CASE 3: 16-YEAR-OLD

KR is a 16-year-old male with a history of severe major depressive disorder, generalized anxiety disorder, predominantly inattentive type ADHD, and PTSD. His mother had recently regained custody of him following foster placement at the age of 5 after she had been found to physically harm him numerous times as a child when she was intoxicated on drugs and alcohol. She had maintained sobriety for one year at which point she regained custody of KR when he was 15.

KR had been in numerous foster home systems in different districts which often resulted in frequently changing schools. He had frequent detentions for incomplete homework and suspensions for fighting. He had a loosely affiliated peer group in each school placement and noted most of his friendships centered around drug use. His foster parents would complain about his daily cannabis use starting at age 12, and frequent arguments often resulted in him leaving foster homes. He refused to attend therapy regularly but did connect briefly with a psychiatric rehabilitation worker who helped him with homework and social connectedness.

After moving in with his mother, she noted he often appeared paranoid that he was being watched. She was concerned his cannabis use was causing him to be paranoid, anxious, and restless, but collateral from his caseworker indicated he had demonstrated these symptoms since he was placed in foster care. KR reported he felt safe with his mother and while he did recall some abuse from her, he attributed this to his mother's own struggle with drugs and alcohol. He felt happier he was able to live in a home with his mother as opposed to frequently moving. He reported his anxiety was largely due to learning gangs were in the area and being afraid of attack. He reported restless sleep with nightmares that he could not recall the following day. His mother noticed he continued to have detention for incomplete school work but since he moved in with her, he had been fighting less with peers and more with her over school work and chores. KR's mother did not feel he avoided her or have a particular trigger for his anxiety, anger, or irritability.

Though he was in his mother's custody, KR continued to have access to social services. He agreed to try group therapy to reduce his cannabis use and was able to taper his smoking to once a week. Despite his reduction in use, his irritability, low mood, anxiety, sleep difficulties, and difficulties with focus continued to interfere with his academic and social functioning. He was prescribed fluoxetine 10 mg which was titrated to 20 mg after one month due to its FDA approval for major depressive disorder. KR reported improvement in mood and feeling more energetic initially but continued to struggle with nightmares. Prazosin 1 mg was added to his regimen, and he noted restful sleep. After several months of trauma-focused therapy along with his existing medication regimen, KR continued to demonstrate some residual paranoia and suspicion of strangers but his focus improved, allowing him to complete school assignments. He no longer fought peers and he had less frequent arguments with his mother.

Comment: This case discusses a common presentation in the foster system where children with TSRDs and other mental health conditions may experience symptoms for several years. They are also at risk for substance use, but complete sobriety is not necessary prior to initiating treatment. The adolescent in this case did have some benefit from social services improving service access once he was able to remain in the same location for a sustained period of time.

PRESCRIBING TO REFUGEE CHILDREN AND ADOLESCENTS

Given the necessity for structure and family involvement in children associated with the welfare system, clinicians should execute the same caution and consideration when treating refugee children who experience and demonstrate symptoms of trauma in a shifting sociocultural framework (Weine, 2011). The United Nations estimates there are over 244 million people living outside of their country of origin (United Nations Population Fund, 2016). The United Nations High Commissioner for Refugees (UNHCR) estimated over 1 million refugees of all ages fleeing to Europe by boat during the year 2015 (UNHCR, 2016) due to war and violence (Turner, 2015). By the very nature of a traumatic and forced migration, refugee communities are at risk for depression, anxiety, and PTSD (Lindert et al. 2009) during three key phases: premigration, transit, and postmigration (Zimmerman et al., 2011). Children and adolescents exposed to trauma in this continuum benefit from cultur ally considerate psychotherapeutic treatment interventions to assist them with acculturation, but this process requires ongoing research (Hall & Olff, 2016). Though health systems vary between nations, the cultural barriers for refugees accessing and adhering to care are ubiquitous. A study in South Australia, a region that resettled 151,134 refugees between 2004 and 2014, found refugee youths are more likely to demonstrate comorbid mental health and substance abuse issues but had reduced access to care. A qualitative evaluation and survey of 15 refugee youth and 15 service providers revealed the most commonly reported barriers for refugee care related to four major areas: (a) organizational and structural, (b) access and engagement, (c) treatment and service delivery, and (d) training and resources (Colucci et al., 2015). A 2015 meta-analysis of refugee care issues by Bellamy and colleagues of refugee care in the United Kingdom, the United States, and Australia noted specific cultural barriers to care including paucity of interpreters; understanding the Western health care system; cultural beliefs about illness; the use of traditional medicine; the need for community, family, and peer support; and medication nonadherence. The authors recommended prioritization of appropriate interpreter and translation services to assist in a prescriber's cross-cultural communication with a patient in order to increase access and adherence (Bellamy et al., 2015). Slobodin and DeJong (2015) also stressed the importance of family interventions for traumatized immigrants and refugees. Their systematic reviews of treatment of traumatized families found school-based and multifamily interventions had some effect but they lack structured outcome measures to validate their effectiveness in this population (Slobodin et al., 2015). Psychopharmacological treatment may be indicated for refugee children with comorbid psychiatric conditions, but there are no medication trials for this population to date. Canadian guidelines on refugee child care specifically discourage the use of psychotropics due to pervasive lack of evidence base treatment and the need for culturally sensitive interventions prior to other types of treatment (Rousseau et al., 2012). Research in the UK has shown that refugee children are more frequently referred by nonmedical sources and that children who receive services that are culturally and linguistically adapted are no more likely to drop out of treatment than host-country youth (Howard & Hodes, 2000).

Refugee children display resilience which aids in their recovery though there continues to be limited research on effective treatment interventions for them. Refugee children benefit through a multitiered and culturally accessible approach of care for their families that provide broad screening and preventive treatments for PTSD and specialized therapeutic interventions for significantly functionally impaired youth. Refugee care continues to be a growing field requiring a strong evidence base of effective interventions that can treat the psychological sequelae of violence, displacement, migration, and transitions (Pacione et al., 2013).

FUTURE PSYCHOPHARMACOLOGICAL CONSIDERATIONS

Existing psychopharmacological trials for TSRD in children and adolescents has focused on interventions from antipsychotics, anticonvulsants, antidepressants, and antiadrenergic medications. Though dopaminergic, serotonergic, and adrenergic systems are established aspects of the development of TSRDs, the HPA axis is implicated as well. This creates potential use for corticotrophin release factor antagonists (Cohen, 2010).

Additionally, though ADHD is often mistakenly given as a diagnosis for children with PTSD, there is potential for the assistance of stimulant medication in children struggling with PTSD and postconcussive symptoms. Stimulants are the most frequently prescribed psychoactive medications to children as they are considered relatively safe, though they pose risks for cardiac arrhythmia, transient growth slowing, and bone mineral density reduction (Hennissen et al., 2017, Poulton et al., 2016). Child and adult studies have found psychostimulants as opiate adjuvants in treating children with mood disorders reduced somnolence in palliative care settings. Despite caution about cardiovascular side effects, they are often well tolerated and have an advantage of rapid onset unlike SSRIs. Immediate-release methylphenidate is commonly used in children because of its rapid onset and short half-life (Stoddard et al., 2006).

Ketamine, an N-methyl-d-aspartate receptor antagonist, produces transient dissociative and psychotic states in healthy humans that resemble symptoms shown by subjects with acute and chronic PTSD. Since ketamine is widely used as an analgesic and sedative, it was once thought of as a factor-triggering, modulating, or exacerbating acute phase trauma for accident victims as they noted retrospective symptoms of trauma following ketamine use with surgery (Schönenberg et al., 2005). This perception has since changed as ketamine has been evaluated in adults for treatment of PTSD and can be a consideration for future research in children and adolescents. A 2008 study by McGhee and colleagues of 119 patients who received ketamine during surgery and 28 who did not found the prevalence of PTSD was 27% in the group who received ketamine versus 46% who did not. In 2014, Feder and colleagues compared intravenous ketamine (0.5 mg/kg) to midazolam (0.045 mg/kg) in treatment of chronic PTSD in adults, finding ketamine resulting in a rapid reduction in PTSD symptom severity 24 hours after infusion. While ketamine has not been studied for TSRDs in children and adolescent, there are several ongoing trials to evaluate the utility of ketamine in child and adolescent depression. Most recently, Dwyer and colleagues (2017) published a single case report on a 16-year-old with ADHD and depression who failed multiple levels of treatment and medication trial. The adolescent in the case received three infusions of ketamine 0.5 mg/kg over 40 minutes for one week followed by weekly treatments for a month that resulted in significant reduction of rated symptoms in the Montgomery–Åsberg Depression Rating Scale, Children's Depression Rating Scale, Beck Hopelessness Scale, and Scale for Suicidal Ideation. Following a residential stay during the early phases of recovery, the patient returned home and attended school full-time. While no adverse events were reported in this case report, the authors cautioned prolonged ketamine infusions due to high risk of adverse neurocognitive effects (Dwyer et al., 2017).

As evidenced by the differences in trials, symptom severity is a significant factor in the decision-making for whether or not a medication is truly effective. Multiple raters such as patient, therapist, and family member are advised for a more comprehensive assessment of symptom remission (Keeshin & Strawn, 2014). Presently, there is scant evidence to guide psychopharmacological treatment of children with TSRDS. Given the variety of symptomatology in childhood TSRDs, the rating scales, comorbid conditions, and importance of psychosocial supports, future areas of research in psychopharmacology for TSRDS may benefit from a focus on medication responsiveness to symptoms after controlling for comorbid conditions and ensuring first-line psychotherapeutic treatment modalities are in place.

CONCLUSIONS

All psychopharmacological interventions discussed in this chapter require ongoing long-term efficacy and RCT research to be considered appropriate evidence-based adjunct treatments for children with TSRD. Even with barriers to creating RCTs, there is potential for prospective or case control studies of psychopharmacological interventions of PTSD through the commonplace use of electronic medical records. This will allow for monitoring of treatment and response to increase the practical empiric evidence base, including efficacy and safety (March et al., 2004). Such child and adolescent psychopharmacological studies are an urgent priority in order to provide evidence-based treatment options which are sorely needed for pediatric PTSD.

Psychotherapeutic interventions remain the first-line treatment for TSRD in children and adolescents. However, existing psychopharmacological interventions have some promise in acute management following trauma exposure through pain management (e.g., early opiates for injured children) and reduction of physiologic hyperarousal with adrenergic agents such as prazosin, clonidine, guanfacine, or propranolol. Pharmacological agents for TSRD in children and adolescents have received little empirical investigation that allow them to be used as first-line interventions or monotherapy rather than psychotherapeutic interventions, although sertraline, fluoxetine, and citalopram could be considered as second-line interventions. Regardless, comorbidities of TSRDs such as ADHD, generalized anxiety disorder, bipolar disorder, and major depressive disorder may warrant pharmacological treatment to improve outcomes related to all conditions. Psychopharmacological agents that can be confidently recommended for TSRD should not only improve the quality of life of the child but also prove to target disabling symptoms and allow children to tolerate the emotionally distressing material as a way to enhance psychotherapeutic experiences (Donnelly et al., 2002).

REFERENCES

Akinsanya, A., Marwaha, R., & Tampi, R. R. (2017). Prazosin in children and adolescents with posttraumatic stress disorder who have nightmares: A systematic review. *Journal of Clinical Psychopharmacology*, *37*(1), 84–88.

American Psychiatric Association. (2013). *Diagnostic and statistical manual of mental disorders* (5th ed.). Washington, DC: American Psychiatric Association.

Bellamy, K., Ostini, R., Martini, N., & Kairuz, T. (2015). Access to medication and pharmacy services for resettled refugees: A systematic review. *Australian Journal of Primary Health*, *21*(3), 273–278.

Birmaher, B., Ryan, N. D., Williamson, D. E., Brent, D. A., & Kaufman, J. (1996). Childhood and adolescent depression: A review of the past 10 years. Part II. *Journal of the American Academy of Child & Adolescent Psychiatry*, *35*(12), 1575–1583.

Brent, D. A., & Gibbons, R. (2014). Initial dose of antidepressant and suicidal behavior in youth: Start low, go slow. *JAMA Internal Medicine, 174*(6), 909–911.

Briere, R. (2001). *Crossing the quality chasm*. Washington, DC: Institute of Medicine.

Bushnell, G. A., Stürmer, T., Swanson, S. A., White, A., Azrael, D., Pate, V., & Miller, M. (2015). Dosing of selective serotonin reuptake inhibitors among children and adults before and after the FDA black-box warning. *Psychiatric Services, 67*(3), 302–309.

Casey, P. (2014). Adjustment disorder: New developments. *Current Psychiatry Reports, 16*(6), 1–8.

Center for Drug Evaluation and Research. (2013, August 14). Postmarket drug safety information for patients and providers—information for healthcare professionals: Dangerous or even fatal skin reactions—carbamazepine (marketed as Carbatrol, Equetro, Tegretol, and generics). Retrieved from https://www.fda.gov/Drugs/DrugSafety/PostmarketDrugSafetyInformationforPatientsandProviders/ucm124718.htm

Christiansen, E., Agerbo, E., Bilenberg, N., & Stenager, E. (2016). SSRIs and risk of suicide attempts in young people—a Danish observational register-based historical cohort study, using propensity score. *Nordic Journal of Psychiatry, 70*(3), 167–175.

Clein, P. D., & Riddle, M. A. (1995). Pharmacokinetics in children and adolescents. *Child and Adolescent Psychiatric Clinics of North America, 4*(1), 59–75.

Cohen, J. A. (2008). Treating PTSD and related symptoms in children: Research highlights. *PTSD Research Quarterly, 19*(2), 1–3.

Cohen, J. A., Bukstein, O., Walter, H., Benson, S. R., Chrisman, A., Farchione, T. R., . . . AACAP Work Group on Quality Issues. (2010). Practice parameter for the assessment and treatment of children and adolescents with posttraumatic stress disorder. *Journal of the American Academy of Child & Adolescent Psychiatry, 49*(4), 414–430.

Cohen, J. A., Mannarino, A. P., Perel, J. M., & Staron, V. (2007). A pilot randomized controlled trial of combined trauma-focused CBT and sertraline for childhood PTSD symptoms. *Journal of the American Academy of Child & Adolescent Psychiatry, 46*(7), 811–819.

Cohen, J. A., Mannarino, A. P., Jankowski, K., Rosenberg, S., Kodya, S., & Wolford, G. L. (2016). A randomized implementation study of trauma-focused cognitive behavioral therapy for adjudicated teens in residential treatment facilities. *Child Maltreatment, 21*(2), 156–167.

Colville, G., Kerry, S., & Pierce, C. (2008). Children's factual and delusional memories of intensive care. *American Journal of Respiratory and Critical Care Medicine, 177*(9), 976–982.

Colucci, E., Minas, H., Szwarc, J., Guerra, C., & Paxton, G. (2015). In or out? Barriers and facilitators to refugee-background young people accessing mental health services. *Transcultural Psychiatry, 52*(6), 766–790.

Connor, D. F., Grasso, D. J., Slivinsky, M. D., Pearson, G. S., & Banga, A. (2013). An open-label study of guanfacine extended release for traumatic stress related symptoms in children and adolescents. *Journal of Child and Adolescent Psychopharmacology, 23*(4), 244–251.

Corbin, J. R. (2007). Reactive attachment disorder: A biopsychosocial disturbance of attachment. *Child and Adolescent Social Work Journal, 24*(6), 539–552.

Correll, C. U., Manu, P., Olshanskiy, V., Napolitano, B., Kane, J. M., & Malhotra, A. K. (2009). Cardiometabolic risk of second-generation antipsychotic medications during first-time use in children and adolescents. *JAMA, 302*(16), 1765–1773.

De Bellis, M. D., Keshavan, M. S., Clark, D. B., Casey, B. J., Giedd, J. N., Boring, A. M., & Ryan, N. D. (1999). Developmental traumatology part II: Brain development. *Biological Psychiatry, 45*(10), 1271–1284.

De Bellis, M. D., Keshevan, M. S., & Harenski, K. A. (2001). Case study: Amterior cingulated N-acetylaspartate concentrations during treatment of a maltreated child with PTSD. *Journal of Child and Adolescent Psychopharmacology, 11*, 311–316.

De Hert, M., Dobbelaere, M., Sheridan, E. M., Cohen, D., & Correll, C. U. (2011). Metabolic and endocrine adverse effects of second-generation antipsychotics in children and adolescents: A systematic review of randomized, placebo controlled trials and guidelines for clinical practice. *European Psychiatry, 26*(3), 144–158.

Domon, S. E., & Andersen, M. S. (2000). Nefazodone for PTSD. *Journal of the American Academy of Child & Adolescent Psychiatry, 39*(8), 942–943.

Donnelly, C. L., & Amaya-Jackson, L. (2002). Post-traumatic stress disorder in children and adolescents. *Pediatric Drugs, 4*(3), 159–170.

Drury, S., & Cuthbert, B. (2015). Advancing pediatric psychiatry research: linking neurobiological processes to novel treatment and diagnosis through the Research Domain Criteria (RDoC) project. *Therapeutic Innovation & Regulatory Science, 49*(5), 643–646.

Dwyer, J. B., Beyer, C., Wilkinson, S. T., Ostroff, R. B., Qayyum, Z., & Bloch, M. H. (2017). Ketamine as a treatment for adolescent depression: A case report. *Journal of the American Academy of Child & Adolescent Psychiatry, 56*(4), 352–354.

Famularo, R., Kinscherff, R., & Fenton, T. (1988). Propranolol treatment for childhood posttraumatic stress disorder, acute type: A pilot study. *American Journal of Diseases of Children, 142*(11), 1244–1247.

Feder, A., Parides, M. K., Murrough, J. W., Perez, A. M., Morgan, J. E., Saxena, S., . . . Iosifescu, D. (2014). Efficacy of intravenous ketamine for treatment of chronic posttraumatic stress disorder: A randomized clinical trial. *JAMA Psychiatry, 71*(6), 681–688.

Federal Drug Administration. Center for Drug Evaluation and Research. List of drugs receiving a boxed warning pertaining to pediatric suicidality. Retrieved from www.fda.gov/cder/foi/label/2005/20031s045,20936s020lbl.pdf.

Foa, E. B., Keane, T. M., Friedman, M. J., & Cohen, J. A. (Eds.). (2008). Effective treatments for PTSD: Practice guidelines from the International Society for Traumatic Stress Studies. New York: Guilford Press.

Foa, E. B., McLean, C. P., Capaldi, S., & Rosenfield, D. (2013). Prolonged exposure vs supportive counseling for sexual abuse–related PTSD in adolescent girls: A randomized clinical trial. *JAMA, 310*(24), 2650–2657.

Food and Drug Administration. (2014, September 10). Consumer updates FDA: Don't leave childhood depression untreated. Retrieved from https://www.fda.gov/ForConsumers/ConsumerUpdates/ucm413161.htm

Fraguas, D., Correll, C. U., Merchán-Naranjo, J., Rapado-Castro, M., Parellada, M., Moreno, C., & Arango, C. (2011). Efficacy and safety of second-generation antipsychotics in children and adolescents with psychotic and bipolar spectrum disorders: Comprehensive review of prospective head-to-head and placebo-controlled comparisons. *European Neuropsychopharmacology, 21*(8), 621–645.

Garland, E. J., Kutcher, S., & Virani, A. (2009). 2008 position paper on using SSRIs in children and adolescents. *Journal of the Canadian Academy of Child and Adolescent Psychiatry, 18*(2), 160.

Gibbons, R. D., Brown, C. H., Hur, K., Marcus, S. M., Bhaumik, D. K., Erkens, J. A., . . . Mann, J. J. (2007). Early evidence on the effects of regulators' suicidality warnings on SSRI prescriptions and suicide in children and adolescents. *American Journal of Psychiatry, 164*(9), 1356–1363.

Gleason, M. M., Egger, H. L., Emslie, G. J., Greenhill, L. L., Kowatch, R. A., Lieberman, A. F., . . . Stafford, B. (2007). Psychopharmacological treatment for very young children: Contexts and guidelines. *Journal of the American Academy of Child & Adolescent Psychiatry, 46*(12), 1532–1572.

Goldbeck, L., & Jensen, T. K. (2017). The diagnostic spectrum of trauma-related disorders in children and adolescents. In M. A. Landolt, M. Schnyder & U. Cloitre (Eds.), *Evidence-based treatments for trauma related disorders in children and adolescents* (pp. 3–28). New York: Springer.

Goldston, D. B., Daniel, S. S., Reboussin, B. A., Reboussin, D. M., Kelley, A., & Frazier, P. H. (1998) Psychiatric diagnoses of previous suicide attempters, first-time attempters and repeat attempters on an adolescent inpatient psychiatry unit. . *Journal of the American Academy of Child & Adolescent Psychiatry, 37*, 924–932

Gould, M. S., Greenberg, T., Velting, D. M., & Shaffer, D. (2003) Youth suicide risk and preventive interventions: a review of the past 10 years. *Journal of the American Academy of Child & Adolescent Psychiatry, 42*, 386–405.

Greenberg, W. M., Rosenfeld, D. N., & Ortega, E. A. (1995) Adjustment disorder as an admission diagnosis. *American Journal of Psychiatry, 152*, 459–461.

Gupta, S., Popli, A., Bathurst, E., Hennig, L., Droney, T., & Keller, P. (1998). Efficacy of cyproheptadine for nightmares associated with posttraumatic stress disorder. *Comprehensive Psychiatry, 39*(3), 160–164.

Guyatt, G. H., Oxman, A. D., Vist, G. E., Kunz, R., Falck-Ytter, Y., Alonso-Coello, P., & Schunemann, H. J. (2008). GRADE: An emerging consensus on rating quality of evidence and strength of recommendations. *British Medical Journal, 336*(7650), 924.

Hall, B. J., & Olff, M. (2016). Global mental health: Trauma and adversity among populations in transition. *European Journal of Psychotraumatology, 7*, 1–3.

Hammad, T. (2004). *Results of the analysis of suicidality in pediatric trials of newer antidepressants.* US Food and Drugs Administration Psychopharmacologic Drugs Advisory Committee and the Pediatric Advisory Committee. Washington, DC: Food and Drug Administration.

Harmon, R. J., & Riggs, P. D. (1996). Clonidine for posttraumatic stress disorder in preschool children. *Journal of the American Academy of Child & Adolescent Psychiatry, 35*(9), 1247–1249.

Hetrick, S. E., McKenzie, J. E., & Merry, S. N. (2010). The use of SSRIs in children and adolescents. *Current Opinion in Psychiatry, 23*(1), 53–57.

Hennissen, L., Bakker, M. J., Banaschewski, T., Carucci, S., Coghill, D., Danckaerts, M., . . . Nagy, P. (2017). Cardiovascular effects of stimulant and non-stimulant medication for children and adolescents with ADHD: A systematic review and meta-analysis of trials of methylphenidate, amphetamines and atomoxetine. *CNS Drugs, 31*(3). 199–215.

Holbrook, T. L., Galarneau, M. R., Dye, J. L., Quinn, K., & Dougherty, A. L. (2010). Morphine use after combat injury in Iraq and post-traumatic stress disorder. *New England Journal of Medicine, 362*(2), 110–117.

Horrigan, J. P. (1996). Guanfacine for PTSD nightmares. *Journal of the American Academy of Child & Adolescent Psychiatry, 35*(8), 975–976.

Horrigan, J. P., & Barnhill, L. J. (1999). Risperidone and PTSD in boys. *Journal of Neuropsychiatry and Clinical Neuroscience, 11*, 126–127.

Howard, M., & Hodes, M. (2000). Psychopathology, adversity, and service utilization of young refugees. *Journal of the American Academy of Child & Adolescent Psychiatry, 39*(3), 368–377.

Hudak, M. L., & Tan, R. C. (2012). Neonatal drug withdrawal. *Pediatrics, 129*(2), e540-e560.

Ipser, J. C., Stein, D. J., Hawkridge, S., & Hoppe, L. (2009). Pharmacotherapy for anxiety disorders in children and adolescents. *Cochrane Database of Systematic Reviews, 3*.

Janicak, P. G., Marder, S. R., & Pavuluri, M. N. (2010). *Principles and practice of psychopharmacotherapy*. Philadelphia: Lippincott Williams & Wilkins.

Kassam-Adams, N., & Winston, F. K. (2004). Predicting child PTSD: The relationship between acute stress disorder and PTSD in injured children. *Journal of the American Academy of Child & Adolescent Psychiatry, 43*(4), 403–411.

Kovacs, M., Gatsonis, C., Pollock, M., & Parrone, P. L. (1994) A controlled prospective study of DSM-III adjustment disorder in childhood. *Archives of General Psychiatry, 51*, 535–541.

Kovacs, M., Ho, V., & Pollock, M. H. (1995). Criterion and predictive validity of the diagnosis of adjustment disorder: A prospective study of youths with new-onset insulin-dependent diabetes mellitus. *The American Journal of Psychiatry, 152*(4), 523.

Kryzhanovskaya, L., & Canterbury, R. (2001). Suicidal behavior in patients with adjustment disorders. *Crisis: The Journal of Crisis Intervention and Suicide Prevention, 22*, 125–131.

Kryzhanovskaya, L., & Canterbury, R. (2001). Suicidal behavior in patients with adjustment disorders. *Crisis: The Journal of Crisis Intervention and Suicide Prevention, 22*(3), 125.

Lakhan, S. E., & Hagger-Johnson, G. E. (2007). The impact of prescribed psychotropics on youth. *Clinical Practice and Epidemiology in Mental Health, 3*(1), 21.

Lake, M. B., Birmaher, B., Wassick, S., Mathos, K., & Yelovich, A. K. (2000). Bleeding and selective serotonin reuptake inhibitors in childhood and adolescence. *Journal of Child and Adolescent Psychopharmacology, 10*(1), 35–38.

Lee, T., Fouras, G., & Brown, R. (2015). Practice parameter for the assessment and management of youth involved with the child welfare system. *Journal of the American Academy of Child & Adolescent Psychiatry, 54*(6), 502–517.

Lehmann, S., Breivik, K., Heiervang, E. R., Havik, T., & Havik, O. E. (2016). Reactive attachment disorder and disinhibited social engagement disorder in school-aged foster children—a confirmatory approach to dimensional measures. *Journal of Abnormal Child Psychology, 44*(3), 445–457.

Leonard, H. L., March, J., Rickler, K. C., & Allen, A. J. (1997). Pharmacology of the selective serotonin reuptake inhibitors in children and adolescents. *Journal of the American Academy of Child & Adolescent Psychiatry, 36*(6), 725–736.

Lexicomp Online®, Pediatric & Neonatal Lexi-Drugs® (2017). Hudson, OH: Lexi-Comp.

Lindert, J., von Ehrenstein, O. S., Priebe, S., Mielck, A., & Brähler, E. (2009). Depression and anxiety in labor migrants and refugees—a systematic review and meta-analysis. *Social Science & Medicine, 69*(2), 246–257.

Looff, D., Grimley, P., Kuller, F., Martin, A., & Shonfield, L. (1995). Carbamazepine for PTSD. *Journal of the American Academy of Child & Adolescent Psychiatry, 34*(6), 703–704.

Luby, J. L. (2013). Treatment of anxiety and depression in the preschool period. *Journal of the American Academy of Child & Adolescent Psychiatry, 52*(4), 346–358.

March, J. S., Silva, S. G., Compton, S., Anthony, G., DeVeaugh-Geiss, J., Califf, R., & Krishnan, R. (2004). The Child and Adolescent Psychiatry Trials Network (CAPTN). *Journal of the American Academy of Child & Adolescent Psychiatry, 43*(5), 515–518.

Martsenkovsky, I., Martsenkovska, I., & Martsenkovsky, D. (2015). Fluoxetine in the treatment of children with PTSD. *European Psychiatry, 30*, 1537.

Marttunen, M., Aro, H., & Lönnqvist, J. (1993) Adolescence and suicide. A review of psychological autopsy studies. *European Child & Adolescent Psychiatry, 2*, 10–18, 22.

Marttunen, M. J., Aro, H. M., Henriksson, M. M., & Lönnqvist, J. K. (1994). Adolescent suicides with adjustment disorders or no psychiatric diagnosis. *European Child & Adolescent Psychiatry, 3*, 101–110.

Masi, G., Milone, A., Veltri, S., Iuliano, R., Pfanner, C., & Pisano, S. (2015). Use of quetiapine in children and adolescents. *Pediatric Drugs, 17*(2), 125–140.

McGhee, L. L., Maani, C. V., Garza, T. H., Gaylord, K. M., & Black, I. H. (2008). The correlation between ketamine and posttraumatic stress disorder in burned service members. *Journal of Trauma and Acute Care Surgery, 64*(2), S195–S199.

Meiser-Stedman, R., McKinnon, A., Dixon, C., Boyle, A., Smith, P., & Dalgleish, T. (2017). Acute stress disorder and the transition to posttraumatic stress disorder in children and adolescents: Prevalence, course, prognosis, diagnostic suitability and risk markers. *Depression and Anxiety*, *34*(4), 348–355.

Miller, M., Swanson, S. A., Azrael, D., Pate, V., & Stürmer, T. (2014). Antidepressant dose, age, and the risk of deliberate self-harm. *JAMA Internal Medicine*, *174*(6), 899–909.

Mitka, M. (2003). FDA alert on antidepressants for youth. *JAMA*, *290*(19), 2534.

Mitrev, I. (1996) A study of deliberate self-poisoning in patients with adjustment disorders. *Folia Medica*, 38, 11–16.

Nathan, P. E., & Gorman, J. M. (Eds.). (2015). *A guide to treatments that work*. New York: Oxford University Press.

National Institute for Health and Care Excellence. (2005, March). Post-traumatic stress disorder: Management. Retrieved from https://www.nice.org.uk/guidance/CG26

Newacheck, P. W., & Stoddard, J. J. (1994). Prevalence and impact of multiple childhood chronic illnesses. *The Journal of Pediatrics*, *124*(1), 40–48.

Nugent, N. R., Christopher, N. C., Crow, J. P., Browne, L., Ostrowski, S., & Delahanty, D. L. (2010). The efficacy of early propranolol administration at reducing PTSD symptoms in pediatric injury patients: A pilot study. *Journal of Traumatic Stress*, *23*(2), 282–287.

O'Brien, P. L., Cummings, N., & Mark, T. L. (2017). Off-Label Prescribing of Psychotropic Medication, 2005–2013: An Examination of Potential Influences. *Psychiatric Services*, *68*(6), 549–558.

Ohring, R., Apter, A., Ratzoni, G., Weizman, R., Tyano, S., & Plutchik, R. (1995) State and trait anxiety in adolescent suicide attempters. *Journal of the American Academy of Child & Adolescent Psychiatry*, *35*, 154–157.

Olfson, M., Marcus, S. C., & Shaffer, D. (2006). Antidepressant drug therapy and suicide in severely depressed children and adults: A case-control study. *Archives of General Psychiatry*, *63*(8), 865–872.

Olfson, M., Shaffer, D., Marcus, S. C., & Greenberg, T. (2003). Relationship between antidepressant medication treatment and suicide in adolescents. *Archives of General Psychiatry*, *60*(10), 978–982.

Pacione, L., Measham, T., & Rousseau, C. (2013). Refugee children: Mental health and effective interventions. *Current Psychiatry Reports*, *15*(2), 341.

Pelkonen, M., Marttunen, M., Henriksson, M., & Lönnqvist, J. (2005). Suicidality in adjustment disorder. *European Child & Adolescent Psychiatry*, *14*(3), 174–180.

Perry, B. D. (1994). Neurobiological sequelae of childhood trauma: post-traumatic stress disorders in children. In M. M. Murburg (Ed.), *Catecholamine function in post traumatic stress disorder: Emerging concepts* (pp. 253–276). Washington, DC: American Psychiatric Press.

Polyakova, I., Knobler, H. Y., Ambrumova, A., & Lerner, V. (1998). Characteristics of suicidal attempts in major depression versus adjustment reactions. *Journal of Affective Disorders*, *47*, 159–167.

Poulton, A. S., Bui, Q., Melzer, E., & Evans, R. (2016). Stimulant medication effects on growth and bone age in children with attention-deficit/hyperactivity disorder: A prospective cohort study. *International Clinical Psychopharmacology*, *31*(2), 93.

Robb, A., Cueva, J., Sporn, J., Yang, R., & Vanderburg, D. (2010). Sertraline treatment of children and adolescents with posttraumatic stress disorder: a double-blind, placebo-controlled trial. *Journal of Child and Adolescent Psychopharmacology*, *20*(6), 463–471.

Robert, R., Blakeney, P. E., Villarreal, C., Rosenberg, L., & Meyer, W. J. (1999). Imipramine treatment in pediatric burn patients with symptoms of acute stress disorder: A pilot study. *Journal of the American Academy of Child & Adolescent Psychiatry*, *38*(7), 873–882.

Rothenberger, A., & Rothenberger, L. G. (2013). Psychopharmacological treatment in children: Always keeping an eye on adherence and ethics. *European Child & Adolescent Psychiatry*, *22*(8), 453–455.

Rousseau, C., Pottie, K., Thombs, B. D., Munoz, M., & Jurcik, T. (2012). Canadian collaboration for immigrant and refugee health guidelines for immigrant health, Appendix 11: Post traumatic stress disorder, evidence review for newly arriving immigrants and refugees. Canadian Collaboration for Immigrant and Refugee Health. Retrieved from http://phstwlp2.partners.org:2327/content/suppl/2010/06/07/cmaj.090313.DC1/imm-ptsd-11-at.pdf.

Rubin, D. M., Kreider, A. R., Matone, M., Huang, Y. S., Feudtner, C., Ross, M. E., & Localio, A. R. (2015). Risk for incident diabetes mellitus following initiation of second-generation antipsychotics among Medicaid-enrolled youths. *JAMA Pediatrics*, *169*(4), e150285–e150285.

Sakolsky, D. J., Perel, J. M., Emslie, G. J., Clarke, G. N., Wagner, K. D., Vitiello, B., . . . McCracken, J. T. (2011). Antidepressant exposure as a predictor of clinical outcomes in the Treatment of Resistant Depression in Adolescents (TORDIA) study. *Journal of Clinical Psychopharmacology*, *31*(1), 92

Saxe, G., Stoddard, F., Courtney, D., Cunningham, K., Chawla, N., Sheridan, R., & King, L. (2001). Relationship between acute morphine and the course of PTSD in children with burns. *Journal of the American Academy of Child & Adolescent Psychiatry, 40*(8), 915–921.

Scheeringa, M. S., Peebles, C. D., Cook, C. A., & Zeanah, C. H. (2001). Toward establishing procedural, criterion, and discriminant validity for PTSD in early childhood. *Journal of the American Academy of Child & Adolescent Psychiatry, 40*(1), 52–60.

Scheeringa, M. S., Zeanah, C. H., Myers, L., & Putnam, F. (2004). Heart period and variability findings in preschool children with posttraumatic stress symptoms. *Biological Psychiatry, 55*(7), 685–691.

Scheeringa, M. S., Zeanah, C. H., Myers, L., & Putnam, F. W. (2003). New findings on alternative criteria for PTSD in preschool children. *Journal of the American Academy of Child & Adolescent Psychiatry, 42*(5), 561–570.

Scheeringa, M. S., Zeanah, C. H., Myers, L., & Putnam, F. W. (2005). Predictive validity in a prospective follow-up of PTSD in preschool children. *Journal of the American Academy of Child & Adolescent Psychiatry, 44*(9), 899–906.

Schönenberg, M., Reichwald, U., Domes, G., Badke, A., & Hautzinger, M. (2005). Effects of peritraumatic ketamine medication on early and sustained posttraumatic stress symptoms in moderately injured accident victims. *Psychopharmacology, 182*(3), 420–425.

Seedat, S., Stein, D. J., Ziervogel, C., Middleton, T., Kaminer, D., Emsley, R. A., & Rossouw, W. (2002). Comparison of response to a selective serotonin reuptake inhibitor in children, adolescents, and adults with posttraumatic stress disorder. *Journal of Child and Adolescent Psychopharmacology, 12*(1), 37–46.

Sharp, S., Thomas, C., Rosenberg, L., Rosenberg, M., & Meyer, W. III. (2010). Propranolol does not reduce risk for acute stress disorder in pediatric burn trauma. *Journal of Trauma and Acute Care Surgery, 68*(1), 193–197.

Sharp, S., Thomas, C., Rosenberg, L., Rosenberg, M., & Meyer III, W. (2010). Propranolol does not reduce risk for acute stress disorder in pediatric burn trauma. *Journal of Trauma and Acute Care Surgery, 68*(1), 193–197.

Slobodin, O., & de Jong, J. T. (2015). Family interventions in traumatized immigrants and refugees: A systematic review. *Transcultural Psychiatry, 52*(6), 723–742.

Sijbrandij, M., Kleiboer, A., Bisson, J. I., Barbui, C., & Cuijpers, P. (2015). Pharmacological prevention of post-traumatic stress disorder and acute stress disorder: A systematic review and meta-analysis. *The Lancet Psychiatry, 2*(5), 413–421.

Spalletta, G., Troisi, A., Saracco, M., Ciani, N., & Pasini, A. (1996) Symptom profile, Axis II comorbidity and suicidal behavior in young males with DSM-III-R depressive illnesses. *Journal of Affective Disorders, 39*, 141–148.

Spirito, A., Valeri, S., Boergers, J., & Donalson, D. (2003) Predictors of continued suicidal behavior in adolescents following a suicide attempt. *Journal of Clinical Child & Adolescent Psychology, 32*, 284–289.

Stathis, S., Martin, G., & McKenna, J. G. (2005). A preliminary case series on the use of quetiapine for posttraumatic stress disorder in juveniles within a youth detention center. *Journal of Clinical Psychopharmacology, 25*(6), 539–544.

Stein, D., Apter, A., Ratzoni, G., Har-Even, D., & Avidan, G. (1998) Association between multiple suicide attempts and negative affects in adolescents. *Journal of the American Academy of Child & Adolescent Psychiatry, 37*, 488–494.

Steiner, H., Warren, B. L., Van Waes, V., & Bolaños-Guzmán, C. A. (2014). Life-long consequences of juvenile exposure to psychotropic drugs on brain and behavior. *Progress in Brain Research, 211*, 13.

Steinhausen, H. C., & Erdin, A. (1991). A Comparison of ICD-9 and ICD-10 diagnoses of child and adolescent psychiatric disorders. *Journal of Child Psychology and Psychiatry, 32*(6), 909–920.

Stoddard, F. J., Sorrentino, E. A., Ceranoglu, T. A., Saxe, G., Murphy, J. M., Drake, J. E., . . . Tompkins, R. G. (2009). Preliminary evidence for the effects of morphine on PTSD symptoms in one-to four-year olds with burns. *Journal of Burn Care & Research, 30*(5), 836–843.

Stoddard, F. J. Jr., Luthra, R., Sorrentino, E. A., Saxe, G. N., Drake, J., Chang, Y., . . . Sheridan, R. L. (2011). A randomized controlled trial of sertraline to prevent posttraumatic stress disorder in burned children. *Journal of Child and Adolescent Psychopharmacology, 21*(5), 469–477.

Stoddard, F. J. Jr., Sorrentino, E. A., Ceranoglu, T. A., Saxe, G., Murphy, J. M., Drake, J. E., . . . Sheridan, R. L. (2009). Preliminary evidence for the effects of morphine on posttraumatic stress disorder symptoms in one-to four-year-olds with burns. *Journal of Burn Care & Research, 30*(5), 836–843.

Stoddard, F. J., Usher, C. T., & Abrams, A. N. (2006). Psychopharmacology in pediatric critical care. *Child and Adolescent Psychiatric Clinics of North America, 15*(3), 611–655.

Strawn, J. R., & Geracioti, T. D. (2008). Noradrenergic dysfunction and the psychopharmacology of posttraumatic stress disorder. *Depression and Anxiety, 25*(3), 260–271.

Keeshin, B. R., & Strawn, J. R. (2014). Psychological and pharmacological treatment of youth with posttraumatic stress disorder: An evidence-based review. *Child and Adolescent Psychiatric Clinics of North America*, *23*, 399–411.

Turner, S. (2015). Refugee blues: A UK and European perspective. *European Journal of Psychotraumatology*, *6*, 1–9.

United Nations High Commissioner for Refugees. (2016). Refugees/migrants emergency response—Mediterranean. Retrieved from http://data.unhcr.org/mediterranean/regional.php

United Nations Population Fund. (2016). Retrieved from http://www.unfpa.org/migration

Wagner, K. D., Robb, A. S., Findling, R. L., Jin, J., Gutierrez, M. M., & Heydorn, W. E. (2004). A randomized, placebo-controlled trial of citalopram for the treatment of major depression in children and adolescents. *American Journal of Psychiatry*, *161*(6), 1079–1083.

Wang, G. J., Belley-Coté, E., Burry, L., Duffett, M., Karachi, T., Perri, D., & Rochwerg, B. (2015). Clonidine for sedation in the critically ill: A systematic review and meta-analysis (protocol). *Systematic Reviews*, *4*(1), 154.

Weinberg, H. A. (2010). Improved functioning in children diagnosed with reactive attachment disorder after SSRI therapy. *Journal of the Canadian Academy of Child and Adolescent Psychiatry*, *19*(1), 48.

Weine, S. M. (2011). Developing preventive mental health interventions for refugee Families in resettlement. *Family Process*, *50*(3), 410–430. doi:10.1111/j.1545-5300.2011.01366.x.

World Health Organization. (2013). Guidelines for the management of conditions that are specifically related to stress. Geneva: World Health Organization.

Yorbık, Ö., Dikkatli, S., Cansever, A., & Söhmen, T. (2001). The efficacy of fluoxetine treatment in children and adolescents with posttraumatic stress disorder symptoms. *Klinik Psikofarmakoloji Bulteni-Bulletin of Clinical Psychopharmacology*, *11*(4), 251–256.

Zeanah, C. H., & Gleason, M. M. (2015). Annual research review: Attachment disorders in early childhood-clinical presentation, causes, correlates, and treatment. *Journal of Child Psychology and Psychiatry*, *56*(3), 207–222.

Zeanah, C. H., Chesher, T., & Boris, N. W. (2016). Practice parameter for the assessment and treatment of children and adolescents with reactive attachment disorder and disinhibited social engagement disorder. *Journal of the American Academy of Child & Adolescent Psychiatry*, *55*(11), 990–1003.

Zimmerman, C., Kiss, L., & Hossain, M. (2011). Migration and health: A framework for 21st century policy-making. *PLoS Medicine*, *8*(5), e1001034.

Zuckerman, M. L., Vaughan, B. L., Whitney, J., Dodds, A., Yakhkind, A., MacMillan, C., . . . Gonzalez-Heydrich, J. (2007). Tolerability of selective serotonin reuptake inhibitors in thirty-nine children under age seven: A retrospective chart review. *Journal of Child and Adolescent Psychopharmacology*, *17*(2), 165–174.

24

Complementary and Alternative Medicine for Trauma- and Stressor-Related Disorders

GARY H. WYNN* AND DAVID M. BENEDEK

INTRODUCTION

The past decade has seen a substantial increase in the use of complementary and alternative medicine (CAM) throughout the United States and abroad. This rise in use has been particularly high for those with mental health issues such as trauma- and stressor-related disorders. Increasing use and consideration by clinicians stems from a combination of increased perceived therapeutic benefit, patient preference for these approaches, recognition of CAM as a low-risk augmentation strategy, and the need for options when traditional approaches are insufficient (Benedek & Wynn, 2016). These factors are especially relevant in trauma- and stressor-related disorders where evidence-based treatment options are particularly limited. The problem facing many providers will be familiarization with the very broad range of modalities potentially considered CAM. Currently there is no generally accepted list of what treatments constitute CAM, nor is there likely to be such given the complexity of creating definitional coherence across a broadly inclusive spectrum of modalities. Presently, instead of any comprehensive list of what CAM is, there are a number of very generalized definitions that attempt to provide some structure to the concept. The chapter uses a clinically focused definition—that is, a definition from the perspective of the clinician rather than the patient. This definition is based on the terms "complementary" and "alternative" and their meaning in a clinical setting. For the purposes of this chapter, complementary treatments are those modalities that are intended to augment more traditional approaches but are not likely to replace standard practices as a monotherapy approach (Wynn, 2015). A good example of a complementary treatment is recreational therapy. While hiking and other outdoor and recreational activities may have therapeutic benefit for some individuals with trauma- and stressor-related disorders, it is quite unlikely that recreational therapy will become a stand-alone treatment or the primary focus of the clinician-patient relationship. Alternative therapies, as a broad category, include alternative treatments and alternative delivery methods which may be intended supplant traditional medication treatment or psychotherapy. Alternative treatments are modalities that have the potential to be the primary focus of a patient-provider interaction (Benedek & Wynn, 2016). An excellent example of an alternative treatment is acupuncture. Acupuncture has a growing body of evidence for use in a number of mental disorders including trauma- and stressor-related disorders. It is also more readily foreseeable that providers (and, in some cases, current practice) suggest a stand-alone course of acupuncture for one of the trauma- and stressor-related disorders (e.g., posttraumatic stress disorder [PTSD]) instead of other treatments options. Even these definitions are somewhat arbitrary as alternative treatments, much like most available therapies in mental health including evidence-based treatments, may also be used as complementary approaches. Alternative delivery methods include means of providing care in new and unique ways through the use of advances in technology such as smartphone apps, the Internet, or telebehavioral health devices. These alternative delivery methods present the real possibility of significant disruption

* Corresponding author: Center for the Study of Traumatic Stress, Department of Psychiatry, Uniformed Services University, School of Medicine, Bethesda, MD. Phone 301-295-3293. Email: gary.wynn@usuhs.edu

to the classic model of behavioral health care by facilitating the relationship between patient and provider and overcoming access to care barriers through technology or in some cases removing the provider entirely.

For the majority of the modalities discussed in this chapter there exists only limited evidence of benefit in treating trauma- and stressor-related disorders. A couple of CAM treatments have shown some efficacy in PTSD, but beyond these few there is very little in the way of science supporting their use. Studies of these modalities specifically for the treatment of adjustment disorder or acute stress disorder have not been published.

This chapter is divided in to three sections as depicted in Table 24.1: (a) complementary medicine which covers animal therapy, recreational therapy, yoga, creative arts therapy, and meditation; (b) alternative therapies which describes alternative pharmacology and acupuncture; and (c) alternative delivery methods which provides a brief overview of the concept. While the chapter is not exhaustive, it does highlight the evidence supporting the use of some CAM treatments for trauma- and stressor related disorders.

COMPLEMENTARY MEDICINE

Animal Therapy

The strong bond between humans and animals is apparent throughout society whether these animals are domestic companions or working animals. Much work has been done showing the positive health benefits of connections with animals. Animal therapies fall in to three major categories—service animals, animal-assisted therapy (AAT), and animal care activities. Of note, there are definite overlaps between these categories and no official definitions exist which delineate the boundaries between these modalities.

The most common practice among these, the provision of service animals (primarily dogs), focuses on animal activities in support of disabilities across a wide spectrum of physical and psychological conditions. The 2010 update to the Americans with Disabilities Act guidance on service animals added language specific to mental illness by including animal activities such as reminding individuals to take medication and calming a person with PTSD (U.S. Department of Justice, 2010). While considerable therapeutic benefit from service animals may stem from the companionship they engender, their primary purpose is in support of the needs of the individual rather than for therapy and as such are not specifically addressed in this chapter.

AAT utilizes the relationship between person and animal (e.g., companion dogs, therapeutic horseback riding) to facilitate progress toward specific therapeutic goals (Fine, 2000). Animal-care activities focus on the tasks of caring for an animal (primarily horsemanship) as the means of therapy. While AAT has been shown to be beneficial in a range of ages and mental illnesses, it has not been well studied in trauma- and stressor-related disorders. Animal-care activities have received less attention in research to date although there have been a number of programs focused on exploring the therapeutic benefit of horsemanship in recent years. To date there are no known

TABLE 24.1. CATEGORIES OF COMPLEMENTARY AND ALTERNATIVE MEDICINE

CAM Type	Definition[a]	Examples[b]
Complementary	Practices that, primarily, augment traditional interventions and are not likely to replace standard practices	Animal therapy Recreational therapy Yoga Creative arts therapy Meditation
Alternative	Nonmainstream treatments that are either already being used or have the potential to be used as monotherapy within typical western medical practice	Alternative pharmacology Acupuncture Neurostimulation
Alternative Delivery Methods	Primarily the use of new technologies and communication platforms to deliver traditional interventions such as psychotherapy	Telemental health Smartphone apps Virtual reality

[a]Definitions from Benedek and Wynn (2016). [b]Examples listed should not be considered exhaustive.

randomized controlled trials (RCTs) evaluating AAT or animal-care activities for any of the trauma- and stressor-related disorders. There has been one small exploratory study and one case study looking at AAT in trauma survivors (Nevins et al., 2013; Earles et al., 2015) as well as one exploratory study evaluating animal-care activities (Lanning & Krenek, 2013). None of these studies defined outcomes in terms of remission of specific symptoms of trauma- and stressor-related disorders. All three found modest benefits, but further research is needed in order to assess the benefit of AAT or animal-care activities for trauma- and stressor-related disorders. While the clinical evidence is lacking, there is science supporting the notion that animals are helpful across a number of domains potentially relevant to trauma- and stressor-related disorders. Interactions with animals are known to decrease blood pressure (Katcher, 1981), may calm individuals with dissociative disorders (Arnold, 1995), and decrease subjective psychological distress (Lass-Henneman et al., 2014).

Beyond the assessment of benefit there is the additional consideration of cost associated with AAT or animal-care activities, especially equine-related therapies (ERT). Over the past decade there has been a considerable increase in the number of non-profit ERT programs throughout the United States. These programs offer ERT for little or no cost to patients. If available locally and at a manageable cost, clinicians should consider recommending an AAT (e.g., dog, horse) to patients dealing with a trauma- and stressor-related disorder. At current, these therapies should be utilized as an augmentation to evidenced-based treatments such as medication or psychotherapy.

Recreational Therapy

Recreational therapy refers to a broad group of activities, primarily conducted outdoors in small groups or one on one, typically involving a trained therapist or facilitator, and often with specific therapeutic goals. These activities can include activities commonly considered sports and leisure such as hiking, gardening, bird watching, skiing, fishing, or hunting. While millions participate in, and find personal benefit from, these activities every year, there has been little rigorous research done on the therapeutic benefit with regard to trauma- and stressor-related disorders. The two recreational activities that have some measure of research supporting their use are wilderness therapy and fly-fishing (Duvall & Kaplan, 2014; Vella et al., 2013). The fact that these two have relatively more research is likely related to investigator or institutional interest rather than theoretical therapeutic benefit.

Adventure therapy programs, such as Outward Bound, are typically brief excursions into nature where participants engage in activities such as hiking, climbing, and whitewater rafting. These programs have gained prominence over the past several decades though little research on their utility in trauma- and stressor-related disorders has been performed to date. One study of adventure therapy which included veterans with PTSD found posttreatment improvements in psychological well-being, social functioning, and outlook on life but did not specifically assess changes in any trauma- and stressor-related disorder (Duvall & Kaplan, 2014). A study by Hyer, Boyd, Scurfield, Smith, and Burke (1996) showed that adventure therapy was associated with improved self-esteem, emotional control, and social connectedness but failed to show improvements in specific PTSD symptoms. This limited data suggests that there may be benefit or at least sufficient reason for further investigation into the utility of adventure therapy in the treatment of trauma- and stressor-related disorders. Given the low risk associated with these activities that millions of individuals participate in every year, it seems appropriate for a clinician to consider recommending adventure therapy in conjunction with a more traditional intervention. Clinicians should be aware that one common concern in the research into adventure therapies is degradation of benefit within a relatively brief period of time (Benedek & Wynn, 2016). Given this degradation it would be of value to consider how patients might incorporate these activities into their life on a regular basis in order to maximize potential value.

Yoga Therapy

Yoga, as practiced in the Western world, is primarily physical, incorporating postures and movements into a routine used to improve fitness and well-being. Originating in India, the broad term "yoga" includes meditation, physical movement, controlled breathing, chanting, and even singing in order to promote physical and mental health (Feuerstein, 1998). Yoga's spiritual and meditative focus may not be as prominent in modern-day Western yoga, but the threads of these foci remain evident. Yoga has been employed in a variety of physical and mental health disorders as well as various settings. From depression to cancer and located within the hospital or in remote locations post-disaster, there has been significant interest in the potential benefits of yoga over the past decade.

Yoga has been used outside the health care arena primarily in disaster survivors. This implementation, while potentially broadly beneficial to all survivors, is best considered a preventive measure against the development of trauma- and stressor-related disorders post-disaster. These studies have evaluated yoga as an intervention to help manage elevated anxiety and distress in individuals who have experienced earthquakes, floods, and tsunamis (Descilo et al., 2010; Telles et al., 2010; Thordardottir et al., 2014). Studies to date have not been statistically significant compared to wait-list controls but have trended toward positive. The lack of positive findings is not entirely surprising given the use of convenience samples and the relatively small sample sizes in these studies.

Yoga delivered in health care settings is most often as a treatment rather than as a preventive measure or for general wellness. The breadth of research on yoga in hospital settings is substantial when considering all disorders but is relatively limited for trauma- and stressor-related disorders. More specifically, health care setting–delivered yoga has been studied exclusively for PTSD, though extrapolations about utility across the range of trauma- and stressor-related disorders is common among yoga practitioners. This potential benefit across trauma- and stressor-related disorders has readily apparent theoretical underpinnings. Yoga incorporates social interaction, physical activity, and meditation, all of which are known to decrease stress. Recent research has further substantiated this benefit, but the research remains relatively limited and is complicated by the variation in yoga practices used by different studies. As with other CAM treatments, yoga is most well studied in PTSD with no specific studies in adjustment disorder or acute stress disorder. Most notable among these is a recent study by Rhodes and colleagues (2016). Rhodes and colleagues performed a long-term follow-up on 49 of 60 women with chronic PTSD roughly 1.5 years after participation in a RCT of 10 sessions of yoga versus supportive women's health education. While group assignment in the original study was not a significant predictor, frequency of continuing yoga significantly predicted decreased PTSD and depressive symptoms and increased likelihood of a loss of PTSD diagnosis (Rhodes et al., 2016). This finding is particularly compelling given a long-standing criticism of most CAM modalities is the lack of evidence for sustained benefit. Similarly, a recent study of a 12-week yoga-based group psychotherapy in 8- to 12-year-old boys with a history of trauma showed clinically and statistically meaningful improvements on parental ratings of interpersonal strength, intrapersonal strength, and family involvement scores (Beltran et al., 2016). Prior to these studies, Macy and Colleagues (2015) performed a meta-review of existing literature that pointed to yoga for trauma and related mental health problems. This comprehensive look at the body of literature for yoga found that the evidence for yoga is encouraging but preliminary and recommends yoga as an ancillary treatment. It is unlikely that the two studies subsequent to this review would significantly alter the overall findings beyond reinforcing the term "encouraging." For clinicians treating individuals with trauma- and stressor-related disorders, the utility of yoga is likely greatest within an overall treatment plan inclusive of evidence-based treatments and as an activity that can be continued long after clinician-involved treatments have been concluded.

Creative Arts Therapy

Creative arts therapy is an umbrella term that captures a wide variety of therapies including art, drama, singing, dancing, and writing, among others. These therapies utilize the chosen medium, for example art, as a means of facilitation toward a therapeutic goal and are a very well-liked form of therapy (Forzoni et al., 2010). The creative arts therapies, like the majority of CAM treatments, have very limited evidence of benefit in trauma- and stressor-related disorders. To date there is only one study evaluating any of the creative arts therapies in a trauma- and stressor-related disorder. This study, by Wang and colleagues (2015), found no difference between creative art therapy and wait-list control for the treatment of PTSD. While research to date has not found evidence of benefit, these activities may provide a compelling space for individuals to explore meaning within the context of their traumatic experiences as well as their broader lives both before and after trauma. Arguably, creative arts therapy provides a unique means of expression and communication (Arvahami, 2005) separate from the traditional verbal and narrative forms of therapy. For trauma- and stressor-related disorders more broadly, further research is warranted, and indeed some ongoing research efforts aim to change this deficit in our understanding. Currently there is little evidence suggesting that clinicians should recommend any of the creative arts therapy given the lack of evidence, but the low risk combined with the theoretical benefit argues that integration into a broader treatment plan may be warranted for those individuals interested in such activities.

Meditation

Meditation has been defined as mental training through regimented practice that facilitates well-being and emotional regulation. These practices have been around nearly as long as the written record of humanity and are frequently integral parts of religious practices. Two of the most notable types of meditation are mantra meditation and mindfulness meditation. "Mantra" comes from Sanskrit origins and means to cross the mind and is the most common form of meditation in religious practices. Mantra meditation is most often the practice of purposeful repetition of a chosen word or phrase (silently or aloud) in order to achieve a state of inner peace.

The most well-studied form of mantra meditation is the mantram repetition program (MRP). This program is meant to facilitate a transformative sense of peace (Easwaran, 2008). Individuals are encouraged to use MRP frequently (e.g., at least daily) in order to achieve a level of skill with their mantra and then uses their mantra as a means of re-establishing the sense of peace when confronted with stressors or when symptoms arise. The research to date has focused on the use of MRP as an adjunctive therapy rather than as a stand-alone treatment and primarily on the treatment of PTSD rather than the broader group of trauma- and stressor-related disorders. For individuals with PTSD, MRP has been shown to divert attention away from triggering events (Borman et al., 2013), increase well-being (Lang et al., 2012), and increase self-efficacy (Oman & Bormann, 2015). The research to date combined with the portability, tolerability, and very low risk make MRP a compelling option for those clinicians seeking an adjunctive approach to an individual's primary treatment regimen.

Mindfulness meditation, often referred to simply as mindfulness, is the use of meditation strategies to achieve a present-centered, open-minded, nonjudgmental awareness. These meditation strategies include myriad ancient traditions as well as more recent systematized approaches to mental health care. Mindfulness-based stress reduction (MBSR), developed originally for individuals with chronic pain, is an eight-week course of two-hour sessions followed by a day-long retreat all focused on learning to maintain a kind and nonjudgmental attitude in one's present centered awareness. Through focused awareness MBSR allows individuals with PTSD to manage unpleasant thoughts or sensations (Kearney et al., 2013). Mindfulness-based relapse prevention, developed for substance disorders, uses meditation techniques in conjunction with cognitive behavioral skills to increase an individual's ability to sustain abstinence. Mindfulness-based cognitive therapy (MBCT) focuses on awareness of thoughts and emotions, viewing these as moments or events rather than an accurate assessment of reality. MBCT has been shown to be beneficial in depressive disorders but has yet to be sufficiently studied in trauma- and stressor-related disorders. In addition to these mindfulness meditation strategies, there are more general meditation approaches that have been used in trauma- and stressor-related disorders. Notably, one of the only CAM studies in adjustment disorders is a study investigating the use of meditation in adjustment disorder with anxiety and depression. The study used a model of yoga meditation with weekly sessions for 28 weeks and found significant difference between the experimental and control groups (Srivastava et al., 2011). In general, the mindfulness approaches should be considered as potential adjunctive treatments for trauma- and stressor-related disorders. Further research is needed before a more firm comment about efficacy can be made regarding mindfulness therapies.

ALTERNATIVE THERAPIES

Alternative Pharmacology

Alternative pharmacology includes off-label use of Food and Drug Administration (FDA)-approved medications, substances of abuse, nutraceuticals, synthetic versions of naturally occurring substances, and herbal supplements. Given the breadth of this topic, readers interested in a more thorough discussion of alternative pharmacology for trauma- and stressor-related disorders (i.e., PTSD) are directed to McLay et al. (2016). This section reviews two medications with off-label use for trauma- and stressor-related disorders with recent research.

Cycloserine (Seromycin) is a cyclic analogue of D-alanine approved for the treatment of tuberculosis secondary to its inhibition of bacterial wall synthesis enzymes. Cycloserine also appears to be a partial agonist of glycine receptors and enhancer of N-methyl-D-aspartate receptor transmission. This second mechanism of action is likely the relevance to treatment of trauma- and stressor-related disorders. There have been several animal studies evaluating the effect of cycloserine on fear conditioning models. These studies showed enhanced stress-induced behavior extinction (Anthony & Nevins, 1993) and normalization of fear-induced learning (Yamamoto et al., 2008). In addition, several studies have shown that cycloserine facilitated fear extinction in humans as well (Ressler et al., 2004; Hofman et al., 2006). These findings of facilitated fear extinction led researchers to investigate whether cycloserine could also facilitate fear extinction in psychotherapy. The hope was that adding this compound would increase the overall effect of psychotherapy. The general approach in studies to date has been to give 50 to 100mg of cycloserine roughly one hour prior to the start of psychotherapy. Results to date have been mixed at best with only one study showing clearly positive results. A study of cycloserine prior to virtual reality exposure therapy showed earlier and greater improvements compared to controls (Difede et al., 2014). A similar trial by Rothbaum et al. (2014) found no difference between cyclosporine and placebo. De Kleine et al. (2012) also found no difference between cyclosporine and placebo though their study augmented imaginal exposure rather than virtual reality. The most negative study to date comes from Litz and colleagues (2012) which showed that participants receiving cycloserine did significantly worse compared to controls during a shortened course of imaginal exposure. Given these mixed results, clinicians should be very deliberate when considering this medication for PTSD or the other trauma- and stressor-related disorders. Cycloserine is best considered as a second-line treatment for patients who do not respond to psychotherapy alone or have a limited initial response to therapy but are hesitant about medication as a primary means of treatment.

Ketamine, an FDA-approved anesthetic agent, similar in structure to phencyclidine, with known abuse potential, has been of substantial interest to the trauma- and stressor-related disorders community in recent years. The first studies regarding the use of ketamine were observational studies that found worsened PTSD in trauma victims who were given ketamine as a part of their anesthetic regimen (Schonenberg et al., 2005). This worsening was in line with the known ketamine side effect of increased dissociation. Despite these concerns and this early observational research, there was data arising from depression research suggestive of significant improvements with ketamine. Several studies further investigated the use of ketamine in trauma- and stressor-related disorders and found improved outcomes in those who received ketamine (McGhee et al., 2008; Pokorny 2012; Zeng et al., 2013). To date there has been only one RCT of ketamine in PTSD though a number are underway. Feder et al. (2014) demonstrated that a single dose of intravenous ketamine was associated with rapid and significant reduction in PTSD symptom severity in comparison to midazolam. These effects showed some diminishment over time. While compelling data, there is much remaining to understand about the use of ketamine before regular clinical use is warranted. The most pressing of these questions is what follow-up administration of ketamine will be required, if any, to maintain the benefits seen after the initial single-dose administration. Currently there is no evidence that ketamine is warranted for any trauma- and stressor-related disorder other than PTSD, and even in PTSD clinicians should take care in recommending this treatment until further research can clarify remaining uncertainties.

Acupuncture

Acupuncture is the practice of needle insertion into specific body points, often referred to as meridian acupuncture points, as a means to alleviate suffering or treat a variety of disorders. Acupuncture has shown benefit in a number of mental health disorders including anxiety disorders and substance abuse disorders, though the mechanism behind this benefit remains unknown. Recently acupuncture has received much attention for the treatment of trauma- and stressor-related disorders. This interest has resulted in several reviews, a few small trials, and most importantly one substantive RCT. In the 2013 review by Kim et al., the authors rightly conclude that the evidence for acupuncture in PTSD is encouraging but requires further research. Subsequent to that review there was a well-designed RCT by Engel et al. (2014). This trial evaluated acupuncture for PTSD in eight sessions over four weeks compared to treatment as usual. Engel et al. found significant improvements after 4 weeks of treatment at 12 weeks after treatment completion. These improvements were in PTSD symptoms, depression ratings, pain, and overall physical and mental health functioning. One limitation of this study was that the population was a primarily male, young, and otherwise healthy military population. Thus, the generalizability of the findings to other traumatized populations is somewhat limited. In general, the findings are supportive of the use of acupuncture, and, when taken in conjunction with the other research showing benefit in anxiety and substance use, there is a compelling case for consideration of this treatment for PTSD.

Alternative Delivery Methods

Alternative delivery methods are best defined as the use of new technologies and communication platforms for delivery of traditional interventions such as psychotherapy. This group is unique in that some of the interventions are evidence-based treatments with significant research and evidence, but the means in which these treatments are provided is different enough to consider these almost entirely new treatments. Telemental health, probably the most widely used of these methods, has seen substantial increases in use along with a growing body of evidence for use in a number of mental health conditions including depression and anxiety (Andrews et al., 2010). The form of telemental health can vary widely from videoconferencing where the communication between therapist and patient is live to computerized interventions with varying levels of therapist engagement. The more limited the interaction with the therapist, the more this form of telemental health is computerized and provides engagement with patient by the software itself. A number of these computerized therapies have been developed for the treatment of PTSD including Interapy (Lange et al., 2003) and DE-STRESS (Engel et al., 2015). With the increasing use of smartphones has come the creation of smartphone apps for the treatment of a variety of mental health disorders including PTSD. While these means of treatment are still under study, it appears that they are acceptable alternatives to traditional in-clinic care, especially when patients have significant difficulties making it to the clinic or live in remote areas with limited mental health support. With each advance in technology and each new platform for communication, we will see attempts to use that communication means to further address mental health and extend the reach of care to additional patients.

CONCLUSION

For trauma- and stressor-related disorders, the CAM treatments have, across the board, been proposed as a potential means of treating PTSD. Among these treatments proposed as potentially effective for PTSD, the evidence is limited though some have ongoing investigations which may shed light on the question of efficacy. Few have been considered for acute stress disorder or adjustment disorder. As a group, these modalities have little to no rigorous evidence of efficacy in any of the trauma- and stressor-related disorders, but conversely there is no evidence that they should not be considered as an augmentation strategy or as an alternative when many of the well-established therapies have failed or when a patient is resistant to traditional psychotherapy or pharmacotherapy. Despite the limited evidence, these treatments remain compelling options for both clinicians and patients in part because they are very low risk and quite a few are enjoyable activities.

REFERENCES

Andrews G, Cuijpers P, Craske MG, McEvoy P, & Titov N. (2010). Computer therapy for the anxiety and depressive disorders is effective, acceptable, and practical health care: A meta-analysis. *PLoS One*. 5(10):e13196.

Anthony EW, & Nevins ME. (1993). Anxiolytic like effects of N-Methyl-D-Aspartate associated glycine receptor ligands in the rat potentiated startle test. *Eur J Pharmacol*. 250(2):317–324.

Arnold JC. (1995). Therapy dogs and the dissociative patient: Preliminary observations. *Dissociation*. 8:247–252.

Avrahami D. (2005). Visual art therapy's unique contribution in the treatment of post-traumatic stress disorders. *J Trauma Dissocation*. 6(4):5–38.

Beltran M, Brown-Elhillali AN, Held AR, Ryce PC, Ofonedu ME, Hoover DW, & Ensor KM, Belcher HM. (2016). Yoga-based psychotherapy groups for boys exposed to trauma in urban settings. *Altern Ther Health Med*. 22(1):39–46.

Benedek DM & Wynn GH (Eds.). (2016). *Complementary and alternative medicine for PTSD*. New York: Oxford University Press.

Bormann JE, Hurst S, & Kelly A. (2013). Responses to mantram repetition program from veterans with posttraumatic stress disorder: A qualitative analysis. *J Rehabil Res Dev*. 50(6):769–784.

de Kleine RA, Hendriks GJ, Kusters WJ, Broekman TG, & van Minnen A. (2012). A randomized placebo-controlled trial of D-cycloserine to enhance exposure therapy for posttraumatic stress disorder. *Biol Psychiatry*. 71(11):962–968.

Descillo T, Vedamurtachar A, Gerbarg P, et al. (2010). Effects of a yoga breath intervention alone and in combination with an exposure therapy for post-traumatic stress disorder and depression in survivors of the 2004 South-East Asia tsunami. *Acta Psychiatr Scand*. 121(4):289–300.

Difede J, Cukor J, Wyka K, et al. (2014). D-cycloserine augmentation of exposure therapy for post-traumatic stress disorder: A pilot randomized clinical trial. *Neuropsychopharmacology*. 39(56): 1052–1058.

Duvall J & Kaplan R. (2014). Enhancing the well-being of veterans using extended group-based nature recreation experiences. *J Rehab Res Dev.* 51(5):685–696.

Earles JL, Vernon LL, & Yetz JP. (2015). Equine-assisted therapy for anxiety and posttraumatic stress symptoms. *J Trauma Stress.* 28(2):149–152.

Easwaran, E. (2008). *The mantram handbook* (5th ed.). Tomales, CA: Nilgiri Press.

Engel C, Cordova E, Benedek DM, et al. (2014). Randomized effectiveness trial of a brief course of acupuncture for posttraumatic stress disorder. *Med Care.* 52(12):S57–S64.

Engel CC, Litz B, Magruder KM, et al. (2015). Delivery of Self Training and Education for Stressful Situations (DESTRESS-PC): A randomized trial of nurse assisted online self-management of PTSD in primary care. *Gen Hosp Psychiatr.* 37(4):323–328.

Feder A, Parides MK, Murrough JW, et al. (2014). Efficacy of intravenous ketamine for treatment of chronic posttraumatic stress disorder: A randomized clinical trial. *JAMA Psychiatry.* 71(6):681–688.

Fine AH. (ed.). (2000). *Handbook on animal-assisted therapy: Theoretical foundations and guidelines for practice.* San Diego, CA: Academic Press.

Feuerstein G. (1998). *The yoga tradition: Its history, literature, philosophy, and practice.* Prescott, AZ: Hohm Press.

Forzoni S, Perez M, Martignetti A, Crispino S. (2010). Art therapy with cancer patients during chemotherapy sessions: An analysis of the patients' perception of helpfulness. *Palliat Support Care.* 8(1):41–48.

Hofman SG, Meuret AE, Smits JA, et al. (2006). Augmentation of exposure therapy with D-cycloserine for social anxiety disorder. *Arch Gen Psychiatry.* 63(3):298–304.

Hyer L, Boyd S, Scurfield R, Smith D, & Burke J. (1996). Effects of Outward Bound experience as an adjunct to inpatient PTSD treatment of war veterans. *J Clin Psychol.* 52:263–278.

Katcher AH. (1981). Interactions between people and their pets: Form and function. In B Fogle (Ed.). *Interrelations between people and pets.* Springfield, IL: Thomas Press.

Kearney D, Malte C, McManus C, et al. (2013). Loving-kindness meditation for posttraumatic stress disorder: A randomized controlled pilot study. *J Clin Psychol.* 69(1):14–27.

Kim YD, Heo I, Shin BC, et al. (2013). Acupuncture for posttraumatic stress disorder: A systematic review of randomized controlled trials and prospective clinical trials. *Evid Base Complement Alternat Med.* 2013:615857

Lang A., Strauss J, Bomyea J, et al. (2012). The theoretical and empirical basis for meditation as an intervention for PTSD. *Behav Modif.* 36(6):759–786.

Lange A, Rietdijk D, Hudcovicova M, van de Ven JP, Schrieken B, & Emmelkamp PM. (2003). Interapy: A controlled randomized trial of the standardized treatment of posttraumatic stress through the internet. *J Consult Clin Psychol.* 71(5):901–909.

Lass-Henneman J, Peyk P, Streb M, et al. (2014). Presence of a dog reduces subjective but not physiological stress response to an analog trauma. *Front Psychol.* 5:1–7.

Lanning BA, & Krenek N. (2013). Guest editorial: Examining effects of equine-assisted activities to help combat veterans improve quality of life. *J Rehabil Res Dev.* 50(8):vii–xii.

Litz BT, Salters-Pedneault K, Steenkamp MM, et al. (2012). A randomized placebo-controlled trial of D-cycloserine and exposure therapy for posttraumatic stress disorder. *J Psychiatr Res.* 46(9):1184–1190.

Macy RJ, Jones E, Graham LM, & Roach L. (2015). Yoga for trauma and related mental health problems: A meta-review with clinical and service recommendations. *Trauma Violence Abuse.* Pii: 1524838015620834.

McGhee LL, Maani CV, Garza TH, Gaylord KM, & Black IH. (2008). The correlation between ketamine and posttraumatic stress disorder in burned service members. *J Trauma Inj Infect Crit Care.* 64(2):S195–S199.

McLay RN, Miletich DM, Brown NA, & Ross L. (2016). Alternative medicine pharmacology. In DM Benedek & GH Wynn (Eds.), *Complementary and alternative medicine for PTSD.* New York: Oxford University Press.

Nevins R, Finch S, Hickling EG, & Barnett SD. (2013). The Saratoga WarHorse project: A case study of the treatment of psychological distress in a veteran of Operation Iraqi Freedom. *Adv Mind Body Med.* 27(4):22–25.

Oman D, & Bormann J. (2015). Mantram repetition fosters self-efficacy in veterans for managing PTSD: A randomized trial. *Psychol Relig Spirit.* 7(1):34–45.

Pokorny ME. (2012). Experiences of military CRNAs with service personnel who are emerging from general anesthesia. *AANA J.* 80(4):260–261.

Ressler KJ, Rothbaum BO, Tannenbaum L, Anderson P, Graap K, Zimand E, Hodges L, & Davis M. (2004). Cognitive enhancers as adjuncts to psychotherapy: use of D-cycloserine in phobic individuals to facilitate extinction of fear. *Arch Gen Psychiatry.* 61(11):1136–1144.

Rhodes A, Spinazzola J, & van der Kolk B. (2016). Yoga for adult women with chronic PTSD: A long-term follow-up study. *J Altern Complement Med.* 22(3):189–196.

Rothbaum BO, Price M, Jovanovic T, et al. (2014). A randomized, double-blind evaluation of D-cycloserine or alprazolam combined with virtual reality exposure therapy for posttraumatic stress disorder in Iraq and Afghanistan war veterans. *Am J Psychiatry.* 171(6):640–648.

Schonenberg M, Reichwald U, Domes G, Badke A, & Hautzinger M. (2005). Effects of peritraumatic ketamine medication on early and sustained posttraumatic stress symptoms in moderately injured accident victims. *Psychopharmacology.* 182(3):420–425.

Srivastava M, Talukdar U, & Lahan V. (2011). Meditation for the management of adjustment disorder anxiety and depression. *Complement Ther Clin Pract.* 17(4):241–245.

Telles S, Singh N, Joshi M, et al. (2010). Post traumatic stress symptoms and heart rate variability in Bihar flood survivors following yoga: A randomized controlled study. *BMC Psychiatry.* 10:18.

Thordardottir K, Gudmundsdottir R, Zoega H, et al. (2014). Effects of yoga practice on stress-related symptoms in the aftermath of an earthquake: A community-based controlled trial. *Complement Ther Med. 22*(2):226–234.

U.S. Department of Justice (2011). ADA requirements: Service animals. Retrieved from https://www.ada.gov/service_animals_2010.pdf

Vella EJ, Milligan B, & Bennett JL. (2013). Participation in outdoor recreation program predicts improved psychosocial well-being among veterans with post-traumatic stress disorder: A pilot study. *Mil Med.* 178(3):254–260.

Wang X, Lan C, Chen J, Wang W, Zhang H, Li L. (2015). Creative arts program as an intervention for PTSD: A randomized clinical trial with motor vehicle survivors. *Int J Clin Exp Med. 8*(8):13585–13591.

Wynn GH (2015). Complementary and alternative medicines approaches in the treatment of PTSD. *Curr Psychiatry Rep.* 17:62.

Yamamoto S, Morinobu S, Fuchikami M, Kurata A, Kozuru T, & Yamawaki S. (2008). Effects of single prolonged stress and D-cycloserine on contextual fear extinction and hippocampal NMDA receptor expression in a rat model of PTSD. *Neuropsychopharmacology.* 33(9):2108–2116.

Zeng MC, Niciu MJ, Luckenbaugh DA, et al. (2013). Acute stress symptoms do not worsen in posttraumatic stress disorder and abuse with a single subanesthetic dose of ketamine. *Biol Psychiatry.* 73(12):e37–e38.

25

Device-Based Treatment for PTSD

MENG-CHEN LO, MARIE-FRANCE MARIN, ALIK S. WIDGE, AND MOHAMMED R. MILAD

INTRODUCTION

Previous chapters have discussed the various treatment modalities for posttraumatic stress disorder (PTSD) including medication, exposure-based therapy, and cognitive behavioral therapy. Device-based neuromodulation is an emerging tool with great potential for significant scientific and clinical implications for a number of mental disorders. Major advantages of neuromodulation over pharmacological treatments include target specificity to induce localized effects and affecting brain functions at the circuit level by modulating connectivity between brain regions (Likhtik, Stujenske, Topiwala, Harris, & Gordon, 2013; Quinn et al., 2015). This latter advantage is particularly useful given that most psychiatric disorders appear to result from a malfunction of multiple brain regions within the same functional circuit. One common feature of the various neuromodulation techniques is that they all deliver electro-magnetic pulses into the brain via invasive or noninvasive electrodes and with various timing and stimulation parameters (Marin & Milad, 2015). The stimulation is thought to work as a "brain pacemaker" that either activates or inactivates targeted brain regions to restore normal homeostasis. There have been significant recent efforts to explore the clinical utility of device-based approaches for the treatment of mood, anxiety disorders, and to a limited extent PTSD (Burger et al., 2016; Osuch et al., 2009). This chapter outlines the scientific underpinnings and rationale for various device-based treatments of PTSD, highlights positive results of studies in other mental disorders, and summarizes the limited clinical data related specifically to the treatment of PTSD and other trauma- and stressor-related disorders (TSRD) to date.

A key aspect of the success of device-based neuromodulation is knowing when and where to stimulate. It is therefore important to study PTSD pathology and to identify methods to implement device-based treatments. A Pavlovian fear conditioning paradigm has been often used to study fear-related disorders including PTSD as well as the basic mechanisms of fear acquisition and extinction, and has been reviewed in prior chapters in this book. Briefly, in a classical fear conditioning experiment, the subject learns that a tone (conditioned stimuli [CS+]) predicts an aversive event (unconditioned stimulus [US]). During this phase, the subject expresses a conditioned fear response to the CS+. In the following session, the CS+ is no longer paired with the US, which leads to gradual extinction of the conditioned response. This is the extinction learning phase. The memory of this extinction can be further assessed after a delayed period of time in a phase referred to as extinction recall or retention. The paradigm has been widely used to study the underlying mechanism of PTSD (Rougemont-Bücking et al., 2011) as several pathological markers from PTSD can be measured using the paradigm. First, one key feature of PTSD is the failure to extinguish fear (Hermans, Craske, Mineka, & Lovibond, 2006; Milad, Rauch, Pitman, & Quirk, 2006; Shvil et al., 2014). Patients with PTSD are unable to dissociate the conditioned cue from the aversive event and repeatedly express fear in the absence of the aversive event. Behavioral exposure therapy treats patients with PTSD by helping them to gradually reduce fear toward the conditioned stimuli (Foa, 2011). This process parallels the fear extinction paradigm described. Second, studies also showed that patients with PTSD suffer from deficient extinction memory recall, where the formed extinction memory fails to consolidate and transfer to the long-term memory system (Marin et al., 2016; Milad et al., 2009). This behavior can also be modeled from the fear extinction recall phase of the fear conditioning paradigm.

The fear conditioning paradigm provides a way to measure fear-related behaviors and to evaluate the effects of device-based treatments. Since multiple brain regions play roles in fear conditioning, the optimal location for the application of electrical stimulus of device-based treatments remains an open question. From neuroimaging studies, it was observed that brain structures involved in fear are similar between humans and animals. Some key regions in the fear circuits are the amygdala, hippocampus, ventromedial prefrontal cortex (vmPFC; human homolog of infralimbic cortex [IL] in rat) and dorsal anterior cingulate cortex (dACC; human homolog of prelimbic cortex [PL] in rat). The amygdala modulates the acquisition and extinction of fear (LeDoux, 2003). The hippocampus modulates contextual information relevant to both fear learning and extinction (Bouton, Westbrook, Corcoran, & Maren, 2006). The PL and the dACC are essential for encoding and expressing fear (Burgos-Robles, Vidal-Gonzalez, Santini, & Quirk, 2007; Lebrón, Milad, & Quirk, 2004) whereas the IL and the vmPFC are essential for the acquisition and consolidation of fear extinction and retention (Baker, Bisby, & Richardson, 2016; Milad & Quirk, 2002). Human neuroimaging studies have also provided useful observations on the pathological features within those brain regions for patients with PTSD. Compared to trauma-exposed healthy controls, patients who suffer from PTSD exhibit higher activation of the amygdala and lower activation in the vmPFC during the late phase of extinction learning (Milad et al., 2009). During extinction recall phase, patients with PTSD show impaired recall (Marin et al., 2016; Milad et al., 2009). Functional imaging results demonstrated hypoactivation of the vmPFC and the hippocampus as well as hyperactivation of the amygdala and the dACC during extinction recall (Milad et al., 2009; Rougemont-Bücking et al., 2011).

Recent efforts have targeted strengthening memory consolidation during extinction learning as a possible treatment principle for PTSD. Device-based interventions have been paired with the fear conditioning paradigm to assess their effects in improving fear responses (Marin, Camprodon, Dougherty, & Milad, 2014). In this chapter, we discuss several device-based intervention modalities and discuss how they can provide a deeper understanding of the fear circuits associated with PTSD. Table 25.1 summarizes several device-based treatments that are discussed in the chapter.

DEEP BRAIN STIMULATION

Deep brain stimulation (DBS) is an invasive neuromodulation technique in which electrodes are implanted in the brain region of interest and deliver chronic, high-frequency electrical pulses (Rosa et al., 2012). Outside of psychiatry, DBS has been safely implemented to treat pain relief (Schultz et al., 2012), seizure (Heck et al., 2014) and Parkinson's disease (Little et al., 2013; Rosin et al., 2011). DBS is of interest for treating psychiatric disorders because it can target very specific brain regions and is able to reach subcortical areas, where most of the key structures in the fear circuit are located (Gross & Lozano, 2000). To date, DBS has been most extensively studied in depression and obsessive-compulsive disorder (OCD; Dougherty & Widge, 2017; Widge, Arulpragasam, Deckersbach, & Dougherty, 2015; Widge & Dougherty, 2015). The majority of published DBS studies target two regions: the ventral capsule/ventral striatum (VC/VS; Bergfield et al.,2016; Dougherty et al.,2015;

TABLE 25.1. DEVICE-BASED TREATMENTS FOR MOOD DISORDERS

Device-Based Interventions	Surgery Required?	Stimulation Location	Form of Stimulation	Tested in Humans?
Deep brain stimulation	Yes	Deep brain structures (e.g., ventral striatum; subgenual cingulate gyrus)	Electrical	Yes
Vagus nerve stimulation	Yes	Vagus nerve	Electrical	Yes
Transcranial direct current stimulation	No	Dorsolateral prefrontal cortex	Electrical	Yes
Transcranial magnetics stimulation	No	Dorsolateral prefrontal cortex	Magnetic	Yes
Optogenetics	Yes	Any brain structures	Optical	No

Greenberg et al., 2010) and the subgenual cingulate gyrus (Cg25; Holtzheimer et al., 2017, Mayberg et al., 2005). The initial open-label clinical study targeting Cg25 was positive with a 43% remission rate after six years of patient follow-up for major depressive disorder (MDD; Kennedy et al., 2011; Mayberg et al., 2009). DBS targeting the VC/CS also showed positive results in an open-label clinical trial with a 72% response rate in OCD patients (Greenberg et al., 2010). In fact, the only invasive brain stimulation treatment available today in the US market is VC/VS DBS for OCD patients. The treatment holds a Humanitarian Device Exemption from the Food and Drug Administration (FDA), which demonstrates the safety and feasibility of using DBS in the clinic (Garnaat et al., 2014).

The positive results of DBS in relieving symptoms of OCD and MDD in humans have provided motivation to study whether DBS can also be used for PTSD. Recently, DBS has been combined with the fear conditioning paradigm to induce changes in fear extinction response in rats (Rodriguez-Romaguera, Monte, & Quirk, 2012). The results demonstrated that stimulation of the dorsal ventral striatum (VS; the rat homolog of human VS/VC) during extinction training reduced fear expression and strengthened extinction memory, whereas DBS in the ventral VS impaired fear extinction. Follow-up experiments showed that the ventral-VS and dorsal-VS projected to different brain subregions in the prefrontal cortex, which is one of the key structures in the fear circuits identified from both animal and human research (Vidal-Gonzalez, Vidal-Gonzalez, Rauch, & Quirk, 2006). Furthermore, several studies also demonstrated that the improved extinction memory recall was only observed when DBS was given during the extinction learning phase (Rodriguez-Romaguera, Do-Monte, Tanimura, Quirk, & Haber, 2015). The results implied that DBS might help potentiate extinction memory formation and that extinction memory can last longer and be retrieved after an extended period of time.

Other than DBS in the ventral striatum, researchers have also applied DBS directly in several key structures in the fear circuits using animal models. DBS applied to the hippocampus during extinction training enhanced extinction learning, as indicated by improved recall performance (Farinelli, Deschaux, Hugues, Thevenet, & Garcia, 2006). Likewise, DBS in amygdala modulated fear behavior in rats (Stidd, Vogelsang, Krahl, Langevin, & Fellous, 2013). Results from animal studies are promising, having demonstrated that DBS can improve fear extinction and retention, which is a common deficit in patients with PTSD. However, currently, there are no clinical trials using DBS in PTSD. Recently, a case report has been published describing the design of a Phase I pilot study (Koek et al., 2014). More studies such as these are needed to refine the DBS approach for PTSD, including optimizing the stimulation parameters and identifying suitable targets, before these techniques can be safely translated into the clinic.

VAGUS NERVE STIMULATION

Vagus nerve stimulation (VNS) is an invasive procedure where electrodes are surgically placed in the extracranial portion of the left vagus nerve at the neck level. The mechanism by which VNS works is not fully understood, but the hypothesized mechanism of action is that the stimulation indirectly influences the activation of specific brain regions such as the nucleus of the solitary tract (NTS) through the primary afferent pathway of the nerve (Frisina, Haroutunian, & Libow, 2009; Rosa & Lisanby, 2012). The NTS relays information to other brain regions through different routes. Within the fear circuits, for example, there have been indications that NTS projects directly to the amygdala and the hippocampus (George et al., 2000). Stimulation in the vagus nerve increases norepinephrine release in the cortex, hippocampus, and amygdala through the NTS projections. Several studies have shown that norepinephrine infusion in the amygdala induces better fear extinction learning in rats and amygdala-potentiated hippocampus activity, which enhances memory consolidation (McGaugh, McIntyre, & Power, 2002; McGaugh & Roozendaal, 2002). These early findings have suggested that VNS could be a promising approach to alter fear behavior by modulating adrenergic activity in the fear circuits.

Using animal models, researchers have investigated the effects of VNS in combination with the fear conditioning paradigm (Peña, Engineer, & McIntyre, 2013). One study used VNS during fear extinction learning and studied whether VNS could promote retention of fear extinction memory (Peña et al., 2013). The rats were trained on an auditory fear-conditioning task and went through fear extinction training. One group of rats received VNS paired with CS whereas the other group received VNS without being paired with CS. The results showed that VNS paired with CS potentiated fear extinction memory, as indicated by the lower freezing levels in response to the CS. The results suggested that VNS could alter fear behaviors and how VNS is applied (i.e., in pairing with the CS or not) is essential to achieve such effects.

In humans, VNS has been evaluated and approved as a treatment for drug-resistant depression and epilepsy (Bajbouj et al., 2010; George et al., 2008; Rush et al., 2005). Despite promising results from animal research in the fear circuits, it is still unclear whether VNS can promote extinction learning and retention in humans. One human pilot study used VNS in patients with treatment-resistant mental disorders such as OCD, panic disorders, and PTSD (George et al., 2008). The results showed some improvement, but the response rates were low. Furthermore, the sample size of the study was too low (<10) to draw any statistically significant conclusions. A more recent study assessed whether transcutaneous VNS can accelerate fear extinction learning and retention in healthy subjects (Burger et al., 2016). The subjects received either VNS or sham VNS stimulation during the extinction learning phase. The results demonstrated that VNS-treated subjects exhibited accelerated fear extinction learning, but this did not lead to better retention of the extinction memory the next day. These mixed results raise concerns of using VNS for fear-related disorders in humans. More studies in both humans and animals will be needed to investigate the mechanisms of VNS in the brain and to confirm its feasibility as a therapeutic tool for psychiatric disorders.

TRANSCRANIAL DIRECT CURRENT STIMULATION

Transcranial direct current stimulation (tDCS) is a noninvasive intervention that delivers extremely low currents (1–2 mA) through the scalp and skull to modulate cortical excitability (Gandiga et al., 2006; Philip et al., 2017; Scholfield, 1990). The system consists of two electrodes soaked with saline solution and placed on the head. The currents flow from one electrode (anode) to another (cathode). Although the polarity of the electrical current seems to be an important factor in determining the therapeutic effects of tDCS, the mechanism by which tDCS alters cortical excitability are not well characterized. It is believed that anodal current increases brain excitability via neuron depolarization whereas cathodal current decreases brain excitability via neuron hyperpolarization (Nitsche et al., 2003; Philip et al., 2017).

The application of tDCS has been explored extensively in human cognitive domains and has been found to enhance learning, attention, and working memory (Coffman, Clark, & Parasuraman, 2014; Reis et al., 2009). Those studies highlighted the possibility of tDCS in modulating emotional memories. Motivated from those studies, tDCS in fear has also been explored. One study assessed tDCS in fear (Asthana et al., 2013) from healthy human subjects. The group tested whether applying tDCS on the left dorsolateral prefrontal cortex (dlPFC) after the fear acquisition phase could alter fear consolidation. They found that the cathodal tDCS impaired fear memory consolidation because the subjects failed to recall of the fear memory on the following day. Another study applied anodal tDCS on the right dlPFC after providing a conditioned fear reminder in healthy subjects. The stimulation resulted in an increase in fear expression on the following day compared to the sham group (Mungee et al., 2014). More recently, another group applied tDCS during fear extinction learning. The tDCS was delivered either before and during the first extinction block or before and during the second extinction block. Participants who received tDCS during the first extinction block displayed significantly lower skin conductance reactivity during the late extinction of the second extinction block in comparison to participants who received tDCS during and before the second extinction block. The findings suggested that the timing of the tDCS when paired with the extinction paradigm can affect fear response (Van't Wout et al., 2016). Those studies provide promising results regarding tDCS's ability to affect fear response and suggest that this technique may be useful as a therapeutic intervention for fear-related diseases such as PTSD.

Taking lessons learned from studies in healthy subjects, researchers and clinicians have started to investigate the possibility of using tDCS to treat patients. One randomized, double-blinded clinical trial for depression combined tDCS with an antidepressant drug and observed increased efficacy compared to the standalone treatments (Brunoni et al., 2013). Only one study has investigated the effects of tDCS in patients with PTSD and showed improvement in various emotional performance measures; however, the study size was small (four patients; Saunders et al., 2015). tDCS is advantageous over other device-based neuromodulation methods because it is inexpensive, is easy to use, has fewer side effects, and is relatively safe. However, for these methods to be applied in the clinic, a better understanding of how different tDCS parameters affect fear circuitry are needed, as are clinical trials that evaluate safety and efficacy.

TRANSCRANIAL MAGNETIC STIMULATION

Transcranial magnetic stimulation (TMS) is another noninvasive procedure used to stimulate small brain regions. During TMS, an electromagnetic coil is placed against the patient's scalp (Rossi et al., 2009). The coil produces small electrical currents that activate targeted brain regions under the coil through electromagnetic induction. TMS gained FDA approval as a treatment in the clinic for depression in 2008 (O'Reardon et al., 2007). Another TMS device with deeper stimulation coils was approved later in 2013 (Bersani et al., 2013), particularly for PTSD. To date, TMS has not been approved as a treatment (Osuch et al., 2009).

The mechanism of TMS limits the depth through brain tissue that can be reached. Nevertheless, although TMS might not be able to exert effects directly into subcortical brain regions, it can target more superficial brain regions, where the effects are transmitted transynaptically. In animal research, the IL and PL have been shown to modulate fear. Activation of the IL is particularly important for extinction learning and recall (Fontanez-Nuin, Santini, Quirk, & Porter, 2011; Herry & Garcia, 2002; Milad & Quirk, 2002). Given the well-established consensus of the literature of the human onto analog of the IL, the vmPFC was proposed as a first target for TMS intervention. However, the vmPFC is too deep for TMS to reach. In human research, functional imaging studies have helped to identify an alternative target, the dlPFC. A specific region of dlPFC is linked to the regulation of the conditioned fear response and there is a functional coupling between dlPFC and vmPFC (Delgado, Nearing, LeDoux, & Phelps, 2008), suggesting that the dlPFC might be a promising target to modulate the activity in vmPFC.

Several human studies have been conducted using TMS in dlPFC to treat anxiety or PTSD. One study delivered daily treatments of 10 Hz repetitive TMS (rTMS) to the right dlPFC (Cohen et al., 2004) and demonstrated improved anxiety and avoidance behaviors in PTSD patients. Another study showed more profound effects of TMS in right dlPFC using a 20 Hz stimulation frequency (Boggio et al., 2010). Positive effects have also been reported when delivering low stimulation frequency (1 Hz) to the right dlPFC (Nam, Pae, & Chae, 2013). There are also studies combining TMS with exposure therapy. One group used deep TMS to target the medial prefrontal cortex in patients with PTSD followed by exposure to the traumatic event via the script-driven imagery procedure. The group who received TMS followed by the traumatic event script showed a significant decrease of the intrusive symptom compared to the sham group (Isserles et al., 2013). An exploratory meta-analysis suggested that TMS in dlPFC is an effective treatment for PTSD; however, all the studies only had small numbers of subjects (10 to 20 per group; Boggio et al., 2010; Isserles et al., 2013) and lacked a consensus on the optimal TMS dosages needed to induce therapeutic effects. One pilot randomized study have demonstrated that delivering rTMS to suicidal patients was possible and safe with no worsening of suicidal thinking (George et al., 2014). Future larger scale studies will be required to confirm the safety, feasibility, and underlying mechanisms of TMS as a PTSD treatment option.

OPTOGENETICS AND CLINICAL APPLICABILITY

Optogenetics has attracted extensive attention in recent years as a new device-based neuromodulation intervention (Aston-Jones & Deisseroth, 2013; Steinberg, Christoffel, Deisseroth, & Malenka, 2015). Optogenetics is a biological technique that provides precise control of brain activities through light. The greatest advantage of optogenetics-based techniques is the significant increase in temporal and spatial specificity. In contrast to electrical brain stimulation, which is nonspecific and activates many different cell types within a single nucleus, optogenetics uses genetic tools to introduce nonmammalian ion channels, making specific cells or pathways of interest sensitive to light. Pulses of laser or LED light can then excite or inhibit those cells specifically.

Optogenetics provides a valuable tool to study various structures in the fear circuits, such as amygdala (Andero et al., 2016), hippocampus (Liu et al., 2012), and prefrontal cortex (Do-Monte, Manzano-Nieves, Quiñones-Laracuente, Ramos-Medina, & Quirk, 2015). For example, one study paired optical stimulation of the lateral amygdala (LA) pyramidal neurons with an auditory sensory cue instead of a commonly used aversive stimulus (Andero et al., 2016). Results showed that activation of the LA pyramidal cells served as an US and produced fear. The group suggested that fear learning is instructed by aversive stimulation of the LA pyramidal cells. It has been known in the field that basolateral amygdala (BLA) consists of different subgroups of neurons that modulate differently fear expression and extinction (Herry et al., 2008). One study used optogenetics to target a specific subpopulation of pyramidal neurons within the BLA. Optogenetic stimulation of the neurons during fear training disrupted the fear memory, while stimulation during extinction training enhanced fear memory consolidation (Jasnow et al., 2013). Those studies show how optogenetics can be a useful tool to study the role of the individual neuron population on the overall fear circuit.

To date, optogenetics-based studies have only been carried out in rodents. There is still a long way to go before one can bring optogenetics into the clinic, mainly because the technique requires the genetic modification of cells using viral transfection. Thus, significant safety and ethical concerns still need to be addressed. Even though optogenetics may not be a feasible treatment in humans in the near future, the technique provides a more sophisticated tool to advance our understanding of the fear circuitry. The insights and knowledge learned can then indirectly help improve the applications of those devices described for better and more efficient parameter titrations such as stimulation locations, dosages, and timing.

CONCLUSION

In this chapter, we reviewed several device-based interventions that have potential implications for PTSD. Specifically, evidence from both human and animal studies are emerging and show that these techniques are effective in enhancing fear extinction learning and memory. Despite promising results with each of these techniques, several challenges remain. First, there is still much that is not known about the exact mechanisms by which these techniques operate. Until these mechanisms are more thoroughly investigated, clinical translation will be difficult due to safety concerns. Furthermore, understanding the mechanistic underpinnings of these techniques will be critical to designing appropriate intervention recipes and titrating more suitable parameters such as stimulation dosages and timing. In PTSD, deficits in extinction recall have been widely studied, and therefore studies have attempted to apply stimulation interventions during extinction recall. However, several studies have also tried to apply stimulation during the fear conditioning or recall phases, with promising results (Jasnow et al., 2013). The fear circuit is a complex and heterogeneous system, and therefore more efforts will be needed for optimal treatment. Second, from a clinical perspective, it remains a question as to who, exactly, should receive device-based treatments. Currently, most of the device-based treatments are given to patients who do not respond to pharmacological or behavioral treatments, because the device-based treatments exhibit more severe side effects. However, as the techniques improve over time and prove to be increasingly effective, the decision becomes less clear. Finally, of all of the device-based treatments cited in this chapter, most of them have shown preliminary positive results in PTSD in humans. However, the patient sizes of those studies were small, and therefore it is hard to confirm clinical safety and feasibility of the treatments. Collaboration between neuroscientists and clinicians will be needed to address those questions. These combined efforts will help to provide guidance for effective device performance while keeping safety and ethical concerns in mind to maximize the therapeutic potential of each interventional approach.

REFERENCES

Andero, R., Daniel, S., Guo, J.-D., Bruner, R. C., Seth, S., Marvar, P. J., . . . Ressler, K. J. (2016). Amygdala-dependent molecular mechanisms of the Tac2 pathway in fear learning. *Neuropsychopharmacology*, *41*(11), 2714–2722. http://doi.org/10.1038/npp.2016.77

Asthana, M., Nueckel, K., Mühlberger, A., Neueder, D., Polak, T., Domschke, K., . . . Herrmann, M. J. (2013). Effects of transcranial direct current stimulation on consolidation of fear memory. *Frontiers in Psychiatry*, *4*. http://doi.org/10.3389/fpsyt.2013.00107

Aston-Jones, G., & Deisseroth, K. (2013). Recent advances in optogenetics and pharmacogenetics. *Brain Research*, *1511*, 1–5. http://doi.org/10.1016/j.brainres.2013.01.026

Bajbouj, M., Merkl, A., Schlaepfer, T. E., Frick, C., Zobel, A., Maier, W., . . . Heuser, I. (2010). Two-year outcome of vagus nerve stimulation in treatment-resistant depression. *Journal of Clinical Psychopharmacology*, *30*(3), 273–281. http://doi.org/10.1097/JCP.0b013e3181db8831

Baker, K. D., Bisby, M. A., & Richardson, R. (2016). Impaired fear extinction in adolescent rodents: Behavioural and neural analyses. *Neuroscience & Biobehavioral Reviews*, *70*, 59–73. http://doi.org/10.1016/j.neubiorev.2016.05.019

Bergfeld, I. O., Mantione, M., Hoogendoorn, M. L. C., Ruhé, H. G., Notten, P., Van Laarhoven, J., . . . Denys, D. (2016). Deep brain stimulation of the ventral anterior limb of the internal capsule for treatment-resistant depression. *JAMA Psychiatry*, *73*(5), 456–464. http://doi.org/10.1001/jamapsychiatry.2016.0152

Bersani, F. S., Minichino, A., Enticott, P. G., Mazzarini, L., Khan, N., Antonacci, G., . . . Biondi, M. (2013). Deep transcranial magnetic stimulation as a treatment for psychiatric disorders: A comprehensive review. *European Psychiatry*, *28*(1), 30–39. http://doi.org/10.1016/j.eurpsy.2012.02.006

Boggio, P. S., Rocha, M., Oliveira, M. O., Fecteau, S., Cohen, R. B., Campanhã, C., . . . Fregni, F. (2010). Noninvasive brain stimulation with high-frequency and low-intensity repetitive transcranial magnetic stimulation treatment for posttraumatic stress disorder. *The Journal of Clinical Psychiatry*, *71*(8), 992–999. http://doi.org/10.4088/JCP.08m04638blu

Bouton, M. E., Westbrook, R. F., Corcoran, K. A., & Maren, S. (2006). Contextual and temporal modulation of extinction: Behavioral and biological mechanisms. *Biological Psychiatry*, *60*(4), 352–360 http://doi.org/10.1016/j.biopsych.2005.12.015

Brunoni, A. R., Valiengo, L., Baccaro, A., Zanão, T. a, de Oliveira, J. F., Goulart, A., . . . Fregni, F. (2013). The sertraline vs. electrical current therapy for treating depression clinical study: Results from a factorial, randomized, controlled trial. *JAMA Psychiatry*, *70*(4), 383–391. http://doi.org/10.1001/2013.jamapsychiatry.32

Burger, A. M., Verkuil, B., Van Diest, I., Van der Does, W., Thayer, J. F., & Brosschot, J. F. (2016). The effects of transcutaneous vagus nerve stimulation on conditioned fear extinction in humans. *Neurobiology of Learning and Memory*, *132*, 49–56. http://doi.org/10.1016/j.nlm.2016.05.007

Burgos-Robles, A., Vidal-Gonzalez, I., Santini, E., & Quirk, G. J. (2007). Consolidation of fear extinction requires NMDA receptor-dependent bursting in the ventromedial prefrontal cortex. *Neuron*, *53*(6), 871–880. http://doi.org/10.1016/j.neuron.2007.02.021

Coffman, B. A., Clark, V. P., & Parasuraman, R. (2014). Battery powered thought: Enhancement of attention, learning, and memory in healthy adults using transcranial direct current stimulation. *NeuroImage*, *85*(Pt 3), 895–908. http://doi.org/10.1016/j.neuroimage.2013.07.083

Cohen, H., Kaplan, Z., Kotler, M., Kouperman, I., Moisa, R., & Grisaru, N. (2004). Repetitive transcranial magnetic stimulation of the right dorsolateral prefrontal cortex in posttraumatic stress disorder: A double-blind, placebo-controlled study. *American Journal of Psychiatry*, *161*(3), 515–524. http://doi.org/10.1176/appi.ajp.161.3.515

Delgado, M. R., Nearing, K. I., LeDoux, J. E., & Phelps, E. A. (2008). Neural circuitry underlying the regulation of conditioned fear and its relation to extinction. *Neuron*, *59*(5), 829–838. http://doi.org/10.1016/j.neuron.2008.06.029

Do-Monte, F. H., Manzano-Nieves, G., Quiñones-Laracuente, K., Ramos-Medina, L., & Quirk, G. J. (2015). Revisiting the role of infralimbic cortex in fear extinction with optogenetics. *The Journal of Neuroscience*, *35*(8), 3607–3615. http://doi.org/10.1523/JNEUROSCI.3137-14.2015

Dougherty, D. D., Rezai, A. R., Carpenter, L. L., Howland, R. H., Bhati, M. T., O'Reardon, J. P., . . . Malone Jr., D. A. (2015). A randomized sham-controlled trial of deep brain stimulation of the ventral capsule/ventral striatum for chronic treatment-resistant depression. *Biological Psychiatry*, *78*(4), 240–248. http://doi.org/10.1016/j.biopsych.2014.11.023

Dougherty, D. D., Widge, A. S. (2017). Neurotherapeutic interventions for psychiatric illness. *Harvard Review of Psychiatry*, *25*(6), 253–255. http://doi.org/10.1097/HRP.0000000000000174

Farinelli, M., Deschaux, O., Hugues, S., Thevenet, A., & Garcia, R. (2006). Hippocampal train stimulation modulates recall of fear extinction independently of prefrontal cortex synaptic plasticity and lesions. *Learning & Memory*, *13*(33), 329–334. http://doi.org/10.1101/lm.204806

Foa, E. B. (2011). Prolonged exposure therapy: Past, present, and future. *Depression and Anxiety*, *28*(12), 1043–1047. http://doi.org/10.1002/da.20907

Fontanez-Nuin, D. E., Santini, E., Quirk, G. J., & Porter, J. T. (2011). Memory for fear extinction requires mGluR5-mediated activation of infralimbic neurons. *Cerebral Cortex*, *21*(3), 727–735. http://doi.org/10.1093/cercor/bhq147

Frisina, P. G., Haroutunian, V., & Libow, L. S. (2009). The neuropathological basis for depression in Parkinson's disease. *Parkinsonism and Related Disorders*, *15*(2), 144–148. http://doi.org/10.1016/j.parkreldis.2008.04.038

Gandiga, P. C., Hummel, F. C., & Cohen, L. G. (2006). Transcranial DC stimulation (tDCS): A tool for double-blind sham-controlled clinical studies in brain stimulation. *Clinical Neurophysiology*, *117*(4), 845–850. http://doi.org/10.116/j.clinph.2005.12.003

Garnaat, S. L., Greenberg, B. D., Sibrava, N. J., Goodman, W. K., Mancebo, M. C., Eisen, J. L., & Rasmussen, S. A. (2014). Who qualifies for deep brain stimulation for OCD? Data from a naturalistic clinical sample. *The Journal of Neuropsychiatry and Clinical Neurosciences*, *26*(1), 81–86. http://doi.org/10.1176/appi.neuropsych.12090226

George, M. S., Sackeim, H. A., Rush, A. J., Marangell, L. B., Nahas, Z., Husain, M. M., . . . Ballenger, J.

C. (2000). Vagus nerve stimulation: a new tool for brain research and therapy*. *Biological Psychiatry*, *47*(4), 287–295. http://doi.org/10.1016/S0006-3223(99)00308-X

George, M. S., Raman, R., Benedek, D. M., Pelic, C. G., Grammer, G. G., Stokes, K. T., . . . Stein, M. B. (2014). A two-site pilot randomized 3 day trial of high dose left prefrontal repetitive transcranial magnetic stimulation (rTMS) for suicidal inpatients. *Brain Stimulation*, *7*(3), 421–431. http://doi.org/10.1016/j.brs.2014.03.006

George, M. S., Ward, H. E., Ninan, P. T., Pollack, M., Nahas, Z., Anderson, B., . . . Ballenger, J. C. (2008). A pilot study of vagus nerve stimulation (VNS) for treatment-resistant anxiety disorders. *Brain Stimulation*, *1*(2), 112–121. http://doi.org/10.1016/j.brs.2008.02.001

Greenberg, B. D., Gabriels, L. A., Malone, D. A., Rezai, A. R., Friehs, G. M., Okun, M. S., . . . Nuttin, B. J. (2010). Deep brain stimulation of the ventral internal capsule/ventral striatum for obsessive-compulsive disorder: worldwide experience. *Molecular Psychiatry*, *15*(1), 64-79. http://doi.org/10.1038/mp.2008.55

Gross, R. E., & Lozano, A. M. (2000). Advances in neurostimulation for movement disorders. *Neurological Research*, *22*(3), 247–258.

Heck, C. N., King-Stephens, D., Massey, A. D., Nair, D. R., Jobst, B. C., Barkley, G. L., . . . Morrell, M. J. (2014). Two-year seizure reduction in adults with medically intractable partial onset epilepsy treated with responsive neurostimulation: Final results of the RNS System Pivotal trial. *Epilepsia*, *55*(3), 432–441. http://doi.org/10.1111/epi.12534

Hermans, D., Craske, M. G., Mineka, S., & Lovibond, P. F. (2006). Extinction in human fear conditioning. *Biological Psychiatry*, *60*(4), 361–368. http://doi.org/10.1016/j.biopsych.2005.10.006

Herry, C., Ciocchi, S., Senn, V., Demmou, L., Müller, C., & Lüthi, A. (2008). Switching on and off fear by distinct neuronal circuits. *Nature*, *454*(7204), 600–606. http://doi.org/10.1038/nature07166

Herry, C., & Garcia, R. (2002). Prefrontal cortex long-term potentiation, but not long-term depression, is associated with the maintenance of extinction of learned fear in mice. *The Journal of Neuroscience*, *22*(2), 577–583. http://doi.org/22/2/577 [pii]

Holtzheimer, P. E., Husain, M. M., Lisanby, S. H., Taylor, S. F., Whitworth, L. A., McClintock, S., . . . Mayberg, H. S. (2017). Subcallosal cingulate deep brain stimulation for treatment-resistant depression: a multisite, randomised, sham-controlled trial. *The Lancet Psychiatry*, *4*(11), 839–849. http://doi.org/10.1016/S2215-0366(17)30371-1

Isserles, M., Shalev, A. Y., Roth, Y., Peri, T., Kutz, I., Zlotnick, E., & Zangen, A. (2013). Effectiveness of deep transcranial magnetic stimulation combined with a brief exposure procedure in post-traumatic stress disorder—a pilot study. *Brain Stimulation*, *6*(3), 377–383. http://doi.org/10.1016/j.brs.2012.07.008

Jasnow, A. M., Ehrlich, D. E., Choi, D. C., Dabrowska, J., Bowers, M. E., McCullough, K. M., . . . Ressler, K. J. (2013). Thy1-expressing neurons in the basolateral amygdala may mediate fear inhibition. *Journal of Neuroscience*, *33*(25), 10396–10404. http://doi.org/10.1523/JNEUROSCI.5539-12.2013

Kennedy, S. H., Giacobbe, P., Rizvi, S. J., Placenza, F. M., Nishikawa, Y., Mayberg, H. S., & Lozano, A. M. (2011). Deep brain stimulation for treatment-resistant depression: Follow-up after 3 to 6 years. *American Journal of Psychiatry*, *168*(5), 502–510. http://doi.org/10.1176/appi.ajp.2010.10081187

Koek, R. J., Langevin, J.-P., Krahl, S. E., Kosoyan, H. J., Schwartz, H. N., Chen, J. W. Y., . . . Sultzer, D. (2014). Deep brain stimulation of the basolateral amygdala for treatment-refractory combat post-traumatic stress disorder (PTSD): Study protocol for a pilot randomized controlled trial with blinded, staggered onset of stimulation. *Trials*, *15*, 356. http://doi.org/10.1186/1745-6215-15-356

Lebrón, K., Milad, M. R., & Quirk, G. J. (2004). Delayed recall of fear extinction in rats with lesions of ventral medial prefrontal cortex. *Learning & Memory*, *11*(5), 544–548. http://doi.org/10.1101/lm.78604

LeDoux, J. (2003). The emotional brain, fear, and the amygdala. *Cellular and Molecular Neurobiology*, *23*(4–5), 727–738. http://doi.org/10.1023/A:1025048802629

Likhtik, E., Stujenske, J. M., A Topiwala, M., Harris, A. Z., & Gordon, J. A. (2013). Prefrontal entrainment of amygdala activity signals safety in learned fear and innate anxiety. *Nature Neuroscience*, *17*(1), 106–113. http://doi.org/10.1038/nn.3582

Little, S., Pogosyan, A., Neal, S., Zavala, B., Zrinzo, L., Hariz, M., . . . Brown, P. (2013). Adaptive deep brain stimulation in advanced parkinson disease. *Annals of Neurology*, *74*(3), 449–457. http://doi.org/10.1002/ana.23951

Liu, X., Ramirez, S., Pang, P. T., Puryear, C. B., Govindarajan, A., Deisseroth, K., & Tonegawa, S. (2012). Optogenetic stimulation of a hippocampal engram activates fear memory recall. *Nature*, *484*(7394), 381–385. http://doi.org/10.1038/nature11028

Marin, M. F., Camprodon, J. A., Dougherty, D. D., & Milad, M. R. (2014). Device-based brain stimulation to augment fear extinction: Implications for PTSD treatment and beyond. *Depression and Anxiety*, *31*, 269–278. http://doi.org/10.1002/da.22252

Marin, M. F., & Milad, M. R. (2015). Neuromodulation approaches for the treatment of post-traumatic stress disorder: Stimulating the brain following exposure-based therapy. *Current Behavioral Neuroscience Reports, 2*, 67–71. http://doi.org/10.1007/s40473-015-0042-5

Marin, M. F., Song, H., Vanelzakker, M. B., Staples-Bradley, L. K., Linnman, C., Pace-Schott, E. F., . . . Milad, M. R. (2016). Association of resting metabolism in the fear neural network with extinction recall activations and clinical measures in trauma-exposed individuals. *American Journal of Psychiatry, 173*(9), 930–938. http://doi.org/10.1176/appi.ajp.2015.14111460

Mayberg, H. S., Lozano, A. M., Voon, V., McNeely, H. E., Seminowicz, D., Hamani, C., . . . Kennedy, S. H. (2005). Deep brain stimulation for treatment-resistant depression. *Neuron, 45*(5), 651–660. http://doi.org/10.1016/j.neuron.2005.02.014

Mayberg, H. S., McKenna, M. T., Michaud, C. M., Murray, C. J., Marks, J. S., Warden, D., . . . Eidelberg, D. (2009). Targeted electrode-based modulation of neural circuits for depression. *Journal of Clinical Investigation, 119*(4), 717–725. http://doi.org/10.1172/JCI38454

McGaugh, J. L., McIntyre, C. K., & Power, A. E. (2002). Amygdala modulation of memory consolidation: interaction with other brain systems. *Neurobiology of Learning and Memory, 78*(3), 539–552. http://doi.org/10.1006/nlme.2002.4082

McGaugh, J. L., & Roozendaal, B. (2002). Role of adrenal stress hormones in forming lasting memories in the brain. *Current Opinion in Neurobiology, 12*(2), 205. http://doi.org/10.1016/S0959-4388(02)00306-9

Milad, M. R., Pitman, R. K., Ellis, C. B., Gold, A. L., Shin, L. M., Lasko, N. B., . . . Rauch, S. L. (2009). Neurobiological basis of failure to recall extinction memory in posttraumatic stress disorder. *Biological Psychiatry, 66*(12), 1075–1082. http://doi.org/10.1016/j.biopsych.2009.06.026

Milad, M. R., & Quirk, G. J. (2002). Neurons in medial prefrontal cortex signal memory for fear extinction. *Nature, 420*(6911), 70–74. http://doi.org/10.1038/nature01138

Milad, M. R., Rauch, S. L., Pitman, R. K., & Quirk, G. J. (2006). Fear extinction in rats: Implications for human brain imaging and anxiety disorders. *Biological Psychology, 73*(1), 61–71. http://doi.org/10.1016/j.biopsycho.2006.01.008

Mungee, A., Kazzer, P., Feeser, M., Nitsche, M. A., Schiller, D., & Bajbouj, M. (2014). Transcranial direct current stimulation of the prefrontal cortex: A means to modulate fear memories. *Neuroreport, 25*, 480–484. http://doi.org/10.1097/WNR.0000000000000119

Nam, D.-H., Pae, C.-U., & Chae, J. (2013). Low-frequency, repetitive transcranial magnetic stimulation for the treatment of patients with posttraumatic stress disorder: A double-blind, sham-controlled study. *Clinical Psychopharmacology and Neuroscience, 11*(2), 96 102. http://doi.org/10.9758/cpn.2013.11.2.96

Nitsche, M., Fricke, K., Henschke, U., Schlitterlau, A., Liebetanz, D., Lang, N., . . . Paulus, W. (2003). Pharmacological modulation of cortical excitability shifts induced by transcranial direct current stimulation in humans. *The Journal of Physiology, 553*(1), 293–301. http://doi.org/10.1113/jphysiol.2003.049916

O'Reardon, J. P., Solvason, H. B., Janicak, P. G., Sampson, S., Isenberg, K. E., Nahas, Z., . . . Sackeim, H. A. (2007). Efficacy and safety of transcranial magnetic stimulation in the acute treatment of major depression: A multisite randomized controlled trial. *Biological Psychiatry, 62*(11), 1208–1216. http://doi.org/10.1016/j.biopsych.2007.01.018

Osuch, E. A., Benson, B. E., Luckenbaugh, D. A., Geraci, M., Post, R. M., & McCann, U. (2009). Repetitive TMS combined with exposure therapy for PTSD: A preliminary study. *Journal of Anxiety Disorders, 23*(1), 54–59. http://doi.org/10.1016/j.janxdis.2008.03.015

Peña, D. F., Engineer, N. D., & McIntyre, C. K. (2013). Rapid remission of conditioned fear expression with extinction training paired with vagus nerve stimulation. *Biological Psychiatry, 73*(11), 1071–1077. http://doi.org/10.1016/j.biopsych.2012.10.021

Philip, N. S., Nelson, B. G., Frohlich, F., Lim, K. O., Widge, A. S., & Carpenter, L. L. (2017). Low-intensity transcranial current stimulation in psychiatry. *American Journal of Psychiatry, 174*(7), 628–639. http://doi.org/10.1176/appi/ajp.2017.16090996

Quinn, E. J., Blumenfeld, Z., Velisar, A., Koop, M. M., Shreve, L. A., Trager, M. H., . . . Brontë-Stewart, H. (2015). Beta oscillations in freely moving Parkinson's subjects are attenuated during deep brain stimulation. *Movement Disorders, 30*(13), 1750–1758. http://doi.org/10.1002/mds.26376

Reis, J., Schambra, H. M., Cohen, L. G., Buch, E. R., Fritsch, B., Zarahn, E., . . . Krakauer, J. W. (2009). Noninvasive cortical stimulation enhances motor skill acquisition over multiple days through an effect on consolidation. *Proceedings of the National Academy of Sciences of the United States of America, 106*(5), 1590–1595. http://doi.org/10.1073/pnas.0805413106

Rodriguez-Romaguera, J., Do-Monte, F. H., Tanimura, Y., Quirk, G. J., & Haber, S. N. (2015).

Enhancement of fear extinction with deep brain stimulation: Evidence for medial orbitofrontal involvement. *Neuropsychopharmacology*, *40*(7), 1726–1733. http://doi.org/10.1038/npp.2015.20

Rodriguez-Romaguera, J., Monte, F. H. M. Do, & Quirk, G. J. (2012). Deep brain stimulation of the ventral striatum enhances extinction of conditioned fear. *Proceedings of the National Academy of Sciences of the United States of America*, *109*, 8764–8769. http://doi.org/10.1073/pnas.1200782109/-/DCSupplemental.www.pnas.org/cgi/doi/10.1073/pnas.1200782109

Rosa, M. A., & Lisanby, S. H. (2012). Somatic treatments for mood disorders. *Neuropsychopharmacology*, *37*(1), 102–116. http://doi.org/10.1038/npp.2011.225

Rosa, M., Giannicola, G., Marceglia, S., Fumagalli, M., Barbieri, S., & Priori, A. (2012). Neurophysiology of deep brain stimulation. *International Review of Neurobiology*, *107*. https://doi.org/10.1016/B978-0-12-404706-8.00004-8

Rosin, B., Slovik, M., Mitelman, R., Rivlin-Etzion, M., Haber, S. N., Israel, Z., . . . Bergman, H. (2011). Closed-loop deep brain stimulation is superior in ameliorating Parkinsonism. *Neuron*, *72*(2), 370–384. http://doi.org/10.1016/j.neuron.2011.08.023

Rossi, S., Hallett, M., Rossini, P. M., Pascual-Leone, A., Avanzini, G., Bestmann, S., . . . Ziemann, U. (2009). Safety, ethical considerations, and application guidelines for the use of transcranial magnetic stimulation in clinical practice and research. *Clinical Neurophysiology*, *120*(12), 2008–2039. http://doi.org/10.1016/j.clinph.2009.08.016

Rougemont-Bücking, A., Linnman, C., Zeffiro, T. A., Zeidan, M. A., Lebron-Milad, K., Rodriguez-Romaguera, J., . . . Milad, M. R. (2011). Altered processing of contextual information during fear extinction in PTSD: An fMRI study. *CNS Neuroscience and Therapeutics*, *17*(4), 227–236. http://doi.org/10.1111/j.1755-5949.2010.00152.x

Rush, A. J., Marangell, L. B., Sackeim, H. A., George, M. S., Brannan, S. K., Davis, S. M., . . . Cooke, R. G. (2005). Vagus nerve stimulation for treatment-resistant depression: A randomized, controlled acute phase trial. *Biological Psychiatry*, *58*(5), 347–354. http://doi.org/10.1016/j.biopsych.2005.05.025

Saunders, N., Downham, R., Turman, B., Kropotov, J., Clark, R., Yumash, R., & Szatmary, A. (2015). Working memory training with tDCS improves behavioral and neurophysiological symptoms in pilot group with post-traumatic stress disorder (PTSD) and with poor working memory. *Neurocase*, *21*(3), 271–278. http://doi.org/10.1080/13554794.2014.890727

Scholfield, C. N. (1990). Properties of K-currents in unmyelinated presynaptic axons of brain revealed by extracellular polarisation. *Brain Research*, *507*(1), 121–128. http://doi.org/10.1016/0006-8993(90)90530-O

Schultz, D. M., Webster, L., Kosek, P., Dar, U., Tan, Y., & Sun, M. (2012). Sensor-driven position-adaptive spinal cord stimulation for chronic pain. *Pain Physician*, *15*(1), 1–12. Retrieved from http://www.ncbi.nlm.nih.gov/pubmed/22270733

Shvil, E., Sullivan, G. M., Schafer, S., Markowitz, J. C., Campeas, M., Wager, T. D., . . . Neria, Y. (2014). Sex differences in extinction recall in posttraumatic stress disorder: A pilot fMRI study. *Neurobiology of Learning and Memory*, *113*, 101–108. http://doi.org/10.1016/j.nlm.2014.02.003

Steinberg, E. E., Christoffel, D. J., Deisseroth, K., & Malenka, R. C. (2015). Illuminating circuitry relevant to psychiatric disorders with optogenetics. *Current Opinion in Neurobiology*, *30*, 9–16. http://doi.org/10.1016/j.conb.2014.08.004

Stidd, D. A., Vogelsang, K., Krahl, S. E., Langevin, J.-P., & Fellous, J.-M. (2013). Amygdala deep brain stimulation is superior to paroxetine treatment in a rat model of posttraumatic stress disorder. *Brain Stimulation*, *6*(6), 837–844. http://doi.org/10.1016/j.brs.2013.05.008

Van 't Wout, M., Mariano, T. Y., Garnaat, S. L., Reddy, M. K., Rasmussen, S. A., & Greenberg, B. D. (2016). Can transcranial direct current stimulation augment extinction of conditioned fear? *Brain Stimulation*, *9*(4), 529–536. http://doi.org/10.1016/j.brs.2016.03.004

Vidal-Gonzalez, I., Vidal-Gonzalez, B., Rauch, S. L., & Quirk, G. J. (2006). Microstimulation reveals opposing influences of prelimbic and infralimbic cortex on the expression of conditioned fear. *Learning & Memory*, *13*(6), 728–733. http://doi.org/10.1101/lm.306106

Widge, A. S., Arulpragasam, A. R., Deckersbach, T., & Dougherty, D. D. (2015). Deep brain stimulation for psychiatric disorders. In R. A. Scott & S. M. Kosslyn (Eds.), *Emerging trends in the social and behavioral sciences: An interdisciplinary, searchable, and linkable resource* (pp. 1–17). Hoboken, NJ: John Wiley.

Widge, A. S., & Dougherty, D. D. (2015). Deep brain stimulation for treatment-refractory mood and obsessive-compulsive disorders. *Current Behavioral Neuroscience Reports*, *2*(4), 187–197. http://doi.org/10.1007/s40473-015-0049-y

26

Public Sector, Disaster, and Military Population-Based Responses to Trauma and Disaster

ELSPETH CAMERON RITCHIE AND KEVIN O'BRIEN

INTRODUCTION

This chapter focuses on systems issues and the implementation of disaster mental health outreach and intervention, illustrating systems issues across the public and military (including US military and the Veteran's Health Administration [VHA]) public health and mental health systems. The chapter focuses on how systems are organized for disasters and how community interventions are aimed to prevent or mitigate trauma-and stressor-related disorders and enhance community resilience at the population level. The chapter reviews briefly the military and associated elements of the Veterans Administration (VA) federal systems which helped shape disaster response in the 21st century. Key innovations in disaster mental health response, including refining the nature of population-based interventions and focused needs assessments are outlined. The chapter describes the health care systems in the military, the VA, and the public health sector. The authors first focus on the military, noting military resources are often called upon in civilian disasters when local response capabilities are overwhelmed. The ways in which military experience with mental health response to disaster has shaped the development of the approach to disaster response in public health systems are then described.

The VHA often has a substantial role in disaster response, and collaborative efforts between the Department of Defense, the VA system, and state and local agencies are discussed. The chapter illustrates the behavioral health response of the military, using two prominent mass violence events: the 9/11 attacks on the Pentagon and a mass shooting at Fort Hood, Texas. In addition, the chapter outlines the disaster mental health trauma office and training of personnel for Washington, DC's Department of Behavioral Health (DBH).

INSTITUTIONAL RESPONSE TO COMMUNITY TRAUMA

Public health and specifically public mental health systems respond to community trauma and to the needs of both healthy populations and to those special populations at increased risk including those with serious mental and physical illness, children and women (Chapter 16), the elderly (Chapter 9), and sexual, ethnic, and racial minorities. These systems also respond to community trauma including childhood trauma (see Chapter 3), trauma from rape and violence, motor vehicle injuries, and trauma from disasters. The mental health disaster literature usually focuses on the overall population of healthy individuals and concentrates on trauma-related stressors. However, the population served by the public mental health system nearly always also includes the seriously mentally ill. In a disaster, the public mental health system also treats survivors and first responders.

EARLY INTERVENTION IN THE AFTERMATH OF MASS VIOLENCE: A PARADIGM SHIFT

Because of concerns about the efficacy of debriefing, especially Critical Incident Stress Debriefing (CISD) stemming from evidence-based reviews, a conference in 2001, focused on the principles of—and evidence for—early intervention after mass violence and disasters. At that time CISD was a frequently encouraged modality for intervention at the small group or community level, but there was concern that it could do more harm than good (Bisson et al., 1993, Hammond & Brooks, 2001, Kagee, 2002, Norris et al., 2002, Raphael & Wilson, 2000, Rose et al., 2001). The conference was a joint effort of the Departments of Defense and Justice, the

National Institute of Mental Health (NIMH), the VA, and the American Red Cross. Despite travel difficulties related to 9/11, nearly a hundred behavioral health clinicians, scientists, and policy developers gathered at a conference center at Airlie House in Virginia and NIMH published the results (Ritchie & Friedman, 2002). This was a pivotal shift away from CISDs and toward evidence-based early interventions. In addition, a *Military Medicine* supplement on the Mental Health Response to the Pentagon was published in September of 2002 (Ritchie & Hoge, 2002, Cox et al., 2002). Other publications, webinars, and other training events followed (Ritchie et al, 2006). The field turned from CISD to a more balanced set of interventions including psychological first aid as derived from a comprehensive review of empirical evidence for early intervention after mass violence (Hobfall, 2007; Psyhcological First Aid Field Operations Guide, 2006; Schreiber 2006: Schreiber 2008).

NEEDS ASSESSMENT AND PUBLIC MENTAL HEALTH INTERVENTIONS

The importance of a needs assessment prior to public mental health intervention has also been stressed (Ritchie & Hamilton, 2004; Katz, 2011). This assessment includes both physical and mental health needs and resources. The physical assessment includes (a) estimates of the extent of lethality including the number of killed and wounded, (b) assessment of environmental factors, including continuing threats, (c) availability of medical resources, (d) immediate needs for food and shelter, and (e) capacity for communication between responders and to victims about all these issues. The mental health assessment includes related factors, such as (a) the number of people (e.g., surviving, loved ones, close friends, co-workers, neighbors) indirectly linked to those killed and wounded; (b) the number of those traumatized (e.g., surviving the event[s] directly witnessing violence or loss of life); (c) environmental factors, including continuing threats and environmental contamination; (d) availability of mental health resources; (e) availability of food and shelter; and (f) ability to communicate about all of these issues. Physical and mental health needs are closely related. and systemic capacity to rapidly identify and treat physical injury and address basic needs of food, shelter, and so on can contribute to a more favorable mental health response at the population level.

HEALTH CARE SYSTEMS IN THE US MILITARY AND RELATED TERMINOLOGY: A BRIEF DESCRIPTION

The military health care system (MHS) and the VHA must, in times of crisis, effectively interact with other response agencies including the National Guard, state public health and state mental health systems, emergency medical personnel, the American Red Cross, and police, fire, and civil defense departments. An appreciation of the "language and culture" of these systems facilitates such interaction. A military "service" refers to the branch of service (i.e., Army, Navy, Air Force, or Marines, which are part of the Department of the Navy). Correspondingly, the personnel are called soldiers, sailors, airmen, or Marines, respectively. The term "service members" refers to all the military personnel.

The term "veteran" has several meanings. It usually describes service members who are no longer on active duty. However, the term "combat veteran" is used for both current service members as well as those no longer on active duty who have served in conflict zones, such as Iraq and Afghanistan. Active duty service members are those who wear the military uniform full time and receive care generally through the MHS. TRICARE is the Department of Defense Health insurance that covers both those who seek care in military hospitals (commonly referred to as the "direct care system") and via the civilian provider network, formerly referred to as CHAMPUS. The term "reservist" describes several categories of reserve service members, including the Army and Air National Guard. Reservists may serve a weekend a month and two weeks a year, although there are many variations. The National Guard is organized at the state level, and members may be mobilized in event of state emergencies or be called up to full-time active duty status and deployed for war. Reservists may transition between active duty and veteran status (Ritchie 2014).

MILITARY RESPONSE TO DISASTERS

The military responds to emergencies on their own bases, such as the Pentagon after 9/11, and to the Fort Hood (Texas), Washington, D.C., Navy Yard shootings. They are occasionally called to assist in international natural disasters, such as the tsunami in 2004, earthquakes, or, the Ebola outbreak in West Africa. The National Guard is often called to assist in local domestic emergencies, such as Hurricane Katrina or other floods and disasters.

The VHA cares for many, but not all, veterans. VHA facilities and personnel are often involved with disaster response at the local level but usually focus on their established veteran patients rather than the larger public. One benefit of enrollment in the VA system at the time of disaster is the VA's use of the electronic medical record, which includes all patients who have sought care in the VA. For example, after Hurricane Katrina, when many veterans were relocated from the Gulf, they could more easily re-establish care (including mental health care) through other VA hospitals. Medical records which would have been destroyed if they were only stored locally as hard-copy documents were obtainable at any VA facility to which a relocated veteran presented.

EXAMPLES OF THE MILITARY POPULATION HEALTH RESPONSE TO TRAUMATIC EVENTS

Two significant example of the military systemic response to disaster are (a) the response to the 9/11 attacks on the Pentagon and (b) the response to the Fort Hood shooting in 2009. These events were separated by eight years, two major wars, and an evolving approach to disasters, both local and foreign.

The Pentagon Attack of 9/11: A Military/Civilian Community Disaster

The Pentagon, nestled in Arlington, Virginia, is near many military bases with mental health staff, including the Walter Reed Army Medical Center, in Washington, D.C., Fort Myers, Fort Belvoir, and Andrews Force Base. On September 11, 2001, when the United Flight #77 left Dulles Airport and crashed into the Pentagon, mental health staff from the medical facilities at each of these bases rapidly responded. They established work sites at the Pentagon, the Family Assistance Center in Crystal City, and within the affected surrounding community. Shortly after the plane crash, the first author (ECR) went to Walter Reed Army Medical Center to develop a plan, along with local military mental health leadership. Initial focus was necessarily dedicated to identifying and treating those severely injured by the crash and fire. But there were relatively few wounded survivors and many more deceased. Responders then focused on doing outreach to people who worked at the Pentagon and surrounding military facilities. The initial plan was changed and evolved many times in the following weeks. As new medical and behavioral health leadership arrived, new perspectives led to a revised approach. However, when air travel to the DC area resumed, the Army senior mental health leadership converged on the Office of the Army Surgeon General to further assist the outreach efforts. While there was risk of a theme common to many disaster responses (i.e., "Who is in charge?") arising here, unlike many organizations responding to communities impacted by disasters, within the Department of Defense, a common command structure formed the basis of the assignment of responsibilities. One author of this chapter (ECR) was then stationed at the Department of Defense Health Affairs and eventually coordinated the outreach efforts in the Washington, D.C., area. Shortly after 9/11, a twice-daily telephone conference was established to allow communication between responders as to locations of mental health resources and needs. In military parlance, such briefings describing the nature of threats and responses are often called a "battle rhythm" (Milliken, 2002). This concept of the battle rhythm is now widely used by state emergency disaster systems in the days following a crisis. The robust military mental health outreach to the events of 9/11, especially to the Pentagon and surrounding areas in Washington, D.C., is laid out in articles in Ritchie and Hoge (2002).

Another common theme to many disasters is that concerned persons from many disciplines converge at the place of the disaster or crash site in an effort to render assistance. For example, there had been a chaplain's conference at the Pentagon on 9/11. The chaplains all went to help. Thus, a frequently heard complaint was that you could not move "without tripping over a chaplain." However, clergy offering pastoral care were those most commonly turned to by the public after 9/11 and other community crises such as the shootings at Sandy Hook Elementary School, highlighting the importance of their training and integration into community health interventions.

Because of the coordinating efforts, the resources could be matched to the needs, including at outlying Department of Defense facilities around the Pentagon and at the Family Assistance Center (FAC). In 2001, there was little guidance on setting up a FAC. The centers for the families of Pentagon workers and United Airlines victims, like the center later established for families in Boston at Logan Airport after the terrorist attack there, functioned well, partially because there was a single chain of command (the Department of Defense) and because the military knows well how to mobilize resources after mass disasters and recognized the importance of establishing a centralized resource to provide updated information and assistance in access to medical, mental health care, support, and legal and financial guidance (Bartone et al., 1989). After 9/11 separate assistance centers for each service were considered (and yet a separate one at Dulles Airport for families of the airline victims of Flight 77). A decision was made to consolidate family assistance at the Sheraton in Crystal City, near the Pentagon. This FAC served the military community, civilians, and contractors. It was jointly staffed by all the services and aided by VA personnel and nongovernmental organizations such as the Red Cross. A host of services was provided there, including metal health outreach, DNA identification, child therapy, animal-assisted (pet) therapy, and massage therapy, relaxation, and respite for the victims and responders. Resources were mobilized to reach out to (a) the family members of the deceased, (b) the wounded victims and their families, (c) the affected populations of the Pentagon and nearby buildings, and (d) the larger military and civilian populations (Ritchie & Hoge, 2002).

Military Response to an On-Base Disaster

The nation went to war in Afghanistan in 2001 and in Iraq in 2003. The Department of Defense became very busy in the efforts to support the mental health needs of the troops, both in the theaters of war (Iraq and Afghanistan) and after return. The focus on local/civilian disaster response, at least in the Department of Defense, took a back seat to addressing the mental health needs related to combat. However, there were many other examples of mass shootings and other traumatic events which required responses, such as the Camp Liberty shooting in 2009 and the mass shooting at Fort Hood in 2009.

On November 5, 2009, an Army psychiatrist, Major Nidal Hasan, opened fire at the Soldier Readiness Processing station at Fort Hood. He killed 13, and many more were wounded. When security guards responded to the attack, he was wounded and paralyzed from the neck down. Although this event stunned the military community—a mass shooting by one of their own—a response plan was quickly developed. A team of 12 experts, both military and civilian, came in to craft and initiate the long-term response. A plan addressing the various subpopulations affected by the event was conceptualized and developed as concentric circles originating at the location of the attack. This approach was first identified through observations of an evolving mental health response to a military plane crash. In that incident, although the plane crashed in Gander, Newfoundland, most immediate family members of the deceased were concentrated at Fort Campbell, Kentucky (Bartone et al., 1989).

In Fort Hood, although the initial focus was at the shooting site and on the dead and wounded, there were many others traumatized. These included (a) those who witnessed the shootings but were not physically injured, (b) first responders to the shootings, (c) children in the schools that were locked down, (d) Major Hasan's patients, (e) the medical staff at Fort Hood, (f) the broader Fort Hood community, (g) the entire military, and (h) the nation.

This approach of looking at the concentric circles of those affected is applicable to most disasters. (see Figure 26.1). Again, the response is conceptualized as broader than the crash or disaster site, to encompass the entire community near and far of those affected. Another feature of the response plan was the time-phased approach. It included the initial response with a recognition that response over weeks and months would be necessary. A needs assessment as to the affected communities and the local resources was initiated. The ongoing plan included phased introduction of mental health professionals from other regional Department of Defense facilities over time. Importantly, the plan called for periodic epidemiologic surveillance of the affected community to assess the extent to which needs were matched with resources and to assist in projecting needs over time.

THE PUBLIC MENTAL HEALTH SYSTEM: WASHINGTON, DC

While the Federal Emergency Management Agency, the military, and MHS have evolved in their response to traumatic events such as disaster, so too have local public health and mental health agencies. Washington, D.C., like all the states, has a public mental health care system, now the DBH. Most of the recipients of government-subsidized mental health services are on Medicaid (the financing system to low-income residents). In practice, that means most are poor and have

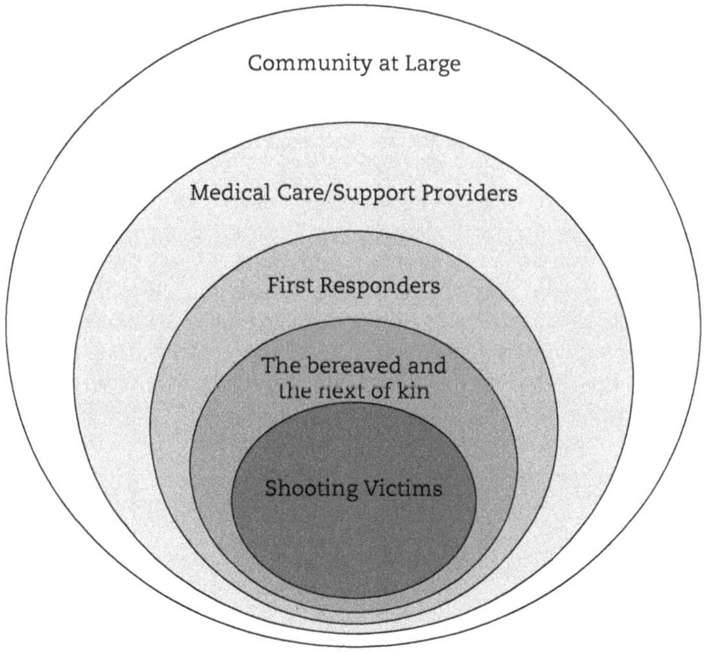

FIGURE 26.1. Concentric circles model of disaster community.

a combination of severe mental illness (schizophrenia and schizoaffective disorder) and drug abuse. Many are at high risk for comorbid trauma- and stressor-related disorders, including PTSD, whether or not these are diagnosed. There is one public psychiatric hospital, Saint Elizabeth's Hospital. Acute psychiatric hospitalization is contracted out to local hospitals.

Much of the outpatient care for the mentally ill in Washington, D.C., is through private Core Service Agencies. These focus on serious mental disorders, to include schizophrenia, bipolar illness, and substance abuse disorders. Of course, many with serious mental illness are also traumatized. Their traumatic events may include combat experiences, violence on the street, domestic violence, and other forms of trauma. Data is not available as to the prevalence of trauma. However, many DBH providers and Core Service Agencies use trauma-informed practices such as cognitive processing therapy.

DISASTER BEHAVIORAL HEALTH SERVICES IN WASHINGTON, DC

The disaster response is informed by the information previously discussed but is tailored for the District of Columbia (DC). DC is heavily influenced by the numerous federal agencies within and around its boundaries and is a prime terrorist target.

Disaster behavioral health has been conceptualized as the provision of mental health, substance abuse, and stress management services to disaster survivors and responders (https://www.phe.gov/Preparedness/planning/abc/Pages/disaster-behavioral.aspx accessed 3/27/2017). Like many other state disaster mental health systems, DBH provides prevention, intervention, and treatment services and support for children, youth, and adults with mental and/or substance use disorders including emergency psychiatric care, community services, and residential treatment services. DBH's Office of Disaster Behavioral Health Services formally began in 2007 to coordinate the agency in its emergency preparedness efforts for internal, localized, city-wide, and regional disasters and emergencies.

Disaster behavioral health is an integral part of the overall public health and medical preparedness, response, and recovery system (All Hazards Response Plan for the DC Department of Behavioral Health, 2009.). Behavioral factors directly and indirectly influence individual and community risks, health, resilience, and the success of emergency response strategies and public health directives (U.S. Department of Health and Human Services, Office of the Assistant Secretary for Preparedness and Response, 2017). Disaster Behavioral Health Services develops and implements plans to ensure that DBH is prepared to quickly mobilize and provide mental health services in the event of a disaster or emergency. Services provided in response to disaster are overlaid on those services routinely provided by the public mental health system. The mental health resources are mainly for persons with schizophrenia or other related disorders. Although trauma-related disorders are very prevalent in the homeless population, for better or worse, current public mental health services concentrate on the psychotic disorders. While many child and adult patients in the DC mental health system have pre-existing trauma- and stressor-disorder related symptoms, their incidence and prevalence are not known. Their experience of prior trauma exposure renders them at risk for PTSD, other related disorders, other mental illnesses, and distress reactions following disaster (Chapters 1, 3, 8, and 10). When services are disrupted because of a disaster, not only psychosocial support systems but also the pharmaceutical supply chain may be disrupted. The lack of available medications means that severely mentally ill persons may be withdrawn from antipsychotic or other medications in an unsupervised manner. Thus, they may become impaired and potentially disruptive to responders or community members. Similarly, those addicted to opioids and other substances may not be able to get their narcotics and may become unruly. Especially in the public mental health system, police and emergency medical services are a critical first line to taking care of the mentally ill.

THE VETERANS HEALTH ADMINISTRATION

In Washington, D.C., there is a major VA facility. There are also Veterans Centers, Community Based Outpatient Clinics, and the Community Resource and Referral Center, with its focus on addressing mental health and medical needs in homeless veterans. Thus, for veterans with honorable discharges, there are extensive resources available for those who are eligible for those services. However, gaps exist for veterans with other than honorable (OTH) discharges. The VA has recently decided to provide care for those with OTH discharges: implementation details are still to be worked out. In addition, some veterans do not want to access those VA services.

CONTINUITY OF OPERATIONS

The response to any sudden onset or gradually emerging catastrophic event must be managed in addition to delivery of basic services provided as part of routine behavioral health care delivery (*Crisis Standards of Care: A Toolkit for Indicators and Triggers*, 2013). Events may seriously impact and disrupt patient care in both hospital- and community-based settings. While the impact of a crisis within DBH itself cannot be predicted, planning for operations under such conditions can reduce the impact of the emergency on its employees, facilities, and mission.

The DBH COOP plan supports the District Response Plan, DBH's Response Plan, and DBH's internal Emergency Operating Procedures, such as any evacuation plan, Designated Assembly Areas, and Shelter-in-Place plans. The plan provides overall guidance for continued operations during an event that may impact the agency's ability to function.

The plan is an "all-hazards" plan, meaning it allows the agency to continue its essential functions after any type of emergency, large or small. The key purposes of this COOP plan are to:

- Ensure continuous performance of and mitigate disruptions to essential functions and operations;
- Identify COOP personnel responsible for carrying out essential functions;
- Ensure the succession of the director and other key personnel, if required, on a temporary basis, and maintain or re-establish control and direction of DBH;
- Maintain communications capabilities within DBH as well as with other district, state, and federal agencies;
- Identify vital records, databases, systems and equipment needed to carry out essential functions;
- Designate alternate facilities, from which DBH operations can be conducted; and
- Achieve a timely and orderly recovery from the emergency and resumption of normal operations.

ALL HAZARDS BEHAVIORAL HEALTH RESPONSE PLAN AND TEAM

The All Hazards Behavioral Health Response Plan is DBH's overarching plan to establish the preparedness framework for localized, district-wide, or catastrophic emergencies affecting DC, the DBH, or its consumers. It is a comprehensive emergency management tool prepared in coordination with the DC Emergency Response Plan and consistent with the Federal Response Framework of the Federal Emergency Response Agency (FEMA). It provides guidance, direction, and coordination for the DBH's emergency and crisis behavioral health support to first responders, survivors, families, or visitors during disasters, emergencies, or city-wide emergencies.

Within the guidance of the COOP and all hazards plans, all DBH behavioral health response team members are trained and certified by DBH to provide disaster and emergency behavioral health assessments, interventions, and referrals for long-term treatment offer service in a variety of settings. The 20 hour certification training is based upon: (a) competencies established by a stakeholder experts working collaboratively through the Association of Public Health Schools and the Centers for Disease Control and Prevention in FEMA Region III; (b) identification of regional and national training resources; (c) best practices research, including a survey of disaster behavioral health stakeholders nationwide; (d) incorporation of Incident Command System/National Incident Management System training; and (e) collaborative input from the disaster behavioral health state agency leads in FEMA Region III. This training has been informed by all the aforementioned information, including many disaster and mass shootings scenarios.

THE CRISIS INTERVENTION OFFICER PROGRAM

The Crisis Intervention Officer (CIO) program is a collaboration between the DC Metropolitan Police Department (MPD) and the DBH. The CIO program is an effort between law enforcement, mental health, and community stakeholders to improve outcomes of police interactions with people experiencing mental health crises. Launched in April 2009, as a collaboration between MPD, DBH, and National Alliance on Mental Illness, Distric of Columbia Chapter, the program was modeled after the Memphis Police Department's Crisis Intervention Team program and best practices from law enforcement jurisdictions across the country (City of Memphis, 2017). CIOs do not work within a specialized mental health response team; instead they perform regular police duties unless dispatched as a CIO to a mental health call, where they often lead the response. CIOs also collaborate with other community service providers, including crisis and homeless outreach teams.

The program has been customized to meet the changing needs of the citizens of DC. At the heart of the initiative is the identification and development of experienced patrol officers skilled in interacting effectively with mentally ill consumers and promoting collaboration with other emergency services, hospitals, and community mental health resources. The two primary goals of the program are safety and the diversion of nonviolent mentally ill offenders away from the criminal justice system to more appropriate mental health services.

Key components of the program are as follows:

1. Training for law enforcement officers includes basic mental health training for all incoming recruits, 40 hours of CIO training for approximately 150 officers annually, and refresher training for existing CIOs to ensure continued skill development. Topics include mental health and substance use concepts and symptoms, local resources and applicable laws, suicide prevention, and verbal de-escalation.
2. Collaboration between MPD, DBH, community providers, emergency services, family, and consumer advocates are crucial to the success of the program and DC service delivery system. Such collaboration is critical nationwide within each state and community. This is fostered through their participation in the training components and forums such as monthly CIO program meetings.
3. Consumer and family involvement in planning and training sessions is coordinated by DBH to ensure officers and consumers have opportunities to engage with each other and improve future interactions.

CONCLUSION

This chapter has described the way systems (or institutions) are organized for disasters and how community-level interventions may be developed to prevent or mitigate trauma-and stressor-related disorders and enhance community resilience. A review of how the military and VA federal systems worked to develop population-based disaster response in the 21st century provided a precursor to plans developed by civilian population centers such as Washington, DC. A focus on systemic response, rather than a focus on small groups of directly exposed persons or individual patients, is presented as a mechanism for reducing the burden of potential trauma- and stressor-related disorders across the population. The roots of this paradigm were traced to a conference of disaster mental health experts that recognized a need to shift from debriefing to more nuanced and psychological first aid based on early interventions at the population level. The military mental health response (as influenced by this new approach) following 9/11 and the Fort Hood shootings, the collaborative role of the VA, and the public mental health response plan of a large city were outlined using the DC DBH as an example of an evolved "state" public mental health system. Although the disaster mental health response systems described have become relatively robust, there is clearly more to be done, including developing systems of monitoring training and measuring preparedness, identifying population (rather than patient-level) outcomes to be measured, and clarifying the specific roles for city, state, and federal responders.

REFERENCES

All Hazards Response Plan for the DC Department of Behavioral Health. Washington, DC: Braintree Solution Consulting, 2009.

Bartone PT, Ursano RJ, Wright KM, Ingraham LH. The impact of a military air disaster on the health of assistance workers: A prospective study. *J Nerv Ment Dis*. 1989;177(6):317–328.

Bisson JI, Jenkins PL, Alexander J, Bannister C. Randomised controlled trial of psychological debriefing for victims of acute burn trauma. *Br J Psychiatry*. 1993;171:78–81.

City of Memphis. Crisis Intervention Team, 2017. Retrieved from http://www.memphistn.gov/Government/PoliceServices/CrisisIntervention-Team.aspx

Crisis standards of care: A toolkit for indicators and triggers. Washington, DC: National Academy of Sciences, 2013.

Hammond J, Brooks J. Helping the helpers: The role of critical incident stress management. *Crit Care*. 2001;5:315–317.

Hobfoll SE, Watson P, Bell CC, et al. Five essential elements of immediate and mid-term mass trauma intervention: Empirical evidence. *Psychiatry*. 2007;70(4):283–315.

Hoge CW, Orman DT, Robichaux RJ, et al. Operation Solace: Overview of the mental health intervention following the September 11, 2001 Pentagon attack. *Milit Med*. 2002;167(9)Suppl: 44–47.

Kagee A. Concerns about the effectiveness of critical incident stress debriefing in ameliorating stress reactions. *Crit Care*. 2002;6(1):88. doi:10.1186/cc1459.

Katz CL. Needs assessment. In: FJ Stoddard, A Pandya, CL Katz, eds. *Disaster psychiatry: Readiness, evaluation and treatment*. Washington, DC: American Psychiatric Publishing, 2011, pp. 49–70.

Milliken CS. Principles guiding implementation of the operation solace plan: "Pieces of PIES," therapy by walking around, and care management. *Milit Med*. 2002;167(9)Suppl:48–57.

Norris MJ, Friedman, PJ Watson, 60,000 disaster victims speak: Part II. Summary and implications of the disaster mental health research. *Psychiatry*. 2002;65(3):240–260.

Norris FH, SP Stevens, B Pfefferbaum. Community resilience as a metaphor, theory, set of capacities, and strategy for disaster readiness. *Am J Commun Psychol*. 2008;41:127–150.

Psychological first aid: Field operations guide, 2nd ed. National Child Traumatic Stress Network and National Center for PTSD, 2006. http://www.ptsd.va.gov/professional/manuals/manual-pdf/pfa/PFA_2ndEditionwithappendices.pdf

Raphael B, J Wilson. *Psychological debriefing: Theory, practice and evidence*. Cambridge, UK: Cambridge University Press, 2000.

Ritchie EC. The Department of Defense and VA health care system overview. In S Cozza & M Goldenberg, eds. *Clinical manual for the care of military service members, veterans and their families*, APPI, Feb 2014. American Psychiatric Press, Arlington VA.

Ritchie EC, Friedman MJ. *Mental health and mass violence—Evidence based early psychological intervention for victims/survivors of mass violence: A workshop to reach consensus on best practices*. National Institute of Mental Health. Washington, DC: U.S. Government Printing Office, 2002.

Ritchie EC, Friedman M, Watson P, eds. *Interventions following mass violence and disasters: Strategies for mental health practice*. New York: Guilford Press, 2006.

Ritchie EC, Hamilton S. Early interventions & risk assessment following disaster. *Psychiatr Ann*. 2004 Sep;

Ritchie EC, Hoge CW, eds. The mental health response to the 9/11 attack on the Pentagon. *Milit Med*. 2002;167(9)Suppl.

Ritchie EC, Watson PJ, Friedman MJ. *Interventions following mass violence and disasters*. New York: Guilford Press, 2006.

Rose S, Bisson J, Wessely S. Psychological debriefing for preventing post traumatic stress disorder (PTSD). *Cochrane Database Syst Rev*. 2001;3.

Schreiber M, Gurwitch R. Listen, protect, connect: Psychological first aid for children and parents. 2006. Retrieved from http://www.cdms.uci.edu/PDF/PFA_Parents.pdf

Schreiber M, Gurwitch R. Listen, protect, and connect: Psychological first aid for children and parents online module. 2008. Retrieved from http://www.cdms.uci.edu/lpc

Walter Reed Army Institute of Research. Contributions during operations Iraqi Freedom and Enduring Freedom form U.S. Department of Health and Human Services Office of the Assistant Secretary for Preparedness and Response Office of Policy and Planning Division for At-Risk Individuals, Behavioral Health, and Community Resilience. 2017. Retrieved from http://www.phe.gov/

27

Trauma- and Stress-Related Issues in the Workplace

BRIAN FLYNN

Trauma and stress respect no boundaries. If any differentiation exists at all between life domains, such as work/occupational domains and personal/family life, they are extremely permeable membranes. That said, there is merit in exploring how trauma and stress impact the workplace, how the workplace impacts trauma and stress, and roles physicians and others play.

While this introduction to trauma- and stress-related workplace issues is primarily targeted to medical students, the content has applicability to many professional disciplines including psychologists, social workers, and others. A wide variety of disciplines perform many diverse workplace roles. These include clinical, administrative, educational, and consultative roles.

Understanding these dynamics and how they impact physicians and others is like hitting a moving target. Medical students will be familiar with the challenges as science is rapidly emerging and practice is variable across both time and context. Psychological factors in the workplace are no different.

Mental health in the workplace is not an unimportant or secondary consideration (World Health Organization [WHO], 2000). The costs of mental disorders are staggering. The World Economic Forum asked health economists to estimate the global cost of mental disorders. They estimated worldwide costs of $6.0 trillion by 2030. They estimated the 2012 cost in the United States to be at least $467 billion (Bloom et al., 2011).

Cost estimates are comprised of many factors, and many costs relate directly to workplace concerns. Harder, Wagner, and Rash (2016) describe factors such as obtaining and maintaining employment, absenteeism, presenteeism (a term applied to workers who are physically present but not attending to tasks or their environment), and workplace accidents, all contributing to productivity declines.

Another method of assessing and describing the impact of diseases, including mental disorders, is illustrated by the landmark Global Burden of Disease 2013 study (Vos et al., 2015). Mental disorders are expressed in disability adjusted life years (DALYs) which constitutes years lost as a result of premature death as well as living with disability. The WHO (2011) reports that mental illnesses are the leading causes of DALYs worldwide, accounting for 37% of the life years lost from noncommunicable diseases. At the same time, the payoff for prevention and treatment is significant. The WHO has concluded that, worldwide, every $1 governments spend on treatment for mental disorders, there is a $4 return on investment (Chisholm et al., 2016).

Other chapters demonstrate that evidence-based treatment of mental disorders has improved dramatically in the past several decades. Simultaneously, appreciation for the positive impact effectively treating disorders has increased. In the United States and most developed countries, stigma has been reduced.

There are three major challenges and opportunities for workplaces, and physicians and others working in and with them, with respect to mental disorders, including stress and trauma:

- Understanding the range of factors contributing to the reduction or exacerbation of mental disorders;
- Providing creative and positive leadership in addressing these issues; and
- Developing and sustaining a variety of approaches to enhancing mental health and preventing and reducing mental disorders.

CHANGING AND MOVING DEFINITIONS

Trauma and Stress

Most health (including behavioral health) professionals are trained in pathology-based models. The links between this training model and practice are neither accidental nor science based. Practice is, and always has been, strongly driven by reimbursement systems. Increasingly, health provider services are based on diagnosing illnesses or disorders. Other services and approaches, such as subclinical and preventive efforts, at least in the United States, receive limited or no reimbursement. More in-depth discussion of this topic is outside the scope of this chapter, but students and early career mental health professionals should understand that training models and reimbursement patterns have a significant impact on shaping the lenses through which practitioners see their work, patients, and clients.

Why is this important in the workplace? Depending on the health professional's (physician or others) role(s), discussed later in the chapter, there may be variable degrees of freedom to focus on different trauma- and stress-related workplace sequelae. For example, if the nature of the services provided is based primarily upon reimbursement through recipient health insurance, the provider will most certainly be drawn toward diagnosing and treating primarily cases in which a clinical diagnosis can be applied. If a physician (or other professional) is hired to consult to an organization's leadership, as occurs in community psychiatry (Caplan & Caplan, 2000), or as a salaried member of an occupational health unit, there may be opportunities to provide a broader array of services, to be discussed later.

Defining the Workplace

The diversity of workplace types and the types of stress and trauma people experience make generalization extremely difficult. Workplaces come in many types and sizes with corresponding challenges and resources. Also, the nature of work and workplaces is in flux, heavily influencing what health care providers do for and in the workplace.

Consider a few examples of the range of workplace size. Think about what types of stressors workers might experience and what level and type of resources might be available to them. Examples include the single self-employed worker, the small business with three to four workers, the small business or corporation with a single or multiple locations, the non-profit organizations, large domestic corporations, multinational corporations, and governmental organizations,

There are considerable differences in workplace types. Again, think about the wide diversity in types of stress workers experience and what types of services might be available to them. Examples include manufacturing, marine/agricultural, service organizations, national/international corporations, educational institutions, and public services.

Work and Workplace Trends

Over the past several decades, trends in both the nature of work and workplaces have impacted workers' stress. These changes present both challenges and opportunities in many areas including preventing workplace disabilities of many types (Ekburg et al., 2016). Trends include

Multiple careers: There is a trend away from single life-long careers. In the United States, the average person born between 1957 and 1964 held 11.7 jobs between ages 18 and 48. Half of these jobs were held between the ages of 18 and 24 (Bureau of Labor Statistics, 2015). Career change can be a positive strategy to mitigate stress or create and exacerbate stress.

Workplace loyalty: There is a trend away from long-term/same-company employment as a result of a general decline in both employer loyalty to employees and vice versa. This trend can both exacerbate or mitigate stress. Workers may feel more freedom to leave employers without as much stigma as before. At the same time, job uncertainty is a stressor (Sverke, Hellgren, & Näswall, 2002).

From traditional employment to nonstandard work: There is a trend away from the historic notion of employment, that is, employment that comes with benefits such as vacation, sick leave, child care, health insurance, and other benefits. More workers are being hired on a nonstandard basis (e.g., part-time and on contract) where employers can reduce costs for providing benefits (Rosenberg & Lapidus, 1999). The absence of such benefits can be stressful to workers who have needs such as health or child care, and they may struggle to access and afford these services. The provision of worker benefits varies greatly among countries, and some organizations are enhancing their reputations by providing services and benefits to their workers that go well beyond most (Black & Lynch, 2004).

Flexible time and flexible location: In the United States, there is a trend toward more flexible work hours and increased flexibility in work location (e.g., working from home). The circumstances of the individual will determine whether this increases or reduces stress. For example, working the same hours in fewer days may reduce commuting and child care costs, and working from home some or all of the time may allow workers more flexibility in managing personal or family needs. For others, working primarily from home with the absence of workplace socialization and increased isolation becomes a stressor.

Changing the nature of concepts of mental/behavioral health: As noted, the world of health care, including behavioral health, is changing, and emerging science and health care financing are drivers for change. Dramatic developments in brain science and imaging have led to medicine, especially psychiatry, moving strongly toward pharmaceutical and other medical intervention with a decline in emphasis on relationships and other environmental and contextual factors. What does this mean for stress in the workplace? Newly trained physicians and others, especially psychiatrists, will likely find themselves better trained for, and more comfortable with, diagnosing psychopathology and medical treatments than they will be with approaches that involve exploring relational and contextual factors related to stress. They may be far more comfortable with diagnosis and treatment than consultation and likely to have had little or no training and orientation to community psychiatry. To admittedly oversimplify, many recent graduates are more likely to be better versed in diagnosis and medical treatment of illness than in promoting and sustaining behavioral health, especially in the workplace.

This discussion is not intended to be critical but rather to constructively remind readers that there are opportunities and limitations resulting from the confluence of contemporary contextual factors. Consequently, it is especially important for providers to know the contributions to which they are best suited, the limits of their expertise, and where, when, and how to engage others with different skill sets when facing complex workplace stress challenges.

Conversely, there are several trends that may work to the advantage of providers involved in workplace stress. These include

- Decreased stigma related to behavioral health issues (Carter, Satcher, & Coelho, 2013);
- Enhanced focus on occupational health and safety (WHO, 1994);
- Enhanced knowledge of the environmental impact on biological and neurological function (U.S. Department of Health and Human Services, 2010); and
- Enhanced knowledge of the interaction of genetics, biology, and environment, especially in psychiatry (Caspi & Moffitt, 2006).

SOURCES OF TRAUMA AND STRESS

As noted, the membrane that separates stress in the various domains of one's life is permeable. The metaphor of a permeable membrane is especially useful here. A membrane is a barrier. It denotes separation and differentiation that depicts the real differences among workplace, personal and family, and community environmental factors. At the same time, the notion of permeability acknowledges that factors inside these domains move among and influence what occurs in another. Viewing these domains as entirely separate misses the importance of cross-influence. Overconflationing domains risks appreciating the special and unique stress-exacerbating and mitigation characteristics of each. Stresses originating in the workplace are brought home and vice versa. Community stressors are brought to both home and work.

Box 27.1 illustrates the separate but overlapping nature of stressors in these three domains.

IMPACT OF TRAUMA AND STRESS IN THE WORKPLACE

As noted, the cost of mental disorders is massive (Bloom et al., 2011) but also difficult to precisely measure. At the same time, prevention and effective intervention can reduce costs significantly. Costs of disorders include

- Reduced productivity (decreased attention, increased sick leave, presentism);
- Increased workplace accidents and errors;
- Reduced retention (increasing recruitment and training costs);
- Increased use of health care resources;
- Increased potential for workplace disruption and violence; and
- Erosion of interpersonal environment (adversely impacting teamwork and commitment to tasks);

> **BOX 27.1. THREE DOMAINS OF STRESSORS**
>
> Illustrative examples (not comprehensive) follow:
>
> **WORKPLACE FACTORS**
> - Personal danger/risk/exposure
> - Interpersonal stress
> - Stressful working conditions
> - Stress-inducing personnel policies and procedures
> - Quality of leadership/management
> - Harassment/bullying
>
> **PERSONAL/FAMILY FACTORS**
> - Health/medical problems
> - Mental illness
> - Poverty/negative economic factors
> - Marital/family conflict
>
> **COMMUNITY/ENVIRONMENTAL FACTORS**
> - Disaster/crisis
> - Epidemic/pandemic
> - Environmental pollution
> - Economic and social justice challenges

STRATEGIES FOR REDUCING WORKPLACE STRESS

Stress in the workplace, including traumatic stress, can result from many factors, some more obvious than others.

- Job description/definition—The nature of the job itself may create risk for stress and/or traumatic stress. Examine what is expected and required for the job to explore what factors might mitigate or exacerbate stress. For example, alternating shifts may disturb sleep cycles. Are alternations necessary?
- Worker selection—Optimizing the match between the worker and the job is the art and science of employee selection. One factor for determining the goodness of this match is the history and temperament of the worker and the type of personality or temperament required by the job. For example, some workers require predictability and stability in their work. These workers may excel in jobs with consistent pace and task. Others thrive on novelty and unpredictability, so they are stressed by positions where work is routine and predictable.

In my work in the field of disaster behavioral health, I have seen both the benefits and the challenges of matching worker temperament with the task. For example, it is helpful to inquire of health, especially behavioral health, of workers interested in becoming involved in disaster preparedness and response and investigate their problem-solving/decision making styles. Those who require significant time, information, and interactive processes are better suited for roles in the preparedness phase than in the response phase where decisions need to be made quickly based on little and conflicting information.

- Worker training—All work requires training and orientation. Does worker training includes anticipating and managing the stresses involved in the job? Ironically, professions (such as police and firefighters) that involve high stress and require ongoing certification of various skills seldom view identifying and managing stress as a necessary job skill.
- Worker support—Regardless of how exceptional selection and training are, stress and trauma occur. When it does, what types of support are available to workers? Peer support? Employee assistance programs(EAP)? Professional help through health insurance?
- Work environment—Characteristics of the work environment impact stress and trauma. Physical characteristics include level of danger, physical demands, light, air quality, exposure to toxic agents, and so on.
- Organizational culture—I strongly believe that an organization's culture and organizational leadership are two of the most important, and under-considered, factors in determining psychosocial impact of workplaces (Flynn & Lane, 2008). People know when the organizations they work in and for respect, value, and care about them and when they do not. A healthy and caring organizational culture identifies problems

early, responds quickly and appropriately, and minimizes barriers to identifying and helping workers who are experiencing stress- and trauma-related problems.
- Leadership—Healthy organizational cultures don't just happen. They are the product of capable and enlightened leadership at all levels. Quality leadership will consider all the factors in a certain situation, monitor their impact, and respond quickly and appropriately when changes are needed.

ROLES FOR ORGANIZATIONAL CONSULTANTS

Organizational consultants play a variety of roles for, and within, organizations, depending on their profession (e.g., psychiatrist, psychologist, social worker, or other consultant). The nature of these roles are strong determinants in what can, should, and should not be done in this context.

- Organizational leaders—Physicians and other consultants often play leadership roles within organizations. The most common leadership roles are within health and medically related organizations where their central role is obvious. However, in other types of organizations, physicians and other behavioral science professionals may play other leadership roles at various places in the organization. Physicians and others may enjoy leadership roles within organizations that exceed their official job description, title, or organizational location.
- Workers within an organization—Physicians and others may find themselves working in many capacities within organizations ranging from line direct service to senior executive positions and everywhere in between. They may also find themselves in staff roles (as compared to line positions) or as special advisors to senior executives where they may have easy and powerful access to key decision-makers while not being in direct supervisory positions.
- Occupational/employee health—Larger corporations often have specialized components dedicated to employee health. These operations can be part of the organization itself or operate by contract. Behavioral health professionals in these components often have responsibilities for direct services to employees and/or advising the larger organization on factors influencing worker health and safety.
- Training and education—Physicians and others may be called upon to provide education and training to all administrative levels on a variety of topics including identification and management of stress, trauma, and other psychosocial topics.
- Consultant (to EAP, leadership, management, etc.)—Physicians and others frequently find themselves in the role of consultant to organizations. As noted, it is important that the consultant understand the role of the consultant, its limits and opportunities, and a variety of consultation techniques and strategies. Knowledge about consultation from medical education is a helpful start. However, that training likely focused more on consultation regarding specific patient clinical topics rather than content about consulting to organizations and leaders regarding the cultural, organizational, and policy aspects of stress-related issues.

Case Example

A psychiatrist colleague and I were asked to provide a consultation that had been requested by a major manufacturing plant in a rural area where "everybody knows everybody." The request originated from plant management's concerns regarding impact of worker stress on a variety of problems including perceived excess sick leave, injuries, and productivity problems. The consultation involved spending time in several different areas of the plant to determine common and unique stressors and meetings with line staff, supervisors, and managers. Especially important were meetings with top management as well as the plant physician, who also served as the community's only physician. As one might anticipate, stress issues involved major environmental factors (e.g., noise, heat, and physical danger), job security, and potential for compromised confidentiality of health and medical issues as a result of minimal care options for workers/patients in and outside the plant.

As consultants, great care was needed in areas including

- Clarification of who was the "client"
- Clarifying and respecting the nature and limits of confidentiality

- Assuring access to people, records, policies, and procedures
- Crafting recommendations that were tailored to the unique circumstances of the organization, plant management and workers, and the community.

- Evaluation of workplace conditions—Consultants may be called upon to evaluate not only individuals but organizations, organizational components, and/or organizational systems. As noted, it is important that the scope and limits of evaluation are clear. What is being evaluated and how? Does evaluation include recommendations? Who receives the completed evaluation?
- Evaluation of workers—Physicians may be called upon to perform medical evaluation of workers at any organizational level. The circumstances of these evaluations will be determined largely by the circumstances of the request and role of the physician. The nature of the request, goals of the evaluation, nature of recommendations, and distribution of the completed evaluation are important factors to clarify prior to beginning the evaluation.

One circumstance that warrants special mention because of its delicacy, complexity, and blending of roles is the physician's role with respect to an impaired leader. As before, the role played by the physician will depend heavily on whether the physician is inside or outside the organization and what options are available to the physician.

Suggestions include

- Analyze the problem's origin. Is the problem the result of a diagnosable disorder (physical or mental)? Is the leader simply unpleasant or difficult? Is the problem recent or long standing?
- What are the consequences of the problem? Depressed morale of the organization's personnel, decreased productivity? Increased adverse actions (e.g., employees' grievances, legal action, etc.)? Increased staff turnover, absenteeism, presentism?
- What are the sources of authority to deal with the leader (e.g., supervisor, board of directors, human resources, labor unions)?
- What actions might solve or reduce the problem (e.g., transfer, treatment, coaching, termination, etc.)?
- What is your role? What actions are you comfortable with and/or prepared to take? Is there someone with whom you can consult?

Some readings on specialized leadership situations may also be helpful. These include Einarsen, Skogstad, and Glasø (2013) on leaders who bully, Goldman (2006) on leaders with borderline personality disorder, and Kets de Vries (2014) on the use of coaching with toxic leaders.

Referral

In many situations involving stress and trauma, referral for services outside the workplace may be appropriate and necessary. Even in organizations with EAPs, there are typically limits to the nature and duration of these services. Physicians and other direct service providers making referrals must be aware of, and current in their knowledge of, referral resources. What are the referral resources? What is known about them? Are there financial or procedural barriers to be dealt with?

I have always believed that referral is an art, not a failure. In too many cases, behavioral health and other providers see facilitating a referral as a shortcoming in their skills or abilities. Instead, referral is a healthy acknowledgment of the limits of our expertise and an acknowledgment of the valuable contributions of others. Above all, it represents a commitment to placing the needs of our patients/clients above all else.

The referral is also an art. Making a successful referral involves assuring that the patient/client is prepared for the referral; that the process is made as smooth as possible; and that the connection to the referral is accomplished.

GETTING STARTED

As in medicine, there are several common, fairly standard questions to be asked and data to be gathered before going into diagnosis and development of workplace intervention strategies. Consider the following:

- Type of workplace—As noted, workplaces come in all shapes and sizes. These factors will have significant impact on all roles played by a physician or other professionals. Is the organization small or large, centralized or decentralized? What is the nature of the workforce, leadership structure, and governance?

- Types of stressors—What is the nature of the stressors? Do they vary by levels and locations? Have there been critical incidents that impacting the organization (e.g., workplace violence, toxic exposure, community unrest, etc.)?
- Resources available—What resources are available to line workers and leadership for stress- or trauma-related problems? Are unions involved? Is there an EAP? Are there appropriate referral resources?
- Your role/resources/task—What is appropriate and feasible for you to do is heavily dependent on the role you play, resources available to you, and nature of the task.
- What resources are available to you? Are there adequate and appropriate human and financial resources to do the job? What are the time frames for accomplishing the job?
- Is the task appropriate and reasonable? Are goals and expectations clear and mutually agreed upon?

Consulting for and Working with Organizations

I have done organizational diagnosis and consultation with many organizations, as well as working within a variety of types of organizations, and can share several of the lessons learned from these experiences. Some of these lessons have been learned through successes and unfortunately some by less than successful ventures:

- Help leadership shape the questions/problems—Consultants are brought into organizations to respond to and or solve particular challenges. Ironically, more often than not, the initial question is not the most important or relevant question. A key role for a consultant is to help the requester shape or reshape the question in order to achieve optimal results and value from the consultation. This might involve setting limits, recommending other consultants, or, at times, walking away from the consultation.

Case Example

I have been asked by several organizations to write their emergency plans. In all cases, reshaping of the request was attempted. These attempts were based on the strong belief that outside consultants can be very helpful in *assisting* organizations in developing their own plans but that consultants should not write plans *for* organizations. Consultants can never know an organization as well as its members and, if plans are written by consultants, there is little organizational investment in the outcome. In most cases, this reshaping of the request from "do it for me" to "do it with me" has been successful. In a few cases, it has not, and the request was politely declined.

- Diagnose the motivation for the request—Every consultant knows that things are often not as they seem. What may seem a benign and simple request may be the product or hidden motivations or goals. These may not necessarily be nefarious, but it is wise to gain the most accurate and comprehensive view possible of the request's context. Who really wants this and why? Are there other internal and external factors at play (e.g., new legislative requirements, pending litigation, test of leadership, etc.)?
- Know the role of consultant and don't do the work of the consultee—As noted, being a consultant is very different than being an member of the organization. In addition, organizational consultation is different than case or clinical consultation. Consultants have credibility by virtue of whatever skills, expertise, or experiences resulted in being asked to consult. Remember, consultants have no direct authority in organizational decision-making or operational control. Those wanting more detail on the scope, limits, and unique opportunities through consultation will find rich theory and practice guidelines in the seminal early work of Gerald Caplan (Caplan & Caplan, 1993), a pioneer in America psychiatry.
- Assure access to all necessary levels organizational levels and components—Providing an effective consultation may require access to and information gathering from parts of the organization different than the requesting entity. At the start, it is important to assure that this access will be provided. There is a high probability that the consultation will be compromised if the consultant is unable to gather information necessary to formulate findings and recommendations. In many

cases, reluctance to provide a consultant with access to necessary sources is an indicator of organizational problems and/or should prompt closer examination of the motivation for the consultation request.

- Look at the organizational chart—This suggestion may surprise some consultants. However, the organizational chart, and how it is described and explained, can be invaluable to consultants. Think of it as a combination of an x-ray and Rorschach inkblot test. The organizational chart displays the inner structure of an organization; relationships among components; relative power, status, and authority within the structure; or, at least, how the organization *wishes* to be perceived. At a minimum, it raises important additional questions.

A multidisciplinary mental health services agency was frustrated by its inability to recruit and retain psychiatrists. In day-to-day operations, the non-clinical director was frustrated by what was seen as manipulative behavior by a series of staff psychiatrists. A look at the organizational chart found the psychiatrist several levels down from the top. Interviews with the psychiatrist indicated his persistent perception that he did not enjoy adequate authority in clinical cases while feeling a burden of disproportional responsibility and liability. The consultation resulted in a different organizational location for the psychiatrist and a heightened sensitivity by the administrator regarding issues of appropriately aligning authorities and responsibilities.

Look at the personnel policies and practices—Some of the simplest solutions to worker stress lie in the most obvious, yet often overlooked, places. When assessing worker stress, a look at an organizations personal policies and practices are often very illuminating. What do they reflect about the organizations culture (discussed earlier)? They can reveal policies that impact stress such as working hours and conditions, grievance procedures, supervisory mechanisms, and worker suggestions, to name a few.

A large government entity requested consultation regarding increased worker stress that was creating performance problems in serving the public. While many factors are at play in this situation, review of the personnel policies and practices revealed a very strong monetary incentive to work overtime. Many of these relatively low-paid workers worked extraordinarily long hours and did so continuously as they had come to depend on the resulting higher income. As a result of the consultation, overtime policies were modified. Initially the workers were unhappy with these changes. However, the long-term result was reduced stress in the workforce and reduction in stress-related illnesses.

It is important to understand the cascading and interactive impact of organizational policies, treatment of psychological disorders, and how these interactive effects impact both workers and organizations. These can be complex and not always obvious.

A large law enforcement organization had a policy that workers could not carry weapons while taking psychotropic medications. Many, if not most, workers would not be allowed to perform their roles without carrying a weapon. As a result, many workers rejected needed treatment, resulting in exacerbation in their disorders. Others self-medicated with alcohol or illicit medications. Others took medication but stopped before regularly scheduled medical evaluations and resumed after. None of these behavioral outcomes helped workers or accomplished the desired goals of the organizations.

For those interested in further exploring organizational diagnosis and consultation, psychologist Harry Levinson's landmark text (Levinson, 2002) is a valuable resource, reflecting Levinson's over 40 years of organizational consulting. It is often used by behavioral health consultants as well as the organizations for which they consult.

Another set of well-respected resources for those wanting to explore group relations especially applicable to organizational diagnosis and consultation is the A. K. Rice Institute (A.K. Rice Institute, 2017; Cytrynbaum & Noumair, 2004). This organization in the United States is affiliated with London's well-known Tavistock Institute of Human Relations (Abraham, 2013).

Finally, the American Psychiatric Association Foundation (APA; 2017a) has an ongoing program to address workplace mental health issues, especially those impacting employee health, work performance, and productivity. That program also produces a quarterly publication *Mental Health*

Works (APA, 2017b) that provides regular workplace mental health research, implementation strategies, and tools.

LEGAL AND ADMINISTRATIVE FACTORS

Dealing effectively with workplace stress and trauma is not limited to clinical or organizational climate consideration. A wide variety of legal and administrative factors are always present and must be considered. These factors are often guided by national legislation and policy while others may be determined by state and local requirements. Other considerations result from agreements with labor unions.

Because of these factors, this chapter does not attempt to provide specifics on these factors but instead provides overall guidance and a sampling of the types of considerations that may need attention.

- Employment law—What are the applicable laws that govern employment in general and specifically mental health and substance use and abuse? Such requirements may include, but are certainly not limited to, disabilities law and discrimination statutes. Examples of relevant federal laws include:

  —Americans with Disabilities Act of 1990 (1990)

  —Mental Health Parity and Addiction Equity Act of 2008 —Health Care and Education Reconciliation Act of 2010 (*Pub.L.* 111–152, 124 Stat. 1029)

  —Occupational Safety and Health Act of 1970 (Public Law 91-596) and its amendments

- Employee rights/union factors—Employer organizations operate under policies and procedures that are guided by laws and agreements concerning the rights of employees. In addition, agreements with labor unions frequently include factors such as employment and retention rights and procedures, union involvement in personnel actions, and working conditions.
- Health insurance requirements—Workers may or may not be covered by health insurance. When it is in place, coverage and options are quite variable. Where no such insurance exists, the availably and costs of receiving services are often barriers to receiving appropriate health and medical services.
- Personnel policies and practices—Personnel policies and practices may have a significant impact on workers in the context of medical practice. This is especially true for psychiatric conditions. For example, recommended sick leave may or may not result in reduced worker pay. Physicians and other organizational consultants should be aware that requiring treatment, especially as a requirement for continued employment, has many ramifications for both employers and employees. Certain medical interventions have performance and career implications. For example, policies regarding workers being on psychotropic medications may preclude workers from preforming specific tasks, carrying weapons, or operating certain machinery. Physicians and others should be fully aware of these factors.
- Medical/health professional and licensing rules and ethics—Licensing is typically handled by states. However, national guild organizations frequently determine the scope of practice and ethical considerations. Obviously, all licensed providers must practice within the scope of their license and the requirements of their professional organizations. When these requirements or their applicability are unclear, it is wise to seek guidance and advice from appropriate parties.

WORKPLACES WITH SPECIAL STRESS-RELATED CONSIDERATIONS

- Public safety workplaces—Some occupations have special characteristics that represent a higher risk of stress and trauma than others by with the nature of the requirements of the work itself. Public safety is a prime example, but such characteristics can be found in other occupational groups such as the military. Special characteristics that tend to exacerbate stress and trauma include

  —Physical danger to workers (e.g., physical assault, working in hostile environments)

—Uncertain nature of work situations (e.g., traffic stops, responding to domestic disturbances)

—Constant observation (e.g., cell phone videos, surveillance cameras, body cameras)

—Highly variable public perception of performance and social value

—Highly variable training

—Variable organizational, community, and political support

Physicians and other behavioral health professionals working with the stress and trauma of workers in these types of work and work environments should be aware of these factors and have specialized training regarding their roles in serving these types of workers.

- Public health and medical workplaces—These types of workplaces have unique and complex challenges, opportunities, and characteristics. Ideally, these should be most sensitized and prepared to deal with workplace stress and trauma. This is not always the case. In these organizations, physicians frequently serve as both workers and leaders. They face unique stressors such as exposure to contagious disease; occupational injury; and high and sometimes unrealistic individual, family, community, and political expectations. At the same time, these workplaces often benefit from having more resources than most for anticipating and responding to worker stress and trauma. Physicians in these environments have special opportunities, and obligations, to appropriately and adequately address these types of worker challenges.
- Toxic exposure—Workers of various types may experience exposure to toxic agents either in their usual workplaces (e.g., asbestos exposure by welders in shipyards) or through episodic exposure due to the nature of their work (e.g., exposure of rescue/recovery workers at the 9/11 World Trade Center's collapse (Smith et al., 2004). These exposures and their intersection with workplace stress are serious and complex. For example, in disaster research it has been long noted that events causing adverse or unknown health effects increase risk for adverse psychosocial consequences (Norris et al., 2002). In the case of rescue and recovery workers in New York following 9/11, psychosocial impact was serious and long lasting and intertwined with physical consequences (Centers for Disease Control and Prevention, 2014).

  Identifying and responding to the psychosocial consequences of toxic exposure is not only a health challenge. These issues frequently are fraught with confounding political, legal, and financial factors.
- Homeland security/emergency preparedness workplaces—These types of workplaces also often experience unique workplace stressors. They anticipate and respond to low-probability, high-impact events. Workers are exposed to highly stressful actual and simulated events with little tolerance for failure. Workers often have high -level security clearances resulting in the requirements that their knowledge and stressors not be shared with others, even behavioral health or other health providers.

  Physicians and other behavioral health professionals working in these types of environment should be well versed in the unique stresses of this type of work as well as special considerations regarding implications of security clearance for themselves and those served.
- Fitness for duty considerations—Behavioral health professionals, and especially physicians, may be asked to make *fitness for duty* evaluations and recommendations regarding workers. In effect, they may be asked to assess if an experience, condition, or disorder would render a worker unable to do his or her duties without endangering themselves or others.

While some of these situations are clear and obvious, many are not. These types of evaluations are enmeshed with factors such as longer-term career impact, stigma, and the potential for seeking secondary gain. When fitness for duty evaluations are part of a behavioral health professional's workplace role, special training and understanding is recommended.

SUMMARY

Trauma respects no boundaries or domains in the lives of individuals and groups. That includes workplaces. The trauma may occur as a consequence of events and characteristics specific to the workplace environment, natural disaster or mass violence in the larger community, or any number of events that may occur in the lives of individuals and families. The range of effects on workers and organizations is wide and variable. Physicians or other leaders working as clinicians, consultants, and leaders in the aftermath of traumatic exposures must recognize this range, identify factors which may mitigate or reduce the adverse consequences, and practice and model leadership behaviors that reduce workplace stress after trauma. Moreover, they must be prepared to advise others in principles of planning for, and responding to, the traumatic experiences of the workforce to promote continuity of mission and favorable outcomes for affected individuals and organizations.

REFERENCES

Abraham, F. (2013). The Tavistock Group. In M. Nitzel & M. Warner (Eds.), *The Oxford handbook of management theorists* (pp. 155–173). Oxford: Oxford University Press.

A. K. Rice Institute (2017). Home page. Retrieved from http://akriceinstitute.org/

American Psychiatric Association Foundation. (2017a). Mental health works. https://www.psychiatry.org/newsroom/news-releases/american-psychiatric-association-foundation-unveils-the-center-for-workplace-mental-health

American Psychiatric Association Foundation. (2017b). Workplace mental health. http://www.americanpsychiatricfoundation.org/priorities/workplace-mental-health

Americans With Disabilities Act of 1990 (As Amended). (1990). Retrieved from https://www.ada.gov/pubs/adastatute08.htm

Black, S. E., & Lynch, L. M. (2004). What's driving the new economy? The benefits of workplace innovation. *The Economic Journal, 114*(493), 97–116.

Bloom, D. E., Cafiero, E. T., Jané-Llopis, E., Abrahams-Gessel, S., Bloom, L. R., Fathima, . . . Weinstein, C. (2011, September). The global economic burden of non-communicable diseases. Geneva: World Economic Forum. Retrieved from http://www3.weforum.org/docs/WEF_Harvard_HE_GlobalEconomicBurdenNonCommunicableDiseases_2011.pdf

Bureau of Labor Statistics. Number of jobs held, labor market activity, and earnings growth among the youngest baby boomers: Results from a longitudinal survey. (2015, March). Washington, DC: Bureau of Labor Statistics. Retrieved from https://www.bls.gov/news.release/pdf/nlsoy.pdf

Caplan, G., & Caplan, R.B. (1993). *Mental health consultation and collaboration.* Long Grove IL: Waveland Press.

Caplin, G., & Caplin, R. (2000). Principles of community psychiatry. *Community Mental Health Journal, 36*(1), 7–24. doi:10.1023/A:1001894709715

Carter, R., Satcher, D., & Coelho, T. (2013). Addressing stigma through social inclusion. *American Journal of Public Health, 103*(5), 773.

Caspi, A., & Moffitt, T. E. (2006). Gene–environment interactions in psychiatry: Joining forces with neuroscience. *Nature Reviews Neuroscience Perspectives, 7*, 583–590. doi:10.1038/nrn1925

Centers for Disease Control and Prevention. (2014) World Trade Center Health Program, Research Meeting Proceedings, June 17–17. Retrieved from https://www.cdc.gov/wtc/proceedings.html

Chisholm, D., Sweeny, K., Sheehan, P., Rasmussen, B., Smit, F., Cuijpers, P., & Saxena, S. (2016). Scaling-up treatment of depression and anxiety: A global return on investment analysis. *The Lancet Psychiatry, 3*(5), 415–424.

Cytrynbaum, S., & Noumair, D. (2004). *Group relations reader, 3*. Jupiter, FL: A. K. Rice Institute.

Einarsen, S., Skogstad, A., & Glaso, L. (2013). When leaders are bullies: Concepts, antecedents, and consequences. In H. S. Leonard, R. Lewis, A. M. Freedman, & J. Passmore, (Eds.), *Wiley-Blackwell handbook of the psychology of leadership, change, and organizational development* (pp. 129–154). London: John Wiley.

Ekberg, K., Pransky, G. S., Besen, E., Fassier, J. B., Feuerstein, M., Munir, F., & Blanck, P. (2016). New business structures creating organizational opportunities and challenges for work disability prevention. *Journal of Occupational Rehabilitation, 26*(4), 480–489.

Flynn, B. W., & Lane, C. F. (2008). Integrating organizational and behavioral health principles to promote resilience in extreme events. In R. J. Burke & C. L. Cooper. (Eds.), *International terrorism and threats to security: Managerial and organizational challenges* (pp. 185–218). Northampton, MA: Edward Elgar.

Goldman, A. (2006). High toxicity leadership: Borderline personality disorder and the dysfunctional organization. *Journal of Managerial Psychology, 21*(8), 733–746.

Harder, H. G., Wagner, S., & Rash, J. (2016). *Mental illness in the workplace: Psychological disability management.* New York: Routledge.

Health Care and Education Reconciliation Act of 2010. P.L. 111–152, 124 Stat. 1029. http://www.hhs.gov/sites/default/files/reconciliation-law.pdf

Kets de Vries, F. R. (2014, April). Coaching the toxic leader. *Harvard Business Review.*

Retrieved from https://hbr.org/2014/04/coaching-the-toxic-leader

Levinson, H. (2002). *Organizational assessment: A step-by-step guide to effective consulting.* Washington, DC: American Psychological Association.

Norris, F. H., Friedman, M. J., Watson, P. J., Byrne, C. M., Diaz, E., & Kaniasty, K. (2002). 60,000 disaster victims speak: Part I. An empirical review of the empirical literature, 1981—2001. *Psychiatry, 65*(3), 207–239..

Occupational Safety and Health Act of 1970. Retrieved from https://www.osha.gov/pls/oshaweb/owadisp.show document?p table=OSHACT&p_id=2743

Organizational Parity and Addiction Equity Act of 2008. Retrieved from https://www.cms.gov/CCIIO/Programs-and-Initiatives/Other-Insurance-Protections/MHPAEA.html

Rosenberg, S., & Lapidus, J. (1999). Contingent and non-standard work in the United States: Towards a more poorly compensated, insecure workforce. In L. Felstead (Ed.), *Global trends in flexible labour* (pp. 62–83). London: Macmillan Education.

Smith, R. P., Katz, C. L., Holmes, A., Herbert, R., Levin, S., Moline, J., . . . Hurrell, J. J. (2004, September). Mental health status of World Trade Center rescue and recovery workers and volunteers—New York City, July 2002–August 2004. *MMWR, 53*(35). Retrieved from https://www.cdc.gov/Mmwr/preview/mmwrhtml/mm5335a2.htm

Sverke, M., Hellgren, J., & Näswall, K. (2002). No security: A meta-analysis and review of job insecurity and its consequences. *Journal of Occupational Health Psychology, 7*(3), 242–264.

U.S. Department of Health and Human Services. (2010). Healthy people 2020: 2020 topics and objectives, environmental health. Retrieved from https://www.healthypeople.gov/2020/topics-objectives/topic/environmental-health

Vos, T., Barber, R. M., Bell, B., Bertozzi-Villa, A., Biryukov, S., Bolliger, I., . . . Duan, L. (2015). Global, regional, and national incidence, prevalence, and years lived with disability for 301 acute and chronic diseases and injuries in 188 countries, 1990–2013: A systematic analysis for the Global Burden of Disease Study 2013. *The Lancet, 386*(9995), 743–800.

World Health Organization. (1994, October). Global strategy on occupational health for all: The way to health at work. (1994, October). Geneva: World Health Organization. Retrieved from http://www.who.int/occupational_health/globstrategy/en/

World Health Organization (2000). *Mental Health and Work: Impact, Issues, and Good Practices.* Geneva: WHO.

World Health Organization. (2011). *Global status report on non-communicable diseases 2010.* Geneva: Author.

28

Family-Based Interventions for PTSD

STEPHEN J. COZZA

INTRODUCTION

Posttraumatic stress disorder (PTSD) is associated with negative health and mental health effects in those afflicted by the condition (Hidalgo & Davidson, 2000; Kessler, 2000) but also has been shown to have negative effects on relationships with intimate partners and close relatives, including children (Whisman, Sheldon, & Goering, 2000). PTSD resulting from natural disasters or terrorism may affect multiple members of the family, especially when family members have been exposed to the same event, or when homes, neighborhoods, or communities have been broadly affected (North & Pfefferbaum, 2013). Other forms of trauma (e.g., sexual assault or combat exposure) may only be experienced by individuals within the family; however traumatic sequelae (to include resultant PTSD) are also likely to affect close family members. Although different types of trauma will require tailored approaches to family intervention, PTSD broadly affects interpersonal relationships, communication, and family functioning. Most of the existing literature has focused on military and veteran families affected by combat-related PTSD. As a result, this military perspective is used to structure this chapter and to highlight several areas important to our understanding of PTSD and its effect on families with children: framing PTSD from a family systems perspective and recognizing its impact on relationships and family functioning (e.g., marital relationships and partner intimacy, parenting, children); reviewing child developmental considerations, describing unique challenges of childhood traumatic bereavement, and summarizing the developing literature examining family interventions for PTSD. Six strategies are highlighted that can mitigate risk in families affected by PTSD.

FAMILY SYSTEMS AND AN UNDERSTANDING OF THE EFFECT OF PTSD

An ecological framework is helpful in examining the impact of PTSD within families. Bronfenbrenner (1979) defined *ecological systems theory* in order to characterize the interactive effects of smaller and larger systems of relationships and social connections that influence human health and development. The association between child health and wellness and parental health has been well documented in trauma-exposed populations (Wickrama & Kaspar, 2008; Chemtob et al., 2010, Chandra et al., 2010; Lester et al., 2010). Because relationships within the family system bidirectionally impact individual and relationship functioning (Cox & Paley, 1997; Bronfenbrenner & Morris, 2006), service providers caring for patients with PTSD must be aware of its effects within the family and be prepared to engage family members in order to address the complex outcomes that can result.

Several theorists have targeted the interactive skills and routines that can protect family members and therefore promote health in spouses and children during times of stress or trauma. Walsh (2006) outlined the Family Resilience Theory which emphasizes the importance of the following processes to overall family health in traumatic circumstances: the ability to develop and preserve shared beliefs, constructive communication, and healthy patterns of organization. Gewirtz, Forgatch, and Wieling (2008) proposed a preventive framework that incorporates positive parenting practices to achieve important family goals after trauma exposure: by providing a social environment that offers structure, security, and emotional warmth and that can address the traumatic event.

Citing work with military families undergoing the stress of combat deployment and reunification, Saltzman and colleagues (2011) proposed that family interventions should also promote: (a) increased understanding, support, and forgiveness among family members; (b) improved communication and cohesion; (c) coordinated parental leadership; (d) defined but adjustable roles and responsibilities; and (e) development of shared goals and beliefs. Several groups have similarly highlighted the theoretical (Wadsworth et al., 2013) and clinical (Cozza, Holmes, & Van Ost, 2013) importance of family centered approaches to combat-related PTSD.

IMPACT OF PTSD ON MARRIAGES, INTIMATE RELATIONSHIPS, AND FAMILIES

PTSD has toxic effects within the family environment, negatively impacting relationships between intimate partners, as well as relationships with children. Studies consistently relate PTSD with relationship problems (Kessler, 2000; Whisman, Sheldon, & Goering, 2000). The combination of risk behaviors and psychological symptoms that characterize PTSD have been associated with poor intimate relationships, negative marital satisfaction, impaired family functioning, greater family distress, higher levels of family violence, and disrupted parenting and parent-child relationships (for a comprehensive review see Galovski & Lyons, 2004). Avoidance or numbing, hyperarousal, and anger (either service member/veteran or partner) have all been associated with family adjustment problems (Hendrix, Erdmann, & Briggs, 1998; Riggs, Byrne, Weathers, & Litz, 1998; Evans, McHugh, Hopwood, & Watt, 2003; Taft, Schumm, Panuzio, & Proctor, 2008). The negative effects of PTSD broadly impact multiple aspects of marital functioning (including divorce) and are consistent regardless of the type of military mission (Kulka et al., 1990; Gimbel & Booth, 1994; Riggs, Byrne, Weathers, & Litz, 1998; Sherman, Zanotti, & Jones, 2005; Karney & Crown, 2007). In studies of service members from past and current wars, children of service members with PTSD exhibited general distress, depression, lower self-esteem, aggression, impaired social relationships, and school-related difficulties (Rosenheck & Nathan, 1985; reviewed in Galovski & Lyons, 2004). All of these effects undermine family health and functioning and appear to be specific to PTSD, rather than more generally attributable to trauma exposure. For example, veterans suffering with PTSD divorce at a higher rate compared to similarly trauma-exposed veterans without PTSD (Jordan et al., 1992; Cook, Riggs, Thompson, Coyne, & Sheikh, 2004).

Spouses and partners of service members with chronic PTSD are more likely than spouses of nonaffected service members to show higher rates of distress, psychological symptoms (to include depression and suicidal ideation), and poorer adjustment (Calhoun, Beckham, & Bosworth, 2002; Manguno-Mire et al., 2007). Of note, a spouse's mental health problems have been shown to incur greater harm to children's functioning than a service member's, suggesting additive and interactive risk (Herzog, Everson, & Whitworth, 2011). The caustic effect of PTSD on spouse health and couple relationships may also undermine relationship trust. Distrust within a couple is likely to complicate collaborative parenting and decrease available support to children in PTSD-affected families.

More recently, investigators have examined the negative impact of PTSD on other marital or relationship functions. For example, Allen and colleagues (2010) have described the association of PTSD symptoms with poorer marital communication, confidence, relationship dedication, parental alliance, and relationship bonding. Fredman et al. (2014) highlighted the association of veteran PTSD symptoms with distress in both partners, suggesting a dynamic interaction of cognitive, behavioral, and emotional processes requiring further therapeutic attention. These investigators (Fredman, Vorstenbosch, Wagner, Macdonald, & Monson, 2014) introduced the concept of *partner accommodation*, which refers to the modification of a partner's own behavior or enabling of avoidance in the veteran spouse with PTSD, defining a powerful process that can interfere with couple functioning or undermine service member/veteran health. Allen and colleagues (2010) described how such behavior might undermine co parenting when a well-meaning partner might attempt to decrease hostility in the home by attempting to control all interactions between children and the parent suffering with PTSD.

Caregiver burden, or the perceived impact of caring for one with a chronic illness on social, emotional, physical, or financial health, has also been identified as negatively contributing to marital relationship well-being. Since up to one-third of those suffering with PTSD do not fully recover (Kessler, Sonnega, Bromet, Hughes, & Nelson, 1995), partners of veterans with PTSD are likely to face a number of ongoing stressors related to caring for someone with a chronic disease (Calhoun, Beckham, & Bosworth, 2002). Caregiver burden has been associated with distress in partners of veterans with PTSD and with the severity of PTSD symptoms (Beckham, Lytel, & Feldman, 1996). These findings suggest the importance of respite and social support services for families managing with chronic PTSD.

The impact of PTSD on relationship intimacy has recently become an area of interest and investigation. Monson et al. (2009) reported findings identifying the relation between PTSD and intimate partner discord, poorer service member and spouse intimate relationships satisfaction, and spouse's perception of marital distress. They concluded that the available evidence strongly associates PTSD symptoms and intimate relationship problems, with avoidance and numbing more closely associated with relationship dissatisfaction and hyperarousal more closely associated with aggression and spousal abuse (Monson, Taft, & Fredman, 2009).

PTSD AND PARENTING

PTSD has also been shown to undermine parenting behaviors and parenting satisfaction (Samper, Taft, Kind, & King, 2004; Berz, Taft, Watkins, & Monson, 2008). PTSD-affected parenting can be impaired by greater emotional reactivity, loss of cognitive capacity, higher levels of interpersonal aggression or increased avoidance, and disconnection from loved ones. In such circumstances, healthier parenting practices that had been in place prior to the onset of illness can be undermined by a variety of individual, social, family, psychiatric, and other health-related factors impacting the parenting couple.

PTSD can be expected to negatively impact parental cooperation and coordination of efforts that are necessary in raising children. Co-parenting is a term that was developed and initially applied in circumstances of separation or divorce in order to minimize conflict and support cooperation across parent households (Doherty, Beaton, & Wenger, 2013). Since its original usage, the term has been applied to intact families, recognizing the unique and varying contributions of fathers and mothers within a family systems model. Doherty, Beaton, and Wenger (2013) describe multiple influences that impact the co-parenting relationship, including contextual factors (e.g., employment, socioeconomic, community support), individual mother and father factors (e.g., physical and psychological well-being, family of origin parenting models, expectation of spouse), child factors (gender, age, and family size), and the marital relationship. Given changes in parental health and well-being resulting from PTSD, shifts in pre-existing parenting practices are likely to occur, often requiring formal renegotiation of the co-parenting relationship. Mental health problems in the spouse are likely to worsen this effect. Clinical literature contains accounts of the challenges couples face in co-parenting when a spouse has PTSD (Allen, Rhoades, Stanley, & Markman, 2010).

Successful PTSD parenting practices are not likely to be straightforward. Gewirtz and colleagues (2010) found strong negative relationships between PTSD, self-reported couple adjustment, and positive parenting behaviors, highlighting the need for better understanding of these processes. In a study describing the relationship of injured service member father self-reported posttraumatic symptoms, parenting behaviors, and child internalizing and externalizing symptoms, Holmes et al. (2013) reported moderating effects of two positive parenting strategies (monitoring/supervision and involvement/engagement) with PTSD but in opposite directions. Parental monitoring/supervision in the presence of higher posttraumatic symptoms decreased children's internalizing symptoms, whereas parental involvement/engagement in the presence of higher posttraumatic symptoms increased externalizing symptoms (Holmes et al., 2013). These preliminary findings indicate that successful parenting with PTSD may require something different than applying traditional positive parenting strategies. Given the changes that PTSD may have on co-parenting capacity, successful parenting with PTSD likely requires a renegotiation between the parents. Further study is needed that can better outline helpful treatment options.

PTSD AND CHILDREN

In studies of Vietnam combat veterans, children of service members with PTSD exhibit general distress, depression, lower self-esteem, aggression, impaired social relationships, and school-related difficulties (Rosenheck & Nathan, 1985). PTSD-associated aggression and family violence may lead to additional traumas within the family, further undermining child health (Galovski & Lyons, 2004).

A parent's PTSD likely affects children depending upon their age, developmental level, temperament, and pre-existing conditions. Younger children may struggle more than older children to cope and adapt to changes in a parent's behaviors and the parenting relationship, and very young children may have an especially hard time coping with the disorganized parental behavior that can result from PTSD, such as overreaction or disengagement.

Children's reactions should be expected to vary by their age and maturity, and a developmental perspective is critical. For example, infants and toddlers (0–2 years old) often respond negatively to family cues, such as changes in schedule and routines, the physical and emotional availability of important adults, as well as changes in the emotional climate (anxiety, interpersonal abruptness, irritability) in their families. An infant may evidence problems in sleeping or eating or may develop irritability or self-regulatory problems or disturbance of attachment in the face of a distressed or impaired caregiver.

Preschoolers (3–6 years old) often use *magical thinking*, an immature process that can lead them to inappropriately assume responsibility for a parent's anger, reactivity, avoidance, or depression. Preschoolers may become extremely anxious or disorganized by exposure to PTSD symptoms and are likely to demonstrate distress through regressive behaviors, such as loss of previously established developmental milestones (e.g., enuresis or sleep problems), clinginess to adults, or tantrums.

School-aged children possess more mature developmental capacity than younger children but still may harbor similar anxieties. Fear, guilt, and a desire to be helpful can complicate the school-aged child's response. These children may be confused about what is expected of them and be unsure how to act, especially toward a parent with PTSD. They may also be uncomfortable bringing up questions that could help them better understand and respond.

Teenagers can face unique developmental challenges related to their parents' illness. Teens normatively anticipate greater independence from parents and less reliance on family. Given their near-adult maturation and greater physical capacity, teenagers may be responsible for increased chores, care for younger siblings, or caregiving responsibilities with the injured parent. Such demands, in contrast to their desire to be with same age friends, may lead to frustration and conflict with parents.

Parents and health care providers should expect that PTSD will result in greater distress or worsening of symptom in children with preexisting medical, developmental, behavioral, or emotional conditions. Given disruptions in geographical transitions, possible separations from established child care providers and other distractions related to the care of the parent with PTSD, children's health care or educational needs can be neglected or inappropriately delayed. Parents and clinicians should use a lower threshold for referral to appropriate clinical resources for these more vulnerable children.

PTSD AND INTERPERSONAL VIOLENCE

PTSD has been associated with violence or aggression, which can further undermine family safety and stability. Studies with Operation Iraqi Freedom/Operation Enduring Freedom (OIF/OEF) veterans have found that the presence and severity of PTSD symptoms best accounts for veteran aggression (Hoge, Auchterlonie, & Milliken, 2006; Jakupcak et al., 2007; Taft, Vogt, Marshall, Panuzio, & Niles, 2007; Sayers, Farrow, Ross, & Oslin, 2009). A recent systematic review and meta-analyses of 16 studies published in the United States and UK conducted by MacManus and colleagues (2015) described contributions to all forms of veteran aggression and found that PTSD mediated the effect between combat and postdeployment violence. Alcohol misuse strengthens that effect. In a national study of veteran violence, Elbogen et al. (2012) surveyed male and female veterans in two waves of data collection and found that co-occurring PTSD and alcohol misuse was associated with violence, young age, and history of premilitary violence; lack of money to cover basic needs also significantly contributed to the outcome.

The impact of PTSD on domestic violence has been studied in Vietnam veteran families. Petrik, Rosenberg, and Watson (1983) found that combat experience, in the absence of PTSD, was not a strong predictor of violence. Similarly, Jordan et al. (1992) compared the wives of veterans with and without PTSD and found higher level of violence in both veterans and spouses in the PTSD versus non-PTSD group. Taft and colleagues (2005) studied potential risk factors for partner violence in 109 male Vietnam veteran violent offenders comparing those with and without PTSD. They found that traumatic experiences, comorbid psychopathology, and relationship problems associated with PTSD were risk factors for partner violence in their sample.

Elbogen and colleagues (2014) have described protective mechanisms that may serve to diminish community violence in PTSD-affected veterans. They conducted a national longitudinal survey between 2009 and 2011 and randomly sampled 1090 OIF/OEF veterans in two waves of data collection. They found that socioeconomic (money and stable employment), psychosocial (resilience, sense of control over one's life, and social support), and physical (adequate sleep and lack of pain) factors served as protective mechanisms to decrease community violence in veterans (Elbogen et al., 2014). These protective mechanisms may diminish partner aggression as well.

INTERVENTION STRATEGIES

There is a paucity of study of family interventions for PTSD. Two family-centered approaches that target parenting and family processes, Families OverComing Under Stress (FOCUS; Lester et al., 2013) and After Deployment Adaptive Parenting Tools (ADAPT; Gewirtz, Pinna, Hanson, & Brockberg, 2014) have shown promise in supporting military child and family health during and after combat deployments. While neither was designed to address the specific challenges of PTSD in families, both incorporate trauma informed strategies to target military families with deployment-related distress. FOCUS and ADAPT share common core components, including a strength-based approach, and an emphasis on emotion regulation, communication, problem-solving, and understanding and addressing children's developmental needs. In addition, ADAPT highlights several positive parenting practices including parental limit setting, monitoring, and involvement in school and other activities (Gewirtz, Pinna, Hanson, & Brockberg, 2014).

Several couples based treatments have been proposed to target family-related stress resulting from PTSD. Glynn and colleagues (1999) reported mixed results from a trial that included traditional exposure therapy for PTSD with random assignment to exposure combined with couples conjoint behavioral therapy. While improvement in PTSD was noted for exposure therapy, those who also received conjoint behavioral therapy received no additional benefit (Glynn et al., 1999). The most promising work to date is Cognitive Behavioral Conjoint Therapy for PTSD, a 15-session intervention that focuses on behavioral and communication strategies, the impact of traumatic experiences, and associated maladaptive thoughts on the couple, as well as the impact of additional symptoms of PTSD (Monson et al., 2011). Results of a small pilot study of seven couples were mixed with PTSD-affected veterans reporting nonsignificant improvements in relationships satisfaction, whereas partners reported statistically significant and large effect size improvements in relationship satisfaction. Studies in larger samples of younger veterans is required (Monson et al., 2011).

As mentioned, Elbogen et al. (2014) have studied mechanisms that may protect against veteran aggression and could serve as targets for preventive intervention efforts. These researchers found that protective mechanisms played a vital role in understanding and preventing post-deployment violence. They conceptualized an intervention based upon psychosocial rehabilitation theory, which focuses on symptom resolution, promoting collaboration care providers and developing skills for improved social functioning (including work and home). Their study identified several opportunities to reduce aggression, including reducing homelessness, helping with the transition to civilian work, improving financial management, and enhancing social support (Elbogen et al., 2014). In addition, these authors recommended addressing PTSD-associated hyperarousal, sleep disturbance, anger, and comorbid psychiatric and medical conditions (Elbogen et al., 2014). Further study is required.

CHILDHOOD TRAUMATIC BEREAVEMENT

Death may be an additional consequence of trauma, as occurs in natural disasters, terrorist events, and war. Grief is a normative response to the death of loved ones, and it encompasses emotional, physiological, cognitive, and behavioral reactions. These reactions may facilitate the bereavement processes, accepting the loss, coping with emotional reactions to the loss, and adjusting to life and self-identity changes (Brown & Goodman, 2005). The death of a parent or another family member can result in profound crises in children and may be traumatic in itself. When losses are sudden and violent, grief reactions can be further complicated by traumatic stress reactions and children may experience the death of loved ones under horrifying circumstances. Children's environments and experiences following a disaster, such as the loss of homes, schools, and religious institutions, as well as the intensity and content of media coverage, may increase their vulnerability for psychopathology (Dyregrov, Salloum, Kristensen, & Dyregrov, 2015). Childhood traumatic grief is a condition in which children are overwhelmed by the loss, and their abilities to mourn the loss are disturbed by trauma-related avoidance (Cohen, Mannarino, Greenberg, Padlo, & Shipley, 2002). Recently, the *Diagnostic and Statistical Manual of Mental Disorders* (fifth edition) included proposed criteria for persistent complex bereavement disorder in order to better identify clinically impairing grief response in both children and adults (American Psychiatric Association, 2013, pp. 789–790).

The broader literature examining the impact of parental death on children describes grief, distress, and dysphoria (Dowdney, 2000), as well as significant levels of psychopathology present within the two years after the death (when compared to a community sample) but resulting in less impairment than children suffering from depression (Cerel, Firstad, Verducci, Weller, & Weller, 2006). Several risk factors for poorer outcome in bereaved children have been identified, including pre-existing psychiatric illness, elevated levels of psychopathology in the surviving parent, traumatic parental deaths, as well as parental suicides (Brent, Melhem, Donohoe, & Walker, 2009; Cerel, Fristad, Weller, & Weller, 2000; Cerel et al., 2006; Dowdney, 2000). Some investigators have reported prolonged grief responses in suicide-related or other traumatically bereaved children, such as depression, functional impairment, and substance abuse (Brent et al., 2009; Melhem, Porta, Shamseddeen, Payne, & DA, 2011).

Effective family and parenting strategies, to include consistent discipline and parental warmth, have been associated with positive child outcomes after parental death (Kwok et al., 2005; Lin, Sandler, Ayers, Wolchik, & Luecken, 2004). The Family Bereavement Program is a group-based multimodal intervention that incorporates these positive parenting strategies along with other individual and conjoint (parent-child) strengthening activities to support family grief outcomes (Sandler et al., 2003). The program has demonstrated multiple family effects, including positive child mental health outcomes associated with effective parenting (Sandler et al., 2003), and follow-up assessments have shown these benefits have continued six years after intervention delivery (Hagan et al., 2012). Other military culturally relevant programs such as the Tragedy Assistance Program for Survivors (TAPS) help bereaved military spouses address the needs of their children through peer mentorship support. TAPS mentors provide comfort and support, inform newly bereaved families how best to gain access to resources and negotiate the intricate systems of care available to support military families, and share strategies for successfully parenting bereaved children. Sudden and violent deaths add risk for complicated grief outcomes in children (Brent et al., 2009). In circumstances when a child exhibits traumatic responses to a parent's death, for example, when a child is uncomfortable thinking about or talking about the circumstances of death or the lost parent, their avoidance can negatively encumber normative grief processes and has been referred to as childhood traumatic grief (Cohen & Mannarino, 2002). Trauma-focused cognitive behavior therapy (TF-CBT) has been effective in addressing traumatic elements to grief in children (Cohen & Mannarino, 2004). While TF-CBT is not a family intervention for grief, it does incorporate parent-child interactive sessions that facilitate communication and sharing within the family, fostering normative grieving for the child (Cohen & Mannarino, 2004).

CLINICAL APPLICATION AND INTERVENTION GOALS

PTSD can have powerful and defining effects on families. It can generate toxic levels of distress, secondarily undermining parenting and disorganizing family roles and healthy functioning. This challenge requires multisystem approaches to support child and family health. Such approaches call for defined family strategies derived from evidence-based principles to assist families at risk, which in turn must be connected to communities capable of support.

Family interventions should be contextualized within broader systems of care. Holmes, Rauch, and Cozza (2013) described recommendations to support children in military families affected by PTSD. For example, it is important to stabilize the family environment by ensuring access to basic needs, such as housing, education, health care, child care, and jobs throughout postmilitary transition; to identify and promote services that support family organization, communication, coping, and resilience; and to sustain systems of support for those families who might need help for many years. In addition, service members/veterans, spouses, and their children must have ready access to trauma-informed, evidence-based treatments close to where they live. In circumstances where children require clinical intervention, parents can still provide active support through collaborative involvement in their children's treatment. Given the stigma associated with mental disorders and hesitation in seeking help for family problems, military service members, veterans, and family members might not seek treatment or assistance, highlighting the need for enhanced outreach and engagement strategies.

Within this context of community and therapeutic support, the following six strategies are recommended for families with PTSD that incorporate the evidence base discussed throughout this chapter (Walsh 2006; Monson et al., 2011; Saltzman et al., 2011; Lester et al., 2013; Elbogen et al., 2014; Gewirtz, Pinna, Hanson, & Brockberg, 2014). These strategies include (a) maintaining a physically safe and structured environment, (b) engaging required community resources, (c) developing and sharing knowledge within and outside of the family that builds shared understanding, (d) building a positive emotionally safe and warm family environment, (e) mastering and modeling important interpersonal skills, including problem-solving and conflict resolution, and (f) maintaining a vision of hope and future optimism for the family.

Maintaining a Physically Safe and Structured Environment

Families faced with PTSD may contend with transitions from communities, as can be the case of military families or those affected by natural disasters or terrorist events, resulting in moves to new communities. Parents must ensure that children are safely integrated into these new communities and that adequate structure and support is provided to ensure healthy development. Positive parenting practices include monitoring of children's whereabouts; peer group participation; compliance with home, school, and civic rules; and active and successful engagement in academic programs. In addition, consistent family schedules (to include family meals, family recreational time) and clear parental expectations and appropriate consequence-based nonpunitive discipline will ensure supportive structure for children. In general, parents must provide their children with opportunities for normal growth and development that are independent from any at-home struggle the family is having resulting from PTSD.

Ensuring that basic needs are met also provides a sense of order and predictability that allows family members to be less distracted, function more effectively, and be supportive of each other as the family accommodates to life outside of the military. Adults are calmer and the frequency of impulsive, threatening, or disruptive behavior among family members is reduced when there is access to systems for household maintenance, meals, medical care, money management, and child care. Children are calmer when adults provide a predictable daily routine and model restraint.

Engaging Required Resources

Many PTSD-affected families will face challenges that require continued professional or personal support and assistance. Parents can address these challenges by engaging support for themselves, including required mental health care, occupational support, or assistance from community support programs or from neighbors, and for their children. Parents can successfully model resource engagement with their children, who must also learn the importance of asking for help from teachers, coaches, relatives, other caring adults, or friends when they are in need of assistance or instrumental support. Parents and children must recognize any barriers to engagement, such as stigmatization or avoidance resulting from PTSD that can undermine their ability to successfully access help. Last, parents and children should recognize that they live within communities of care that include relatives, neighbors, friends, health care professionals, school personnel, counselors, coaches, spiritual leaders, military and veteran support organizations, as well as local, state, and federal governmental agencies, and they can call upon each for assistance. Modeling the use of resources teaches one's children about the importance of asking for help and support when required and provides a lesson that can be used throughout life.

Developing and Sharing Knowledge Within and Outside of the Family that Builds Shared Understanding

Parents, along with health care providers, must provide appropriate information to children about their parents' PTSD and any of the consequences that they may have experienced as a result of those stressors. Any changed behavior that results from PTSD should be directly attributed to the psychiatric condition, rather than allowing a child to be confused about its origin. Clinicians and parents must provide helpful information about diagnoses, treatment options, and the likely long-term outcomes of the conditions. Adults as well as children may need to be reminded that emotional distance is a common symptom of PTSD and should be attributed to the illness, rather than to a change in an emotional commitment on the part of the parent. A key principle is that everyone, parents and children alike, is affected by the PTSD. Children, especially, must be reminded that the tension they see at home is not their fault and that it is not their responsibility to "fix" it.

Given the associated distress and the amount of information that must be shared among loved ones and with professionals, families may face unique challenges that can compromise communication. A primary goal of effective communication, to be achieved over time through frequent discussion, is to foster the family's *shared understanding* of the impact of PTSD on both adults and children. Effective communication must be ongoing (as situations can change) and include individuals both within and outside of the family. The detail and amount of information to be shared must be tailored to each recipient's "need to know" and "capacity to know." Children should not be provided paintful details about the trauma, but parents should answer children's questions respectfully and honestly. Communication with outside resources (extended family, neighbors, care systems, schools, clergy, etc.) is essential to the family's sense of safety and stability, but it must also respect each family member's need for a measure of privacy.

Children and adults should adopt a brief, clear, easily repeated, and general description of their family's story when speaking with teachers, coaches, and other concerned adults. For example, when speaking with a coach, a child can be taught to say that "my dad would love to see me play but can't be here today because he is a soldier who was in combat and gets bothered by crowds."

Because recovery from PTSD can proceed over a period of years, explanations to children must account for a family member's changing capacities and be commensurate with each child's developmental level. Adults should speak in a calm and matter-of-fact manner using language that is comprehensible to the child and should exclude any unnecessary or frightening information. Older children and teenagers will require more detailed and logical explanations of a military parent's condition, its impact on the family, and reasons for any expansions of their own household responsibilities.

Most importantly, effective communication creates a family atmosphere in which discussion is encouraged. Children should be prompted to express any emotions, either positive or negative, to let parents know when they are confused and encouraged to ask questions. Maintaining family dialogue allows both children and adults opportunities to develop a sense of closeness and shared understanding of how the recovery process affects each of them.

Building a Positive Emotionally Safe and Warm Family Environment

Strength-based family approaches and positive parenting strategies are common to previously discussed interventions (Gewirtz et al., 2014; Lester et al., 2013). Positive strategies include helping children and adults stay identified with strengths that were present prior to the development of PTSD. In the face of their current stress, both adults and children may need to be reminded that while their family may be "changed" by the event, they do not need to be defined by the illness. They continue to possess those prior-held strengths and they can use them effectively in the present and future. In fact, they can build new strengths.

Family distress sometimes undermines what was previously competent parenting. Parents may need to draw their attention to their own preoccupation or irritability or be reminded or trained on the fundamentals of positive parenting, such as expecting positive behaviors from their children, complimenting them when they are in compliance, encouraging cooperative behavior, taking time to listen, helping with problems, and recognizing and responding to their children's emotions. The latter is extremely important as parental sadness or distress may make it difficult for them to recognize or respond to their children's troubled feelings. Given the higher likelihood of emotional dysregulation in PTSD families, children and adults should be taught to practice personally effective stress-reduction strategies. This includes instruction on how to monitor changes or extremes in emotional states by learning to label and express feelings and identifying when and how positive or negative responses are precipitated. Though identifying and sharing feelings is a first step toward the control of emotion, families must also develop and encourage individual and family activities that promote calm and relaxation. Both children and adults can be taught to reduce worry and tension by engaging in positive self-talk, allowing themselves breaks when needed, developing more realistic expectations, and setting priorities. Parents can be particularly helpful as teachers by modeling healthy self-calming behaviors for their children. Families can increase a sense of unity and mutual support by sharing enjoyable activities at times when everyone is relaxed. Similarly, all family members can be encouraged to jointly identify and engage in activities that are calming for all. The more opportunities that the family has to enjoy positive family time together, the more everyone will identify him or herself as healthy and the family as unified.

Mastering and Modeling Important Interpersonal Skills, Including Problem-Solving and Conflict Resolution

Like all families, families affected by PTSD are likely to face problems that require attention and solving, although these families may have more problems than most. Any problem that seems unsolvable can lead to a sense of individual or family frustration or incompetence and can undermine a child's, adult's, or family's sense of confidence. Festering problems can also result in increasing interpersonal conflict, alienation, and family unrest. Parents should remind children that everyone has problems, adults as well as children, and that what helps people feel strong is being able to solve the problems with which they are faced. Parents can model for their children by calmly showing them how solving problems is a series of steps that can be mastered. Basic problem-solving methods have been used in a number of interventions and generally include (a) defining the problem, (b) listing possible solutions, (c) evaluating the pros and cons of the choices, (d) choosing one of the options, and (e) planning how best to enact (Dausch & Saliman, 2009). Successful problem-solving brings a sense of individual and interpersonal confidence and adds to family strength.

Conflict resolution is a critical type of problem-solving, especially when violence is a concern. While all families have "hot spots" or issues that tend to provoke more intense emotional responses when they arise (homework, chores, finances, etc.), PTSD can contribute to greater reactivity and therefore leave these families more easily upset by ordinary stressors. In addition, reminders or "triggers" can prompt memories of previous traumas. For example, the occurrence of an unexpected noise (a child's shout) may agitate a combat veteran who suffered injury due to an IED. A child might become upset at the unannounced absence of his father, because this is a reminder of when the father was deployed. Each family member likely brings sensitivity to mutual interactions that can disrupt their time together. Families must learn to identify hot spots and trauma triggers so that they can anticipate the service member's reactions to such events, as well as their own. For example, family members can be helped to control their reaction to a service member's provoking behavior by not taking the triggered behavior personally and by prompting the service member to employ previously developed strategies for calming or controlling the reaction.

When interpersonal conflicts do occur, adults need to model strategies that promote calm resolution and interpersonal understanding in order to minimize hurt feelings. Most importantly, both children and adults must recognize that interpersonal conflicts are not likely to be improved when either or both parties are frustrated, angry, or distraught. Taking time to compose oneself and employ reflective listening in order to understand the viewpoint of the other is a way that children can learn that conflict resolution is less about "winning the fight" and more about coming to an understanding with another person. Successful conflict resolution creates patterns of interaction that are more likely to repeat themselves and result in fewer future conflicts, more repaired relationships, and stronger family bonds. In highly volatile families, clinicians should help parents develop violence prevention plans, including seeking help or resources or making use of family "timeout" options before violence erupts.

As mentioned earlier in the chapter, co-parenting in families affected by PTSD may create opportunities for shared and balanced parenting contributions but also can be sources of interpersonal conflict. While little evidence exists to provide specific recommendations for co-parenting practices in these families, anecdotal reports suggest that parents benefit by maximizing individual strengths and limiting weaknesses between parents. As an example, if a father with PTSD is both reactive to and avoidant of his teenage daughter and son, respectively, he and his wife might agree that she will take the lead engaging their daughter about the boyfriend relationship, but he will monitor his son's compliance with an established curfew. Such co-parenting decisions can be successful. In contrast, if a parent feels excluded from parenting decisions, it may lead to conflict, dysphoria, or further disconnection.

Maintaining a Vision of Hope and Future Optimism for the Family

Families faced with chronic PTSD must grieve the loss of their previous health and functioning. The changed personality and interpersonal skills of a family member suffering from PTSD can create a sense of loss in family members who mourn previous relationships. Grief over these relationship losses can be further complicated by confusion about whether their loved one will recover over time. Parents can model acceptance of this changed reality while using family-based skills to create a positive vision of the future, helping their children accommodate. If parents are able to sustain a safe and emotionally warm family environment and help their children master skills to address challenges they face both within and outside of their home, then they can all look to the future with greater hope. Families that sustain the capacity to actively engage helpful support also develop a greater sense of self-efficacy and confidence about their ability to shape solutions for future challenges. Sharing new and positive experiences together while recognizing and respecting changes brought about by PTSD can foster a sense of future hopefulness and optimism.

CONCLUSIONS AND FUTURE DIRECTIONS

Families can face many challenges related to PTSD, especially when the condition is chronic. Further study is required to distinguish the parenting and family mechanisms that are likely to promote health and mitigate risk for children in each of these circumstances. Certain parenting strategies are typically considered helpful, such as emotional engagement with children. However, the effect of such "positive parenting" may be different or even problematic when employed by a parent who is suffering with PTSD. For example, children who are actively engaged by unpredictable or emotionally reactive parents may be negatively impacted when a clinician recommends greater parental emotional closeness. As another example, children typically benefit from enhanced communication with parents, but they may become emotionally distressed when parents share too much information about their own traumatic narrative. Future research must better define which parenting strategies are likely to be helpful in differing circumstances, recognizing that the application of traditionally positive parenting approaches may need to be sculpted and contextually applied depending upon family circumstances.

Future research must promote more sensitively and contextually designed interventions for families, including studies of families affected by PTSD resulting from various traumas. Research must also examine unique gender role contributions (i.e., fathers vs. mothers) to successful parenting practices, as well as any unique gender dyadic contributions (i.e., father-son, mother-son, father-daughter, mother-daughter) to child and family outcomes. Finally, family cultural contributions must also be more closely examined, as well as unique needs of nontraditional families, such as single parent or families with lesbian, gay, bisexual, transgender, and queer members.

REFERENCES

Allen, E., Rhoades, G., Stanley, S., & Markman, H. (2010). Hitting home: Relationships between recent deployment, posttraumatic stress symptoms, and marital functioning for Army couples. *Journal of Family Psychology, 24*(3), 280–288.

American Psychiatric Association. (2013). *Diagnostic and statistical manual of mental disorders*, (5th ed.). Washington, DC: American Psychiatric Association.

Beckham, J., Lytel, B., & Feldman, M. (1996). Caregiver burden in partners of Vietnam veterans with posttraumatic stress disorder. *Journal of Consulting and Clinical Psychology, 64*(5), 1068 1071.

Berz, J., Taft, C., Watkins, L., & Monson, C. (2008). Associations between PTSD symptoms and parenting satisfaction in a female veteran sample. *Journal of Psychological Trauma, 7*(1), 37–45.

Brent, D., Melhem, N., Donohoe, M., & Walker, M. (2009). The incidence and course of depression in bereaved youth 21 months after the loss of a parent to suicide, accident or sudden natural death. *Am J Psychiatry, 166*, 786–794.

Bronfenbrenner, U. (1979). *The ecology of human development*. Cambridge, MA: Harvard University Press.

Bronfenbrenner, U., & Morris, P. (2006). The bioecological model of human development. In R. E. Lerner (Ed.), *Handbook of child psychology* (pp. 793–828). New York: Wiley.

Brown, E, & Goodman, R. (2005). Childhood traumatic grief: An exploration of the construct in children bereaved on September 11. *Journal of Clinical Child and Adolescent Psychology, 34* (2), 248–259.

Calhoun, P., Beckham, J., & Bosworth, H. (2002). Caregiver burden and psychological distress in partners of veterans with chronic posttraumatic stress disorder. *Journal of Traumatic Stress, 15*(3), 2015–212.

Cerel, J., Firstad, M., Verducci, J., Weller, R., & Weller, E. (2006). Childhood bereavement: psychopathology in the 2 years postparental death. *J Amer Acad Child Adolesc Psychiatry, 45*(6), 681–690.

Chandra, A., Lara-Cinisomo, S., Jaycox, L., Tanielian, T., Burns, R., Ruder, T., & Han, B. (2010). Children on the homefront: The experience of children from military families. *Pediatrics, 125*(1), 16–25.

Chemtob, C., Nomura, Y., Rajendran, K., Yehuda, R., Schwarz, D., & Abramovitz, R. (2010). Impact of maternal posttraumatic stress disorder and depression following exposure to the September 11 attacks on preschool children's behavior. *Child Development, 81*, 1129–1141.

Cohen, J., & Mannarino, A. (2002). Childhood traumatic grief: concepts and controversies. *Trauma, Violence and Abuse, 3*, 307–327.

Cohen, J., & Mannarino, A. (2004). Treatment of childhood traumatic grief. *Journal of Clinical Child and Adolescent Psychology, 33*(4), 819–831.

Cohen, J., Mannarino, A., Greenberg, T., Padlo, S., & Shipley, C. (2002). Childhood traumatic grief: Concepts and controversies. *Trauma, Violence & Abuse, 3*(4), 307–327.

Cook, J., Riggs, D., Thompson, R., Coyne, J., & Sheikh, J. (2004). Posttraumatic stress disorder and current relationship functioning among World War II ex-prisoners of war. *Journal of Family Psychology*, 36–45.

Cox, M., & Paley, B. (1997). Families as systems. *Annual Review of Psychology, 48*, 243–267.

Cozza, S., Holmes, A., & Van Ost, S. (2013). Family-centered care for military and veteran families affected by combat injury. *Clinical Child and Family Psychology Review, 16*, 311–321.

Dausch, B., & Saliman, S. (2009). Use of family focused therapy in rehabilitation for veterans with traumatic brain injury. *Rehabilitation Psychology, 54*(3), 279–287.

Doherty, W., Beaton, J., & Wenger, L. (2013). Mothers and fathers coparenting together. In A. Vangelisti (Ed.), *The Routledge handbook of family communication* (2nd ed., pp. 225-240). New York: Routledge.

Dowdney, L. (2000). Annotation: childhood bereavement following parental death. *J Child Psychol Psychiatr, 41*(7), 819–830.

Dyregrov, A., Salloum, A., Kristensen, P., & Dyregrov, K. (2015). Grief and traumatic grief in children in the context of mass trauma. *Current Psychiatry Report, 17*(6), 48.

Elbogen, E., Johnson, S., Newton, V., Timko, C., Vasterling, J., Van Male, L., . . . Beckham, J. (2014). Protective mechanisms and prevention of violence and aggression in veterans. *Psychological Services, 11*(2), 220–228.

Elbogen, E., Johnson, S., Wagner, R., Newton, V., Timko, C., Vasterling, J., & Beckham, J. (2012). Protective factors and risk modification of violence in Iraq and Afghanistan war veterans. *Journal of Clinical Psychiatry, 73*(6), e767–e773.

Evans, L., McHugh, T., Hopwood, M., & Watt, C. (2003). Chronic posttraumatic stress disorder and family functioning of Vietnam veterans and their partners. *Australian and New Zealand Journal of Psychiatry, 37*, 765–772.

Flake, E., Davis, B., Johnson, P., & Middleton, L. (2009). The psychosocial effects of deployment on military children. *Journal of Developmental and Behavioral Pediatrics, 30*(4), 271–278.

Fredman, S., Vorstenbosch, V., Wagner, A., Macdonald, A., & Monson, C. (2014). Partner accommodation in posttraumatic stress disorder: Initial testing of the Significant Others' Responses to Trauma Scale (SORTS). *Journal of Anxiety Disorders, 28*, 372-381.

Galovski, T., & Lyons, J. (2004). Psychological sequelae of combat violence: A review of the impact of PTSD on the veteran's family and possible interventions. *Aggression and Violent Behavior, 9*, 477–501.

Gewirtz, A., Forgatch, M., & Wieling, E. (2008). Parenting practices as potential mechanisms for child adjustment following mass trauma. *Journal of Marital and Family Therapy, 34*(2), 177–192.

Gewirtz, A., Pinna, K., Hanson, S., & Brockberg, D. (2014). Promoting parenting to support reintegrating military families: After deployment, adaptive parenting tools. *Psychological Services, 11*(1), 31–40.

Gewirtz, A., Polusny, M., DeGarmo, D., Khaylis, A., & Erbes, C. (2010). Posttraumatic stress symptoms among National Guard soldiers deployed to Iraq: Associations with parenting behaviors and couple adjustment. *Journal of Consulting and Clinical Psychology, 78*(5), 599–610.

Gimbel, C., & Booth, A. (1994). Why does military combat experience adversely affect marital relations? *Journal of Marriage and the Family, 56*(3), 691–704.

Glynn, S., Eth, S., Randolph, E., Foy, D., Urbaitis, M., Boxer, L., . . . Crothers, J. (1999). A test of behavioral family therapy to augment exposure for combat-related posttraumatic stress disorder. *Journal of Consulting and Clinical Psychology, 67*(2), 243–251.

Hagan, M., Tein, J., Sandler, I., Wolchik, S., Ayers, T., & Luecken, L. (2012). Strengthening effective parenting practices over the long term: effects of a preventive intervention for parentally bereaved families. *Journal of Clinical Child and Adolescent Psychology, 41*(2), 177–188.

Hendrix, C., Erdmann, M., & Briggs, K. (1998). Impact of Vietnam veterans' arousal and avoidance on spouses' perceptions of family life. *American Journal of Family Therapy, 26*(2), 115–128.

Herzog, J., Everson, R., & Whitworth, J. (2011). Do secondary trauma symptoms in spouses of combat-exposed national guard soldiers mediate impacts of soldiers' trauma exposure on their children? *Child and Adolescent Social Work Journal, 28*(6), 459–473.

Hidalgo, R., & Davidson, J. (2000). Posttraumatic stress disorder: Epidemiology and health-related considerations. *Journal of Clinical Psychiatry, 61*(Suppl. 7), 5–13.

Hoge, C., Auchterlonie, J., & Milliken, C. (2006). Mental health problems, use of mental health service, and attrition from military service after returning from deployment to Iraq or Afghanistan. *JAMA, 295*(9), 1023–1032.

Holmes, A., Cozza, S., Anderson, A., Sullivan, J., Fullerton, C., & Ursano, R. (2013). *Child functioning in combat-injured military families: The moderating effects of injured service member parenting and PTSD symptoms.* Seattle, WA: Society for Research in Child Development.

Holmes, A., Rauch, P., & Cozza, S. (2013). When a parent is injured or killed in combat. *The Future of Children, 263*(2), 143–162.

Jakupcak, M., Conybeare, D., Phelps, L., Hunt, S., Holmes, H., Felker, B., & McFall, M. (2007). Anger, hostility, and aggression among Iraq and Afghanistan war veterans reporting PTSD and subthreshold PTSD. *Journal of Traumatic Stress, 20*(6), 945–954.

Jordan, B., Marmar, C., Fairbank, J., Schlenger, W., Kulka, R., Hough, R., & Weiss, D. (1992). Problems in families of male Vietnam veterans with posttraumatic stress disorder. *Journal of Consulting and Clinical Psychology, 60*(6), 916–926.

Karney, B., & Crown, J. (2007). *Families under stress: An assessment of data, theory, and research on marriage and divorce in the military.* Santa Monica, CA: RAND.

Kessler, R. (2000). Posttraumatic stress disorder: The burden to the individual and to society. *Journal of Clinical Psychiatry, 61*(Suppl. 5), 4–12.

Kessler, R., Sonnega, A., Bromet, E., Hughes, M., & Nelson, C. (1995). Posttraumatic stress disorder in the National Comorbidity Survey. *Archives of General Psychiatry*, 1048–1060.

Kulka, R., Schlenger, W., Fairbank, J., Hough, R., Jordan, B., Marmar, C., & Weiss, D. (1990). *Trauma and the Vietnam war generation: Report of findings from the National Vietnam Veterans Readjustment Study.* Philadelphia: Brunner Mazel.

Kwok, O., Haine, R., Sandler, I., Ayers, T., Wolchik, S., & Tein, J. (2005). Positive parenting as a mediator of the relations between parental psychological distress and mental health problems of parentally bereaved children. *Journal of Clinical Child and Adolescent Psychology, 34*, 260–271.

Lester, P., Peterson, K., Reeves, J., Knauss, L., Glover, D., Mogil, C., . . . Beardslee, W. (2010). The long war and parental combat deployment: effects on military children and at-home spouses. *Journal of the American Academy of Child & Adolescent Psychiatry, 49*(4), 310–320.

Lester, P., Stein, J., Saltzman, W., Woodward, K., MacDermid, S., Milburn, N., . . . Beardslee, W. (2013). Psychological health of military children: Longitudinal evaluation of a family-centered prevention program to enhance family resilience. *Military Medicine, 178*(8), 838–845.

Lin, K., Sandler, I., Ayers, T., Wolchik, S., & Luecken, L. (2004). Resilience in parentally bereaved children and adolescents seeking preventive services. *Journal of Clinical Child and Adolescent Psychology, 33*, 673–683.

MacManus, D., Rona, R., Dickson, H., Somaini, G., Fear, N., & Wessely, S. (2015). Aggressive and violent behavioral among military personnel deployed to Iraq and Afghanistan: Prevalence and link with deployment and combat exposure. *Epidemiologic Reviews, 37*(1), 196–212.

Manguno-Mire, G., Sautter, F., Lyons, J., Myers, L., Perry, D., Sherman, M., . . . Sullivan, G. (2007). Psychological distress and burden among female partners of combat veterans with PTSD. *Journal of Nervous and Mental Disease, 195*(2), 144–151.

Melhem, N., Porta, G., Shamseddeen, W., Payne, M., & DA, B. (2011). Grief in children and adolescents bereaved by sudden death. *Arch Gen Psychiatry, 68*(9), 911–919.

Monson, C., Fredman, S., Adair, K., Stevens, S., Resick, P., Schnurr, P., . . . McDonald, A. (2011). Cognitive-behavioral conjoint therapy for PTSD: Pilot results from a community sample. *Journal of Traumatic Stress, 24*(1), 97–101.

Monson, C., Taft, C., & Fredman, S. (2009). Military-related PTSD and intimate relationships: From description to theory-driven research and intervention development. *Clinical Psychology Review, 29*, 707–714.

North, C., & Pfefferbaum, B. (2013). Mental health response to community disasters: A systematic review. *JAMA, 310*(5), 507–518.

Petrik, N., Rosenberg, A., & Watson, C. (1983). Combat experience and youth: Influences on reported violence against women. *Professional Psychology, Research and Practice, 14*(6), 895–899.

Riggs, D., Byrne, Weathers, F., & Litz, B. (1998). The quality of the intimate relationships of male Vietnam veterans: Problems associated with posttraumatic stress disorder. *Journal of Traumatic Stress, 11*(1), 87–101.

Rosenheck, R., & Nathan, P. (1985). Secondary traumatization in children of Vietnam vetrerans. *Hospital and Community Psychiatry, 36*(5), 538–539.

Saltzman, W., Lester, P., Beardslee, W., Layne, C., Woodward, K., & Nash, W. (2011). Mechanisms of risk and resilience in military families: Theoretical and empirical basis of a family-focused resilience enhancement program. *Clinical Child and Family Psychological Review, 14*, 213–230.

Samper, R., Taft, C., Kind, D., & King, L. (2004). Posttraumatic stress disorder symptoms and parenting satisfaction among a national sample of male Vietnam veterans. *Journal of Traumatic Stress, 17*(4), 311–315.

Sandler, I., Ayers, T., Wolchik, S., Tein, J., Kwok, O., Haine, R., . . . Griffen, W. (2003). The Family Bereavement Program: efficacy evaluation of a theory-based prevention program for parentally bereaved children and adolescent. *Journal of Consulting and Clinical Psychology, 71*(3), 587–600.

Sayers, S., Farrow, V., Ross, J., & Oslin, D. (2009). Family problems among recently returned military veterans referred for a mental health evaluation. *Journal of Clinical Psychiatry, 70*(2), 163–170.

Sherman, M., Zanotti, D., & Jones, D. (2005). Key elements in couples therapy with veterans with combat-related posttraumatic stress disorder. *Professional Psychology: Research and Practice, 36*(6), 626–633.

Taft, C., Pless, A., Stalans, L., Koenen, K., King, L., & King, D. (2005). Risk factors for partner violence among a national sample of combat veterans. *Journal of Consulting and Clinical Psychology, 73*(1), 151–159.

Taft, C., Schumm, J., Panuzio, J., & Proctor, S. (2008). An examination of family adjustment among Operation Desert Storm veterans. *Journal of Consulting and Clinical Psychology, 76*(4), 648–656.

Taft, C., Vogt, D., Marshall, A., Panuzio, J., & Niles, B. (2007). Aggression among combat veterans: Relationships with combat exposure and symptoms of posttraumatic stress disorder, dysphoria, and anxiety. *Journal of Traumatic Stress, 20*(2),135–145.

Wadsworth, S., Lester, P., Marini, C., Cozza, S., Sornborger, J., Strouse, T., & Beardslee, W. (2013). Approaching family-focused systems of care for military and veteran families. *Military Behavioral Health, 1*, 31–40.

Walsh, F. (2006). *Strengthening family resilience* (2nd ed.). New York: Guilford Press.

Whisman, M., Sheldon, C., & Goering, P. (2000). Psychiatric disorders and dissatisfaction with social relationships: does type of relationship matter? *Journal of Abnormal Psychology, 109*(4), 803–808.

Wickrama, K., & Kaspar, V. (2008). Family context of mental health risk in tsunami-exposed adolescents: findings from a pilot study in Srik Lanka. *Social Science & Medicine, 64*, 713–723.

29

Ethical Issues in the Forensic Assessment of Posttraumatic Symptoms

EDMUND G. HOWE

INTRODUCTION

Traumatic exposures that result in acute stress disorder or clinically significant stress reactions lead to the longer-term symptoms of posttraumatic stress disorder (PTSD) about 10% to 20% of the time (Mezey, 2006). As a result of the social and occupational dysfunction of PTSD, sufferers may commit crimes or lose their ability to continue to be able to work (Stojakovic, 2011). This may occur even when persons have only some PTSD symptoms and not the full-fledged disorder. Psychiatrists and other mental health experts then may be called upon to assess these persons for the relationship between their posttraumatic symptoms and dysfunctional behavior. They may be asked to determine, for example, their criminal responsibility, or whether they should receive financial compensation for being occupationally disabled as a result of the impairment resulting from traumatic stress.

Each of these determinations raises ethical and legal questions. In this chapter some of the core challenges and questions forensic psychiatrists may encounter when making each of these determinations are discussed. While a variety of medical and mental health professionals may be asked to render opinions on such matters, this chapter refers to psychiatrists and other professionals who carry out these evaluations as "psychiatrists" or "examiners" throughout this discussion.

This chapter first addresses considerations that trauma-related symptoms and behaviors might raise in all legal contexts, such as whether all the diagnostic criteria should be required to render a diagnosis in a medico-legal assessment. Psychiatrists may, for example, consider the effects of traumatic experience as resulting from PTSD only when the history of symptoms obtained through evaluation meet all of the criteria for this diagnosis, or they may consider the impact of trauma on those they examine whose symptoms do not meet the full criteria. As has been explained in detail elsewhere in this volume and is highlighted here, the criteria for making this diagnosis recently have been expanded. This expansion raises questions regarding what diagnosis should apply to those who no longer meet criteria but used to do so under the previous diagnostic definition. Further, although people may have only a few of these symptoms, these symptoms may affect them profoundly. Thus the magnitude of symptoms rather than the number of symptoms present is addressed as a relevant consideration in assessing the impact of this disorder on social or occupational function.

In the second section of this chapter, ethical and legal questions that may arise during evaluations for criminal responsibility and disability are discussed. These two types of examinations are, perhaps, the two most common. In this section, ethical considerations in the assessment of children and adolescents are also highlighted as children and adolescents find themselves caught in the midst of medico-legal assessments as part of custody evaluations or in determinations relating to their status (adult vs. minor) in adjudication of criminal matters. There are, of course, other legal determinations that psychiatrists may make as well, but the ethical and legal concerns raised here should be sufficiently paradigmatic of most concerns in other contexts.

One additional consideration raised in this chapter represents a departure from conventional forensic psychiatric practice. Historically, psychiatrists conducting forensic exams have viewed themselves as adopting a different allegiance (i.e., as one to the state or the court rather than to the person whom they have been asked to evaluate). It has recently been proposed that psychiatrists doing forensic work might instead seek to find ways to retain their first loyalty to even these patients (Candilis et al., 2007).

Regardless of their primary allegiance, psychiatrists may be able to alter past habits and skills to improve the patient/examiner relationships even in forensic contexts. Specifically how they might do this, if they can at all, remains unclear. Arguments justifying such alteration and examples of where—if not how—this might be operationalized are noted in the final section of this chapter.

GENERAL CONSIDERATIONS

Two aspects of the diagnosis of PTSD are particularly relevant to forensic examiners. The first is that many of the criteria for making this diagnosis are imprecise. The second is that many of these criteria are based on patients' self-reports. These characteristics may much affect how examiners make these forensic assessments.

Ethical Problems Posed by Unclear Diagnostic Boundaries

Some psychiatrists may make forensic conclusions only when persons have full-blown PTSD (i.e., meet minimum threshold diagnostic criteria across all four symptom clusters specified by the fifth edition of the *Diagnostic and Statistical Manual of Mental Disorders* [DSM-5]). Others may make forensic conclusions when the persons they evaluate have only "partial disorders." This, then, is in all legal contexts a first ethical question that forensic examiners must answer: Should they consider making a legal conclusion only when examinees have PTSD or also when they have only subthreshold conditions?

The strongest ethical argument for rendering forensic opinions in persons with only partial disorders is that of justice or fairness. Even when the disorder is only partially present and a person demonstrates or reports only some of the symptoms required to make the diagnosis of PTSD, the symptoms a person does experience may affect him or her more than others who experience all the symptoms necessary for a "full" diagnosis. If, however, examiners adopt this latter approach and consider evaluating for forensic purposes even a person with only one symptom of PTSD, this decision will be further affected by recent changes in DSM-5 that have greatly expanded these criteria. Specifically, the number of examinees considered would be greatly increased. The impact of changes in diagnostic definition or "case-ness" is illustrated by the example of the fourth edition of the DSM (DSM-IV), where significant differences existed between the diagnostic criteria specified by the predecessor to the current DSM-5 definition and the International Classification of Diseases (10th revision [ICD-10]). In one study, almost twice the number of people were diagnosed with PTSD under ICD-10 than were under DSM-IV (Mezey, 2006, p. 244).

The criteria in DSM-5 have been broadened such that mild stresses may suffice. Examples are the stress of separating from a partner, losing a job, and even just witnessing a frightening event or learning of the details of events that occurred in close others may qualify as traumas (Levin et al., 2014). The example going furthest and thus most representative of this current approach is the stress people may have fearing inappropriate sexual behavior. PTSD may be deemed as resulting from this stress even when there has been no physical contact. Due to this broadening, Levin (2014) has referred to this change as "bracket creep" (p. 149). The division of opinion regarding what is or is not PTSD poses then an initial ethical decision that forensic examiners now must make.

This difficulty of deciding when to allow fewer than all PTSD symptoms to "count" is further complicated by two additional possibilities: these symptoms may fluctuate and thus re-occur, and they may be delayed. These possibilities, like the broader criteria for diagnosing PTSD, increase the discretion examiners may exercise when they decide whom they will evaluate for forensic purposes.

This decision-making is still further complicated by examiners also having to decide what to make of findings that are less objective, evidence-based, or guided by diagnostic criteria. An example illustrating this is Eiser's (2015) suggestion that there is now a need for a new entity of PTSD which he calls a "post-modern" stress disorder. This disorder could be caused, he believes, by a person's overexposure to exceptionally violent video games that now are, of course, readily available. Eiser suggests that these games include graphic scenes that may stimulate people's amygdala in a way that lessens their capacity to inhibit their violent impulses. Their electronic digital overload, he proposes, may lead to sleep deprivation and fatigue, and this combination may then cause these persons to engage in otherwise inexplicable violent acts.

This claim, whether sound or not, illustrates the extent to which the diagnosis and consequences of PTSD can be extended. This, in turn, poses for examiners a greater risk that when deciding whom they will assess, they may be affected by their underlying emotional biases, whether they are aware of this or not. They may, for example, attempt to avoid this risk by not assessing these persons even when, from the standpoint of fairness, they should.

A specific example of such a question that this may pose for examiners is how they should respond when they encounter an examinee with "eggshell-like" emotions. This term is intended to convey a kind of examinee that psychiatrists may encounter that is extrapolated from a closely related concept of persons having an "eggshell-like skull" in tort law (McQuade, 2001). The term suggests that some people may be more vulnerable to negative effects of stress than others. This may be due to past events such as child abuse or their genetics, but beyond this, why some persons remain relatively unaffected (or resilient) in the aftermath of traumatic experience but others become chronically symptomatic after the same event is not well understood.

Persons with eggshell-like emotions may respond most profoundly to even minimal stress. This possibility is analogous to the notion already existing within the law that some persons may have "eggshell-like skulls." If so, this leaves them exceptionally vulnerable to blows to their head. If, then, an offender delivers such a blow, this offender is responsible for the consequences even though the offender had no way of knowing that his or her victim's skull was this "thin."

In a like way, minor stresses may cause exceptional and unexpected emotional harm to some victims, because they, like those with "eggshell-like skulls," are unusually emotionally vulnerable. Ethically, examiners knowing that a stress victim may have eggshell-like emotions may further increase the risk that they may again be at greater risk of responding to their biases.

A specific example exemplifying this is a person's becoming significantly impaired as a result of "just" witnessing a traumatic event. Rare patients may even be "traumatized" by what they hear or see on YouTube or television. An example is the mother of a young child. She saw in a TV show a gangster who threatened a mother who had a young child like hers. This gangster threatened to give this child a grisly death if this mother later reported him to legal authorities. The mother who watched this show had repeated intrusive flashbacks of this television scene that disrupted her ability to concentrate after seeing this for several months.

Examiners may then consider taking into account stresses such as this which lie at the borders of the diagnosis of DSM-V. They may be overly inclined to want to include some examples because they want to be just, or overly likely to not include these examples to avoid being too inclusive. Ethically, their seeking above all to be just as by including people with eggshell-like emotional responses would perhaps most fulfill the true intent of the law. This could allow, however, determinations that are more speculative and thus that would vary more greatly. Examiners evaluating these people would differ to a greater extent. This would introduce more inconsistency into these determinations, and judgments might veer more toward being even arbitrary, which would be ethically problematic. Whether these untoward results should be outweighed by allowing greater justice for those with more eggshell-like emotions is open to debate. Still, it may be that psychiatrists making this call can do no better that judging each case on its individual merits as they see it as opposed to their adopting either all-or-none approach.

The Uncertainty Caused by Self-Report

The diagnosis of PTSD and the forensic implications of its symptoms, full or partial, is still more difficult to determine because many of the symptoms of PTSD are based on patients' self-reports (Frierson, 2013). Thus this diagnosis and its symptoms are easier to feign than orthopedic injuries or even organ damage (which may be quantified by laboratory evaluations).

Since these persons' self-reports may be invalid, corroboration is considered the best means and indeed a gold standard for making forensic assessments, in that this may greatly aid examiners to increase the validity of their forensic findings. This practice of contacting others who have known and know these "patients" may itself raise a significant ethical dilemma. This dilemma involves how much forensic examiners should tell potential informants when they contact them prior to asking them for more information. How those they contact respond to their questions may confirm or refute the self-reports of those they are examining.

It is generally considered mandatory for examiners to try to corroborate the findings they discern to the degree that they can (Giorgi-Guarnieri et al., 2002; Knoll et al., 2006). It is standard practice for forensic examiners to identify themselves to the persons they call (Giorgi-Guarnieri, 2002; Knoll, 2006); however, this limited guideline does not say how far in this regard examiners should go.

Let us suppose, for example, that the examiner contacts a partner or parent. Should the psychiatrist just ask questions, or say, through using other words, "I am calling to discern whether your partner or adult child is lying?" Should examiners be still more respectful of these parties' autonomy and their interests by indicating the possible consequences that could come about as a result of the answers they give? In the most extreme case, this might be the death of their loved one. Thus to fully respect the autonomy of a party, psychiatrists might need to say, again through other words, "Your loved one may face the death penalty for first-degree murder if it is found that he is faking his mental illness and what you say serves to confirm this."

The result of the examiner's saying this may be of course that the other person will no longer disclose key information. Yet, again, if the examiner withholds this information, this involves at least implicit deception. A possible argument in favor of this deception by omission is that the contacted parties are likely to know that these are possible consequences already, once the examiner identifies him- or herself. While this may be true, the argument remains flawed. It is therefore an example of the kind of rationalization forensic psychiatrists should eschew. If these psychiatrists' basis for not sharing this information is that these parties should know already, these examiners logically should tell them to make sure. Further, if examiners will not give all informants this information, some will surely know this more than others. This will violate equality for both these persons called and those the psychiatrist is examining. For the latter, the result of this in equality may be profound. This difference may result, for instance, in their prolonged imprisonment or even death.

Means to Increase Objectivity

There are several screening measures that may help detect malingering. One, the SIRS exam has even been designed particularly for this purpose (Mezey, 2006). Still, no test nor combination of tests is conclusive in this regard (Ali et al., 2015; Kleinman et al., 2015).

In making these forensic assessments, there are no definitive ways by which malingering can be determined. Accordingly, some have sought to enhance their ability to accurately make this diagnosis by employing more objective measures. One has, for example, suggested showing those they examine pictures or other reminders of the stress they claim to have experienced and then measuring the degree to which they show physiological distress (Levin, 2014).

Other providers have found ways to try to lure these individuals into making false statements, thus adding, arguably at least, to the probability that they are malingering. This too raises ethical questions. Psychiatrists trying to trick such patients are themselves, engaging in deception. Should they?

Deceit

It has just been noted that examiners evaluating persons whom they suspect of malingering may want to deceive them to better determine whether they are malingering. The ethical question this raises is whether examiners should go this far (or even engage in deceit at all) to try to add to the validity of their inferences. Ethically, perhaps the most important way of viewing this question is to ask whether the ends sought are justified by this means.

Generally, the common assumption in ethics is that means should be often limited even when this allows unwanted losses. Examiners eliciting information know specific ways in which those they examine may indicate that they are lying. Examiners having this information but not disclosing it are deceiving those they examine by omission. Examiners may, accordingly, ask themselves seriously whether they should engage in this or any deception, or where they should draw this line.

There are ways other than using deception by which examiners may suspect those they examine are malingering. A clue, for example, may be such persons often using words that are rarely used in lay conversations but more frequently appear in diagnostic manuals or medical texts such as "hypervigilant." If examinees do this, this may suggest that they may have read before and "boned-up" on the current PTSD diagnostic criteria in the manual itself or some other psychiatric text. This inference may, however, on the other hand, be wrong and misleading. These persons may be merely much more knowledgeable than most others.

An ethical concern this latter possibility raises again involves equity. Examiners should evaluate all those they see equally to the degree possible. Those who know more about psychiatric disorders, such as mental health or other medical professionals, may be much better at feigning this emotional illness than others. If providers see such "expertise" as more likely to be malingering, they may also be unjustly using these persons' exceptional knowledge against them. On the other hand, if they consider malingering only among persons who lack mental health training, this would also involve treating these people unequally.

Examiners may take other special measures to try to determine whether patients are faking their symptoms. They may ask about symptoms they know that the examined persons are most likely to *not* have or are not associated or rarely reported by patients with the diagnosis in question. If those they examine acknowledge that they have these symptoms, examiners may conclude that this increases the likelihood that the examined person is malingering. Here, again, this may be misleading. Examinees may endorse such symptoms because they wish inordinately to please their examiner, or because they are scared, or simply because they truly experience rare or unusual symptoms.

Finally, in some cases, examiners may be able to discern feigning only if they know more about a psychiatric illness than the examinee and are able to outwit them. This is exemplified by Orne et al.'s (1984) examination of a man who killed several others and then feigned having what was then called a multiple personality, a condition considered to be associated with persons being highly hypnotizable.

Orne, an expert on hypnosis, used hypnosis to try to discern whether this defendant's portrayal of a multiple personality was feigned. This defendant had read up on hypnosis and apparently hoped to persuade Orne that he was indeed highly hypnotizable. Orne, however, used his knowledge of two less well-known responses that persons in hypnotic states tend to have to detect that this defendant was just trying to simulate this dissociative disorder. People in a hypnotic state can accept experiences that make no sense. Thus, if and when they encounter such experiences while hypnotized, they are unlikely to show alarm.

In this particular case, Orne asked the defendant to positively hallucinate a person already in the room at the other side of the room. This defendant, seeing this same person at two places, showed surprise and alarm. First clue. Orne, then, again, utilized this same little-known propensity of persons in a hypnotic state to be at ease with logical contradictions. He told the defendant that he would feel nothing in one hand. He then asked this defendant to tell him every time that Orne touched this hand. Orne then touched it repeatedly. This defendant said nothing. It would of course be most illogical if he did. But those in a true hypnotic state are not concerned with illogical reactions. They would have answered. Thus clue number two. Both gave this defendant away. Orne knew he was faking.

Orne said later that "fortunately" he knew a bit more about hypnosis than the person he examined. The unmasking of this defendant's attempt to simulate mental illness depended, in this case, on Orne's having greater knowledge regarding hypnosis and then deceiving this defendant successfully. Efforts such as Orne's may be ethically both justifiable and preferable to their not discerning defendants' faking in every way that they can. Still, it is at least open to question when, if ever, this should not be the case and discomfiting in any event that discerning an examinee's deception may depend upon the examiners knowing more than he or she does.

Psychiatrists Taking Initiative to Convey the Certainty or Lack Thereof of Their Findings

When psychiatrists do forensic work, they offer their findings in an adversarial legal system (Giorgi-Guarnieri, 2002). They may believe in telling the whole truth and nothing but, but they may be working with attorneys who work for one side or the other. These attorneys may want them to limit their testimony, as by leaving out the lack of certainty of some inferences they make so that it is up to the "other side" to bring this out. Legal theory supports this. If there are weaknesses in either side, as in an expert's testimony, it is up to the other side and their experts to bring these out. Through this clashing the most truth may be gleaned.

This practice makes it more likely that the outcomes of those examined may be determined not by the truth but according to the skills the opposing experts have relative to each other. If so, this is unjust. This undermines the intent of the law to arrive at the truth. Psychiatrists cannot state their conclusions (Giorgi-Guarnieri, 2002). They can try to indicate the relative certainty of each of their inferences, however, to the degree that they can.

This practice ethically may be especially important to increase justice because in addition to experts' skills differing, lawyers may differ also in the degree to which they will take steps to help those for whom they are working. They may, for example, "coach" plaintiffs on how to feign PTSD. In one study, for instance, 70 attorneys were asked whether they believed in giving their clients information regarding tests they could face when they would be evaluated for PTSD. Forty-two percent of these lawyers said that they did (Kleinman, 2015, p. 81).

One person going to court disclosed that his lawyer had in addition showed him the testimonies of previous clients who had gone to court claiming that they had what he would claim, namely, that he had "classical PTSD." This attorney in addition sent all these clients to the same psychologist for evaluation (Kleinman, 2015, p. 81). Again, if legal outcomes reflect not the truth but these differences between lawyers, they are unjust. One court, accordingly, has declared that psychologists who will test people for forensic purposes need not disclose in advance the tests that they will use (Kleinman, 2015, p. 81).

Lawyers, as well as plaintiffs, may also now seek information on the Internet. Lawyers, having researched the criteria for diagnoses on their own, may then suggest to their clients what they should say. Examinees may construe such suggestions as legal advice and either embellish or lie about their symptoms, even though they would not and/or even could not do this on their own.

Examiners who testify generally know which parts of their statement are most open to rebuttal. Their specifying each of their inference's strengths and weaknesses to the greatest degree possible may place before the judge or jury the truer picture of what they can reasonably infer than they could acquire in any other way.

An illustrative example is one of a mother who may have been exaggerating or even faking some PTSD symptoms. She then described with strong feeling the shame she had felt when for the first time her children saw her "fall apart" in response to a flashback. Her having and indeed "showing" this shame response made more credible her claim of PTSD to the psychiatrist who was examining her. He made sure to include this in his testimony though he was working at this time for the state and believed her to be embellishing her presentation.

Prioritizing Examinees More Than We Have

One final question following these general considerations is the one alluded to in the introduction to this chapter: Can and should psychiatrists take initiatives in these legal contexts to try to remain more compassionate and caring as they would with their patients in therapy?

In some contexts as when assessing persons for disability, they might do this by indicating that they understand the bind they are in. As an example, when patients are seeking disability compensation, examiners may say that it is most understandable to them why these examinees might want to exaggerate their symptoms; namely, they might then gain greater financial rewards (Ali, 2015, p. 16; Knoll, 2006). This show of understanding would in one sense be validating and supportive. This, therefore, would be one way in which psychiatrists might successfully carry out the quest to retain a greater alliance with even these patients, as some have proposed is both warranted and desirable.

Examiners making this statement might also move these persons to tell less embellished truths. Thus the interviewer's motivation in saying this may be either to help themselves and the state, or to help the patient, or a combination. Should this intention matter?

Examiners may want to assess this within themselves. If they sense that they would want to do this for the sake of their evaluation, not these patients, they could add to what they have said. They could add that the reason they are saying this is to serve the state, not them.

This effect may be paradoxical. This statement is of course harsh. Yet it may result in the examinee's sense of greater trust. This could result in the person examined saying something against his or her best interests that is in some way self-incriminating.

ETHICAL AND LEGAL CONSIDERATIONS IN SPECIFIC CONTEXTS

Ethical and forensic considerations also differ, depending on the legal context. This section considers different questions that arise when determining criminal issues and disability.

Determining Criminal Responsibility

PTSD may form the basis of an insanity defense when people commit crimes while experiencing dissociation or having flashbacks (Mezey, 2006, p. 244). The legal assumption here is that during this time, they may not have known that what they were doing was wrong. In legal terms, they may not be able to appreciate the nature and quality or the wrongfulness of their criminal act. They may also be seen as acting reflexively. This latter phenomenon is referred to as an "automatism" (Mezey, 2006, p. 244).

In some states defendants may be excused from criminal responsibility also on a second ground. These states continue to use the so called "volitional" prong of the Model Penal Code. This code was developed by the American Law Institute in 1955 and was adopted in the Federal Courts from 1972 until

1984. This second prong allows defendants to be excused from their crimes if, at the time of their alleged offense, they were "unable to control or conform their conduct to the requirements of the law" (Ali, 2015). The use of PTSD as an insanity defense is, however, uncommon. In one study this figure is, for example, only 0.3% of insanity defenses (Frierson, 2013, p. 80).

An example illustrating such a defense that succeeded is that of a combat veteran who had a nightmare. During this nightmare, he grabbed his gun and fired at a door jam. He was charged with a criminal offense but no one was injured. This is what he had been trained to do as a soldier. He then hid under a car until the police came, pointing their guns. Then, he surrendered without incident to these authorities. He was reenacting at this time, the court felt, what he had learned before without at the time of this crime having sufficient awareness of what he was doing. He also had no motive and had subsequent amnesia for this event. Both of these findings were consistent with his not being aware and thus were important supporting factors (Frierson, 2013).

A more atypical and perhaps controversial case is the following: A man's best friend had been taken away to a concentration camp when he was just a small child living in Europe. In his adult years he went yearly to concentration camps in the hope of finding some trace of his childhood friend. His wife went with him on these trips and verified this.

Later, he came to be under extreme work stress. He went into a room and allegedly tried to light himself on fire. This was, of course, how he believed his friend had probably died. He was prosecuted for arson.

He had before this been a most responsible citizen, and he had no prior illegal behavior. The court concluded that his behavior was a consequence of this traumatic loss he had experienced as a child. It inferred that at the time he tried to kill himself by fire, he lacked sufficient control of his behavior and was acting, in essence, in response to an irresistible impulse. Under the second prong of the American Law Institute (ALI) standard (American Academy of Psychiatry and the Law, 2014; Allen, 1962) then in effect there, he was acquitted.

His disorder, if what the court determined was true, might be construed as an example of the psychiatrist who testified "for" him applying the concept discussed earlier of an eggshell-like vulnerability of his emotions and of the jury believing this. This happening, if true, may have been especially likely because when he experienced this loss of his friend, he was a child. Another contextual factor which bore no relevance to the determination of his criminal responsibility but may still have contributed to jury acceptance of the diagnosis and his acquittal, was the fact that no other parties were injured and the nature of his traumatic experience itself—the loss of a dear childhood friend to the horrors of the Holocaust.

This case might particularly illustrate how in many legal contexts, criminal and civil, that involve a PTSD claim, examiners may confront the ethical question raised earlier in this chapter: how far should they go in a legal proceeding to consider whether a person's behavior might have been due to prior stress.

In the criminal arena, though PTSD is used only rarely as a responsibility defense, it is used commonly in other ways. It is used, for example, to show diminished capacity and to wholly negate an offender's having had a specific intent. It is also used in sentencing. As one author has described this, extending how PTSD may connect with the law still further, "PTSD can be present before and/or after the crime, separately in the victim or perpetrator or both and it may be present in the witness of the proceedings" (Stojakovic, 2011, p. 47).

As discussed earlier, partial or subthreshold states may also have a place (Levin, 2014). Reckless driving is an example. People may react after stress by thrill-seeking. Reckless driving may result from stress. Thus PTSD or partial PTSD may be used to excuse or at least mitigate the penalties for persons accused of this crime (Levin, 2014, p. 150).

Here, as described in more general terms previously, there are numerous ways in which examiners may seek to assess whether alleged offenders are malingering. The example used to illustrate this in regard to crime is examiners' evaluation of amnesia. In one study, 20% to 30% of defendants who committed violent offenses claimed to have amnesia (Scott, 2012, p. 797; Evans et al., 2009). In another study, 20% of those who claimed to have amnesia later acknowledged that they were faking this. (Scott, 2012; Hopwood, 1933).

Examiners assessing these claims know that many emotional states may cause amnesia, ranging from extreme anger to dissocation (Scott, 2012). As is consistent with this, those who commit impulsive violent acts claim to have amnesia more often than those whose violence is planned (Scott, 2012, p. 801; Evans, 2009).

Memory loss occurring in a crime of passion is known as a "red out" (Scott, 2012). This memory loss occurs at the peak of the violent act and lasts until this violent response has ended (Swihart et al., 1999). Examiners aware of this must assess carefully when amnesia is feigned.

In some cases, there are better grounds for inferring this. An example is when a defendant claims to have retrograde amnesia from a blow to the head. Older memories should come back sooner than later ones. Thus if this does not occur, the defendant's claim of amnesia is more suspect (Scott, 2012). Psychiatrists should be more careful about giving inferences less factually based than this weight. When factual bases such as the above finding are not present, examiners' inferences are also more subject to their bias, as has been indicated more generally.

As an example of this risk, persons may, after reacting violently, whether dissociated or not, come to. Then, after they regain their usual awareness, they may recognize what they have done and take steps to cover their crime.

Examiners may tend to reflexively regard this history as added and even conclusive evidence that these persons had clear awareness of what they were doing at the time they committed their crime. They may not have. They alternatively may have emerged from a dissociated state or an automatism, realized what they had done, and then taken self-exculpatory actions.

This example illustrates an ethical question examiners should routinely consider—how much weight they should place on such less likely but plausible possibilities, and then share them in court. They may fear that if they report these possibilities, they will be perceived as unduly biased or, as may be worse for them, gullible.

Their sharing this may more importantly work against their ability to credibly convey other "truths." Judges or juries may see them as less trustworthy.

Ethically, this risk is probably not a sound ground for not sharing these possibilities. Again, they rather, to be most fair to those they examine, should share what they infer as they see this. They *can* also say, however, if and when they share this, that they know that in most cases, their or anyone's seeing this self-exculpatory behavior as "separate" is a stretch. They can add why they think that in the instance before them, this may or may not be the case.

Disability

Post-traumatic stress disorder, unlike many other psychiatric disorders, involves a causal connection between the stressful event and emotional symptoms (Mesey, 2006). Thus people are particularly likely to use this disorder as a claim for disability compensation (Levin, 2014). Fourteen percent of occupational injury claims have been reported as being based on PTSD or other stress-related disorders (Ali, 2015).

Since many of the symptoms of PTSD are based on self-report, malingering, is more easily accomplished relative to most other disorders. Estimates of malingering in personal injury cases have ranged from 1% to 50% (Mezey, 2006).

As with criminal responsibility, there is no clinical tool available for identifying malingering in personal injury cases with great certainty (Ali, 2015, p. 15). This raises the previously discussed ethical question : what should psychiatrists say to third persons they call when they seek to confirm the reports of those they have interviewed (Knoll, 2006)?

If comparing the ethical considerations of examiners seeking corroboration in criminal assessments to those doing so in the context of disability evaluations, one difference looms. The former group may pose a direct threat to others in the future. This consideration may justify to some degree examiners informing those third parties they contact differently. Those in the latter group who malinger may also harm others in the future by draining public resources, but the harm from this is enormously less.

Persons claiming disability also may much suffer. They may, for example, be partially disabled and, as suggested, "merely" be exaggerating their symptoms for secondary and maximal compensatory gain. Further, they may as a result of their interactions and even those with their forensic examiners get worse. They may develop increased and then unmet dependency needs. It has been reported, for example, that some persons may undergo, in part as a result of their initial disabilities, a progressive erosion of their confidence and their independent living skills (Mezey, 2006).

Children

Children may be exceptionally harmed due to trauma because they are still developing. They also are less likely to understand what they are experiencing and why. For particularly these reasons, ethically, they are considered more vulnerable. As a result, research on children which could be most beneficial to them has often not been carried out.

This past practice of not doing research on children has, while well-intentioned, been at a price. Evidence-based knowledge needed to help these children has not been available. Consequently, one of the ethical problems that exists when child psychiatrists testify in the courts regarding the effects of trauma on these children is that these doctors' conclusions may be based on less objective beliefs. This may leave these outcomes more open to arbitrary and even specious results.

Illustrative examples have recently been reported. In one case, for example, a 3-year-old boy testified in response to his mother's accusing his father of sexual abuse. This child's report was open to question. He reported, for example, that his father hammered his penis with a shovel (Bernet, 2011). While this abuse may have occurred in this instance, this and other cases reported by Bernet illustrate how difficult it may be to make valid forensic inferences regarding children, especially in the absence of better data.

Fortunately, this has begun to change. Measures are now available, for example, to give child care providers better means of predicting how children will respond after trauma over both the shorter and longer runs (Corwin & Keeshin, 2011). Fortunately, too, researchers are now exploring how to best help these patients from the time they are born though late adolescence. They have studied, for example, how mothers may parent better after having experienced traumatic deliveries, how parents can most help their children after they have been injured, and how adolescents fare when they travel to other countries alone to seek asylum (Furuta et al., 2016; Alisic et al., 2015; Newman, 2013).

The ethical issues that arise in regard to treating children may be the same as those with adults in many contexts. These include, for example, the extent to which psychiatrists should respect these patients' confidentiality, as by insisting on their privacy (Joshi et al., 2008). These answers may depend on these patients' culture. For example, psychiatrists in the United States may not hesitate to ask a parent to leave the examining room. In other cultures, all information may, much more, "belong" to the family.

A final, special concern that may arise when children are traumatized is the effect on psychiatrists' feelings. People often respond more to seeing pain in children than to seeing it in adults. These providers' requirement to handle their feelings adequately when assessing these children may be greatest when they assess children for child abuse and when they help determine custody. For example, a social worker whose job was to help determine when children should be taken away from their parents remained depressed despite all psychiatric treatments. When she switched jobs, however, her depression spontaneously and immediately remitted.

A child psychiatrist assessing a child to determine custody was informed that this child's father, whose interests she would be testifying against, had hid outside her office behind a tree and had a gun. She elected then to not see this child again and to not testify in any way.

The moral angst children can evoke when psychiatrists see them in forensic contexts can, as these cases illustrate, be most extreme. This particularly may be the case when these children have experienced trauma.

This may be also be said of those accused of crime. They too may suffer greatly. This raises again the question whether psychiatrists can continue to relate to people in both these legal situations more empathically and if so, how. If, however, examiners are more empathic, the party examined may be more likely to incriminate him or herself. Thus, examiners may here most respect these examinees' personhood and autonomy most by reiterating their allegiance to the state when evaluating these criminal defendants so as not to allow their skills in developing rapport overwhelm the accused party's decision **to** not incriminate him or herself. This warning is initially required.

HOW MIGHT PSYCHIATRISTS RELATE BETTER EVEN IN THESE CONTEXTS? OR SHOULD THEY?

The question arises in both criminal and disability exams how psychiatrists should warn those they interview. Psychiatrists working for the state are wearing a different "hat." How should they say that they are working for the state? How many times? And should they initially and throughout the**se**ir interviews be maximally warm or try to appear distant?

Greater warmth may be implicitly misleading as it may suggest that examiners will support their interests more than they will. This could result in these persons disclosing self-incriminating truths against their best interests. This, in turn, ethically, should require the examiner to give this same warning if necessary again and again.

A further concern regarding psychiatrists evaluating people for disabilities is whether they should advise them to have therapy at this same time. It is often presumed in these circumstances that patients are less likely to get better from PTSD and other disabling disorders if they are simultaneously seeking to legally recover damages. This belief logically makes sense, but data supporting this is mixed. Some findings support this belief, others do not. (Blanchard, 1996; Ehlers et al., 1998; Miller, 1961).

Ethically, in light of this mixed data, providers who believe they should not treat or encourage these patients to get treatment when they are still "suing" may be mistaken. It may be more ethically enlightened to share maximally with all such patients the recommendation that they seek treatment while concomitantly assessing them. This asymptotic orientation to remain as committed to patients as possible even when serving other parties—as acting for the state—raises a final representative issue of whether psychiatrists should take initiative to offer to testify in support of their patients and particularly those they are seeing for psychotherapy.

Traditional psychiatric thinking often has held that therapists should generally not go to court for their patients because this may undermine their therapy. If, for instance, patients anticipate this potential secondary gain, they might say in therapy whatever they think could increase their financial gain. If they hoped to gain compensation from a disability, for example, they might elaborate on this disability in therapy in the hope that their therapist might then later on say this on their behalf.

This again may be short-sighted. Psychiatrists seeing patients in therapy may have insights regarding them that no one else knows. There are, it would seem, at least times at which therapists should make exceptions to this general theoretical prohibition against testifying for patients they treat in both criminal and civil settings.

Providers may justifiably *offer* to testify out of compassion. This possibility, more than any, represents a way in which psychiatrists might specifically seek to continue to value their priority to these patients, as opposed to continuing to see themselves as having mutually exclusive, conflicting roles as they have in the past.

A patient whose circumstances exemplify this possibility is the mother described earlier who reported feeling intense shame when her children first saw her falling apart. In response to the recommendation that she seek treatment for her PTSD, she was pursuing many kinds of therapy while seeking relief through the courts.

The ethical question was posed whether it made sense to tell her that it was "understandable" why she might *not* want at this time to get better. This was true and in one sense empathic. In another sense, however, it would also risk being demeaning. The psychiatrist chose therefore not to say this.

These last examples merely perhaps hint at a range of largely unprecedented interventions psychiatrists conducting forensic exams could newly consider. Using these, they could perhaps come closer to wearing one hat, rather than two. To the degree, if any, that they can do this they may be able to maintain some of even their chief loyalty and commitment to these patients.

CONCLUSION

When psychiatrists and other mental health workers assess people for criminal responsibility or disability, they may be asked to do so when these persons have either full-blown or partial PTSD. This chapter has discussed ethical and legal questions as a result of this and other difficult forensic decisions posed to those who conduct forensic assessments in patients with posttraumatic symptoms.

Some general ethical and legal concerns these evaluations pose are common to all. The influence of stress may apply widely, many of its symptoms are subjective, and thus they are easy to feign. Among the difficult questions posed here in response to these challenges is the extent (if any) to which examiners should engage in deceit.

A core question raised here in regard to psychiatrists being *more caring* regardless of whether they wear a clinical or forensic "hat" is this: should they validate what examinees may feel by saying that they can understand why they may want to exaggerate or why they may not want to get well from their symptoms until their legal quests are complete? This intervention is but one among many psychiatrists in these contexts may be able to newly imagine. Whether they choose to do so or not, asking this question (even if only to themselves) as opposed to seeking forensic and caring roles as entirely separate may be a challenge worth pursuing.

REFERENCES

Ali, S., Jabeen, S., & Alam, F. (2015). Multimodal approach to identifying malingered posttraumatic stress disorder: A review. *Innovations in Clinical Neuroscience, 12* (1–2), 12–20.

Alisic, E., Barrett, A., Bowles, P., Babl, F. E., Conroy, R., McClure, R. J., . . . Mehl, M. R. (2015). Ear for recovery: Protocol for a prospective study on parent-child communication and psychological recovery after paediatric injury. *BMJ Open, 5*(2), e007393. doi:10.1136/bmjopen-2014-007393

Allen, F.A. (1962). The rule of the American Law Institute's Model Penal Code. *Marquette Law Review*, *45*(4), 494–505.

American Academy of Psychiatry and the Law. (2014). AAPL practice guideline for forensic evaluation of defendants raising the insanity defense. *Journal of the American Academy of Psychiatry and the Law*, *42*(4 Suppl.), S3–S76.

Bernet W. (2011). Ridiculous statements by mental health experts. *Child and Adolescent Psychiatric Clinics of North America*, *20*(3), 557–564.

Blanchard, E. B., Hickling, E. J., Barton, K. A., Taylor, A. E., Loos, W. R., & Jones-Alexander, J. (1996). Who develops PTSD from motor vehicle accidents? *Behaviour Research and Therapy*, *34*, 1–10.

Candilis, P. J., Weinstock, R., & Martinez, R. (2007). *Forensic ethics and the expert witness*. New York: Springer.

Corwin, D. L., & Keeshin, B. R. (2011). Estimating present and future damages following child maltreatment. *Child and Adolescent Psychiatric Clinics of North America*, *20*(3), 505–18.

Ehlers, Q., Mayou, R. A., & Bryant, B. J. (1998). Psychological predictors of chronic posttraumatic stress disorder after motor vehicle accidents. *Journal of Abnormal Psychology*, *107*, 508–519.

Eiser, A. R. (2015). Postmodern stress disorder (PMSD): A possible new disorder. *American Journal of Medicine*, *128*(11), 1178–1181. doi:10.1016/j.amjmed.2015.04.030

Evans, C., Mezey, G., & Ehlers, A. (2009). Amnesia for violent crime among young offenders. *Journal of Forensic Psychiatry and Psychology*, *20*(1), 85–106.

Frierson, R. L. (2013). Combat-related post-traumatic stress disorder and criminal responsibility determinations in the post-Iraq era: A review and case report. *Journal of the American Academy of Psychiatry and the Law*, *41*, 79–84.

Furuta, M., Spain, D., Bick, D., Ng, E. S., & Sin, J. (2016). Effectiveness of trauma-focused psychological therapies compared to usual postnatal care for treating post-traumatic stress symptoms in women following traumatic birth: A systematic review protocol. *BMJ Open*, *6*(11), e013697. doi:10.1136/bmjopen-2016-013697

Giorgi-Guarnieri, D., Janofsky, J., Keram, E., Lawsky, S., Merideth, P., Mossman, E. D., . . . Zonana, H. (2002). AAPL practice guideline for forensic evaluation of defendants raising the insanity defense. *Journal of the American Academy of Psychiatry and the Law*, *30*, S3–S40.

Hopwood, J. S., & Snell, H. K. (1933). Amnesia in relation to crime. *Journal of Mental Science*, *79*, 27–41.

Joshi, P. T., Dalton, M. E., O'Donnell, D. A. (2008). Ethical issues in local, national, and international disaster psychiatry. *Child and Adolescent Psychiatric Clinics of North America*, *17*(1), 165–185.

Kleinman, S. B., & Martell, D. (2015). Failings of trauma-specific and related psychological tests in detecting post-traumatic stress disorder in forensic settings. *Journal of Forensic Sciences*, *60*(1), 76–83.

Knoll, J. & Resnick, P. J. (2006). The detection of malingered posttraumatic stress disorder. *Psychiatric Clinics of North America*, *29*, 629–647.

Levin, A. P., Kleinman S. B., & Adler, J. S. (2014). DSM-5 and posttraumatic stress disorder. *Journal of the American Academy of Psychiatry and the Law*, *42*, 146–158.

McQuade, J. S. (2001).The Eggshell Skull Rule and related problems in recovery for mental harm in the Law of Torts. *Campbell Law Review*, *24*(1), 1–45.

Mezey, G. (2006). Post-traumatic stress disorder and the law. *Psychiatry*, *5*(7), 243–247.

Miller, H. (1961). Accident neurosis. *British Medical Journal*, *5230*, 919–925.

Newman, L. (2013). Seeking asylum—trauma, mental health, and human rights: An Australian perspective. *Journal of Trauma & Dissociation*, *14*(2), 213–223.

Orne, M. T., Dinges, D. F., & Orbe, E. C. (1984). On the differential diagnosis of multiple personality in the forensic context. *International Journal of Clinical and Experimental Hypnosis*, *32*, 118–169. doi:10.1080/00207148408416007

Scott, C. L. (2012). Evaluating amnesia for criminal behavior: A guide to remember. *Psychiatric Clinics of North America*, *35*, 797–819.

Stojakovic, M. B. (2011). Forensic psychiatric expertise: Posttraumatic stress disorder. *Srpski Arhivza Celokupno Lekarstvo*, *139*(Suppl. 1), 46–51. PMID 22352203.

Swihart, G., Yuille, Y., & Porter, S. (1999). The role of state-dependent memory in "red-outs." *International Journal of Law and Psychiatry*, *22*, 199–212.

30

Future Directions in Clinical Care, Research, and Nosology

FREDERICK J. STODDARD JR., DAVID M. BENEDEK,
MOHAMMED R. MILAD, AND ROBERT J. URSANO

The science of the study of trauma and stress has accelerated as never before, due to increased recognition of the need, greater capabilities for the research, expanding knowledge, and increased numbers of investigators and funding. There has also been significant advancement in our understanding of the neural circuits underlying fear and anxiety and the relationship of trauma and stress to these circuits. The increased understanding of underlying mechanisms of psychopathology may lead to better diagnostics that are biologically based and to improving the development of novel therapeutics, especially in the device-based neurotherapeutics. Genetics and genomics may also further our understanding of the neurochemistry and mechanisms of traumatic stress disorders that can also lead to new methods and drugs to prevent disorders due to trauma and stress. The recent call by the National Institute of Mental Health (NIMH) to develop Research Domain Criteria (RDoC) approaches for psychopathology in general and posttraumatic stress disorder (PTSD) and anxiety disorders more specifically is likely to continue to push the field to rely more on neurobiological basis for diagnosis, intervention, and prevention of PTSD. While the acceleration of scientific discovery is exciting, much more is needed as well to address the global burden of trauma and stress across all age groups.

The field of neuropsychiatry is pushing forward with NIMH's call for RDoC approach to trauma and stress. This approach, combined with past studies and other non-RDoC studies have resulted in an extensive number of brain-based studies focusing on the neural correlates of fear, stress, and anxiety. These studies give hope for the discovery of more individualized care and linkage to genetics and genomics.

The RDoC frames dimensional constructs (concepts) relevant to mental disorders with multiple metrics, developmental trajectories, and environmental influences. Constructs are grouped in domains of human behavior and functioning reflecting knowledge of systems of emotion, cognition, motivation, and social behavior. Methods to investigate constructs span molecular, genetic, neural circuits based, and behavioral. The RDoC matrix includes the constructs, domains, and units of analysis that collectively establish this framework. The five domains in its matrix are (a) negative valence systems (e.g., potential threat/fear, anxiety, loss); (b) positive valence systems (e.g., approach motivation, reward learning, habit); (c) cognitive systems (e.g., attention, perception, language, working memory); (d) systems for social processes (e.g., affiliation and attachment, social communication, perception of self and others); and (e) arousal/regulatory systems (e.g., arousal, circadian rhythms, sleep, and wakefulness). [https://www.nimh.nih.gov/research-priorities/rdoc/index.shtml] This matrix opens pathways to additional translational research for example on potential threat (Rosso et al., 2015). The RDoC criteria for PTSD have not gone unchallenged. While some disagree with this approach outright, others argue that it is incomplete. For example, Schmidt and Vermetten (2017) suggest adding two more domains: stress and emotional regulation, and maintenance of consciousness. Nonetheless, the RDoC approach is providing a different pathway to merging the fields of neuroscience, psychology, and psychiatry to conceptualize emotions, behaviors and their consequences as all biologically based and occurring across a continuum of quantifiable outcomes.

Where to go from here? There will continue be struggles regarding whether to ground nosology more in basic science, genetics and genomics, and neuroscience or in the more practical applications of diagnosis (e.g., clusters of observable signs and or reported symptoms) most relevant to current clinical care and public health practices. Categorical diagnoses are "traditional" in the *Diagnostic and Statistical Manual of Mental Disorders* (DSM) and International Classification of Diseases, but the fifth edition of the DSM moves us toward future dimensional diagnoses relating activations of neural circuits and genomics than traditional symptom-based categorical diagnoses. For instance there is much interest in identifying and preventing the psychopathological outcomes of childhood trauma (Stoddard, 2014), the symptomatic and biological underpinnings of comorbid depression and PTSD (Flory & Yehuda, 2015), comorbid substance use disorders and PTSD (Fareed et al., 2013; Korte et al., 2017), and, as discussed already, increased Parkinson's disease (Chan et al., 2017) and possibly increased dementia associated with chronic PTSD.

THE FUTURE IN DIAGNOSIS, TREATMENT, AND PREVENTION USING NEUROBIOLOGY

New methodologies in the laboratory, at the bedside, and in communities are adding approaches to the trauma- and stress-related disorder (TSRD) mental health problems and disorders. Neuropsychology and especially its interface with neuroimaging is identifying operative brain circuits even for basic brain functions under stress, psychotherapies, and the full range of psychopharmacology.

Novel therapeutic approaches are appearing that use pharmacological agents as adjuncts to exposure therapy or other traditional psychosocial interventions. For example, d-cycloserine (DCS) held initial promise for facilitating therapy; others now being studied in the treatment of PTSD include THC, estrogens, cortisol, and dexamethasone. These are ongoing explorations. Others are likely to emerge over the next decade. The idea behind these approaches is to augment the efficacy of exposure therapy or hasten the effectiveness of such intervention. Their efficacy and safety in treating PTSD is yet to be determined but neuroscience will continue to produce new agents to be tested.

Device-based approaches to the treatment of TSRD are also among the most novel areas of active exploration. There are several device-based approaches presently being studied including vagus nerve stimulation, deep brain stimulation, transcranial magnetic stimulation, and transcranial direct current stimulation. TMS is already an Food and Drug Administration (FDA)-approved for treating depression and some initial studies suggest efficacy for PTSD. Others are being explored and their use is being optimized for PTSD treatment, either alone or as adjuncts to exposure therapy. More focused and patient-specific applications of these technologies (e.g., as targeted by functional neuroimaging) is an exciting area of research that is likely to continue to expand based on our developments in neuroscience. Further advances in neuroimaging may enable us to better optimize and implement personalized approaches to the treatment of PTSD and other TSRD.

Sleep is another prime area of research given its relevance to PTSD and its impact on the etiology, diagnosis, and treatment for PTSD. Nightmares have, at times, been termed the "hallmark" of PTSD with some justification. Disturbance in sleep interferes with memory consolidation, so better understanding (and targeting) of sleep dysfunction may prove to be key in improving diagnosis and treatment of PTSD. This area has not had sufficient focus in research to date. Germaine (2013) proposes the study of "the chronic sleep disruption" connected to nightmares which may affect outcomes of first-line PTSD treatments. She advises "prospective and longitudinal studies" of sleep physiology and neurobiology of high-risk groups, to identify the parameters which contribute to improved or worsened outcomes of treatments. There is much more to come in this area of research in the upcoming decades that will impact future treatment and diagnosis of PTSD.

Studies of the neural circuits of fear extinction and PTSD and the interactions between prefrontal cortical areas and subcortical regions including the amygdala and hippocampus have made significant contributions to our understanding of the pathophysiology of PTSD. This area of research has informed drug-development and device-based strategies to improve on identifying additional brain areas to target and refine existing target engagement parameters for clinical interventions.

In addition to the current and well-established models, Ledoux and Pine (2016) have most recently provided a strong case for restructuring the translational science of PTSD research. In order to do that, they advocate for a two-system neural circuit model of fear and anxiety elicited by threats. They distinguish cortical from subcortical circuits, with the cortical being conscious feeling states reflected in self-reports of fear and anxiety and the subcortical being behavioral responses of defensive behaviors and accompanying physiological changes in the brain and body. They believe that the failure to emphasize this distinction has interfered with research into effective pharmacological and psychological treatments. This call has received much attention, and several groups are testing this approach, and outcome measures and proposed treatments targeting these distinct circuits will certainly follow.

Additional areas of nascent research in TRSDs involve neuroimmunology and gut-brain interactions. These preliminary studies point to neurochemical, neuroinflammatory, and immunological linkages (Danese & Lewis, 2017) with trauma and stressor disorders. The gut-brain axis involves millions of organisms in the gut and their relation to brain centers stress responses with bidirectional communication influencing cognition, anxiety, and depression (Burokas et al., 2017; Rieder et al., 2017; Wallace & Milev, 2017).

Advanced computing techniques are also influencing TSRD research. An area appearing in the field is the use of machine learning. Neuroimaging tools, high throughput sequencing, and other multimodal approaches used in the past three decades have generated massive data sets. Researchers are more willing and able to share data with other colleagues. This is leading to developing novel analytic approaches to handle massive data sets. The significant advantage of this approach is the combination of brain activation with neuropsychmetrics, psychophysiological, and behavioral data to identify of variables that are most salient to early diagnosis or treatment response prediction for PTSD. More focus is being placed on studying the interactions of a brain areas rather than the correlation between two brain areas in a given task. This domain of research will likely generate critical data that can propel the field forward. Beyond computing capacity, other advances in information technology offer great potential. Developing and fielding handheld devices and powerful/portable methods for data gathering, data analysis, and sharing as well as for training people in the recognition of and treatments for TRSDs are important to early intervention and provision of care outside of hospitals or clinics. The literature highlights this rapid growth (Acierno et al., 2017; Anthes, 2016; Battaglia et al 2016; Franklin et al., 2017; Gilmore et al., 2016; Gros et al., 2016; Lindsay et al., 2015; Miller et al., 2016; Nassan et al., 2015; Olden et al., 2017; Radovic et al., 2016; Wierwille et al., 2016; Whealin et al., 2016; Wood et al., 2017). A plethora of treatment applications, some of them apps providing health information technology (HIT) for TSRD, are emerging with various names such as telemedicine, telemental health (Augusterfer et al., 2015), and others. Use of telepsychiatry is rapidly evolving to provide direct HIT for psychiatric screening, to identify vulnerabilities, and to provide evaluation, consultation, and treatment for rural health, child psychiatry, disaster psychiatry, and international mental health.

STRENGTHENING THE EVIDENCE BASE FOR INTERVENTION

As noted in this volume, across all TSRD the strongest evidence base exists for psychotherapy, particularly cognitive behavioral therapy (CBT) in adults and children, with the use of exposure therapy, which has been called a "gold standard" (Rauch et al., 2012; Clapp et al., 2016). A limitation is that many people cannot tolerate exposure therapy or do not complete treatment. Eye movement desensitization and reprocessing has also achieved a place in treatment, reflecting its CBT associations. The evidence for psychopharmacology with adults is limited, but studies have been replicated to varying degrees in various trauma-exposed populations. For children (and specific adult populations including combat-exposed veterans), the evidence is much more limited and only slowly developing. Despite the relative lack of evidence compared to other areas of medicine and their treatments, medications are widely used for both adults and children. Conducting evidence-based research remains difficult, expensive, and time-consuming. As a result much psychotherapeutic and psychopharmacological treatment of patients is conducted on a limited or absent evidence base, and treatment with medications is often as an "off label" use, meaning without specific approval for that use by the FDA. Moving forward, future research must include a critical evaluation of these practices as well.

Complementary and alternative medicine approaches including mind-body interventions such as meditation or yoga have minimal evidence for treatment of PTSD or other TSRD yet they are widely recommended and practiced. Other approaches including animal-assisted or recreation-based therapies, like novel agents, or new device-based treatments may achieve an evidence-based place in treatment, but this has not yet occurred.

PUBLIC HEALTH AND HEALTH CARE POLICY

Providing treatment to more of those who would benefit—in the United States and internationally—raises a substantial set of challenges. Access to care is a significant problem, not easily solved either in the United States or in the rest of the world, but many are seeking solutions. Continued strengthening of the evidence base for mental health treatment of TSRDs must also remain a priority as widespread acknowledgement of efficacy also promotes access.

Advances in scientific understanding and treatment should foster and support preventive approaches and policies at the individual and population level. Global mental health priorities require scaling up resources and methods of communication and intervention, including telemedicine, to reach populations impacted by TSRDs (Becker & Kleinman, 2013; Raviola et al., 2011; Baingana et al., 2015). The global burden of mental disorders is enormous, especially in low and middle-income countries. Climate change and its health and mental health risks, including the TSRDs that may emerge as a consequence of extreme weather and natural disaster, are a newly recognized concern and must become a priority (Hunter, Frumkin, & Jha, 2017). A sociocentric approach with increased emphasis on identifying and maintaining social ties may be important too as enhanced as "social connectedness" has been identified as a protective factor in the aftermath of disaster, and increased PTSD risk is associated with social fragmentation (Bryant et al., 2017). More generally, globally, the neglect and marginalization of mental health resources particularly for children, TSRDs, depression, and substance use disorders remains very concerning. Integral to addressing these challenges are improved methods for overcoming stigma, developing primary care screening, and promoting international initiatives to prevent and mitigate trauma, stress, disasters, and war and importantly reducing poverty and gender-based violence, as well as promoting resilience. Workforce issues include how to train, expand, and make resilient the numbers of people needed to provide mental health interventions, and this has begun to occur at various university medical centers in the United States with global outreach (Cancedda et al., 2017).

In the United States, mental health priorities to reduce the burden of TSRD should also include primary care screening and interventions for children, minorities, and the disadvantaged. Here, too, it is necessary to address poverty and gender-based violence and to continue to improve disaster preparedness, including expansion of the availability of resources (surge capacity) for mass trauma, including burns (Dai et al., 2017). Consideration of various efforts to reduce handgun violence in the United States is also important. While obstacles to legislation have been well described by Kalesan et al. (2016), gun safety education and training for families may be a strategy for medical care providers to encourage.

History has taught us that the emotional, psychological, and behavioral consequences of disaster, war, terrorism, and interpersonal violence are far-reaching and likely to continue to exact a substantial burden on society. The labels applied to the observed morbidity—by social commentators, historians, authors, artists, scientists, and physicians have evolved as our understanding of the pathogenesis and neurobiological underpinnings of these phenomena have expanded. The assessment, diagnosis, and treatment of the TSRDs as they are presently termed (and understood) is an important task for medical care as well as communities and nations. As our knowledge expands, the labels attached to these observations will continue to evolve. The DSM-5 acknowledges the inevitability of these changes and has been developed in a manner that will accommodate them. What remains to be answered is the full extent to which such change in the nosology can be accompanied by truly meaningful reductions in psychosocial distress and dysfunction for the individual patient, as well as at the community and the global community of nations. Much progress has been made in recent years, and current efforts hold great promise. While history suggests that trauma and stressors surely lie ahead for our society, it also reminds us that our knowledge, understanding, and hope will continue to foster advances for those who need care. As we focus efforts on primary, secondary, and tertiary prevention we must continue the search for a cure.

There's the sulphury pit, burning, scalding,
Stench, consummation. Fie, fie, fie: pah, pah!
Give me an ounce of civet, good apothecary,*
To sweeten my imagination.
There's money for thee.
[*a perfume]
King Lear (Shakespeare, 2006, Sc. 18, lines 123–127)

REFERENCES

Acierno R, Knapp R, Tuerk P, Gilmore AK, Lejuez C, Ruggiero K, Muzzy W, Egede L, Hernandez-Tejada MA, Foa EB. A non-inferiority trial of Prolonged Exposure for posttraumatic stress disorder: In person versus home-based telehealth. *Behav Res Ther.* 2017 Feb;89:57–65. doi:10.1016/j.brat.2016.11.009. PMID:27894058

Anthes E. Mental health: There's an app for that. *Nature.* 2016 Apr 7;532(7597):20–23. doi:10.1038/532020a. PMID:27078548

Augusterfer EF, Mollica RF, Lavelle J. A review of telemental health in international and post-disaster settings. *Int Rev Psychiatry.* 2015;27(6):540–546. doi:10.3109/09540261.2015.1082985. PMID: 26576720

Baingana, F, al'Absi M, Becker AE, Pringle B. Global research challenges and opportunities for mental health and substance-use disorders. *Nature.* 2015 Nov 19;527(7578):S172–S177. doi:10.1038/nature16032. PMID: 26580324

Battaglia C, Peterson J, Whitfield E, Min SJ, Benson SL, Maddox TM, Prochazka AV. Integrating motivational interviewing into a home telehealth program for veterans with posttraumatic stress disorder who smoke: A randomized controlled trial. *J Clin Psychol.* 2016 Mar;72(3):194–206. doi:10.1002/jclp.22252. PMID:26783736

Becker AE, Kleinman A. Mental health and the global agenda. *N Engl J Med.* 2013 Oct 3;369(14):1380–1. doi:10.1056/NEJMc1309899. PMID: 24088110

Bryant RA, Gallagher HC, Gibbs L, et al. Mental health and social networks after disaster. *Am J Psychiatry.* 2017;174:277–285; doi:10.1176/appi.ajp.2016.15111403. PMID: 27838935

Burokas A, Arboleya S, Moleoney RD, Peterson VL, Murphy K, Clarke G, Stanton C, Dinan TG, Cryan JF. Archival report: Targeting the microbiota-gut-brain axis: Prebiotics have anxiolytic and antidepressant effects and reverse the impact of chronic stress in mice. *Biol Psychiatry.* 2017;82(7):472–487. http://dx.doi.org/10.1016/j.biopsych.2016.12.031

Cancedda C, Riviello R, Wilson K, et al. Building workforce capacity abroad while strengthening global health programs at home: Participation of seven Harvard-affiliated institutions in a health professional training initiative in Rwanda. *Acad Med.* 2017 May;92(5):649–658. doi:10.1097/ACM.0000000000001638. PMID: 28328735

Chan YE, Bai YM, Hsu JW, et al. Post-traumatic stress disorder and risk of Parkinson Disease: A nationwide longitudinal study. *Am J Geriatr Psychiatry.* 2017 Aug;25(8):917-923. doi: 10.1016/j.jagp.2017.03.012.

Clapp JD, Kemp JJ, Cox KS, Tuerk PW. Patterns of change in response to prolonged exposure: Implications for treatment outcome. *Depress Anxiety.* 2016 Sep;33(9):807–815. doi:10.1002/da.22534. PMID:27321062

Dai A, Carrougher GJ, Mandell SP, Fudem G, Gibran NS, Pham TN. Review of recent large-scale burn disasters worldwide in comparison to preparedness guidelines. J *Burn Care Res.* 2017 Jan/Feb;38(1):36–44. doi:10.1097/BCR.0000000000000441. PMID: 27654867

Danese A, Lewis SJ. Psychoneuroimmunology of early-life stress: The hidden wounds of childhood trauma? *Neuropsychopharmacology.* 2017 Jan;42(1):99–114. doi:10.1038/npp.2016.198. PMID: 27629365

Fareed A, Eilender P, Haber M, Bremner J, Whitfield N, Drexler K. Comorbid posttraumatic stress disorder and opiate addiction: a literature review. *J Addict Dis.* 2013;32(2):168–179. doi:10.1080/10550887.2013.795467. PMID: 23815424

Flory JD, Yehuda R. Comorbidity between posttraumatic stress disorder and major depressive disorder: Alternative explanations and treatment considerations. *Dialogues Clin Neurosci.* 2015;17:141–150. PMID: 26246789

Franklin CL, Cuccurullo LA, Walton JL, Arseneau JR, Petersen NJ. Face to face but not in the same place: A pilot study of prolonged exposure therapy. *J Trauma Dissociation.* 2017 Jan-Feb;18(1):116–130. doi:10.1080/15299732.2016.1205704. PMID: 27348462

Germain A. Sleep disturbance and the hallmark of PTSD: Where are we now? *Am J Psychiatry.* 2013; 170:372–382. PMID: 23223954

Gilmore AK, Davis MT, Grubaugh A, Resnick H, Birks A, Denier C, Muzzy W, Tuerk P, Acierno R. "Do you expect me to receive PTSD care in a setting where most of the other patients remind me of the perpetrator?": Home-based telemedicine to address barriers to care unique to military sexual trauma and Veterans Affairs hospitals. *Contemp Clin Trials.* 2016 May;48:59–64. doi:10.1016/j.cct.2016.03.004. PMID:26992740

Gros DF, Lancaster CL, López CM, Acierno R. Treatment satisfaction of home-based telehealth versus in-person delivery of prolonged exposure for combat-related PTSD in veterans. *J Telemed Telecare.* 2016 Sep 26. pii: 1357633X16671096. PMID:27672059

Hunter DJ, Frumkin H, Jha A. Preventive medicine for the planet and its peoples. *N Engl J Med.* 2017;376(17):1605–1608. PMID: 28249124

Kalesan B, Adhikarla C, Pressley JC, Fagan JA, Xuan Z, Siegel MB, Galea S. The hidden epidemic of firearm injury: Increasing firearm injury rates during 2001–2013. *Am J Epidemiol.* 2016:185(7):546–553. doi:10.1093/aje/kww147. PMID: 28338922

Korte KJ, Bountress KE, Tomko RL, Killeen T, Moran-Santa Maria M, Back SE. Integrated treatment of PTSD and substance use disorders: The mediating role of PTSD improvement in the reduction of depression. *J Clin Med.* 2017 Jan 13;6(1). pii: E9. doi:10.3390/jcm6010009. PMID: 28098747

Ledoux JE, Pine DS. Using neuroscience to help understand fear and anxiety: A two system framework. *Am J Psychiatry* 2016;173:1083–1093. doi:10.1176/appi.ajp.2016.16030353

Lindsay JA, Kauth MR, Hudson S, Martin LA, Ramsey DJ, Daily L, Rader J. Implementation of video telehealth to improve access to evidence-based psychotherapy for posttraumatic stress disorder. *Telemed J E Health.* 2015 Jun;21(6):467–72. doi:10.1089/tmj.2014.0114.

Miller CJ, McInnes DK, Stolzmann K, Bauer MS. Interest in use of technology for healthcare among veterans receiving treatment for mental health. *Telemed J E Health.* 2016 Oct;22(10):847–854. PMID:26982279

Nassan M, Frye MA, Adi A, Alarcón RD. Telepsychiatry for post-traumatic stress disorder: A call for action in the Syrian conflict. *Lancet Psychiatry.* 2015 Oct;2(10):866. doi:10.1016/S2215-0366(15)00380-6. PMID:26462214

Olden M, Wyka K, Cukor J, Peskin M, Altemus M, Lee FS, Finkelstein-Fox L, Rabinowitz T, Difede J. Pilot study of a telehealth-delivered medication-augmented exposure therapy protocol for PTSD. *J Nerv Ment Dis.* 2017 Feb;205(2):154–160. doi:10.1097/NMD.0000000000000563. PMID:27441461

Radovic A, Vona PL, Santostefano AM, Ciaravino S, Miller E, Stein BD. Smartphone applications for mental health. *Cyberpsychol Behav Soc Netw.* 2016 Jul;19(7):465–70. doi:10.1089/cyber.2015.0619. PMID:27428034

Rauch SL, Eftekhari A, Ruzek JI. Review of exposure therapy: A gold standard for PTSD treatment. *J Rehabil Res Dev.* 2012;49:679–687.

Raviola G, Becker AE, Farmer P. A global scope for global health—including mental health. *Lancet.* 2011 Nov 5;378(9803):1613–1615. doi:10.1016/S0140-6736(11)60941-0

Rieder R, Wisniewski PJ, Alderman BL, Campbell SC. Microbes and mental health: A review. *Brain, Behav Immun.* 2017;66:9–17. http://dx.doi.org/10.1016/j.bbi.2017.01.016 08889-1591/

Rosso IM, Dillon DG, Pizzagalli DA, Rauch SL. Translational perspectives on anxiety disorders and the research domain criteria construct of potential threat. In: KJ Ressler, DS Pine, and BO Rothbaum, Eds. *Anxiety disorders: Translational perspectives on diagnosis and treatment.* Oxford: Oxford University Press, 2015. pp. 17–32.

Schmidt U, Vermetten E. Integrating NIMH Research Domain Criteria (RDoC) into PTSD research. *Curr Top Behav Neurosci.* 2017 Mar 25. doi:10.1007/7854_2017_1 [Epub ahead of print] PMID:28341942

Stoddard FJ. Outcomes of traumatic exposure. In: SJ Cozza, JA Cohen, JG Doherty, Eds. Special issue: Disaster and trauma. *Child Adolesc Psychiatr Clin N Am.* 2014;23(2)243–256.

Wallace CJK, Milev R. The effects of probiotics on depressive symptoms in humans: A systematic review. *Ann Gen Psychiatry* 2017;16:14. doi:10.11.86/s12991-017-0138-2

Wierwille JL, Pukay-Martin ND, Chard KM, Klump MC. Effectiveness of PTSD telehealth treatment in a VA clinical sample. *Psychol Serv.* 2016 Nov;13(4):373–379. PMID:27657798

Whealin JM, Jenchura EC, Wong AC, Zulman DM. How veterans with post-traumatic stress disorder and comorbid health conditions utilize eHealth to manage their health care needs: A mixed-methods analysis. *J Med Internet Res.* 2016 Oct 26;18(10):e280. PMID:27784650

Wood AE, Prins A, Bush NE, Hsia JF, Bourn LE, Earley MD, Walser RD, Ruzek J. Reduction of burnout in mental health care providers using the Provider Resilience mobile application. *Community Ment Health J.* 2017;53(4):452-459 doi:10.1007/s10597-016-0076-5. PMID: 28070775

INDEX

Page numbers followed by *f*, *t*, and *b* refer to figures, tables, and boxes respectively.